Handbook of Aging and the Social Sciences

The Handbooks of Aging

Consisting of Three Volumes

Critical comprehensive reviews of
research knowledge, theories, concepts, and issues

Editors-in-Chief
Laura L. Carstensen
and
Thomas A. Rando

Handbook of the Biology of Aging, 7th Edition
Edited by Edward J. Masoro and Steven N. Austad

Handbook of the Psychology of Aging, 7th Edition
Edited by K. Warner Schaie and Sherry L. Willis

Handbook of Aging and the Social Sciences, 7th Edition
Edited by Robert H. Binstock and Linda K. George

Handbook of Aging and the Social Sciences

7th Edition

Editors

Robert H. Binstock and Linda K. George

Associate Editors

Stephen J. Cutler, Jon Hendricks, and James H. Schulz

Amsterdam • Boston • Heidelberg • London • New York • Oxford • Paris
San Diego • San Francisco • Singapore • Sydney • Tokyo

Academic Press is an imprint of Elsevier

Academic Press is an imprint of Elsevier
32 Jamestown Road, London NW1 7BY, UK
30 Corporate Drive, Suite 400, Burlington, MA 01803, USA
525 B Street, Suite 1800, San Diego, CA 92101-4495, USA

Seventh edition, 2011

British Library Cataloguing-in-Publication Data
A catalogue record for this book is available from the British Library

Library of Congress Cataloging-in-Publication Data
A catalog record for this book is available from the Library of Congress

ISBN: 978-0-12-380880-6

Typeset by MPS Limited, a Macmillan Company, Chennai, India
www.macmillansolutions.com

Printed and bound in the United States of America

11 12 13 14 15   10 9 8 7 6 5 4 3 2

Contents

Contents

Contributors

Numbers in parentheses indicate the page number on which the author's contribution begins

Jacqueline L. Angel (163), Department of Sociology, Lyndon B. Johnson School of Public Affairs, Population Research Center, University of Texas, Austin, Texas

Camila Arza (251), Latin American School for Social Sciences/CONICET, Buenos Aires, Argentina

Lisa F. Berkman (337), Department of Society, Human Development, and Health, Harvard School of Public Health, Cambridge, Massachusetts

Robert H. Binstock (265), School of Arts and Sciences, Medicine, and Nursing, Case Western Reserve University, Cleveland, Ohio

J. Scott Brown (105), Department of Sociology and Gerontology and Scripps Gerontology Center, Miami University, Oxford, Ohio

Andrea L. Campbell (265), Department of Political Science, Massachusetts Institute of Technology, Cambridge, Massachusetts

Stephen J. Cutler (221), Emeritus, Department of Sociology, University of Vermont, Burlington, Vermont

Dale Dannefer (3), Department of Sociology, Case Western Reserve University, Cleveland, Ohio

Karen A. Ertel (337), Department of Society, Human Development, and Health, Harvard School of Public Health, Cambridge, Massachusetts

Elizabeth Frankenberg (73), Sanford School of Public Policy, Duke University, Durham, North Carolina

Vicki A. Freedman (57), Institute for Social Research, University of Michigan, Ann Arbor, Michigan

Linda K. George (149), Department of Sociology and Center for the Study of Aging, Duke University, Durham, North Carolina

John Gist (353), The George Washington University, Washington, DC

Maria M. Glymour (337), Department of Society, Human Development, and Health, Harvard School of Public Health, Cambridge, Massachusetts

Stephen M. Golant (207), Department of Geography, University of Florida, Gainesville, Florida

Deborah T. Gold (235), Departments of Psychiatry & Behavioral Sciences and Sociology, Duke University Medical Center, Durham, North Carolina

Ishtar O. Govia (91), University of the West Indies, Mona, Jamaica; University of Michigan, Ann Arbor, Michigan

Jon Hendricks (221), Emeritus, Honors College, Oregon State University, Corvallis, Oregon

Pamela Herd (121), Department of Sociology, University of Wisconsin, Madison, Wisconsin

Scott M. Hofer (135), Department of Psychology, University of Victoria, Victoria, British Columbia, Canada

James S. House (121), Department of Sociology and Gerald R. Ford School of Public Policy, University of Michigan, Ann Arbor, Michigan

James S. Jackson (91), University of Michigan, Ann Arbor, Michigan

Martin Kohli (251), Department of Political and Social Sciences, European University Institute, Florence, Italy

Scott M. Lynch (105), Department of Sociology and Office Population Resarch, Princeton University, Princeton, New Jersey

Linda G. Martin (33), RAND Corporation, Arlington, Virginia

Madonna Harrington Meyer (323), Center for Policy Research, Syracuse University, Syracuse, New York

Marilyn Moon (295), American Institutes for Research, Silver Spring, Maryland

Contributors

Stipica Mudrazija (163), Lyndon B. Johnson School of Public Affairs, Population Research Center, University of Texas, Austin, Texas

S. Jay Olshansky (47), School of Public Health, University of Illinois in Chicago, Chicago, Illinois

Greg O'Neill (221), National Academy on an Aging Society, Gerontological Society of America, Washington, DC

Wendy M. Parker (323), Albany College of Pharmacy and Health Sciences, Albany, New York

Virginia P. Reno (175), National Academy of Social Insurance, Washington, DC

Sara E. Rix (193), AARP, Washington, DC

Stephanie A. Robert (121), School of Social Work, University of Wisconsin, Madison, Wisconsin

Michael J. Shanahan (135), Department of Sociology and Center for Developmental Science, University of North Carolina at Chapel Hill, Chapel Hill, North Carolina

Sherrill L. Sellers (91), Miami University, Oxford, Ohio

Duncan Thomas (73), Department of Economics, Duke University, Durham, North Carolina

Ben Veghte (175), National Academy of Social Insurance, Washington, DC

Joshua M. Wiener (309), RTI International, Washington, DC

John B. Williamson (281), Department of Sociology, Boston College, Chestnut Hill, Massachusetts

Yang Yang (17), Department of Sociology & Lineberger Comprehensive Cancer Center, University of North Carolina, Chapel Hill, North Carolina

Foreword

Advances in science and technology in the twentieth century reshaped twenty-first-century life in industrialized nations around the world. Living conditions so improved that infant and childhood mortality were profoundly reduced and medical advances in the prevention and treatment of leading causes of death among adults, such as heart disease and cancer, further extended the lives of older individuals. As a result, in the course of a single century, the average life expectancy in developed countries nearly doubled. For the first time in human history, old age became a normative stage in life. Not only are individuals living longer on average, but populations have begun to age as a result of this increase in life expectancy along with a precipitous drop in fertility rates. Countries in the developed world are rapidly reaching the point where there will be more people over 60 than under 15. Thus, the status of older people holds ramifications for the functioning of entire societies.

Even though the near-doubling of life expectancy was a spectacular achievement, there were not concurrent advances in our ability to alleviate the disabling conditions of later life. Nor were there sociological advances to create a world as responsive to the needs of very old people as to those of the very young. In order to realize the enormous potential of longer life, scientists must come to a more comprehensive understanding of human aging and the social, psychological, and biological factors that contribute to optimal outcomes. Along with the phenomenal advances in the genetic determinants of longevity and susceptibility to age-related diseases has come an awareness of the critical importance of environmental factors that modulate and even supersede genetic predispositions. This series provides a balanced perspective of the interacting factors that contribute to human aging.

The *Handbooks of Aging* series, consisting of three separate volumes, the *Handbook of the Biology of Aging*, the *Handbook of the Psychology of Aging*, and the *Handbook of Aging and the Social Sciences*, is now in its seventh edition and has provided a foundation for an understanding of the issues of aging that are relevant both to the individual and to societies at large. Because discoveries in these fields have been both rapid and broad, the series has played a uniquely important role for students and scientists. By synthesizing and updating progress, they offer state-of-the-art reviews of the most recent advances. By continually featuring new topics and involving new authors, they have pushed innovation and fostered new ideas. With the explosion of information and research on aging in recent decades, there has been a concomitant increase in the number of college and university courses and programs focused on aging and longevity. The *Handbook of Aging* series has provided knowledge bases for instruction in these continually changing fields.

Indeed, the *Handbooks* are resources for teachers and students alike, providing information for didactics and inspiration for further research. Given the breadth and depth of the material covered, they serve as both a source of the most current information and as an overview of the various fields. One of the greatest strengths of the chapters in the *Handbooks* is the synthesis afforded by authors who are at the forefront of research and thus provide expert perspectives on the issues that currently define and challenge each field. The interdisciplinary nature of aging research is exemplified by the overlap in concepts in chapters ranging from basic biology to sociology.

We express our deepest thanks to the editors of the individual volumes for their incredible dedication and contributions. It is their efforts to which the excellence of the products is largely credited. We thank Drs. Edward J. Masoro and Steven N. Austad, editors of the *Handbook of the Biology of Aging;* Drs. K. Warner Schaie and Sherry L. Willis, editors of the *Handbook of the Psychology of Aging;* and Drs. Robert H. Binstock and Linda K. George, editors of the *Handbook of Aging and the Social Sciences.* We would also like to express our appreciation to Nikki Levy, our publisher at Elsevier, whose profound interest and dedication has facilitated the publication of the *Handbooks* through their many editions. And, finally, we extend our deepest gratitude to James Birren for establishing and shepherding the series through the first six editions.

Thomas A. Rando, Laura L. Carstensen
Center on Longevity, Stanford University

Preface

This seventh edition of the *Handbook of Aging and the Social Sciences* provides extensive reviews and critical evaluations of research on the social aspects of aging. It also makes available major references and identifies high-priority topics for future research.

To achieve these purposes, the *Handbook* has presented knowledge about aging through the systematic perspectives of a variety of disciplines and professions: anthropology, bioethics, biology, demography, economics, epidemiology, history, law, medicine, political science, policy analysis, public administration, social psychology, social work, and sociology. Building upon six previous editions (1976, 1985, 1990, 1996, 2001, and 2006), this edition reflects the tremendous growth of ideas, information, and research literature on the social aspects of aging that has taken place during the last five years.

The *Handbook* is intended for use by researchers, professional practitioners, and students in the field of aging. It is also expected to serve as a basic reference tool for scholars, professionals, and others who are not presently engaged in research and practice directly focused on aging and the aged.

When the first edition of this *Handbook* was being prepared by Bob Binstock and Ethel Shanas in the early 1970s, only a small number of social scientists were equipped to address any specific topic in a first-rate fashion. More than a quarter of a century later, the field has burgeoned in such quality and quantity that a great many scholars would be outstanding contributors for each of the various subjects chosen for this volume.

Accordingly, this seventh edition was planned and implemented to enlist predominantly new contributors from among the rich variety of distinguished scholars and path-breaking perspectives now constituting the field. Of the 40 authors and co-authors in this edition, 32 did not contribute to the last edition.

In several respects, the contents of this seventh edition are also substantially different from those in the 2006 edition. Eighteen chapters are on subjects that were not in the sixth edition. Their topics are: Aging, the Life Course, and the Sociological Imagination: Prospects for Theory; Aging, Cohorts, and Methods; Demography and Aging; Trends in Longevity and Prospects for the Future; Disability, Functioning, and Aging; Global Aging; Racial and Ethnic Influences over the Life Course; Stratification and Inequality Over the Life Course; Health Disparities Among Older Adults: Life Course Influences and Policy Solutions; Molecular Genetics, Aging, and Well-Being; Social Factors, Depression, and Aging; Aging, Inheritance, and Gift-Giving; Economic Status of the Aged in the United States; Employment and Aging; The Changing Residential Environments of Older People; Civic Engagement and Aging; Late-Life Death and Dying in 21st-Century America; The Politics of Pension Reform in Europe; Politics and Aging in the United States; Gender, Aging and Social Policy; Aging and Social Intervention; and Fiscal Implications of Population Aging.

Six of the seven topics that were maintained from the previous edition have been addressed by different authors, who bring their own perspectives to bear upon the subject matter. The other chapter, Organization and Financing of Health Care, has been substantially revised and brought up-to-date by its author. The continuing topics dealt with by new authors have been treated from rather different viewpoints than in previous editions. The chapter on long-term care, for example, provides a multi-country cross-national perspective on experiences with financing, service delivery, and quality assurance.

As implied by this design of having continuing topics addressed from new but comple-mentary perspectives, the editors and associate editors regard the earlier editions of the *Handbook* as part of the active literature in the field. The chapters in them remain important reference sources for topics and perspectives not represented in this seventh edition. Indeed, because of the ongoing life of those earlier chapters, it was feasible to introduce new dimen-sions within the limited space available in the present volume. Some of the present chapter authors, in fact, build explicitly and actively upon the work of their predecessors in the ear-lier editions. By the same token, it seemed reasonable to not allocate space in this volume to updating certain subjects that were treated in excellent chapters published in the sixth edition only five years ago.

The 25 chapters of this seventh edition are organized in four sections: Part 1. Theory and Methods; Part 2. Aging and Social Structure; Part 3. Social Factors and Social Institutions; and Part 4. Aging and Society. Each chapter was conceived and written specifically for this volume. The book includes a thorough subject-matter index and a comprehensive bibliog-raphy on the social aspects of aging. The research literature cited and referenced in each chapter is also indexed by author at the end of the volume.

The contributors to this seventh edition successfully met a number of challenges. They organized their chapters in terms of analytical constructs that enabled them to sift through a great deal of literature bearing upon their topics. They provided historical perspectives on these subjects, drawing upon classic and contemporary references in the field, and con-structed their presentations so as to ensure that the usefulness of the volume would not be limited by specific time referents. Most impressively, they were able to present their knowledge and viewpoints succinctly and to relate their treatments to those of their fellow authors.

In developing the subject matter for this volume and in selecting contributors, the edi-tors were assisted by three associate editors: Stephen J. Cutler, Jon Hendricks, and James H. Schulz. They also helped the editors substantially in the process of editorial review, in which critical comments and suggestions were forwarded to the authors for their considera-tion in undertaking revised drafts.

Steve Cutler and Joe Hendricks, who joined our editorial team for the sixth edition, were again tremendous assets. Jim Schulz has been an associate editor throughout six editions of the *Handbook* and has authored five different chapters starting with the first edition; we take this opportunity to express our great appreciation and admiration for his outstanding con-tributions over a thirty-five-year journey with the *Handbook*.

The success of this volume is due primarily to the seriousness with which the chapter authors accepted their assignments and to the good will with which they responded to edi-torial criticism and suggestions. To these colleagues, the editors and associate editors would like to express their special appreciation.

Robert H. Binstock
Linda K. George

About the Editors

Robert H. Binstock

Robert H. Binstock is Professor of Aging, Health, and Society at Case Western Reserve University. A former president and fellow of the Gerontological Society of America, and Chair of the Gerontological Health Section of the American Public Health Association (1996–97), he has served as director of a White House Task Force on Older Americans and has frequently testified before the US Congress. He is currently a member of the MacArthur Foundation's Research Network on an Aging Society. Binstock is the author of about 300 articles, book chapters, and monographs, most of them dealing with politics and policies related to aging. His 25 authored and edited books include *Aging Nation: The Economics and Politics of Growing Older in America* (2008, co-authored with James Schulz) and the six previous editions of the *Handbook of Aging and the Social Sciences*. Among the honors he has received for contributions to gerontology and the well-being of older persons are the Kent and Brookdale awards from the Gerontological Society of America; the Lifetime Achievement and Key awards from the Gerontological Health Section of the American Public Health Association; the American Society on Aging Award; the American Society on Aging's Hall of Fame Award; the Ollie A. Randall Award from the National Council on Aging; and the Clark Tibbitts Award from the Association for Gerontology in Higher Education.

Linda K. George

Linda K. George is Professor of Sociology at Duke University, where she also serves as Associate Director of the Duke University Center for the Study of Aging and Human Development. She is a fellow and past president of the Gerontological Society of America. She is former chair of the Aging and Life Course Section of the American Sociological Association. She is former editor of the *Journal of Gerontology, Social Sciences Section*. She currently is Associate Editor of *Demography* and serves on the editorial board of *Society and Mental Health*. Professor George is the author or editor of seven books and author of more than 250 journal articles and book chapters. She co-edited the third, fourth, fifth, and sixth editions of the *Handbook of Aging and the Social Sciences*. Her major research interests include social factors and illness, stress and coping, and the aging self. Among the honors Professor George has received are Phi Beta Kappa; the Duke University Trinity College Distinguished Teaching Award; the W. Fred Cottrell Award for Outstanding Achievement in the Field of Aging; the Mentorship Award from the Behavioral and Social Sciences Section of the Gerontological Society of America; the Kleemeier Award from the Gerontological Society of America; the Dean's Mentoring Award from Duke University; the Matilda White Riley Award from the American Sociological Association; and the Distinguished Career Contribution Award from the Behavioral and Social Sciences Section of the Gerontological Society of America.

Stephen J. Cutler

Stephen J. Cutler is Professor of Sociology, Emeritus and Emeritus Bishop Robert F. Joyce Distinguished University Professor of Gerontology at the University of Vermont. He is a fellow and past president of the Gerontological Society of America (GSA), a past chair of the GSA's Behavioral and Social Sciences Section, and a past chair of the Aging and Life Course Section of the American Sociological Association. Professor Cutler is also a fellow of the Association for Gerontology in Higher Education (AGHE) and has served as an elected and an appointed member of AGHE's Executive Committee. He is a former editor of the *Journal of Gerontology: Social Sciences* and is on the editorial boards of *Research on Aging*, the *Journal of Applied Gerontology*, the *International Journal of Aging and Human Development*, the *American Journal of Alzheimer's Disease*, and *Social Work Review*. He received the Clark Tibbitts Award from the Association for Gerontology in Higher Education, has been designated as a University Scholar by the University of Vermont, was a Petersen Visiting Scholar at Oregon State University, and has taught and conducted research in Romania as a Senior Fulbright Scholar. His research and publications have been in the areas of caregiving, transportation, household composition, social and political attitude change, voluntary association participation, social aspects of cognitive change, and ethics.

Jon (Joe) Hendricks

Jon (Joe) Hendricks is Dean and Professor Emeritus, Oregon State University. He is a past president of the Association for Gerontology in Higher Education (AGHE) and has served as Chair of the Behavioral and Social Sciences Section of the Gerontological Society of America (GSA) and the Section on Aging and the Life Course of the American Sociological Association. He has been named as a fellow in both organizations. Hendricks is widely published in social gerontology, with over two dozen authored or edited books, and has edited two book series in aging for Little, Brown and for Baywood Publishers. He has been recognized by the GSA with its Kalish Innovative Publication Award (1998) and its Kleemeier Award for outstanding research (2008) as well as the Behavioral and Social Sciences Section Award for Distinguished Career Contributions (1994). He has also received AGHE's Clark Tibbitts Award for Outstanding Contributions to Gerontology (2004). In 1994 he was recognized as Researcher of the Year by Oregon State University's chapter of Sigma Xi, the Scientific Research Society. Hendricks has served on the editorial boards of a number of social gerontological journals and is currently Co-Editor-in-Chief of the *Hallym International Journal of Aging*.

James H. Schulz

James H. Schulz is Professor Emeritus, Brandeis University. He is an economist (Ph.D., Yale, 1966) specializing in the economics and demography of aging, pension and retirement policy, and international aging issues. A former president of the Gerontological Society of America, he received the Society's 1983 Kleemeier Award for outstanding research in aging. He also received the 1998 Clark Tibbitts Award for contributions to the field of gerontology and a 1999 Testimonial Award from the United Nations Secretary General for his international aging research and other activities related to the "International Year of Older Persons." His books include *Aging Nation: The Economics and Politics of Growing Older in America* (co-author); *Providing Adequate Retirement Income* (co-author); *The World Ageing Situation, 1991*; *Economics of Population Aging; When "Life-Time Employment" Ends: Older Worker Programs in Japan; Social Security in the 21st Century* (co-author); and *Older Women and Private Pensions in the United Kingdom*. His best-known book is *The Economics of Aging* (which has been translated into Japanese and Chinese and is currently available in its seventh edition).

Part | 1 |

Theory and Methods

Chapter | 1 |

Age, the Life Course, and the Sociological Imagination: Prospects for Theory

Dale Dannefer,
Department of Sociology, Case Western Reserve University, Cleveland, Ohio

CHAPTER CONTENTS

INTRODUCTION: AGE, LIFE COURSE, AND SOCIOLOGICAL IMAGINATION

Recent years have seen a range of new issues emerging to confront social science approaches to age and the life course (hereafter ALC). These include an expanding array of work on the life course in fields as diverse as health and criminology, the growing body of work on cumulative dis/advantage that problematizes the intersection of age and inequality, break-through understandings of biosocial interactions, and global population aging. In some respects, such issues represent fresh versions of longstanding problems in the study of ALC. Yet they also comprise a range of new phenomena for analysis that may challenge the contours of existing theory, and they cannot be ignored by efforts to develop a theoretical understanding of ALC.

This chapter reviews aspects of these developments in the context of more general theoretical considerations. It begins with a review of the place of theory in life course studies. Although the field of ALC has been subjected to little formal theorizing, insights contributed along several axes of inquiry have had a major impact on the study of age, especially in compelling a recognition of the importance of social circumstances and events in shaping age-related patterns and outcomes. Moreover, despite the lack of formal theory, theoretical assumptions are often implicit in empirical studies and discussions of the life course, and they have consequences for the framing of research questions and the interpretation of findings. This chapter is concerned with such implicit assumptions as well as more explicit theoretical statements.

To organize the discussion, I rely on a refined version of the matrix of ALC research outlined in earlier work (Dannefer & Kelley-Moore, 2009; Dannefer & Uhlenberg, 1999), comprised of typologies of *explananda* (types of phenomena to be explained) and *explanantia* (types of explanations), beginning by offering some general comments about the development of theoretical problems in the study of ALC. It is useful to begin by clarifying what is meant by "theory" – a term with many possible definitions. As defined here, a scientific theory consists of an effort to provide an *account* or *explanation* of a phenomenon of interest, based on empirical evidence. It is the objective of theory to illuminate that which was obscure and simplify that which was complex or bewildering. By showing how seemingly disparate forces may be connected to each other, it gives order to a congeries of disorganized observations.

Developing sound theory has special challenges in fields where unsound beliefs and assumptions abound, which is inevitably the case in the study of age. "Knowledge" of many familiar and seemingly obvious age-related phenomena – often those involving forms of decline – is readily available to everyone. Despite extensive evidence that development and aging are contingent and modifiable processes, even social and behavioral scientists share the popular idea that many kinds of individual change "inevitably happen" with age, and are therefore "explained" by age. From doctor visits to late-night television, such assumptions are part of daily experience in late modern societies, to which gerontologists are not immune.

In the case of age, the problem is complicated not only by an unreflected and culturally defined familiarity with the subject matter, but also by the fact that age itself appears as a property of the *individual* that is anchored largely in the self-contained processes of the *organism*. It is thus inherently a topic that is vulnerable to reductionism, naturalization, and microfication.

Half a century ago, C. Wright Mills called upon social scientists to cultivate and nurture "sociological imagination" – the proactive exploration of the ways in which social forces shape human experience and the values and perspectives that regulate individual lives. As Mills noted, a failure to exercise sociological imagination is an abdication of intellectual responsibility that risks the ceding of conceptual terrain to the explanatory efforts of other disciplines (1959, p. 13–18). This chapter is concerned with the potentials of sociological imagination to illuminate the issues currently facing the study of ALC, from the dynamics of retirement to gene–environment (GE) interactions. We begin with a review of key developments in the establishment of the current field of ALC studies, before focusing on how social science explanations are being mobilized in current work and their potentials for illuminating emerging questions and issues.

THE EMERGENCE OF THE LIFE COURSE IN THE STUDY OF AGE

In the last few decades, the role of circumstances and events in shaping how human beings' age has been increasingly recognized, catalyzed by the emergence of several strands of work that comprise the life course perspective. These themes were given an initial articulation in early statements outlining the life course as a field of study (Cain, 1964; Elder, 1975). Along with cohort analysis (Ryder, 1965) and Riley's initial articulation of the "aging and society" (or "age stratification") framework (Riley et al., 1972, 1994), the life course perspective emerged in the 1970s as a key arena of scholarship for understanding aging. Simultaneously, constructivist approaches provided fresh and powerful insights into the constitution of aging in everyday life (e.g. Gubrium, 1978). The sociological imagination was clearly vibrant during this foundational period, which established life course principles as essential to understanding human aging.

BIOGRAPHY AND STRUCTURE: TWO PARADIGMS OF LIFE COURSE SCHOLARSHIP

From its beginnings, the life course perspective has included two broad, yet distinct, paradigmatic orientations, which may termed the *biographical* and the *institutional*. The term *biographical* encompasses the analysis of life course patterns and outcomes in terms of trajectories and transitions; the *institutional* perspective refers to the organization of social structures and practices in age-graded and age-normalized terms. The distinction represents a refinement of an earlier framework (e.g. Dannefer & Kelley-Moore, 2009) and is also represented in other recent discussions, such as Mayer's contrast of "early conditions and later life outcomes" vs "institutions" as the two major foci of life course research (2009, pp. 417–419). Each of these orientations is focused on a distinct set of explananda, with its own research questions and problems. Both are essential to a full discussion of ALC theory.

The *biographical* perspective is focused on depicting the trajectories and transitions that characterize individual lives. Studies in this tradition have numerous intellectual foci ranging from identifying the impact of individuals' early experiences on subsequent life outcomes to studies that examine historical change in transition behavior. In this tradition, the explananda consist of the empirical patterning and/or outcomes of individual lives. For most research within the biographical tradition, the individual is the unit of analysis (George, 2009). However, the unit of analysis can also be collective. Indeed, the cohort is often the unit of analysis in several important lines of life course research, such as studies of cumulative dis/advantage that rely on measures of inequality, and studies of life transition behavior based on cohort-level measures.

The *institutional* perspective focuses on the life course as a component of social structure and culture. As such, the life course is a property not of individual human actors but of social systems, manifested in rules, practices, law, policy, and operative aspects of social institutions. This approach is prototypically illustrated in the formulation of the institutionalized life course (hereafter ILC) first set forth by Martin Kohli (1986, 2007). The social apparatus that organizes age also includes the realm of ideas – in "expert" knowledge and in norms and aesthetics that serve to legitimate and naturalize age-graded practices. Such pronouncements are often based on age-related notions that are accorded the status of authoritative knowledge (deriving from areas such as science or medicine), and are sometimes used to sanction behavior as well as inform policy formulation. Here, the study of aging intersects with the sociology of science (Dannefer, 1999a). In sum, from the institutional perspective, the set of social institutions, practices, and ideas that defines the life course is itself the central problematic of analysis.

While both biographical and institutional foci are described in the seminal formulations of Cain and of Riley and associates, these two approaches reflect a differential emphasis between North America and Europe. Research on biographical life course outcomes

has characterized life course analysis in North America, whilst European scholars have elaborated the problem of the life course as a structural feature of society (Hagestad & Dannefer, 2001; Mayer, 2009).

STRATEGIES OF EXPLANATION

Within each of these two types of life course phenomenon or problematization, several strategies of explanation – *explanantia* – have been advanced. It is often in the type of explanation a researcher proposes that theoretical ideas enter the analysis, regardless of whether the theoretical claim is explicit or implicit. Strategies of explanation can be generally categorized in to the two encompassing categories of *personological* and *sociological*. *Personological* refers to postulated explanations that locate the presumed cause primarily within the person rather than in the domain of temporally proximate experience and context. Such causal factors may range from general organismic processes of aging to psychosocial processes involving skills, memories, or "choices." *Sociological* explanations, by contrast, are those in which the explanation is located externally to the person, in aspects of the temporally proximate micro-, meso-, or macro-level environment. Within each of these two broad categories, a range of different subtypes can be distinguished. A matrix of life course explananda and explanantia (Figure 1.1) will be used to organize the discussion, including examples for each cell. Emphatically, this is a classification of types of *research*, not of *researchers*. The work of many scholars cannot be confined to just one of these categories.

THE BIOGRAPHICAL PERSPECTIVE

Perhaps the most popular type of problem for life course analysis, especially in North America, concerns *individual life trajectories and outcomes* and their shaping by earlier life circumstances.

EXPLANANDA	EXPLANANTIA	
	Personological	**Sociological**
Biographical Individual	**A1** General age-related change processes Stable individual differences Early life experiences Agency	**B1** Trajectory change via adult opportunity Predictive adaptive response Social effects on physical change
Collective	**A2** Population aging & cognitive change Social change in transition timing/choice	**B2** Inequality, poverty, and social policy Cumulative dis/advantage by opportunity structures
Institutional	**C** Cohort norm formation	**D** Institutionalization of the life course Age norms Naturalization of age by developmental theories

Figure 1.1   Explananda and explanantia of the life course.

Cell A1: Individual Life Course Outcomes Accounted for by Personological Factors

Personological explanations for individual life course outcomes take numerous forms, including: (1) general age-related change processes; (2) putatively stable individual-difference characteristics such as genes, traits, temperament, or personality; (3) prior experience including the development of habits, creative potentials, and coping skills; and (4) "agency" or "choice."

General Age-Related Change Processes

The assumption of an inevitable age-related decline in functioning was, of course, famously formalized in the universalized propositions of disengagement theory (Cumming & Henry, 1961). Like other stage models, disengagement is a version of organismic theory (Dannefer, 1984; Hochschild, 1975). This approach continues to be an influential idea in numerous areas of research such as cognitive aging (Alwin & Hofer, 2008) and in social science applications lifespan theories such as Baltes' Selection-Optimization-Compensation model (e.g. Kahana et al., 2002). Descriptive evidence pointing to age-related decline as a general trend for many individual characteristics probably sustains the plausibility of these ideas, even though they often entail the risk of what Riley (1973) called a "life course fallacy" – mistaking cross-sectional observations for biographical patterns.

Stable Individual Differences

Beyond explanations that focus on species-wide or general age-related factors, some studies take an individual differences approach, focusing on trait-like features of the individual. Whether regarded as innate or as developing early in the life course, such characteristics are often hypothesized to predict later life outcomes.

Some of the work on GE interactions fits within this category, reflecting a growing interest in the "social or environmental influence on the expression of genetic predisposition" (Guo & Stearns, 2002, p. 884; see also Chapter 10). As life course scholars have become concerned with integrating developments from the expanding discourse on GE interactions into their work, one form that such interaction can take is expressed in the simple assumption that genetically determined or constrained characteristics may shape life course outcomes. Shanahan et al. (2003) describe three ways that genetic endowment may "correlate" with environmental influences: passive, reactive, and active. Even the most interactive of these (active) clearly locates the primary explanatory force within the individual, at the genetic level:

> The active correlation refers to the person actively selecting and molding settings that are congruent with his or her genetic endowment.

> For example, a person with a genotype favoring high reasoning ability may choose work that is substantively complex, which tends to provide further opportunities for enhanced intellectual functioning. (2003, p. 605)

Although interactive, the primacy of a postulated genetic cause is clearly articulated here in a straightforward way. Numerous examples of research postulating such a unidirectional logic of causality from genetic endowment to phenotypic characteristics and life course outcomes can be found in research on an array of topics relevant to life course studies (e.g. childbearing and family formation, crime, twin studies). This work represents an important early step in bringing together work on the life course and GE interactions. As will be discussed below, however, such approaches comprise a relatively narrow set of a broader spectrum of ways that GE interactions are currently being conceptualized (see also Chapter 10).

Early Life Experience

Much research in the life course tradition has emphasized the importance of early experience on life course outcomes. Indeed, the prototypical logic of life course research introduced by Glen Elder in *Children of the Great Depression* (1999 (1974)) and related writings is based on a straightforward logic that seeks to account for outcomes later in the life course on the basis of earlier life experiences. By demonstrating the consequences of early experience, this work helped make clear that aging cannot be understood as a purely individual matter. It provided a major catalyst to demonstrate the importance of social science approaches in the study of aging, opening a window onto a horizon of context and social structure.

Such work has clearly extended the reach of the sociological imagination. Nevertheless, in this approach, measurement of the environment is often limited to the initial wave of data collection, so that subsequent circumstances and events are not considered. This practice, called "Time One Encapsulation," means that context only matters at the point of initial data collection and its effects "are thus carried forward through time and assumed to manifest themselves as a characteristic of the individual in middle and later life" (Dannefer & Kelley-Moore, 2009, p. 395).

A second example of Time One Encapsulation is provided by Doblhammer and Vaupel's (2001) longitudinal study of the link between seasonality and mortality. They find that mortality risk at age 50 is related to month of birth, with lower risk for persons born in Autumn than in Spring in both Southern and Northern hemispheres. Despite the strength of the finding, the use of vital statistics records limits exploration of unmeasured social factors that may mediate or underlie the birth-month–mortality connection, thereby encapsulating the primary explanans for the later-life mortality differential in early life.

Agency

Agency is frequently invoked in the discourse on the life course, sometimes nominated to explain what is "left over" as unexplained variance, but in other cases as a central component in a carefully articulated model. For example, in stress research (Pearlin & Skaff, 1996), concepts such as proactive aging and "preventive proactivity" have received increasing attention (Kahana et al., 2002; Ouwehand et al., 2007).

As a second example, consider research on work and retirement. In this area, choice is assumed in economic models that rely on a few predictor variables aligned with rational choice theory (Costa, 1998; Lee, 2001). Such models involve a series of difficult assumptions that invite more careful empirical analysis, including attention to work–family issues (Han & Moen, 1999; Shuey & O'Rand, 2004), the equation of age and disability, and other issues (Kelley-Moore, 2010; O'Rand, 2005; Warner et al., 2010).

Cell B1: Individual Life Course Outcomes Explained by Sociological Factors

Sociological explanantia of individual life course outcomes are those that refer to temporally proximate features of social structure and the dynamics of ongoing social life. There has been no shortage of sociological research that illustrates the impact of the immediate social circumstances on life course outcomes. Often, such circumstances have no explicit connection to age, but in many familiar and relevant instances they do – as in the case of retirement policies, age grading in schools, and the documented salience of the correlated factors of age and time-in-job in the construction of careers (Hermanowicz, 2007; Kanter, 1993; Lawrence, 1996). Indeed, the social meanings and rules assigned to age may themselves become a force that explains life course outcomes. Thus, age-graded social structures such as the ILC are relevant not only as a problem to be explained (to be discussed below) but also as an explanation – as a factor that shapes individual and collective life course trajectories. Whatever the property being studied, the importance of looking at temporally proximate social characteristics is well-illustrated by cases in which circumstances in adulthood change the course of earlier trajectories.

The Potential of Social Circumstances in Adulthood to Modify Life Course Trajectories

The work of Laub and Sampson on crime over the life course (2003; Sampson & Laub, 2005) offers an exemplary set of studies demonstrating the contingency of adult outcomes on recent as well as biographically prior experiences. Based on a follow-up of the participants in the Gluecks' classic study of delinquent boys begun in the 1940s, they demonstrate that changing opportunities and circumstances in adulthood can "reset" what happens earlier. For example, they found that the post-World War II GI Bill disproportionately benefited veterans with a delinquent past (2003, pp. 48–51), demonstrating how emergent opportunity structures can create a dramatic change in what once appeared to be a stable trajectory. Marriage and stable work circumstances also predicted a reduced likelihood of criminal activity. Laub and Sampson demonstrated that these findings cannot be accounted for by a turnaround in delinquent behavior that precedes these work–family changes, and that such life course developments cannot be explained by selection effects. At least in the post-World War II environment, it appeared that military experience combined with the GI Bill led both to a severing of earlier peer relationships and a diminishment of the stigmatization deriving from having earlier been labeled a delinquent.

Predictive Adaptive Response: The Interaction of Fetal Development with Adult Health

Especially in domains related to health, some of the clearest demonstrations of the effects of social forces on individual outcomes have come from outside the social sciences, as discoveries in the health sciences have continued to point to the role of multiple aspects of social experience (e.g. nutrition, toxin exposure, lifestyle factors). Among the consequences of such research has been the establishment of an emerging field of biology: ecological developmental biology (e.g. Gilbert & Epel, 2009). Barker's (1998) work relating birthweight and adult obesity was an important catalyst for this developing field, which emphasizes the interaction of early and subsequent environments in determining the form of gene expression.

The unavoidable necessity of incorporating the analysis of social forces into such research is well illustrated in the work of biologists Peter Gluckman and Mark Hanson, who describe their version of "a life course approach" in remarkably familiar terms: "There are at least three aspects to consider: the various strands of inheritance, the environment experienced during development, and the environment now being faced" (2006a, 2006b, p. 204). Gluckman and Hanson coined the term "predictive adaptive response" to describe components of fetal or early childhood development that "set" the developing organism's pattern of gene expression, with sometimes counterintuitive effects on adult health. The term refers to the capacity of fetus and infant to "sense its environment," and to use nutritional or hormonal signals from the mother to determine key settings for "mobilizing nutrients to support…development" (2006b, p.166).

Two key elements of these processes are relevant to life course theorizing. The first is "epigenesis," or the regulation of genetic expression by environmental conditions (see Chapter 10). Second is the "setting" or stabilization of the epigenetic outcome into a specific set of metabolic and hormonal "habituations" that constitute the organism's prediction of its future environmental circumstances. If, for example, the food supply changes so that nutritional intake does not match predictions made at the very beginning of the life course, severe health problems may ensue. The prototypical example, found in alarming proportions in a growing number of societies, is ready access to high-fat, high-carbohydrate diets of individuals who were undernourished as infants – a recipe for obesity, diabetes, and other health problems. Such a case makes clear that the risk of health problems in adulthood can be understood neither by Time One nor Time Two information alone, but as the product of their interaction (Gluckman & Hanson, 2004). This case makes clear the growing recognition in biology and genetics of the sustained importance of social and environmental forces over the life course. In the context of aging, similar arguments have also been developed concerning life course risks for developing dementia (Douthit, 2006; Douthit & Dannefer, 2007). Such cases illustrate vividly the limitations to knowledge that may accompany Time One Encapsulation.

Efforts to link genetic influence to complex human activity and behavior have shown relatively little success, compared to the powerful effects seen in "Mendelian" outcomes involved in disease processes that are determined or largely determined by one allele (Guo et al., 2009). Findings such as those discussed here suggest that advances in such efforts will require more detailed information on social and environmental factors. Such work has the potential to enhance simultaneously our understanding of the life course, and the value of social science theory and techniques for colleagues working in other disciplines.

Physical and Genetic Effects of Experience During Adulthood

The development of brain imaging techniques has made it possible to show the impact of environmental change on brain growth during childhood. Children who have lived under sustained traumatic or near-feral circumstances have the effects of those experiences inscribed in abnormal patterns of brain development, but such physical abnormalities can be corrected by effective early interventions (see, for example, Perry & Svalavitz, 2006). However, such socially regulated cognitive and physical changes do not appear to be limited to childhood. In a study

utilizing structural MRI brain scans, significantly increased "gray matter volume" was found in both hippocampal lobes of licensed London cab drivers (who must study for a minimum of 10 months, memorizing the city's map to qualify) compared with a control group (Maguire et al., 2000).

Other developments demonstrate that the relevance of the sociological imagination in adulthood also reaches to the genetic level. Here, one promising line of discovery concerns features of social experience, specifically of one's social network. Social isolation and connectedness are of increasing interest to some biologists, who have found effects of the quality of social experience to be correlated with gene expression, with consequences for immune system functioning. For example, in an analysis of 55-year-olds (using the Chicago Health, Aging, and Social Relations Study), differences between individuals reporting high and low levels of social isolation were found in the expression of 209 genes in circulating leukocytes. The authors conclude that the "data identify a distinct transcriptional fingerprint of subjective social isolation in human leukocytes, which involves increased basal expression of inflammatory and immune response genes." (Cole et al., 2007, p. 10). Interestingly, biological researchers began to look at such issues, in part through concern about the societal issues of television and computer usage, and the substitution of such activity for face-to-face social interaction (Sigman, 2009).

Across these several horizons of discovery of the importance of social forces in shaping biosocial interactions and genetic expression, it is interesting to note the extent to which intellectual questions are being driven by biological researchers. Such lines of research suggest that new measures of physical change at both the genetic and cellular levels provide opportunities to link such characteristics to social science measures, and hence to apply the sociological imagination to a much wider range of age-related and life course outcomes than previously envisioned.

Cell A2: Collective Life Course Outcomes Accounted for by Personological Factors

Cells A2 and B2 are concerned with the life course outcomes of a population or other collectivity. Typically, in life course research, the cohort comprises the collective unit of analysis. Examples are distributional characteristics such as intracohort variability or inequality, or measures of cohort transition behavior such as the interquartile range. Cohort size can also be a factor of interest. An example is provided by the analysis undertaken by Alwin and associates, who focus on the societal costs and policy implications of cognitive decline assumed to accompany population aging. In their view, declines in physical and cognitive function are "to some extent intrinsic to the organism rather than brought about by the environment; and they occur in a pattern that is characteristic of all members of a given species" (Alwin, 2010; see also Alwin & Hofer, 2008). Thus, the projected rapid expansion in the numbers of aging individuals likely to experience cognitive decline poses a societal problem that requires attention because of the population-level strains it will place on the social system.

A second example is offered by demographic studies of cohort differences in transition behavior. During the twentieth century, research consistently suggested trends toward increasing homogeneity among age peers in making the transitions to adulthood (e.g. Buchmann, 1989; Hogan, 1981) and retirement (Blossfeld et al., 2006). This increase in conformity in transition behavior has been interpreted as resulting from economic prosperity, which provides greater opportunities for individual expression or choice (Costa, 1998; Modell, 1989). As has been noted earlier, this interpretation is quite paradoxical, in that it presumes greater choice leading to greater conformity (e.g. Dannefer, 1984; Kohli, 2007). More recently, there has emerged some evidence that this trend toward age-based conformity in transition behavior may be showing signs of reversal with the delay of marriage (Harper & Harper, 2004; Lehrer, 2008), extended educational careers, erosion of work life and career stability (Fitch & Ruggles, 2000), and boomerang children. Yet again, choice and individual decision making often figure in the interpretation offered for such changes.

Cell B2: Collective Life Course Outcomes Accounted for by Sociological Factors

A topic of growing interest in the study of ALC has been the process of cumulative dis/advantage, which is concerned with the intersection of age and inequality (e.g. Crystal & Shea, 2003; Dannefer, 1987, 2003a, 2009; Ferraro & Shippee, 2009; O'Rand, 2003). As noted earlier, inequality and variability are inherently properties not of individuals but of cohorts (or other population units), and the outcomes of interest concern the distribution of a characteristic over the specified population unit and the construction of life course trajectories of inequality. Several studies in this tradition present trajectories of inequality (e.g. Crystal & Waehrer, 1996; Dannefer & Sell, 1988), although others examine inequality by comparing subgroup differences (Farkas, 2003; Ferraro & Kelley-Moore, 2003; Mirowsky & Ross, 2005). In this work, the underlying theoretical framework focuses on macro-level social processes believed to amplify inequality as individuals move through age-graded opportunity structures. This argument is supported by related work showing historical (e.g. Leisering & Leibfried, 2000) and

cross-national (Hoffman, 2008) variation consistent with predictions based on policy differences and change, such as the effects of social security and other pension systems in the US and the implementation of more extensive welfare state policies in European societies. Due to the link between resources and health that comprises the socioeconomic gradient, such patterns may also reflect effects on health.

The Institutional Perspective: Cells C and D

Although great variation exists among and within societies over time (e.g. Achenbaum, 1978; Chudacoff, 1989; Ikels & Beall, 2001), the established practices of every society deal with matters of aging. In each society, a particular mode of apprehending aging is an integral feature of language, culture, and social organization. Cells C and D are concerned with this phenomenon – with age as an integral and organizing feature of social structure.

Sociological Accounts of Age and Life Course as Elements of Social Structure

The early North American formulations of the life course (Cain, 1964; Riley et al., 1972) acknowledged the importance of age and life course ideation as a feature of social structure. Yet this idea has been given its most systematic elaboration in several lines of European work, beginning with the pioneering work of Martin Kohli (1986) on the life course as a social institution.

From this perspective, the particular constellation of roles, age-based legal statuses, policies, norms, and expectations that comprises the life course of late modernity can be analyzed as a social institution that is an emergent feature of the modern state, which first institutionalized age grading in childhood (see, e.g. Gillis, 1974; Kett, 1977), and then in later life through the establishment of retirement (Ekerdt & DeViney, 1990; Macmillan, 2005). Such demographic "age homogenization" gave rise to further increases in "age consciousness" and to age norms (Settersten & Hagestad, 1996).

Kohli's framework is not limited to the analysis of the structural and symbolic apparatus of society. An important element of his overall argument concerns the effect of the institutionalization of the life course on individual lives, which was noted earlier. As such, numerous properties related to the hereafter ILC, such as pension policy or age norms, stand as explanantia in relation to biographical life course outcomes. The order provided by such structures, Kohli suggests, is one form of solution to the enduring social problem of order in modernity. *Gemeinschaft* is thus replaced not by some new form of collectivity, but by "individualization" and "temporalization," which bring a sense of orderliness to individual biography – a solution to the threat of anomie never anticipated by the classical theorists:

> *The model of institutionalization of the life course refers to the evolution, during the last two centuries, of an institutional program regulating one's movement through life both in terms of a sequence of positions and in terms of a set of biographical orientations by which to organize one's experiences and plans (Kohli, 2007, p.255).*

For life course scholars, a key point is that these developments rely on chronological age as an organizing criterion. Kohli refers to this process as "chronologization," and it receives support from historical work documenting the development of age awareness and age norms in North America (Chudacoff, 1989). Of course, the ILC can take a variety of forms across as well as within societies (Mayer, 2001). Moreover, it is clear that the generic structure of life course institutionalization is much broader and can be configured in ways that are dramatically different from the dominant narrative form of the ILC as a component of the welfare state.

Consider, for example, the career stages (tiny gangster, li'l homey, homeboy, O.G.) of the abbreviated life course that is institutionalized within the social world of urban street gangs in the US (Bing, 1991; Burton, 2007; Burton et al., 1996; Dannefer, 2003b). The life course of such "marginal" social worlds can easily pass unnoticed by middle-class researchers, but it is enduring and resilient; in the US, street gang culture is older than the culture of schools. It is intriguing to consider whether the life course perspective may add to, or be informed by, an analysis of the structural interdependence of such marginal yet resilient subcultural structures with the official and state-sanctioned versions of the ILC.

Another aspect of the ILC that requires sociological analysis is its *ideological* function in legitimating and naturalizing age. The dominant narrative of the ILC has made specific ideas about "age normality" or "age-appropriateness" widely plausible and popular, giving them a sense of taken-for-granted-ness. This *naturalization* of the life course has been sanctioned by psychological and developmental theories that declare the life stages comprising the ILC to be universal expressions of human nature. In each case, historical and social analysis have shown how such theories are recent innovations that have followed the emergence of an institutional apparatus leading to a social preoccupation with a particular life stage (see, for example, Kett (1977) on adolescence, Hochschild (1975) and Riley (1978) on disengagement, and Dannefer (1984, 1999b) on adult development theory). Thus, such theories can be analyzed as components of an ideological apparatus that supports the ILC by conferring upon it the status of "human nature."

Currently, scholars of the ILC are debating whether the challenges posed to the welfare state by the second demographic transition (Lesthage & Neels, 2002) and globalization are leading to a *de-institutionalization* of the life course, if greater economic uncertainty threatens the stability of the life course regime (Kohli, 2007; Macmillan, 2005; Phillipson & Scharf, 2004).

From the "life course as structure" perspective, the uncritical acceptance of social or psychological theories of individual aging (whether in terms of age-graded roles or "life stages") is a form of naturalization (Dannefer, 1999b) that is content to make general extrapolations about aging from a superficial description of observed life course patterns in the immediate and local present, without probing to understand the causal forces underlying such patterns.

Personological Approaches to the Life Course as Structure

To the extent that discussions of age norms or life course institutions emphasize individual aging as a reality to which social structure must *accommodate*, they provide examples for Cell C – personological explanations for the institutionalization of the life course. That is the implication of selection-based psychological models applied to age (e.g. Baltes & Freund, 2003; Charles & Carstensen, 2007), and of Callahan's "expectable life course," proposed as a rationale for limiting medical care to elders, in response to projections of rising health care costs (1995; for an analysis see Binstock, 2002).

In addition to arguments that presume inevitable organismic change, human agency has also been proposed as an explanation of change in the social-structural organization and meaning of age. That is what Matilda Riley attempted to do with her idea of cohort norm formation (1978). Using as an example age-related changes in women's status in the 1970s, she proposed that changes in age norms – specifically age-related changes in gender expectations – resulted from a large aggregation of individual women simultaneously making similar decisions about their lifestyle. While her depiction is not incorrect, it is inevitably incomplete since it does not address the contextual factors behind the decision making processes of the women in question. Rather than a matter of decontextualized "pure choice," this was seen as a response to the women's movement and the attendant cultural, political, and economic developments of the time.

SOCIAL SCIENCE THEORIES OF AGE AND THE LIFE COURSE AND THE SOCIOLOGICAL IMAGINATION

Although the sociological imagination has been alive and well in the study of ALC, recent developments compel scholars of ALC to think in more interdisciplinary, global, and critical terms. As population aging becomes an increasingly global phenomenon even as globalization challenges the capacities of post-industrial societies to maintain policies that support growing elder populations, the organization and meaning of age may change again. And at the individual level, we are learning more about the extent to which aging is shaped by experience, and hence by the social, political, and economic structures that organize everyday life.

It is ironic that at the same time that social scientists are seeking to integrate concepts from fields such as behavioral genetics and evolutionary biology into their work, biologists are emphasizing the importance of environmental influences on physical change, including the regulation of gene expression, throughout the life course. Such dynamics unavoidably cross disciplinary boundaries and involve multiple kinds of multi-level processes. Within and beyond the study of ALC, efforts to understand and conceptualize such processes are still at an early stage. Clearly, this comprises an important horizon for the sociological imagination.

One way to consider the place of the sociological imagination in theorizing ALC is to contrast two broadly different heuristic postures toward the investigation of individual life course outcomes with social forces: first, a heuristic of *containment*, and second, a heuristic of *openness*. As will be seen, these two heuristic postures or attitudes correspond to two different modes of theorizing – first, the symbiosis of functionalism and developmental theory that has guided much theorizing in social science approaches to ALC and that rests on a modified organismic model of development, and, second, a social critical or constitutionalist approach that begins with a recognition of human development, age, and life course as constituted to the core only in and through social processes (Dannefer, 2008).

Heuristic of Containment

The heuristic of containment refers to explanatory models in which the logic of the analysis implicitly, if not explicitly, limits and contains the effect of social forces. Such logic has a long history in social science approaches to aging. For example, cohort analyses have often been conducted with a heuristic of containment, as when environmental effects are equated with intercohort differences, while ignoring intracohort variability. In such cases, intracohort variation has the conceptual status of noise, or uninteresting error variation.

Another arena in which a heuristic of containment can be discerned is in discussions of GE interactions that credit an unwarranted amount of variation in social practices or outcomes to genotypic variation. Numerous such studies exist in the psychological and social-psychological literatures, dealing with issues as diverse as crime, poverty, sexuality, and even religiosity.

To illustrate the logic of containment in such work, the typology of GE interactions presented by Shanahan and Hofer (2005) offers a useful starting point. In their four-fold typology, social conditions may (1) trigger, (2) control, (3) compensate, or (4) enhance genetic potentials. Except for triggering, each of these four categories entails a heuristic of containment, because in each case one single socio-environmental variable is introduced; everything not accounted for by this single factor is implicitly credited to the genotype.

Consider as an example one popular idea in studies of GE interactions, which is that the amount of repressive control one experiences regulates the influence of the genome. As Guo and Stearns (2002, p.885) contend:

Within a society, individuals may enjoy different levels of opportunities or face different levels of societal constraint with respect to a particular behavior. Individuals who live under greater societal constraint have more difficulty in realizing their genetic potential.

Similar arguments by others have suggested that genetic differences can explain phenomena as diverse as school performance and historical variation in sexual activity (Dunne et al., 1997).

Such discussions acknowledge the importance of social context as an operative factor in regulating activity, including genetic expression, *but only in the matter of social control as indexed by one or two factors, such as long-term social change or family stress.* Remaining variance is assumed to be accounted for at the individual level, and assigned to the genome. The problem with this approach should be obvious: The sociological imagination recognizes that one or a few measured social factors cannot begin to represent the total effect of social forces, nor can all remaining variance properly be ascribed to the genome, for at least two kinds of reasons that respect entirely the importance of genetic differences. First, consider the point – well-established but seldom recognized – that some genetic characteristics (e.g. skin color, height) trigger interactional cues from others that shape behavior (e.g. Jencks, 1980; Joseph, 2004; Marmot, 2004). Thus, the behavioral significance of gene-based traits is socially organized. A second kind of issue concerns what is overlooked in terms of psychosocial dynamics. For example, it can be questioned whether the kinds of change generally depicted in such analyses represent a *reduction* in social control rather than, possibly, a *reconfiguration* of social control – locating it, for example, in the peer group rather than community-level constraints (as regards sexual behavior [Dunne et al., 1997]), or, paradoxically, in community-level constraints rather than the peer group or street gang (as regards intellectual development (Guo & Stearns, 2002)). More generally, scholarship on historical change in the self contends that what is imagined to be an increase in freedom is merely a shift in the mode of control from, for example, religious to commercial regulation of impulses (Ewen, 1976; Schor, 2004; Turner, 1976; Wexler, 1977).

Heuristic of Openness

The heuristic of openness entails a logic that imposes no preconceived foreclosure on the scope of influence of social forces, and considers the possibility of their effects in domains where they may be unexpected. Developing work in areas such as ecological developmental biology make clear that this strategy can be pursued not just by social scientists, but by natural scientists as well, when confronted with clear empirical evidence of the importance of the social, as, for example, in the earlier discussion of the effects of social isolation on gene expression.

The heuristic of openness begins with an explicit recognition that, since before the event of birth, the genetic material contained in each individual has been immersed in a pervasive social and physical environment that regulates the expression of genes, with long-term consequences for the phenotype (Gluckman & Hanson, 2006b; Jablonka & Raz, 2009). Subtle but relentless forces of everyday life, from diet to the quality of social contact, are responsible for setting initial parameters on genetic expression and continue throughout the life course.

In seeking to understand GE interactions, the sociological imagination thus compels the rigorous development of hypotheses concerning how social processes may regulate genetic expression in previously unrecognized ways and in every type of social environment. The power of social life to influence individual development and aging (whether measured at biochemical and cellular levels or through direct measures of, for example, health, cognition, or activity) does not change with a change in social regime. It is a constant of human existence and human development. From this perspective, the idea that social or environmental effects might "enhance" or "compensate" for the genotype (Shanahan & Hofer, 2005) must rely on an assumption of the existence of a "normal" situation against which enhancement or compensation is measured – a "normal" situation that is itself socially constructed. Such an assumption, integral to the functionalist-developmental symbiosis that underlies the heuristic of containment, must be rejected if we are to recognize that social contexts, no less than individuals, are continuously reconstituted in social

activity (Baars, 1991; Berger & Luckmann, 1967; Dannefer, 1999b). Only by recognizing the actual processes through which social relations are constituted will we be in a position to apprehend the multilevel power of social forces in shaping the life course.

Thus, the heuristic of openness begins with the recognition that emphasizes developmental plasticity at every level, beginning with a recognition that the translation of the genome into a phenotype is irreducibly an *epigenetic* process. It recognizes that a human organism will never be formed into a person at all without massive influences upon gene expression by environmental interaction (from chemical to the purely social), and the intricacies of the phenotype that emerges will depend fundamentally on the nature of experience (Cole, 2008; Dannefer, 2008).

SUMMARY: AGE AND THE REACH OF THE SOCIOLOGICAL IMAGINATION

The study of ALC faces an era of new possibilities, and with it new obligations, to exercise sociological imagination. The ideal types of "containment" and "openness" each have their own distinctive posture to approaching research and theory, and offer a distinction that may be useful in clarifying assumptions that underlie postulated explanations that cut across disciplines.

In view of the apprehensions of some social scientists toward physical and biological factors, it is noteworthy that biometric techniques such as brain imaging and gene mapping have provided compelling arguments for the unrecognized reach of social forces, and hence for a heuristic of openness. Failing to press the question of the possibility of an effect of social forces is a betrayal of the sociological imagination and a failure to perform the central task of social science, which is to ensure that the full power of social forces in shaping reality is recognized.

The issues that are at stake in considering these two heuristic postures are not limited to abstract theoretical discussion or debates over how to interpret research findings. They may reach to other domains, ranging from general cultural constructions of age (which, as noted, naturalize differences between and within age groups) to the formulation of research agendas by funders (Falletta, 2010). It may also reach to the arenas of policy and practice. For example, a strategy of containment is integral to the structure and operation of nursing homes, which by their logic assume the passivity and incompetence of residents. Such an assumption can be quite destructive, since it entails a social organization and cultural logic that focuses on the vulnerabilities of frail elders rather than their remaining strengths – a focus that has implications for the goals of care and the structure of opportunities afforded frail elders for engagement and growth in everyday life (Barkan, 2003; Dannefer et al., 2008; Kane et al., 2007; Kayser-Jones, 1990). Despite the proliferation of alternative residential models and culture change initiatives (Kane et al., 2007; Thomas, 1996), the traditional model of containment remains robust.

Across multiple domains of research, policy, practice, and popular constructions, implicit theoretical assumptions organize and guide our understanding and consciousness concerning the nature and possibilities of age, development, and the life course. In some cases, such assumptions may be correct and useful. In many cases, as gerontologists well know, they can be empirically wrong and humanly destructive. Yet to the extent that they are taken for granted as inevitable aspects of aging, they cannot be subjected to careful empirical and intellectual scrutiny. Therefore, a key contribution of efforts to theorize

ALC is to encourage, model, and nurture the careful examination of such assumptions. Such scrutiny can be enhanced by the deliberate thought required by theoretical formulations. Even more fundamentally, however, such scrutiny will require a lively and sustained sociological imagination. Nurturing such imagination is the central task of a social science approach to theorizing and the life course.

ACKNOWLEDGMENTS

The author wishes to thank the editors, Linda George and Joe Hendricks, and Elaine Dannefer, Kathryn Douthit, Lynn Falletta, Gunhild Hagestad, Jessica Kelley-Moore, Michael Shanahan, Robin Shura, Paul Stein, and David Warner for comments on earlier drafts of this chapter. Thanks also to Rachel Bryant and Mary Ellen Stone for comments and for research assistance, and to Debra Klocker for clerical assistance.

REFERENCES

Achenbaum, W. A. (1978). *Old age in the new land: The American experience since 1790*. Baltimore: Johns Hopkins University Press.

Alwin, D. F. (2010). Social structure, cognition and aging. In D. Dannefer & C. R. Phillipson (Eds.), *The Sage handbook of social gerontology*. Thousand Oaks, CA: Sage.

Alwin, D. F., & Hofer, S. (2008). Opportunities and challenges for interdisciplinary research. In S. Hofer & D. F. Alwin (Eds.), *Handbook of cognitive aging*. Thousand Oaks, CA: Sage.

Baars, J. (1991). The challenge of critical gerontology: The problem of social constitution. *Journal of Aging Studies, 5*, 219–243.

Baltes, P. B., & Freund., A. M. (2003). Human strengths as the orchestration of wisdom and selective optimization with compensation. In L. G. Aspinwall & U. M. Staudinger (Eds.), *A psychology of human strengths* (pp. 25–35). Washington DC: American Pyschological Association.

Barkan, B. (2003). The Live Oak Regenerative Community: Championing a culture of hope

and meaning. In A. S. Weiner & J. Ronch (Eds.), *Culture change in long-term care* (pp. 197–221). London: Routledge.

Barker, D. J. P. (1998). In utero programming of chronic disease. *Clinical Sciences, 95*, 115–128.

Berger, P., & Luckmann, T. (1967). *The social construction of reality: A treatise in the sociology of knowledge*. New York: Anchor.

Bing, L. (1991). *Do or die*. New York: Harper Perennial.

Binstock, R. (2002). Age-based rationing of health care. In D. J. Eckerdt, R. A. Applebaum, K. C. Holden, S. G. Post, K. Rockwood, R. Schulz, et al. (Eds.), *Encyclopedia of aging* (pp. 24–28). New York: Macmillan Reference.

Blossfeld, H., Buchholz, S., & Hofacker, D. (2006). *Globalization, uncertainty and late careers in society*. London: Routledge.

Buchmann, M. (1989). *The script of life in modern society: Entry into adulthood in a changing world*. Chicago: The University of Chicago Press.

Burton, L. M. (2007). Childhood adultification in economically disadvantaged families: A conceptual model. *Family Relations, 56*, 329–345.

Burton, L. M., Obeidallah, D. O., & Allison, K. (1996). Ethonographic perspectives on social context and adolescent development among inner-city African American teens. In R. Jessor, A. Colby & R. Shweder (Eds.), *Essays on ethnography and human development* (pp. 395–418). Chicago: University of Chicago Press.

Cain, L. D., Jr. (1964). Life course and social structure. In R. E. L. Faris (Ed.), *Handbook of modern sociology* (pp. 272–309). Chicago, IL: Rand-McNally.

Callahan, D. (1995). *Setting limits: Medical goals in an aging society with "a response to my critics"*. Washington, DC: Georgetown University Press.

Chudacoff, H. (1989). *How old are you? Age consciousness in American culture*. Princeton, NJ: Princeton University Press.

Charles, S. T., & Carstensen, L. L. (2007). Emotion regulation and aging. In J. J. Gross (Ed.), *Handbook of emotion regulation* (pp. 307–327). New York: Guilford.

Cole, S. W. (2008). Social regulation of leukocyte homeostasis: The role of glucocorticoid sensitivity.

Brain, Behavior, and Immunity, 22, 1049–1055.

Cole, S. W., Hawkley, L. C., Arevalo, J. M., Sung, C. Y., Rose, R. M., & Cacioppo, J. T. (2007). Social regulation of gene expression in human leukocytes. *Genome Biology, 8,* R189.

Costa, D. L. (1998). *The evolution of retirement: An American economic history, 1880–1990.* Chicago: University of Chicago Press.

Crystal, S., & Waehrer, K. (1996). Later-life economic inequality in longitudinal perspective. *Journal of Gerontology: Social Sciences, 51B,* S307–S318.

Crystal, S., & Shea, D. (2003). Prospects for retirement resources in an aging society. In S. Crystal & D. Shea (Eds.), *Economic outcomes in later life: Public policy, health, and cumulative advantage* (pp. 271–281). New York: Springer.

Cumming, E., & Henry, W. E. (1961). *Growing old: The process of disengagement.* New York, NY: Basic.

Dannefer, D. (1984). Adult development and social theory: A paradigmatic reappraisal. *American Sociological Review, 49,* 100–116.

Dannefer, D. (1987). Aging as intracohort differentiation: Accentuation, the Matthew Effect, and the life course. *Sociological Forum, 2,* 211–236.

Dannefer, D. (1999a). Freedom isn't free: Power, alienation and the consequences of action. In J. Brandstadter & R. M. Lerner (Eds.), *Action & Development: Origins and functions of intentional self development* (pp. 105–131). New York: Springer.

Dannefer, D. (1999b). Neoteny, naturalization and other constituents of human development. In C. Ryff & V. Marshall (Eds.), *Self and society in aging processes* (pp. 67–93). New York: Springer.

Dannefer, D. (2003a). Cumulative advantage and the life course: Cross-fertilizing age and social science knowledge. *Journal of Gerontology, 58b,* S327–S337.

Dannefer, D. (2003b). Toward a global geography of the life course: Challenges of late

modernity to the life course perspective. In J. T. Mortimer & M. Shanahan (Eds.), *Handbook of the life course* (pp. 647–659). New York: Kluwer.

Dannefer, D. (2008). The waters we swim: Everyday social processes, macrostructural realities, and human aging. In K. W. Schaie & R. P. Abeles (Eds.), *Social structures and aging individuals: Continuing challenges* (pp. 3–22). New York: Springer.

Dannefer, D. (2009). Stability, homogeneity, agency: Cumulative dis/advantage and problems of theory. *Swiss Journal of Sociology, 35,* 193–210.

Dannefer, D., & Kelley-Moore, J. A. (2009). Theorizing the life course: New twists in the path. In V. Bengtson, D. Gans, N. M. Putney & M. Silverstein (Eds.), *Handbook of theories of aging* (pp. 389–411). New York: Springer.

Dannefer, D., & Sell, R. (1988). Age structure, the life course and 'aged heterogeneity': Prospects for research and theory. *Comprehensive Gerontology B, 2,* 1–10.

Dannefer, D., & Uhlenberg, P. (1999). Paths of the life course: A typology. In V. Bengston & K. W. Schaie (Eds.), *Handbook of theories of aging* (pp. 306–326). New York: Springer.

Dannefer, D., Stein, P., Siders, R., & Patterson, R. (2008). Is that all there is? The concept of care and the dialectic of critique. *Journal of Aging Studies, 22,* 101–108.

Doblhammer, G., & Vaupel, J. W. (2001). Lifespan depends on month of birth. *Proceedings of the National Academy of Sciences, 98,* 2934–2939.

Douthit, K. Z., & Dannefer, D. (2007). Social forces, life course consequences: Cumulative disadvantage and "getting Alzheimer's". In J. M. Wilmoth & K. F. Ferraro (Eds.), *Gerontology: Perspectives and issues* (pp. 223–243). New York: Springer.

Douthit, K. Z. (2006). Dementia in the iron cage: The biopsychiatric construction of Alzheimer's Dementia. In J. Baars, D. Dannefer, C. Phillipson & A. Walker (Eds.), *Aging, globalization and inequality: The new critical gerontology.* Amityville, NY: Baywood.

Dunne, M. P., Martin, N. G., Statham, D. J., Slutske, W. S., Dinwiddie, S. H., Bucholz, K. K., et al. (1997). Genetic and environmental contributions to variance in age at first sexual intercourse. *Psychological Science, 8,* 211–216.

Ekerdt, D. J., & DeViney, S. (1990). On defining persons as retired. *Journal of Aging Studies, 4,* 211–299.

Elder, G. H., Jr. (1975). Age differentiation and the life course. *Annual Review of Sociology, 1,* 165–190.

Elder, G. H., Jr. (1999). *Children of the great depression: Social change in life experience* (25th Anniversary Edition). Boulder, CO: Westview Press. (Originally published in 1974, University of Chicago Press.)

Ewen, S. (1976). *Captains of consciousness.* New York: McGraw-Hill.

Falletta, L. (2010). *Re-focusing upstream: Federal research policy related to children's mental health.* Paper presented at Section on Childhood and Youth, Annual Meeting of American Sociological Association, Atlanta.

Farkas, G. (2003). Human capital and the long-term effects of education on late-life inequality. In S. Crystal & D. Shea (Eds.), *Annual review of gerontology and geriatrics: Focus on economic outcomes in later life* (Vol. 22, pp. 138–154). New York: Springer.

Ferraro, K. F., & Kelley-Moore, J. A. (2003). Cumulative disadvantage and health: Long-term consequences of obesity. *American Sociological Review, 68,* 707–729.

Ferraro, K. F., & Shippee, T. P. (2009). Aging and cumulative inequality: How does inequality get under the skin? *The Gerontologist, 49,* 333–343.

Fitch, C. A., & Ruggles, S. (2000). Historical trends in marriage formation: The United States, 1850–1990. In L. J. Waite, C. Bachrach, M. Hindin, E. Thomson & A. Thornton (Eds.), *The ties that bind: Perspectives on marriage and cohabitation* (pp. 59–88). New York: de Gruyter.

George, L. (2009). Conceptualizing and measuring trajectories. In G. H. Elder & J. Z. Giele (Eds.), *The craft of life course research* (pp. 163–186). New York: Guilford.

Gilbert, S. F., & Epel, D. (2009). *Ecological developmental biology*. Sunderland, MA: Sinauer.

Gillis, J. R. (1974). *Youth and history: Tradition and change in European age relations, 1770–present*. New York: Academic Press.

Gluckman, P. D., & Hanson, M. A. (2004). Living with the past: Evolution, development, and patterns of disease. *Science, 305*(5691), 1733–1736.

Gluckman, P. D., & Hanson, M. (Eds.), (2006a). *Developmental origins of health and disease*. Cambridge: Cambridge University Press.

Gluckman, P. D., & Hanson, M. A. (2006b). *Mismatch: The lifestyle diseases timebomb*. New York: Oxford University Press.

Gubrium, J. F. (1978). Notes on the social organization of senility. *Journal of Contemporary Ethnography, 7*, 23–44.

Guo, G., & Stearns, E. (2002). The social influences on the realization of genetic potential for intellectual development. *Social Forces, 80*, 881–910.

Guo, G., Elder, G. H., Cai, T., & Hamilton, N. (2009). Gene–environment interactions: Peers' alcohol use moderates genetic contribution to adolescent drinking behavior. *Social Science Research, 38*, 213–224.

Hagestad, G., & Dannefer, D. (2001). Concepts and theories of aging. In R. H. Binstock & L. K. George (Eds.), *Handbook of aging and the social sciences* (pp. 3–21). New York: Academic Press.

Han, S.-K., & Moen, P. (1999). Work and family over time: A life course approach. *The Annals of the American Academy of Political and Social Sciences, 562*, 98–110.

Harper, S., & Harper, S. (Eds.), (2004). *Families in ageing societies: A multi-disciplinary approach*. New York: Oxford University Press.

Hermanowicz, J. C. (2007). Argument and outline for the sociology of scientific (and other) careers. *Social Studies of Science, 37*, 625–646.

Hochschild, A. (1975). Disengagement theory: A critique and proposal. *American Sociological Review, 40*, 553–569.

Hoffman, R. (2008). *Socioeconomic differences in old age mortality*. New York: Springer.

Hogan, D. P. (1981). *Transitions and social change: The early lives of American men*. New York: Academic Press.

Ikels, C., & Beall, C. M. (2001). Age, aging and anthropology. In R. H. Binstock & L. K. George (Eds.), *Handbook of aging and the social sciences* (pp. 125–138). Burlington, MA: Academic Press.

Jablonka, E., & Raz, G. (2009). Transgenerational epigenetic inheritance: Prevalence, mechanisms and implications for the study of heredity and evolution. *Quarterly Review of Biology, 84*, 131–176.

Jencks, C. (1980). Heredity, environment, and public policy reconsidered. *American Sociological Review, 45*, 723–736.

Joseph, J. (2004). *The gene illusion*. New York: Algora Publishing.

Kahana, B., Lawrence, R. H., Kahana, E., Kercher, K., Wisniewski, A., & Stoller, E. (2002). Long-term impact of preventive proactivity on quality of life of the old-old. *Psychosomatic Medicine, 64*, 382–394.

Kane, R. A., Lum, T. Y., Cutler, L. J., Degenholtz, H. B., & Yu, T. C. (2007). Resident outcomes in small-house nursing homes: A longitudinal evaluation of the initial green house program. *Journal of the American Geriatrics Society, 55*, 832–839.

Kanter, R. M. (1993). *Men and women of the corporation*. New York: Basic Books.

Kayser-Jones, J. S. (1990). *Alone and neglected: Care of the aged in the United States and Scotland*. California: University of California Press.

Kelley-Moore, J. (2010). Disability and aging: Social construction of causality. In D. Dannefer & C. R. Phillipson (Eds.), *Handbook of social gerontology*. London: Sage.

Kett, J. F. (1977). *Rites of passage: Adolescence in America 1790 to the present*. New York: Basic.

Kohli, M. (1986). Social organization and subjective construction of the life course. In A. Sorensen, F. E. Weinert & L. R. Sherrod (Eds.), *Human development and the life course: Multidisciplinary perspectives* (pp. 271–292). Hillsdale, NJ: Lawrence Erlbaum.

Kohli, M. (2007). The institutionalization of the life course: Looking back to look ahead. *Research in Human Development, 4*, 253–271.

Laub, J. H., & Sampson, J. (2003). *Shared beginnings, divergent lives: Delinquent boys to age 70*. Cambridge, MA: Harvard.

Lawrence, B. S. (1996). Organizational age norms: Why is it so hard to know one when you see one? *Gerontologist, 36*, 209–220.

Lee, C. (2001). The expected length of male retirement in the United States, 1850–1990. *Journal of Population Economics, 1*, 641–650.

Lehrer, E. L. (2008). Age at marriage and marital instability: Revisiting the Becker-Landes-Michael hypothesis. *Journal of Population Economics, 21*, 463–484.

Leisering, L., & Leibfried, S. (2000). *Time and poverty in Western welfare states*. Cambridge: Cambridge University Press.

Lesthage, R., & Neels, K. (2002). From the first to the second demographic transition – An interpretation of the spatial continuity of demographic innovation in France, Belgium and Switzerland. *European Journal of Population, 18*, 225–260.

Macmillan, R. (2005). The structure of the life course: Classic issues and current controversies. In R. Macmillan (Ed.), *Advances in Life Course Research: The structure of the life course: standardized? individualized? differentiated?* (Vol. 9, pp. 3–24). Oxford: Elsevier.

Maguire, E. A., Gadian, D. G., Johnsrude, I. S., Good, C. D., Ashburner, J., Frackowiak, R. S., et al. (2000). Navigation-related structural change in the hippocampi of taxi drivers. *Proceedings of the National Academy of Sciences, 97*, 4398–4403.

Marmot, M. (2004). *The status syndrome*. New York: Holt.

Mayer, K. U. (2001). The paradox of global social change and national path dependencies: Life course patterns in advanced societies. In A. E. Woodward & M. Kohli (Eds.), *Inclusions and exclusions in European societies* (pp. 89–110). London: Routledge.

Mayer, K. U. (2009). New directions in life course research. *Annual Review of Sociology, 35*, 413–433.

Mills, C. W. (1959). *The sociological imagination*. New York: Oxford University Press.

Mirowsky, J., & Ross, C. (2005). Education, cumulative advantage and health. *Ageing International, 30*, 27–62.

Modell, J. (1989). *Into one's own: From youth to adulthood in the United States, 1920–1975.* Berkeley, CA: University of California Press.

Ouwehand, C., de Ridder, D. T. D., & Bensing, J. M. (2007). A review of successful aging models: Proposing proactive coping as an important additional strategy. *Clinical Psychology Review, 27*, 873–884.

O'Rand, A. M. (2003). Cumulative disadvantage theory in life-course research. In S. Crystal & D. Shea (Eds.), *Annual review of gerontology and geriatrics: Focus on economic outcomes in later life* (Vol. 22, pp. 14–30). New York: Springer.

O'Rand, A. M. (2005). When old age begins: Implications for health, work and retirement. In R. Hudson (Ed.), *The new politics of old age policy* (pp. 109–128). Baltimore: Johns Hopkins.

Pearlin, L., & Skaff, M. (1996). Stress and the life course: A paradigmatic alliance. *The Gerontologist, 36*, 239–247.

Perry, B., & Svalavitz, M. (2006). *The boy who was raised as a dog: And other stories from a child psychiatrist's notebook: What traumatized children can teach us about loss, love and healing.* New York: Basic Books.

Phillipson, C., & Scharf, T. (2004). *The impact of government policy on social exclusion of older people: A review of the literature.* London: Social Exclusion Unit, Office of the DPM.

Riley, M. W. (1973). Aging and cohort succession: Intepretations and misinterpretations. *Public Opinion Quarterly, 37*, 35–49.

Riley, M. W. (1978). Aging, social change, and the power of idea. *Daedalus, 107*, 39–52.

Riley, M. W., Johnson, M., & Foner, A. (1972). *Aging and society, Volume III: A sociology of age stratification.* New York: Russell Sage Foundation.

Riley, M. W., Kahn, R. L., & Foner, A. (Eds.), (1994). *Age and Structural Lag: Society's failure to provide meaningful opportunities in work, family, and leisure.* New York: Wiley.

Ryder, N. (1965). The cohort as a concept in the study of social change. *American Sociological Review, 30*, 843–861.

Sampson, R. J., & Laub, J. H. (2005). When prediction fails: From crime prone boys to hetero-geneity in adulthood. *Annals of the Academy of Political and Social Sciences, 602*, 73–79.

Schor, J. (2004). *Born to buy.* New York: Scribner.

Settersten, R. A., Jr., & Hagestad, G. O. (1996). What's the latest? Cultural age deadlines for family transitions. *The gerontologist, 36*, 178–188.

Shanahan, M. J., Hofer, S. M., & Shanahan, L. (2003). Biological models of behavior and the life course. In J. T. Mortimer & M. J. Shanahan (Eds.), *Handbook of the life course* (pp. 597–622). New York: Kluwer Academic Publishers.

Shanahan, M. J., & Hofer, S. M. (2005). Social context in gene–environment interactions: Retrospect and prospect. *Journal of Gerontology: Psychological Sciences, 60*, 65–76.

Shuey, K. M., & O'Rand, A. M. (2004). New risks for workers: Pensions, labor markets, and gender. *Annual Review of Sociology, 30*, 453–477.

Sigman, A. (2009). Well connected? The biological implications of "social networking." *Biologist, 56*, 14–20.

Thomas, W. H. (1996). *Life worth living: How someone you love can still enjoy life in a nursing home: The Eden alternative in action.* Acton, MA: Vanderwyk & Burnham.

Turner, R. (1976). The real self: From institution to impulse. *American Journal of Sociology, 81*, 989–1016.

Warner, D. F., Hayward, M. D., & Hardy, M. A. (2010). The retirement life course in America at the dawn of the twenty-first century. *Population Research and Policy Review.*

Wexler, P. (1977). Comment on Ralph Turner's "The real self: From institution to impulse". *American Journal of Sociology, 83*, 178.

Chapter | 2 |

Aging, Cohorts, and Methods

Yang Yang

Department of Sociology & Lineberger Comprehensive Cancer Center, University of North Carolina, Chapel Hill, North Carolina

CHAPTER CONTENTS

INTRODUCTION

Theoretical developments combined with new methodological tools and data sources have contributed to considerable growth in aging research in the social sciences over the past few decades (Elder, 1985). To address key questions of aging and the life course paradigm – how individual lives unfold with age and are shaped by historical time and social context – researchers often need to compare age-specific data recorded at different points in time and from different birth cohorts. A systematic study of such data, termed the age-period-cohort (APC), or simply "cohort analysis," is one of the most useful means to gain a greater understanding of the process of aging within and across human populations.

The challenges posed by cohort analysis are well known. Whether observed time-related differences are related to aging or cohort variation is a question usually deemed conceptually important but empirically intractable for two reasons. The first is data limitations. Using cross-sectional data at one point in time, for example, aging and cohort effects are confounded. Similarly, comparing data from multiple time periods for the same age group precludes distinguishing between period and cohort effects. The second reason is the use of linear regression models that suffer from either specification errors or an identification problem and consequently are incapable of distinguishing age, period, and cohort effects. What should one do to model these effects in empirical research to understand the true social and biological mechanisms generating the data? This chapter aims to provide some useful guidelines on how to conduct cohort analysis. The expository strategy is to provide those guidelines in the context of illustrative empirical analyses. The remainder of this chapter is organized as follows. The next section summarizes the state of knowledge on cohort analysis in aging research in

DOI: 10.1016/B978-0-12-380880-6.00002-2

sociology, demography, and epidemiology. Following on further, the next section synthesizes new developments in cohort analysis, including models, methods, and substantive applications. Finally, the last section outlines new directions for which methods and data are promising, but not yet completely developed.

EARLY LITERATURE

Why Cohort Analysis?

In a classic article, Norman Ryder (1965) made an extended argument for the conceptual relevance of cohorts to an extraordinary range of substantive issues in social research. He argued that cohort membership could be as important in determining behavior as other social structural features such as socioeconomic status (SES). APC analysis is, in this sense, synonymous with cohort analysis (Smith, 2008). Among various cohorts defined by different initial events (such as marriage and college/university entrance), birth cohorts are the most commonly examined unit of analysis in demographic and aging research. A birth cohort shares the same birth year and ages together. Birth cohorts born in different time periods that encounter different historical and social conditions as they age would conceivably have diverse developmental paths. Cohort analysis concerns the precise depiction of such time-related phenomena, is central to the study of aging and the life course, and is crucial for inference. *Age effects* represent aging-related physiological or developmental changes and offer clues to etiology in epidemiologic studies. *Period effects* reflect changes in contemporaneous social, historical, and epidemiologic conditions that affect all living cohorts. *Cohort effects* reflect different formative experiences resulting from the intersection of individual biographies and macrosocial influences. In the absence of period and cohort changes, age effects are broadly applicable across historical eras and different cohorts. Presence of either or both of these changes, however, indicates the existence of exogenous forces or exposures that are period- and/or cohort-specific.

Why is there an APC Identification Problem?

The essence of cohort analysis is the identification and quantification of different sources of variation that are associated with age, period, and/or cohort effects in an outcome of interest. Early investigators developed models for situations in which all three factors account for a substantive phenomenon and in which simpler two-factor models (such as an age-period model) are subject to model specification errors and spurious results (Mason et al., 1973). The "conventional linear regression model," also known as the APC multiple classification/accounting model (Mason et al., 1973), has been widely adopted as the general methodology for cohort analysis, but it also suffers from a well-known model identification problem. Specifically, any two of the constituent factors perfectly predict the third. For example, if date of birth (i.e. birth cohort) and time of measurement are known, age also is known. This produces multiple instead of unique estimates of the three effects.

The Mason et al. (1973) article spawned a large methodological literature in the social sciences beginning with Glenn's critique (1976) and Mason et al.'s reply (1976), followed by Fienberg and Mason's work (1978). Similar debates occurred between Rodgers (1982) and Smith et al. (1982). These early investigations culminated in an edited volume on cohort analysis by Mason and Fienberg in 1985. Limitations of those analytic strategies propelled the search for new approaches. For example, a Bayesian approach was proposed by Saski and Suzuki (1987), which was again critiqued by Glenn, who cautioned against "mechanical solutions" to the problem (1987). APC analysis also took root in biostatistics and epidemiology (e.g. Clayton & Schifflers, 1987; Holford, 1991; Kupper et al., 1985). Several recent reviews provide useful additional material on these and related contributions to cohort analysis (Mason & Wolfinger, 2002; Yang, 2007a, 2009).

Conventional Solutions

Within the framework of linear regression models, three conventional solutions to the identification problem have been used. The purpose of each is to break the linear dependency between the three variables and, thus, to identify the model, but each has limitations.

The *constrained coefficients* approach imposes one or more *equality constraints* on the coefficients of one parameter vector to just-identify (one constraint) or over-identify (two or more constraints) the model (Mason et al., 1973; Yang et al., 2004). For example, in an APC analysis of US tuberculosis mortality, Mason and Smith (1985) placed the constraint by equating the contrasts for ages 0–9 and 10–19. This yielded unique estimates for age, period, and cohort effects. This is the most widely used approach, but is not immune to problems. First, the analyst must rely on prior or external information that rarely exists or cannot be verified to select constraints. Second, different identifying constraints (e.g. two age groups vs two cohorts) can produce widely different estimates of age, period, and cohort effects. And third, all just-identified constrained coefficients models produce the same levels of goodness-of-fit to the data. Thus, model fit cannot be used as the criterion for selecting the best model (Yang et al., 2008).

The *nonlinear parametric (algebraic) transformation approach* defines a nonlinear parametric function for at least one of the age, period, and cohort variables so that its relationship to others is nonlinear (Mason & Fienberg, 1985). For example, one can specify a quadratic or cubic function of age to model the nonlinear rate of change in happiness with age (Yang, 2008a). The drawbacks of this approach are that: (1) specifying a structure of the parameters makes the model less flexible and (2) it may not be clear what nonlinear function should be defined.

The *proxy variables approach* uses one or more proxy variables to replace the age, period, or cohort variable. This is a popular approach because of its substantive appeal. After all, the indicator variables of age, period, and cohort serve as surrogates for different sets of unmeasured structural correlates (Hobcraft et al., 1982). Examples of proxy variables for cohort effects include relative cohort size (O'Brien et al., 1999) and cohort mean years of smoking before age 40 (Preston & Wang, 2006). Unemployment rate, labor force size, and gender role attitudes have been used as proxy variables for period effects (Pavalko et al., 2007). Smith and colleagues (1982, p. 792), however, cautioned that replacing cohort or period with a measured variable "leaves open the question of whether all of the right measured variables have been included in an appropriately wrought specification. Although replacing an accounting dimension with measured variables solves an identification problem, it makes room for others." Thus, assuming that *all* of the variation associated with the A, P, or C dimension is fully accounted for by the chosen proxy, variable(s) may be unwarranted. Winship and Harding (2008) proposed a mechanism-based approach that accommodates a more general set of models. Using the framework of causal modeling described by Pearl (2000) to achieve identification, the approach allows any given measured variable to be associated with more than one of the age, period, and cohort dimensions and provides statistical tests for the plausibility of alternative restrictions. If a rich set of mechanism variables are available and the original age, period, and cohort categories can be conceived as the exogenous elements of a causal chain (Smith, 2008), this is an enriched and sophisticated alternative to the proxy variable approach.

Where does the early literature on cohort analysis leave us today? If a researcher has a temporally ordered data set and wants to tease out its age, period, and cohort components, how should he/she proceed? Can any methodological guidelines be recommended? A problem with much of the extant literature is that there is a lack of useful guidelines on how to conduct an APC analysis. Instead, one is left with the impression that either it is *impossible* to obtain meaningful estimates of the distinct contributions of age, cohort, and time period, or that the conduct of an APC analysis is an *esoteric art* that is best left to a few skilled methodologists (Yang, 2009). I now seek to redress this situation by focusing on recent developments in APC analysis for three research designs commonly used in research on aging.

NEW DEVELOPMENTS: MODELS, METHODS, AND SUBSTANTIVE RESEARCH

In this section, I introduce a new estimation method to solve the identification problem within the context of conventional linear models. Note that the identification problem is not inevitable in all settings – only in the case of linear models that assume additive effects of age, period, and cohort. The text then describes other families of models that are not subject to this problem and are suitable for many research questions. Empirical studies of aging, health, and well-being for each of the three research designs will be use as illustrative examples. Sample codes using standard statistical software packages are available at http://home.uchicago.edu/~yangy/apc.

Research Design I: Age-by-Time Period Tables of Rates/Proportions

In demographic and epidemiologic investigations, researchers are typically interested in aggregate population-level data such as rates of morbidity, disability, or mortality. Using the conventional data structure, rates or proportions are arranged in rectangular arrays with age intervals defining the rows and time periods defining the columns. Age and period are usually of equal interval length (e.g. 5 or 10 years), so the diagonal elements of the matrix correspond to birth cohorts. An example of this data structure is shown in Figure 2.1, where age-specific lung cancer death rates for 14 five-year age groups (30 to 95+) of women are plotted by eight time periods between 1960 and 1999 and for 21 cohorts born between 1870 and 1920 (mid-year).

Guidelines for Estimating APC Models of Rates

Many previous applications of cohort analysis using linear regression models are based on the age-by-period matrix. Among the limitations of conventional solutions to the identification problem is the lack of guidelines for estimating APC models of rates or proportions. A three-step procedure is helpful for this purpose. Step 1 is to conduct descriptive data analyses using graphics. The objective is to provide qualitative understanding of patterns of age,

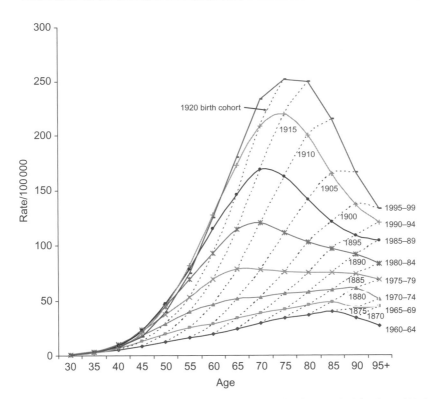

Figure 2.1 US female lung cancer mortality rates per 100 000 by age at death, period of death, and birth cohort.
Source: Yang (2008b).

period, cohort, and two-way age by period and age by cohort variations. Step 2 is model fitting. The objective is to ascertain whether the data are sufficiently well-described by any single factor or two-way combination of age, period, and cohort. If these analyses suggest that only one or two of the three effects are operative, the analysis can proceed with a reduced model that omits one or two groups of variables and there is no identification problem. If, however, these analyses suggest that all three dimensions are at work, Yang and colleagues (2004, 2008) recommend Step 3: applying a new method of estimation of the linear model, the intrinsic estimator (IE). We will now look at these steps using examples from recent analyses of US adult chronic disease mortality change (Yang, 2008b). The example below focuses on lung cancer mortality (see Yang, 2008b for the complete set of analyses of other causes of death).

Temporal Changes of US Adult Lung Cancer Mortality

Figure 2.1 is a graphical presentation of the female lung cancer rate data for the Step 1 descriptive analyses. The age pattern shows much higher rates of deaths due to lung cancers in older ages than young adulthood. Rates of lung cancer deaths in women aged 40 and older also increased dramatically. Large increases in successive cohorts are also evident: more recent cohorts of women had higher death rates than their predecessors at the same ages. Because cohort effects can be interpreted as a special form of interaction effect between age and period, cohort effects can be detected by non-parallel age-specific curves by time period – a pattern evident in Figure 2.1. Peak ages shifted to the left over time, indicating higher death rates at younger ages for more recent female cohorts. The graphical analyses present all available rates, but provide no summary or quantitative assessment of the source of mortality change (Kupper et al., 1985). The curve of age-specific death rates for women in any given time period cuts across multiple birth cohort curves. Therefore, the period curve is affected by both varying age effects is cohort effects. The question of which of these effects is more important in explaining the mortality change can only be addressed using regression modeling.

In Step 2, the relative importance of the A, P, and C dimensions can be determined by comparing overall measures of model fit (e.g. R-squared for linear regression models or deviance statistics/penalized likelihood functions such as Bayes the Information Criterion for generalized linear models). For this analysis, goodness-of-fit statistics for four log-linear

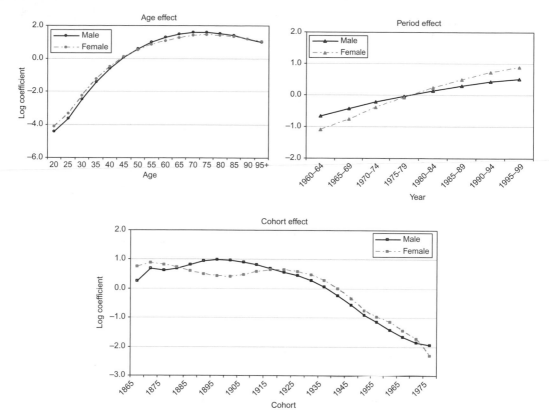

Figure 2.2 Intrinsic estimates of age, period, and cohort effects of lung cancer mortality by sex.
Source: Yang (2008b).

models of female lung cancer mortality were produced: age effects only (A), age and period effects
(AP), age and cohort effects (AC), and age, period,
and cohort effects (APC). The three-factor model best
fit the data, regardless of the statistics used. Thus, all
three sources of variation contribute to the mortality
change and need to be included in the model.

In Step 3, one estimates the APC model coefficients
to reveal the age, period, and cohort effects. The IE is
a new method of estimation that yields a unique solution to the APC model and is the unique estimable
function of both the linear and nonlinear components of the APC model. It has minimal assumptions
and is estimated using principal component regression. The reason why the IE is useful lies in the special constraint it imposes – removing the influence of
the number of age and period groups (which is not
related to the outcome) on coefficient estimates. This
constraint allows the IE to avoid the bias that the conventional equality constraints produce. For the mathematical foundations of the IE see Yang et al. (2004)
and for additional information about its statistical
properties see Yang et al. (2008).

The log coefficient estimates using the IE on the
lung cancer mortality data by sex are shown in
Figure 2.2. Age effects are concave: the mortality

risk increased rapidly from early adulthood, peaked
around ages 80 to 85, and then leveled off. Cohort
mortality curves increased first and decreased for more
recent cohorts, following an inverse-U shape. Period
effects are modest compared to age and cohort effects.

Conclusion

Is the IE a "final" or "universal" solution to the APC
"conundrum"? No. There will never be a solution
within the confine of linear models. Researchers should
never naively apply any estimator to APC data and
expect to get meaningful results. In all cases, APC
analysis should be approached with great caution and
awareness of its many pitfalls. The IE appears to be the
most useful approach to the identification and estimation of these models, but shares some of the limitations of conventional linear models.

Research Design II: Repeated Cross-Sectional Surveys

Repeated cross-sectional surveys, such as the Current
Population Survey (CPS) and General Social Survey
(GSS), provide unique opportunities for cohort
analysis. Pooling data of all survey years yields the

age-by-year data structure needed for cohort analysis. Many researchers previously assumed that the APC identification problem for repeated cross-sectional surveys is the same as that for population rates. But sample surveys are different from aggregate population-level data in two important ways. First, repeated cross-sectional surveys allow age intervals to differ from period intervals. More importantly, the sample size for each age-by-period cell exceeds rather than equals one. This data structure suggests a multi-level data structure. In this design, respondents are *nested in* and *cross-classified simultaneously* by the two higher-level *social contexts* defined by time period and birth cohort. That is, individual members of any birth cohort are interviewed in multiple replications of the survey, and individual respondents in any particular wave of the survey can be drawn from multiple birth cohorts.

Hierarchical Age-Period-Cohort (HAPC) Models

Given these data characteristics, there are two potential solutions to the identification problem in addition to those described in the first section. First, within the framework of the conventional linear regression model, different temporal groupings for the A, P, and C dimensions can be used to break the linear dependency. For example, one can use single year of *age, time periods* corresponding to years in which surveys are conducted (which may be several years apart), and *cohorts* defined either by five- or ten-year intervals, which are conventional in demography, or by application of substantive classification (e.g. War babies, baby boomers, Baby Busters, etc.). Despite the appeal of this approach, it has several problems.

First and foremost, linear models assuming additivity of age, period, and cohort effects not only produce the identification problem, but are poor approximations of the processes generating social changes. Second, simple linear models do not account for multilevel heterogeneity in the data and may underestimate standard errors. Third, the APC accounting model cannot include explanatory variables and test substantive hypotheses. A useful alternative is a different family of models that (1) do not assume fixed age, period, and cohort effects that are additive and therefore avoid the identification problem; (2) can statistically characterize contextual effects of historical time and cohort membership; and (3) can accommodate covariates to aid better conceptualization of specific social processes generating observed patterns in the data.

The Hierarchical APC (HAPC) models approach (Yang, 2006; Yang & Land, 2006) is appropriate for these purposes and can address questions unique to repeated cross-sectional surveys. If there is level-two (period and/or cohort) heterogeneity, assuming fixed period and cohort effects ignores this hetero-geneity and may not be adequate. In this case, cross-classified random effects models (CCREMs), mixed (fixed and random) effects models, can be used to quantify the level-2 heterogeneity. The objectives of CCREM are to (1) assess the possibility that individuals within the same periods and cohorts share unobserved random variance and (2) test explanatory hypotheses of A, P, and C effects by including additional variables at all levels.

Social Inequality of Happiness

To illustrate the application of HAPC models, I will use the example of subjective well-being from a recent study (Yang, 2008a). This study is based on time series data on happiness in the US as reported by people 18 years of age and older from the GSS 1972–2004 (N = 28 869). This study addressed the following questions: Do people get happier with age and over time? How do social inequalities in happiness vary over the life course and by time? Are some people born to be happy? Are there any birth cohort differences in happiness?

The HAPC-CCREM method was applied to estimate fixed effects of age and other individual-level covariates and random effects of period and cohort. Hypotheses about differential sex, race, and SES effects over the life course were tested by entering their interaction terms with age. The level-2 (period- and cohort-level) model was further specified to take into account error terms associated with period and cohort. The simplest specification of a HAPC model, as introduced by Yang and Land (2006), is a *linear mixed effects* model for normally distributed outcomes. *Generalized linear mixed model* specifications need to be used for dichotomous and multiple categorical outcome variables. In this case, the ordinal logit HAPC models of happiness were estimated. These estimates were obtained using the SAS PROC GLIMMIX.

Next came a calculation of the predicted probabilities of being very happy by age, sex, and race, adjusting for all other factors and net of period and cohort effects. The age curves of happiness are quadratic and convex. The J-shaped net age effects suggest that average happiness levels bottom out in early adulthood and then increase at an increasing rate across age. Thus, with age comes happiness. Everything else being equal, women are slightly happier than men at all ages, and the gap converges at older ages. And when other factors are held constant, the race gap shows stronger trends of convergence with reversals at around the age of 70, with blacks becoming slightly happier than whites afterwards. Thus, life course variations in social inequalities in happiness are more consistent with the age-as-leveler hypothesis than the cumulative advantage hypothesis. Longitudinal panel data are needed to sort out whether selective survival of the happier or other processes are more plausible explanations of the stratification of aging and subjective well-being.

Estimates of variance components at level-2 indicated significant period and cohort effects controlling for age and other individual-level variables. The results on period and cohort effects as estimated by the random effect coefficients showed variations in levels of happiness over time for all groups and that sex and race disparities decreased during the last 30 years. The most interesting cohort effect was a dip in happiness levels for cohorts born between 1945 and 1960, i.e. the baby boomers.

What accounts for these period and cohort patterns? One hypothesis is that period effects may reflect changes in macroeconomic variables such as gross domestic product (GDP) and levels of joblessness between the 1970s and 1990s (Di Tella et al., 2003). Exploratory analysis suggests that GDP is concurrent with the period changes in happiness and that the unemployment rate has a lagged effect. The two period-level covariates (GDP per capita and changes in unemployment rate) can be added to the models for the overall mean, sex, and race effects to determine whether the economic environment explains period variations in happiness and sex and race gaps therein. In addition, the cohort analysis proposition emphasizes the exogenous social demographic environments into which cohorts are born and age. The baby boomer pattern is consistent with the Easterlin hypothesis that large cohort sizes have negative consequences on cohort members' socioeconomic and other life course outcomes, such as sense of well-being and mental stress (Easterlin, 1987). Relative cohort size (adopted from O'Brien et al., 1999) can be added to the model for the overall mean to account for cohort-level variance.

Results of the Yang (2008a,b) study indicated that GDP per capita was significantly and positively associated with happiness and larger cohort size reduces happiness significantly, although the residual period effect remains significant. Economic conditions also affect sex and race differences over time. Higher GDP per capita reduces the sex and race differences by 83% and 38%, respectively. Higher unemployment rates, interestingly, decrease the race gap. Relative cohort size not only reduces the cohort variance by 73%, but also diminishes its statistical significance. So the lower levels of happiness in baby boomers are largely due to their large size compared to their predecessors and successors. More competition to go to school and find jobs meant more pressure and strains as the boomers came of age – something that can decrease their positive affect and assessment of quality of life (QOL).

Conclusion and Extensions

The empirical example above suggests that HAPC analysis moves far beyond simply identifying age and cohort trends. It allows us to see how social stratification operates over the life course and historical time and to test the extent to which aging and cohort theories apply to subjective well-being in ways that cannot be achieved by a conventional linear regression analysis. The HAPC model does not incur the identification problem because the age, period, and cohort effects are not assumed to be linear and additive. This analytic technique opens new doors to research on aging by offering a systematic and flexible modeling strategy that takes advantage of the multilevel data structure and rich covariates in repeated cross-sectional surveys.

HAPC models can be extended in various ways to address other research questions. We focus on three extensions here: fixed vs random effects models, an F-test for the presence of random effects, and full Bayesian HAPC models. First, the HAPC-CCREM approach illustrated above uses a *mixed (fixed and random) effects model* with a *random effects* specification for the level-2 variables (period and cohort). A frequently used alternative is a *fixed effects* specification for the level-2 variables in which dummy variables are used to represent cohorts and survey years. This approach may be appropriate when the number of survey replications is relatively small (three to five). In general, however, the random effects specification is preferable to the fixed effects specification for the level-2 variables because (1) it avoids an assumption of fixed effects models that the dummy variables representing the fixed cohort and periods effects fully account for the group effects; (2) it allows group-level covariates to be incorporated into the model and explicitly models cohort characteristics and period events to test explanatory hypotheses; and (3) it is generally more statistically efficient for unbalanced research designs (designs in which there are unequal numbers of respondents in the period-by-cohort cells), which is typical in repeated cross-section surveys (Yang & Land, 2008).

Second, the random effects of level-2 variables in the HAPC models, particularly the variance components of cohort and period, are obtained by using the restricted maximum likelihood (REML) method, which assumes that the level-2 residual or error terms are asymptotic normally distributed, and yields variance estimators with good large sample properties. When the number of level-2 units, in this case cohorts and periods, is not large, this assumption may not be appropriate. Further, the z-scores for the REML estimates of the variance components are only proximate. To test more exactly whether the birth cohort and period effects make statistically significant contributions to explained variance in an outcome variable, a general linear hypothesis may be applied. Specifically, one can use an F test to test the hypothesis of the presence of random effects. The F statistic is preferred over the z-score when the sample sizes for random effects are small (Littell et al., 2006) and can be constructed using sum of squares for the linear mixed effects model and log-likelihood functions for some generalized linear mixed effects models. Interested readers should see Yang et al. (2009) for detail on the formulation of the F-test.

Third, the standard REML-EB (empirical Bayes) estimation algorithm for mixed effects models has other limitations when applied to APC analyses of finite time period survey data. As noted above, the numbers of periods and birth cohorts in surveys usually are too small to satisfy the large sample criterion required by the maximum likelihood estimation of variance components. In addition, the sample sizes within each cohort are highly unbalanced. These result in inaccurate REML estimates of variance-covariance components that further result in inaccurate EB estimates of fixed effects. This is because errors in the REML estimates may produce increased uncertainty in the EB estimates of fixed effects coefficients that will not be reflected in the standard errors. A remedy is to use the full Bayesian approach that, by definition, ensures that inferences about every parameter fully account for the uncertainty associated with all others. To this end, one specifies the level-1 model as the likelihood function, assigns prior probability distributions for all fixed effect parameters and variance components, and uses the Bayes rule to yield the joint model or posterior distribution. Gibbs sampling has been widely used to derive the marginal posterior distributions for each model parameter and can be implemented using the software WinBUGS (freely available at http://www.mrc-bsu.cam.ac.uk/bugs/). For an example of Bayesian HAPC analysis, see Yang (2006).

Research Design III: Accelerated Longitudinal Panels

The former two designs rely on information from synthetic cohorts that contain different cohort members at each point in time. Inferences drawn from such designs, therefore, assume that synthetic cohorts mimic true cohorts, and changes over time across synthetic cohort members mimic the age trajectories of change within true cohorts. If the composition of cohorts does not change over time due to migration or other factors and sample sizes are large, these assumptions are generally met.

However, longitudinal data obtained from the same persons followed over time are increasingly available. The accelerated longitudinal panel design – where multiple birth cohorts are followed over multiple points in time – is an important advance in aging and cohort research. The primary advantage of this design is that it provides cross-time linkages within

individuals and hence information pertaining to true birth cohorts.

Growth Curve Models of Individual and Cohort Change

Hierarchical models are a useful tool for modeling longitudinal data. Because repeated observations over time (level-1 units) can be viewed as nested within individuals (level-2 units), one can specify growth curve models to assess simultaneously the intracohort age changes and intercohort differences. Although the application of two-level hierarchical regression models to standard longitudinal data is relatively straightforward, growth curve analysis of multi-cohort multi-wave data is complicated by two issues.

First, because the observable age trajectories of different cohorts initiate and end at different ages, cohort comparisons are based on different segments of cohort members' life courses. This raises the question of the potential confounding of the age and cohort effects. Two analytic strategies help to resolve this problem. The first is the use of centered age variables (e.g. centered around cohort median). Age centering eases the interpretation of the intercept, stabilizes estimation, and prevents the bias in the estimate that arises from systematic variation in mean age across the cohorts, hence eliminating the confounding of age and cohort variables. Second, the models yield tests of significance of overlapping segments of the life course of adjacent cohorts. As waves of data accumulate, the number of overlapping ages of adjacent cohorts increases, which increases statistical power. In this case, age and cohort will become less and less confounded, making it increasingly possible to compare cohort differences in age trajectories.

The second issue concerns period effects. This model does not explicitly incorporate period effects for both substantive and methodological reasons. First, in contrast to synthetic cohort designs that usually cover several decades, longitudinal designs typically span much shorter time periods (e.g. a decade or so). So, the effects of period can be assumed to be trivial and omitted from the models, especially if the theoretical focus is on aging. Second, it is challenging to estimate a separate period effect in accelerated longitudinal designs. In the framework of the growth curve models, the level-1 analysis reflects within-individual change by modeling the outcome as a function of the time indicator (Singer & Willett, 2003). This means that one can include age *or* wave (period), depending on substantive focus, but not *both* because within individuals age and period are the same. The simultaneous estimation of period effects creates the model identification problem, which requires different data designs and mixed model specifications to resolve (Yang & Land, 2006, 2008). Third, one does not need to estimate period effect per se and can focus instead on the age by cohort interaction effects.

Sex and Race Health Disparities Across the Life Course

This illustrative example comes from a recent analysis of life course patterns and cohort variations in sex and race health gaps (Yang & Lee, 2009). An important question in recent aging research is whether, and how, social status affects health dynamics in later life. Evidence about whether social disparities in health grow or diminish over the life course has been inconsistent (e.g. House et al., 1994; Lynch, 2003; Wilson et al., 2007). Another key unresolved issue concerns the distinct roles of aging and cohort succession. Whether recent birth cohorts show more or less sex and race inequalities in health due to cohort changes in social attainment, health capital, and the roles of women and blacks merits further study.

This study systematically examines intercohort variations and intracohort heterogeneity in health trajectories to shed light on the social mechanisms generating sex and race inequalities in health over the life course. It addresses three questions. First, are there cohort differences in age trajectories of health? It tests the *intercohort change hypothesis* by modeling main cohort and age by cohort interaction effects. Second, how do sex and race health disparities change over the life course within cohorts? The prevailing explanations for decreasing health gaps with age are the age-as-leveler and selective survival processes. The primary explanation for increasing health gaps with age is the cumulative advantage process. The double jeopardy hypothesis has also been proposed as a secondary explanation. Because these theoretical perspectives all emphasize intracohort differentiation in aging, a proper test should control for cohort differences that might otherwise be confounded with aging effects, but this was not previously tested. The current analysis tests the *intracohort inequality hypothesis* by modeling age by sex and age by race interaction effects, net of cohort effects. Third, are there intercohort variations in the intracohort health differentials by sex and race? The study further tests the *intercohort difference in intracohort inequality hypothesis* by incorporating three-way interactions between age, cohort, and social status.

The data are from the Americans' Changing Lives (ACL) study, which uses an accelerated longitudinal design. An initial sample of 3617 adults aged 25 and older from seven 10-year birth cohorts (before 1905 to 1964) were interviewed in 1986, 1989, 1994, and 2001/2002. Three health outcomes were of interest: depressive symptoms as measured by an 11-item CES-D (Center for Epidemiologic Studies – Depression) scale, physical disability as measured by a summary index indicating levels of functional disability (range 1–4),

and self-rated health as measured by a scale indicating levels of perceived general health (range 1–5). The analytic sample consisted of 10 174 person-year observations from black and white respondents at all waves for which data on all variables were available.

Growth curve models are the method of analysis. The level-1 model characterizes within-individual change with age. In this model, the response variable is modeled as a function of linear and quadratic terms of age, where age is centered around the cohort median. The level-2 model assesses individual differences in change with age and determines the associations between the change with age and person-level characteristics including birth cohort and its quadratic function, sex, race, and the interaction effects of sex and cohort and race and cohort. A similar model was tested for the quadratic growth rate and was not significant. Control variables are entered at level-1 for time-varying covariates (family income, marital status, chronic illnesses, body mass index (BMI), and smoking).

The hierarchical linear modeling (HLM) growth curve methodology has the advantage of allowing data that are unbalanced in time (Raudenbush & Bryk, 2002). That is, it incorporates all individuals with data for the estimation of trajectories, regardless of the number of waves s/he contributes to the person-year data set. Compared to alternative modeling techniques, this substantially reduces the number of cases lost to follow-up due to mortality or nonresponse. However, this method does not completely resolve the sample selection problem unless it distinguishes those lost to follow up from those with complete data for all waves. If mortality and nonresponse are significantly correlated with worse health and key covariates of health, such as age and SES, parameter estimates of the health trajectories may be biased if they are not controlled. To account for this, the analysis controls for the effects of attrition by including dummy variables indicating the deceased and nonrespondents in the level-2 models. All statistical analyses are performed using SAS PROC MIXED.

The analysis tested the cohort-based models (full model) against the models combining all cohorts (reduced model with no cohort effect) to determine whether cohort-specific trajectories can actually be represented by a single mean-age trajectory. The hypothesis that there are no cohort differences in age trajectories was rejected.

Results from the growth models yield several significant findings. First, the *intercohort change hypothesis* is supported for all three health outcomes. There are significant cohort differences in health trajectories, with more recent cohorts faring better in physical functioning and self-rated health, but worse in mental health. Second, the *intracohort inequality hypothesis* is supported only for depression. Specifically, there is evidence of a converging sex gap in depression trajectories, but constant sex and race gaps in physical and self-rated health trajectories within cohorts. Third, there is support for the hypothesis of *intercohort variations in intracohort sex and race differences* in mean levels of all health outcomes, but not in the growth rates other than depression. Sex and race gaps in mean levels of health narrowed across cohorts for disability, but widened for depression and perceived health. The predicted mean levels of CES-D scores are plotted in Figure 2.3 by cohort for blacks and whites based on the model estimates, adjusting for age and all other factors. It shows that the black excess in depression has become more pronounced for more recent cohorts. We further find significant intercohort differences in age changes of intracohort sex gaps in depression. Figure 2.4 shows the predicted age trajectories of depressive symptoms by sex for selected cohorts. It suggests that the sex gaps in growth rates of depression are strongly contingent upon cohort membership. We see less convergence in the male–female gap in depression with age in more recent cohorts, suggesting a weaker age-as-leveler process in these cohorts.

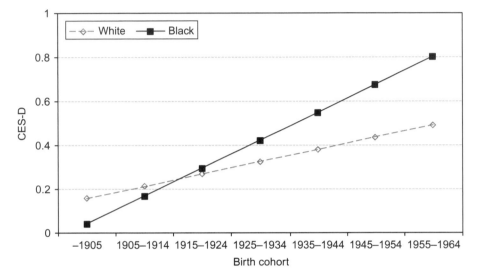

Figure 2.3 Predicted mean levels of CES-D score by birth cohort: race gap.
Source: Yang & Lee (2009).

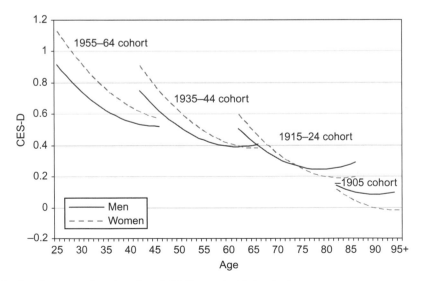

Figure 2.4 Predicted age growth trajectories of CES-D score by birth cohort: sex gap.
Source: Yang & Lee (2009).

Conclusion

This analysis provides an example of how to address some long-standing questions in the stratification of aging from the perspective of cohort analysis. It provides substantial evidence that the process of cohort change is important for the theory, measurement, and analysis of social inequalities in health over the life course. Controlling for cohort effects substantially alters existing explanations of sex and race gaps in health trajectories over the life course. For example, because we do not find any significant changes in the intracohort sex or race gaps in disability or self-rated health with age, but find substantial intercohort variations in sex and race gaps in mean levels of these outcomes, we conclude that any changes with age observed in previous studies are actually due to intercohort differences in disability or self-rated health levels. Furthermore, there is no meaningful cumulative advantage process or age-as-leveler effect at work in later or earlier cohorts' physical and self-rated health when the confounding effects of cohort and other social factors are controlled. The constant intracohort disparities in disability and self-rated health trajectories indicate the persistent disadvantages of women and African Americans.

The analytic framework exemplified above facilitates studies of patterns of inequality within and between birth cohorts that can provide a particularly useful line of inquiry into how individual lives evolve with social change. For example, analyzing five waves of data from the China Health and Nutrition Survey (CHNS) from 1991 to 2004 with growth curve methods, a recent analysis reveals patterns of social stratification in health trajectories for multiple cohorts in the context of an ever-changing macro-social environment in China (Chen et al., 2010). The study found strong cohort variations in SES disparities on health trajectories: the effect of education on mean level of health is smaller for more recent cohorts; the income gap in age trajectories of health increases for earlier cohorts but decreases for most recent cohorts. These cohort effects are in an opposite direction to recent US studies (e.g. Lynch, 2003; Wilson et al., 2007). Thus, this study highlights the uniqueness of China's social, economic, and political structures; China's stage of epidemiologic transition; and the changing impact of the government on health care.

In sum, cohort membership contextualizes aging-related outcomes such as mental and physical well-being, QOL, and longevity, and also conditions social inequalities therein. The significance of cohort change in shaping the individual life suggests that new patterns may emerge for future cohorts as a result of their new life circumstances. The methods and findings illustrated here should prompt future examinations of aging-related hypotheses in a cohort-specific context.

DIRECTIONS FOR FUTURE RESEARCH

Demographic rates and social indicators arrayed over time by age or cohort are canonical organizations of data in research on aging. A vast literature in the social sciences uses linear models methodology for APC analysis. Different solutions to the model identification problem often produce ambiguous and inconsistent results and have ignited continuous debates on whether any solutions exist or which solutions are better. Researchers do not agree on methodological solutions to these problems and have concluded that APC analysis is still in its infancy (Mason & Wolfinger, 2002).

The developments introduced in this chapter highlight new solutions to this problem – or simply new ways of thinking about the problem. They provide an important insight that the identification problem is model-specific rather than data-specific (Fu, 2008). Because the use of linear models (and hence the identification problem) characterizes the majority of previous studies, investigators erroneously concluded that the problem is inherent in APC analysis. In fact, it is the linear models, not the APC data structure, that incur the identification problem. Thus, the most effective way of accounting for aging-related phenomena and social and demographic change is to develop alternative approaches that do not treat age, period, and cohort as independent covariates in an additive fixed effects model. In addition to the new estimator for the conventional models and hierarchical models already discussed above, two approaches – one methodological and the other data design – hold promise for moving cohort analysis to a new era of methodological development and substantive research.

Continuously Evolving Cohort Effects Model

It is well known that the linear model suffers from identification problems. Less appreciated is that the model also suffers from a conceptual problem. The model rests on key assumptions that do not always accurately describe most APC-related phenomena. It assumes that the effect of age is the same for all periods and cohorts (Hobcraft et al., 1982). But the influence of age may change over time and across cohorts. Consider, for instance, the dramatic declines in infant mortality over the past century. It also assumes that the effect of period is the same for people of all ages. But period effects are often age-specific. For example, the influenza epidemic of 1918 caused especially high mortality among people in their teens and twenties. Similarly, it assumes that a cohort effect remains the same as long as the cohort lives. But cohorts must change (Ryder, 1965). That is, cohorts are continuously exposed to events whose influences accumulate over the life course. Wars and epidemics are examples of events that may occur in the middle of a cohort's life and leave an imprint on all of its subsequent behaviors and outcomes. New events constantly occur. A model with unchanging cohort effects is appropriate only if all relevant events occur before the initial observation and only if these events' impacts stay fixed as the cohort ages (Hobcraft et al., 1982). To capture the process of changing cohort effects over time, however, one needs a more general model – a framework that Hobcraft et al. (1982) labeled "continuously accumulating cohort effects."

Schulhofer-Wohl and Yang (2009) addressed this gap in a recent paper. They developed a general model that relaxes the assumption of the conventional additive model. The new model allows age profiles to change over time and period effects to differ for people of different ages. The model also defines cohort effects as an accumulation of age-by-period interactions over all events across the life course. Although a longstanding literature on theories of social change conceptualizes cohort effects in exactly this way, this is the first time that a method of statistically modeling for this more complex form of cohort effects has been presented. This new model was applied to analyze changes in age-specific mortality rates in Sweden over the past 150 years and found that the model fits the data dramatically better than the additive model. The analyses also yield interesting results that show the utility of this model in testing competing theories about the evolution of human mortality. The flexibility of the model, however, comes at a high computational cost because it involves the estimation of a large number of parameters. The inclusion of additional covariates also has not been analytically attempted. So, this new approach presents both opportunities and challenges for future analysts. When further improved, it may find applications in many areas of research.

Longitudinal Cohort Analysis of Balanced Age-by-Cohort Data Structure

The multi-cohort multi-wave data design is especially important for aging and cohort analysis. Although more longitudinal surveys using this design are available, such as the Health and Retirement Survey (HRS) and the National Long Term Care Survey, cohort studies would benefit from further developments in data collection.

The usual accelerated longitudinal design has two limitations: (1) some ages cannot be observed for all cohorts and (2) coverage of the individual life course and historical time is extremely restricted.

The imbalance of the age-by-cohort structure arises from the fact that the baseline survey consists of cohorts of different ages and follow-up surveys occur at the same times. As a result, cohorts age for exactly the same number of years but will remain age-heterogeneous at the end of data collection. The growth curve models applied to these data therefore yield estimates of cohort differences in age trajectories based only on the overlapping age groups of adjacent cohorts rather than the entire possible range of ages. As mentioned above, this could affect the accuracy of the estimates when the number of waves is small or the overlapping age intervals are few. Increasing the number of follow-ups alleviates problems for inference, but is less than perfect for the purposes of disentangling aging effects from birth cohort differences and observing period effects.

A better design is one in which the age-by-cohort data structure is balanced and extends for a long time. Extant secondary data that meet these criteria are exceedingly rare, however. The Liaoning Multigenerational Panel (LMGP) data (Campbell & Lee, 2009) may be an exceptional resource for cohort studies. The LMGP is a database of at least one million observations of 200 000 individuals from eighteenth to early-twentieth Chinese population registers. It provides entire life histories for men and nearly complete life histories for women. The length of the historical period spanned and the sheer number of observations included make it a great candidate for future longitudinal research on aging. It holds the potential for vastly enhancing our ability to estimate various age and cohort models.

Data like these are difficult to collect and compile, but can be highly useful for a variety of substantive investigations. For example, the mechanisms underlying persistent cohort differences in mortality need to be better understood. The "cohort morbidity phenotype" hypothesis has been proposed to link large cohort improvement in survival to reductions in exposures to infections, inflammation, and increased nutrition in early life (Finch & Crimmins, 2004). But evidence of an association between early life conditions and late-life mortality is solely based on aggregate population data from developed countries and needs further testing using individual life histories across multiple birth cohorts in other national populations such as those in the LMGP.

The APC problem has intrigued and frustrated social scientists for decades. Recent developments in techniques for modeling APC data – techniques that avoid the identification problem that has long compromised previous APC analyses – are available and have already generated important substantive findings. These techniques, coupled with new and superior data sources, set the stage for enhancing our understanding of the complex interplay of human aging, cohort characteristics, and historical events and processes.

REFERENCES

Campbell, C., & Lee, J. (2009). Long-term mortality consequences of childhood family context in Liaoning, China, 1749–1909. *Social Science & Medicine, 68,* 1641–1648.

Chen, F., Yang, Y., & Liu, G. (2010). Social change and socioeconomic disparity in health over the life course in China: A cohort analysis. *American Sociological Review, 75,* 126–150.

Clayton, D., & Schifflers, E. (1987). Models for temporal variation in cancer rates. I-II: Age-period and age-cohort models. *Statistics in Medicine, 6,* 449–481.

Di Tella, R., MacCulloch, R. J., & Oswald, A. J. (2003). The macroeconomics of happiness. *The Review of Economics and Statistics, 85,* 809–827.

Easterlin, R. A. (1987). *Birth and fortune: The impact of numbers on personal welfare.* Chicago: University of Chicago.

Elder, G. H. Jr. (Ed.), (1985). *Life course dynamics: Trajectories and transitions, 1968–1980.* Ithaca, NY: Cornell University Press.

Fienberg, S. E., & Mason, W. M. (1978). Identification and estimation of age-period-cohort models in the analysis of discrete archival data. *Sociological Methodology, 8,* 1–67.

Finch, C. E., & Crimmins, E. M. (2004). Inflammatory exposure and historical changes in human life spans. *Science, 305,* 1736–1739.

Fu, W. J. (2008). A smoothing cohort model in age-period-cohort analysis with applications to homicide arrest rates and lung cancer mortality rates. *Sociological Methods and Research, 36,* 327–361.

Glenn, N. D. (1976). Cohort analysts' futile quest: Statistical attempts to separate age, period, and cohort effects. *American Sociological Review, 41,* 900–905.

Glenn, N. D. (1987). A caution about mechanical solutions to the identification problem in cohort analysis: A comment on Sasaki and Suzuki. *American Journal of Sociology, 95,* 754–761.

Hobcraft, J., Menken, J., & Preston, S. H. (1982). Age, period, and cohort effects in demography: A review. *Population Index, 48,* 4–43.

Holford, T. R. (1991). Understanding the effects of age, period, and cohort on incidence and mortality rates. *Annual Review of Public Health, 12,* 425–457.

House, J. S., Lepkowski, J. M., Kinney, A. M., Mero, R. P., Kessler, R. C., & Herzog, A. R. (1994). The social stratification of aging and health. *Journal of Health and Social Behavior, 35,* 213–234.

Kupper, L. L., Janis, J. M., Karmous, A., & Greenberg, B. G. (1985). Statistical age-period-cohort analysis: A review and critique. *Journal of Chronic Disease, 38,* 811–830.

Littell, R. C., Milliken, G. A., Stroup, W. W., Wolfinger, R. D., & Schabenberger, O. (2006). *SAS for mixed models* (2nd edn.). Cary, NC: SAS Institutes, Inc.

Lynch, S. M. (2003). Cohort and life course patterns in the relationship between education and health: A hierarchical approach. *Demography, 40,* 309–331.

Mason, W. M., & Fienberg, S. E. (1985). *Cohort analysis in social research: Beyond the identification problem.* New York: Springer-Verlag.

Mason, W. M., & Smith, H. L. (1985). Age-period-cohort analysis and the study of deaths from pulmonary tuberculosis. In W. M. Mason & S. E. Fienberg (Eds.), *Cohort analysis in social research* (pp. 151–228). New York: Springer-Verlag.

Mason, W. M., & Wolfinger, N. H. (2002). Cohort analysis. In Smelser N. J. & Baltes P. B. (Eds.), *International encyclopedia of the social and behavioral sciences* (pp. 151–228). New York: Elsevier.

Mason, K. O., Mason, W. M., Winsborough, H. H., & Poole, W. K. (1973). Some methodological issues in cohort analysis of archival data. *American Sociological Review, 38,* 242–258.

Mason, K. O., Mason, W. M., & Winsborough, H. H. (1976). Reply to Glenn. *American Sociological Review, 41,* 904–905.

O'Brien, R. M., Stockard, J., & Isaacson, L. (1999). The enduring effects of cohort characteristics on age-specific homicide rates, 1960–1995. *American Journal of Sociology, 104,* 1061–1095.

Pavalko, E. K., Gong, F., & Long, S. (2007). Women's work, cohort change, and health. *Journal of Health and Social Behavior, 48,* 352–368.

Pearl, J. (2000). *Causality: Models, reasoning, and inference.* Cambridge, UK: Cambridge University Press.

Preston, S. H., & Wang, H. (2006). Smoking and sex mortality differences in the United States. *Demography, 43,* 631–646.

Raudenbush, S. W., & Bryk, A. S. (2002). *Hierarchical linear models: Applications and data analysis methods.* Thousand Oaks: Sage.

Rodgers, W. L. (1982). Estimable functions of age, period, and cohort effects. *American Sociological Review, 47,* 774–787.

Ryder, N. B. (1965). The cohort as a concept in the study of social change. *American Sociological Review, 30,* 843–861.

Saski, M., & Suzuki, T. (1987). Changes in religious commitment in the United States, Holland, and Japan. *American Journal of Sociology, 92,* 1055–1076.

Schulhofer-Wohl, S., & Yang, Y. (2009). *Modeling the evolution of age and cohort effects in social research.* Paper presented at the annual meetings of the Population Association of America, Detroit, MI, April.

Singer, J. D., & Willett, J. B. (2003). *Applied longitudinal data analysis: Modeling change and event occurrence.* New York: Oxford University Press.

Smith, H. L. (2008). Advances in age-period-cohort analysis. *Sociological Methods & Research, 36,* 287–296.

Smith, H. L., Mason, W. M., & Fienberg, S. E. (1982). More chimeras of the age-period-cohort accounting framework: Comment on Rodgers. *American Sociological Review, 47,* 787–793.

Wilson, A. E., Shuey, K. M., & Elder, G. H., Jr. (2007). Cumulative advantage processes as mechanisms of inequality in life course health. *American Journal of Sociology, 112,* 1886–1924.

Winship, C., & Harding, D. J. (2008). A mechanism-based approach to the identification of age-period-cohort models. *Sociological Methods & Research, 36,* 362–401.

Yang, Y. (2006). Bayesian inference for hierarchical age-period-cohort models of repeated cross-section survey data. *Sociological Methodology, 36,* 39–74.

Yang, Y. (2007a). Age/Period/Cohort distinctions. In K. S. Markides (Ed.), *Encyclopedia of health and aging* (pp. 20–22). Los Angeles, CA: Sage Publications.

Yang, Y. (2007b). Is old age depressing? Growth trajectories and cohort variations in late life depression. *Journal of Health and Social Behavior, 48,* 16–32.

Yang, Y. (2008a). Social inequalities in happiness in the U.S.

1972–2004: An age-period-cohort analysis. *American Sociological Review, 73,* 204–226.

Yang, Y. (2008b). Trends in U.S. adult chronic disease mortality: Age, period, and cohort variations. *Demography, 45,* 387–416.

Yang, Y. (2009). Age, period, cohort effects. In D. Carr (Ed.), *Encyclopedia of the life course and human development* (pp. 6–10). New York: Gale Publishing.

Yang, Y., & Land, K. C. (2006). A mixed models approach to age-period-cohort analysis of repeated cross-section surveys: Trends in verbal test scores. *Sociological Methodology, 36,* 75–97.

Yang, Y., & Land, K. C. (2008). Age-period-cohort analysis of repeated cross-section surveys: Fixed or random effects? *Sociological Methods & Research, 36,* 297–326.

Yang, Y., & Lee, L. C. (2009). Sex and race disparities in health: Cohort

variations in life course patterns. *Social Forces, 87,* 2093–2124.

Yang, Y., Fu, W. J., & Land, K. C. (2004). A methodological comparison of age-period-cohort models: Intrinsic estimator and conventional generalized linear models. *Sociological Methodology, 34,* 75–110.

Yang, Y., Schulhofer-Wohl, S., Fu, W. J., & Land, K. C. (2008). The intrinsic estimator for age-period-cohort analysis: What it is and how to use it. *American Journal of Sociology, 113,* 1697–1736.

Yang, Y., Frenk, S., & Land, K. C. (2009). *Assessing the significance of cohort and period effects in hierarchical age-period-cohort models.* Paper presented at the annual meetings of the American Sociological Association of America, San Francisco, CA, August.

Part | 2 |

Aging and Social Structure

Chapter | 3 |

Demography and Aging

Linda G. Martin
RAND Corporation, Arlington, Virginia

www.census.gov

INTRODUCTION

Demography is the study of the size, growth, and characteristics of populations, and aging is a growing area of inquiry within it. Demographers are affiliated with many disciplines (sociology, economics, anthropology, to name a few), and they investigate both individual behaviors and macro phenomena. This chapter will focus on the latter; specifically, aging at the level of countries, regions, and the world. In particular, the chapter will highlight the unprecedented population aging of recent decades and projected for the future, demographic changes underlying population aging, alternative demographic indicators of aging, demographic consequences of population aging, and policy responses to population aging that are related to demographic factors.

POPULATION AGING TRENDS AND UNDERLYING DEMOGRAPHIC CHANGE

Population aging is commonly defined as the growth in the proportion of a population that is above a particular age. The age chosen to demarcate the older population often is related to institutions within a society. For example, in the US, from the inception of Social Security in 1935 until 2002, the age of eligibility for full pension benefits was 65 years, so that age has typically been used in examining the proportion of the US population that is older. In other settings in which age of pension receipt or age of typical retirement are lower, 55 or 60 years or some other age may be used to delimit the older population.

DOI: 10.1016/B978-0-12-380880-6.00003-4

Table 3.1 Population ages 65 and over (number in millions and percent of total population) for the world, more-developed countries, and less-developed countries: 1950, 2000, and 2050.

	WORLD		MORE-DEVELOPED COUNTRIES[a]		LESS-DEVELOPED COUNTRIES[b]	
	MILLIONS	%	MILLIONS	%	MILLIONS	%
1950	130.5	5.2	63.9	7.9	66.6	3.9
2000	417.2	6.8	171.5	14.4	245.7	5.0
2050	1,486.9	16.2	334.2	26.2	1,152.7	14.6

Source: Data from United Nations Population Division, 2009, medium variant.
[a]More-developed countries are defined by the United Nations as the countries of Europe and North America, as well as Australia, Japan, and New Zealand.
[b]Less-developed countries are the countries of Africa, the rest of Asia, Latin America and the Caribbean, and the rest of Oceania.

But, by any measure, the current aging of the world's population is rapid in historical terms. As shown in Table 3.1, from 1950 to 2000, the number of people aged 65 and older tripled from 131 million to 417 million, and the proportion of the world population aged 65 and over increased from 5.2% to 6.8%. For historical perspective, consider the experience of Sweden, the proportion of whose population aged 65 and over increased from 8.4% in 1900 to 10.3% in 1950, but then surged to 17.2% in 2000 (Cowgill, 1974; United Nations Population Division, 2009). Going forward, the pace of aging for the world as a whole will accelerate. The United Nations' medium population projection indicates by 2050 another tripling of the population aged 65 and older to 1.5 billion and an increase in the proportion of those aged 65 and over to 16.2% (United Nations Population Division, 2009).

Population aging is occurring in both rich and poor countries or, as they are labeled by the United Nations, both more- and less-developed countries (MDCs and LDCs). Although the proportion aged 65 and older in 2000 is considerably higher in the more-developed countries than the less-developed countries (14.4% vs 5.0%; see Table 3.1), the absolute number of older people is greater in the latter. Moreover, by 2050, the proportion aged 65 and older in the poorer countries will have reached the proportion for the richer countries in 2000. So, population aging is a worldwide phenomenon.

Demographic Components of Population Aging

Population change, and more specifically, population aging, occur as a result of three demographic phenomena: fertility, mortality, and migration. Perhaps, counter-intuitively, the initial primary factor behind population aging typically has been fertility decline (Coale, 1956). As birth rates decline, the proportion of young people in a population declines, and, consequently, the proportion of older people increases. The effect of mortality decline on age composition depends on the ages at which survival improves.

Understanding of the population aging process is informed by the stylized facts of the demographic transition (Notestein, 1945) and the epidemiologic transition (Omran, 1971). Over the course of socio-economic development, populations experience a demographic transition from high fertility and mortality rates to low fertility and mortality rates. The demographic transition begins typically with mortality decline at the youngest ages. Fertility remains high, the population growth rate (birth rate minus death rate in a closed population with no immigration) increases, and the population becomes younger. Subsequently, fertility declines, the population growth rate decreases, and the population ages. At some point, mortality at older ages declines, and further population aging occurs. In the epidemiologic transition, the emphasis is on the shift in predominant causes of death from infectious to degenerative diseases. Omran (1971) noted that children aged one to four years especially benefit from the decline in mortality from infectious pandemics in the early stages of the epidemiologic transition, which is consistent with the rejuvenation of the population at the beginning of the demographic transition. In the later stages, survival is posited to increase for all but the very oldest ages. (See Chapter 6 for more in-depth discussion of the epidemiologic transition.)

The influence of migration on the population aging process in a receiving country is more idiosyncratic, depending on immigrants' age distribution and subsequent fertility in comparison to those of the native-born population. For example, in recent decades, immigrants to the US have tended to arrive at prime working ages, sometimes bringing children with them, thus leading to a younger US population. If the fertility rate of immigrants is higher than that of those born in the US and remains so (which appears to be the case recently; see Swicegood et al., 2006), then there is a further rejuvenating influence. The ultimate effect of immigration on population aging in both sending and receiving countries also depends on the time horizon considered. Immigrants themselves do age, but some immigrants return to their origins, especially as they approach later life (Serow, 1987). Thus, many factors are involved in the immigration and population aging relation, and they may vary over time and across countries. That said, in 2004, 12.2% of the native-born US population was aged 65 and over, whereas only 10.8% of the foreign-born US population was (US Census Bureau, 2005).

Regional Variation in Demographic Change and Population Aging

Most more-developed countries were experiencing gradual but substantial improvements in survival by the turn of the twentieth century, and fertility decline began not long thereafter (Coale, 1987), following the "classic western" transition pattern of Omran (1971). Public health improvements in the late nineteenth century and medical advances in the twentieth century played roles in the demographic change, but the primary driving forces before the turn of the century were socioeconomic in nature; namely, improved standards of living, hygiene, and nutrition (Coale, 1987; Omran, 1971). Many richer countries experienced post-World War II baby booms, but by 2000–2005 the average total fertility rate (TFR) in the more-developed countries was 1.6 children per woman (United Nations Population Division, 2009), which is well below 2.1, the rate at which each couple is replaced in the next generation. Expectation of life at birth was 75.8 years on average in these countries (United Nations Population Division, 2009).

Because the demographic and epidemiologic transitions for nearly all of the more-developed countries occurred over the course of decades, the resulting population aging has been relatively slow. Figure 3.1 shows the speed of population aging for ten countries, defined as the number of years it takes for the proportion of the population aged 65 years and over to increase from 7% to 14%. (This measure of the speed of aging is arbitrary, but has appeared in multiple publications over the years, e.g. Torrey et al., 1987.) Sweden, which along with the other Nordic countries began its demographic transition quite early (Chesnais, 1993), has taken 155 years. France, which had the earliest fertility decline, beginning in the late eighteenth century (Chesnais, 1993), has taken 85 years. The US and the UK began to age much later, with the process slowed considerably in the former by the extended post-World War II baby boom.

A major exception to this pattern among the richer countries is Japan, whose demographic and epidemiologic transitions occurred somewhat later but at a relatively accelerated pace (Chesnais, 1993; Omran, 1971). The eight years of war and seven years of military occupation culminated in very low post-World War II fertility (Taeuber, 1960). Mortality also declined rapidly, and in 2006 Japan had the lowest mortality on earth with males expected to live 79 years on average and females 86 years (Japan Statistics Bureau, 2009). Consequently, it took only 24 years – from 1970 to 1994 – for Japan's proportion of those aged 65 and over to increase from 7% to 14%.

Also diverging from the classic western pattern described by Omran have been the experiences of

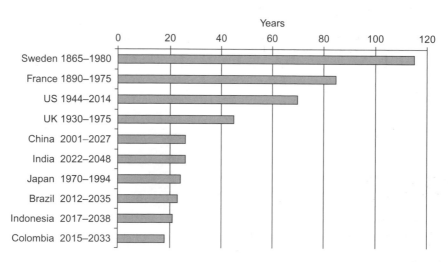

Figure 3.1 Number of years for the proportion aged 65 years and over to increase from 7% to 14%, selected countries.
Sources: Author's graph based on data from Kinsella & Velkoff, 2001, and US Census Bureau, 2009.

the countries of the former Soviet Union (none of these countries are included in Figure 3.1 because time series of vital statistics are not available). Although mortality improvements in these countries have long lagged behind those in Western Europe, absolute increases in mortality rates in Russia and the Ukraine in the 1990s were remarkable (Meslé, 2004). The increases in mortality from cardiovascular disease (CVD), violence, and infectious diseases in Russia have been linked to multiple factors, most prominently alcohol consumption (Leon et al., 2007; Zaridze et al., 2009) and the transition to a market-based economy (Stuckler et al., 2009). Russian working-age males appear to have been the most affected (Meslé, 2004), and fertility is quite low; thus, population aging has continued with the proportion aged 65 years and over in Russia increasing from 10% in 1990 to 14% in 2005 (US Census Bureau, 2009).

Many less-developed countries experienced their demographic and epidemiologic transitions in the last decades of the twentieth century. The pace of change was rapid as a result of the diffusion from richer countries of medical and public health advances. So, these countries have been said to be getting "old" before they are getting rich. In addition, some governments had explicit policies encouraging fertility decline in particular. As a result, many of the countries of Asia and Latin America are expected to experience rapid population aging at a speed matching or surpassing that of Japan. In Asia, the two largest populations of the world, China and India, are expected to take just 26 years to move from 7% to 14% of the total population aged 65 and over. The fourth largest population (after the US in third place), Indonesia, is projected to take only 21 years. In Latin America, Brazil (the fifth largest population in the world) is expected to take 23 years and Colombia 18 years.

As shown in Figure 3.2, the only major region of the world that is still quite young, and is expected to age relatively slowly in the first half of the twenty-first century, is sub-Saharan Africa. Although the population proportion aged 65 years and over is projected to double over the period, it increases from only 3% to 6%. High fertility and high mortality (and in some cases increasing mortality as a result of HIV/AIDS) are common. In 2000–2005, the total fertility rate for the region was 5.4 children per woman, and the expectation of life at birth was 51.2 years (United Nations Population Division, 2009).

So, population aging is a worldwide phenomenon, but there is considerable variation across countries in the level and pace of aging. Europe and North America are clearly in the lead. Indeed, Europe has 19 of the 20 oldest populations on earth (Kinsella & Phillips, 2005). Asia and Latin America are also aging rapidly, but there is considerable diversity within these regions. Asia is home to Japan, which has aged the most rapidly of the richer countries, as well as the population giants of China and India, which are expected to age almost as fast. But other countries in Asia in 2008 still had relatively low proportions aged 65 and over: for example, Afghanistan (2%), Iraq (3%), Pakistan (4%), and the Philippines (4%). Similarly, in Latin America and the Caribbean, the proportion aged 65 and over in 2008 ranged from 4% in Bolivia and Guatemala to 12% in Cuba and 13% in Uruguay (Population Reference Bureau, 2008). Thus, there is variation in population aging across and within regions that reflects past histories of fertility and mortality.

ALTERNATIVE INDICATORS OF POPULATION AGING

Besides the proportion of a population above an age typically associated with retirement, there are multiple other indicators of population aging. Some focus on the proportion of the population at even greater ages, others on broader measures of the population age distribution, and others on the ratio of an older

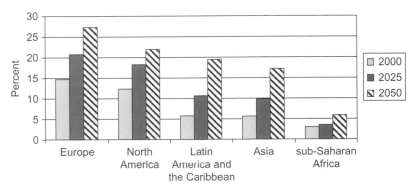

Figure 3.2 Percent of total population aged 65 and over by major region: 2000, 2025, and 2050.
Sources: Author's graph, based on data from United Nations Population Division, 2009, medium variant.

age group to younger groups. Finally, indicators that are defined in terms of average years of remaining life, so-called prospective age, rather than chronological age, have been recently proposed. These new measures are especially important given the changing meaning of specific chronological ages over time.

Percent Aged 80 and Over and Centenarians

Because the need for assistance and risk of health problems typically increase with age, there is particular interest in changes in population proportions at ages more advanced than 65 years. Many data collection agencies publish information on trends in the proportions aged 80 and over (although other ages have been used to define the "oldest old," e.g. age 85 in Suzman et al., 1992). Japan, which in 2008 had the largest proportion of its population aged 65 and over of any country (21.6%; Kinsella & He, 2009), also had the largest proportion aged 80 and over (5.7%; US Census Bureau, 2009). However, the proportion of the 65 and over population that is 80 and older varies considerably across countries and over time, as a result of past fertility and mortality (Kinsella & He, 2009). For example, in the US in 2008, 30% of the 65 and over population was 80 and older, but in 2025 the proportion is projected to be only 23% (US Census Bureau, 2009), as a result of the baby boom cohort being aged 61 to 79 years old. But even though the proportions 80 and older vary over time, the absolute numbers at those ages will generally increase rapidly. For the more-developed countries, the population aged 80 and over is projected to increase at a rate of 2.3% annually from 2000 to 2050, even as their total populations grow at a rate of only 0.1% annually and the population aged 65 and over grows at 1.3% annually (calculations based on data from United Nations Population Division, 2009). This rapid rate of growth implies that the number of oldest old will double in just 30 years.

The number of centenarians also appears to be growing rapidly, although precise estimates should be viewed with some caution because of the potential for age misreporting (Jeune & Vaupel, 1999). The United Nations estimates that the number of centenarians worldwide will increase from 209 000 in 2000 to over four million in 2050 (United Nations Population Division, 2009).

Median Ages and Population Pyramids

A broader characterization of the population aging process is captured by median ages and population pyramids. The median age indicates the age at which half the population is younger and half the population is older, whereas population pyramids present graphically the proportion of the population at each age.

The median age of more-developed countries was almost 39 years in 2005, whereas that of less-developed countries was only 25 years (United Nations Population Division, 2009). In some of the highest fertility countries in the latter group, the median age is even younger. For example, the median age in Pakistan, the sixth largest population in the world with a total fertility rate of over four children per woman, is estimated to have been only 20 years in 2005. The oldest population by this measure is again Japan, whose median age of 43 years in 2005 is projected to increase to 51 years in 2025 and 55 years in 2050 (United Nations Population Division, 2009).

As populations age, their population pyramids change shape from a pyramid (hence the name) to a rectangle. This transformation is shown clearly in Figure 3.3 for age and sex distributions of the more-developed countries from 1950 to 2000 to 2050. In 1950, the largest 10-year age group for both males and females was the 0–9 group, the base of the pyramid. By 2000, the largest group was age 30–39 years, and by 2050 it is expected to be aged 60–69 years. At the later date, the overall age distribution also has taken on a decidedly rectangular shape. One other feature of Figure 3.3 to note is that the female population in all years has an older age distribution. This pattern results both from the greater numbers of males than females at birth and from the female survival advantage throughout life in these countries.

Dependency Ratios

Dependency ratios are used to compare the proportion of younger or older population to the population at prime working ages. The youth dependency ratio (YDR) is defined as the ratio of the population aged 0–14 or 0–19 to the population aged 15–64 or 20–64, respectively. As education has been extended and completion of high school has become the norm in richer countries, the 0–19 v 20–64 comparison is more commonly made. Similarly, the old-age dependency ratio (OADR) can be defined as the ratio of the population aged 65 and over to the population aged 20–64. Depending on typical retirement age in a country, the upper bound of the middle group and the lower bound of the upper group also may vary. The total dependency ratio (TDR) is the sum of the population aged 0–19 and 65 and over divided by the population aged 20–64 years.

As populations go through their demographic transitions, the YDR first increases slightly as a result of improved child survival and then declines as fertility declines (Bongaarts, 2001). The OADR is

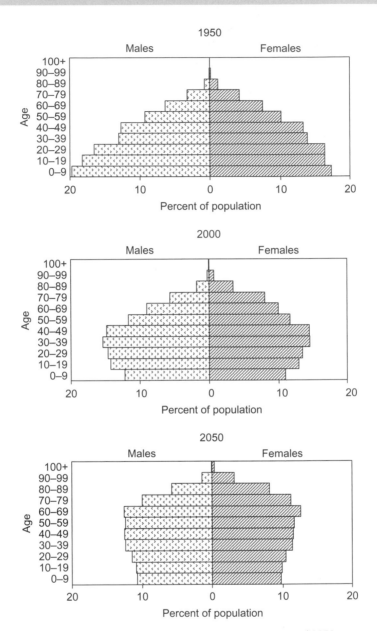

Figure 3.3 Age and sex distributions of more-developed countries: 1950, 2000, and 2050.
Sources: Author's graph, based on analysis of data from United Nations Population Division, 2009, medium variant.

relatively stable, so overall the TDR declines as the transition progresses. This period of declining or low dependency ratio is sometimes referred to as the demographic bonus, dividend, or window (Lee, 2003; United Nations Population Division, 2004). Ultimately, towards the end of the demographic transition, as survival at older ages improves, the OADR increases substantially and the TDR also begins to increase. Figure 3.4 presents trends in the OADR for the more-developed countries from 1955 to 2045.

In 1955, there were roughly 15 people aged 65 and over for every 100 people aged 20 to 64 years. By 2045, the ratio is expected to be 47 to 100, so for every older person there will be only two people in the prime working ages.

Dependency ratios are, at best, rough indicators of the extent to which one group in a population is dependent on another group. For example, labor force participation is by no means universal at ages 20 to 64 years, and older people may continue to

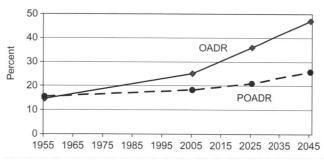

Figure 3.4 Old-age dependency ratios (OADRs) and prospective old-age dependency ratios (POADRs), more-developed countries: 1955, 2005, 2025, and 2045.
Sources: Author's graph, based on data from Sanderson & Scherbov, 2008 (supplemental table).

work well past age 65. Another issue is the extent to which resources flow from one generation to another. In Europe and the US, net financial transfers and social support typically flow from the older to the younger generation (Albertini et al., 2007; US National Institute of Aging, 2007), so the concept of dependency defined grossly in terms of age groups is further undermined. Nevertheless, trends in OADRs may be useful in general characterizations of the implications of population aging for the fiscal viability of public pension programs.

Prospective Age and Changing Meaning of Chronological Age

As life expectancy has increased, the meaning of chronological age has changed. For example, in the US, in 1950, people aged 65 could expect to live an additional 14 years, but by 2005 University of California, that number had increased to almost 19 years (Berkeley & Max Planck Institute, 2009). In 2005, it is 72-year-olds who on average can expect to live an additional 14 years. So, in this example, age 72 is the new 65. Recently, measures of so-called prospective age or forward-looking age have been used to compare aging in populations with different life expectancies. These new measures, as well as other fundamental ways in which the meaning of chronological age is changing, will be discussed below.

Measures of Prospective Aging

Sanderson and Scherbov (2005, 2007, 2008) have suggested that insight into population aging can be enhanced by considering both measures using chronological age and measures using prospective age. For instance, in addition to comparing the proportion of a population at ages 65 and older across countries or within a country over time, one might compare the proportions at or above the age at which remaining

life expectancy (RLE) is a particular number of years, say 15. Because the probabilities of need for care from both formal and informal sources are likely greatest in the last part of life, such a perspective can be especially useful from a policy perspective.

For example, in India, the proportion aged 65 and older increased from 3.4% in 1955 to 5.3% in 2005 and is projected to rise to 8.1% in 2025, showing monotonic growth. However, the proportions at or above the ages at which RLE is 15 years or less (RLE ≤ 15) first decreased from 7.5% in 1955 to 5.8% in 2005, but is expected to increase to 7% in 2025 (Sanderson & Scherbov, 2008, supplemental table). The decline in the population proportion at ages RLE ≤ 15 between 1955 and 2005 reflects the increase in life expectancy at older ages, as well as past fertility and survival at younger ages, as incorporated in the number of people at each age. In India in 1955, the age at which RLE = 15 was only 57 years, but was 64 years in 2005 and is expected to be almost 67 years in 2025. So, from this perspective, the potential old-age burden in terms of care may have been declining over the initial 50-year period, in contrast to the monotonic increase suggested by the changes in the proportion aged 65 and over.

The concept of prospective age can be applied to the other indicators of aging discussed earlier (Sanderson & Scherbov, 2008). For example, if we use the year 2000 as the standard, then the prospective median age in 2025 is the age of a person in 2025 with the same RLE as the median-aged person in 2000. The change in prospective median age over time approximately tracks the change in the median age minus the change in life expectancy at the median age (Lutz et al., 2008). If life expectancy is steadily increasing, then prospective median age rises less rapidly than median age.

Application of prospective age to the calculation of OADRs involves defining the lower boundary of "old age" in the ratio as the age at which there are a given number of remaining years of life on average.

Again, if life expectancy is steadily increasing, prospective OADRs (POADRs) increase more slowly than conventional OADRs, as shown for the more-developed countries in Figure 3.4. In 1955, the OADR and POADR were both approximately 15 to 100, because in that year the age at which RLE was 15 years in the more-developed countries was about 65. By 2045, the path of the POADRs is expected to have diverged considerably from the path of the OADRs. The POADR is only about 26 to 100, in comparison to an OADR of 47 to 100. Thus, taking increases in life expectancy into account, old-age dependency is cut roughly in half, so that there are four people at ages 20 to the age when RLE ≤ 15 (age 73 in 2045) for every older person instead of a ratio of two to one using the OADR.

Use of the POADR instead of the OADR also changes the ranking of the oldest countries in the world. Sanderson and Scherbov (2008) reported that the five oldest countries in the world on the basis of OADRs in 2005 were Italy, Japan, Germany, Belgium, and Greece. But POADRs indicated that the top five were Ukraine, Bulgaria, Belarus, Estonia, and Croatia. The relatively low life expectancies at older ages in these Eastern European countries and differences in the age distributions account for the reordering. For example, in 2005, in Italy and the Ukraine, the proportions aged 65 and older were 20.0% and 16.1%, respectively, and the OADRs were 32.7 and 26.4, so Italy was the older of the two countries by these measures. However, the ages at which RLE = 15 were 70.5 and 63.7 years for Italy and the Ukraine, respectively. The population proportions at RLE ≤ 15 were 13.7% and 17.5% and the POADRs were 20.4 and 29.4, respectively. So the Ukraine is the older of the two by these alternative measures of population aging (Sanderson and Scherbov, 2008, supplemental table).

Changing Meaning of Chronological Age

The preceding discussion of prospective age emphasized just one way in which the characteristics of people of a particular chronological age are changing over time; namely, their average remaining years of life. There are many other ways in which older people of today (defined using chronological age) are different from older people of the past and older people of the future. For example, there is a growing body of evidence for the US that the prevalence of disability among the older population has declined in recent decades (Freedman et al., 2002; Manton et al., 1997; see Chapter 5 for a full discussion). Such change suggests that older people may be able to prolong their labor force participation, if they so desire or if it is necessary financially, and that they may be able to live independently for a longer period. In contrast, in some Asian countries, disability among

older populations has increased in recent decades (Ofstedal et al. 2007; Zimmer et al., 2002). The reasons for this upward trend are not clear; however, there is evidence for Taiwan that expansion of access to health care has been associated with greater increases in survival among those with disabilities. The difference in timing of the epidemiologic transition in richer v poorer countries also may be related to differences in trends in late-life functioning, since the older populations in poorer countries likely experienced greater exposure to infectious diseases earlier in life than did those in the richer countries. Given the relation of infection and inflammation to some late-life chronic diseases (Finch & Crimmins, 2004), one might expect functioning to be affected among survivors. Thus, temporal trends in the disability profiles of richer and poorer countries may differ.

More generally, changes in the composition of the older population over time are not difficult to imagine when one thinks about the rapid socioeconomic development that has occurred worldwide during the lifetimes of many of today's older people and the lifetimes of the future old who are now young. One of the most distinctive and rapid changes of the twentieth century has been the increase in educational attainment. For example, in the US in 1985, 51% of the population aged 65 and over had not graduated from high school (Bruno, 1987), but by 2005, just 20 years later, only 26% were in this least-educated category (US Census Bureau, 2006). This phenomenal increase in educational attainment is occurring around the world, and the implications for the older populations in less-developed countries will be especially manifested in the future (Hermalin, 2002). (Uncertainty surrounding projections of educational attainment of the older population for, say, 50 years from now is minimized by the facts that those people are already alive today and that education is typically completed fairly early in life.) For example, in China, the mean number of years of schooling for the 65 and older population was under three years in 2000, but is projected to increase to almost nine years by 2050 (Samir et al., 2009). Notably, the sex differential in educational attainment among the Chinese older population will be reduced considerably. Average attainment for older males will increase from roughly four to nine years over the period, while for females the increase will be from about 1.5 to over eight years.

. Given the strong associations of educational attainment with income, wealth, and physical and cognitive health, to name just a few indicators of well-being, these projected increases in the educational attainment of the older population augur well for the future and reinforce the earlier observation that the older populations of tomorrow defined in terms of chronological age will likely be quite different from the older populations of today.

DEMOGRAPHIC CONSEQUENCES OF POPULATION AGING

Besides the future changes in the composition of older populations just highlighted, some more fundamentally demographic consequences for entire populations will likely be manifested as a result of population aging and the demographic processes underlying it.

Changes in Sex Ratio

As populations age, the overall ratio of males to females is likely to change. The so-called sex ratio at birth is typically in the range of 104–107 males to 100 females in populations in which there is not sex-selective abortion or infanticide (Chahnazarian, 1991), and, in the richer countries, in which there is not systematic discrimination against females in terms of nutrition and access to health care, female mortality rates are less than male mortality rates at every age. Because of this female survival advantage, by around age 40, females typically outnumber males, and in 2005, the sex ratio for the population aged 65 and over in the more-developed countries was 68 males to 100 females (United Nations Population Division, 2009). The gap between male and female life expectancy in the richer countries began to narrow in the 1990s, and this convergence is expected to continue in the future, so the sex ratio for the population aged 65 and over is projected to increase to 77 males to 100 females in 2050.

In the poorer countries in which the overall female survival advantage is much smaller than in richer countries, females do not outnumber males until about age 60 (United Nations Population Division, 2009). The female survival advantage is expected to increase as overall mortality falls (Hill & Choi, 2004; United Nations Population Division, 2009), in part because of differential trends in tobacco use and accidents (Kinsella & Phillips, 2005). So, the sex ratio of the population aged 65 and older in the less-developed countries is projected to decline slightly from 86 to 100 in 2005 to 83 to 100 in 2050 (United Nations Population Division, 2009).

Given that there are more older females than males and given that husbands are typically older than their wives and thus at greater mortality risk, females are less likely to be married in late life than are males. For example, in the population aged 65 and over in the US in 2006, 72% of males were married, as opposed to only 40% of females (Kinsella & He, 2009). In India in 2001, the proportions were 79% for males and 41% for females. Marital status has important implications for well-being in later life. In both richer and poorer countries, there is evidence that females who become widows are more likely to become impoverished (Martin, 1990; United Nations Division for the Advancement of Women, 2001; Zick & Holden, 2000).

Changes in Kin Availability

Besides having implications for changes in sex ratio and marital status, population aging and the underlying demographic phenomena influence broader kin availability. As mortality declines, more generations of a family may be alive at the same time. However, fertility decline reduces the number of immediate offspring who potentially could provide assistance in late life, if it is needed. Billari (2005) found that, for 13 of the richer countries, the proportion of females in the 1940 birth cohort who were childless ranged from 8% to 15%. Currently, the overall proportion of older people who are childless in the richer countries is low in comparison to historical levels, but it is likely to increase in the coming decades (Kinsella & He, 2009). There also are early indications that childlessness in old age may increase in the future in Latin America (Rosero-Bixby et al., 2009). (See Chapter 6 for a more detailed discussion of kin availability and living arrangements.)

Population Decline

Some populations in Europe and Asia are not only experiencing rapid population aging, but are also facing the prospect of population decline; that is, a decrease in the absolute number of people in the total population. Population growth in a given year is equal to births minus deaths plus net migration. If net in migration is relatively small and deaths outnumber births, then population decline occurs. Decline has already begun or soon will in such countries as Germany, Italy, Japan, Russia, and the Ukraine (United Nations Population Division, 2009). Russia represents the extreme case; it is projected to lose 27 million people, or almost 20% of its population, between 2005 and 2050.

But other countries in which over 15% of their populations are already aged 65 or over, such as France, Sweden, and the UK, are not projected to experience population decline by 2050. These countries have total fertility rates that, although below the replacement level of 2.1 children per woman, are roughly 1.85. In contrast, many of the countries experiencing decline have total fertility rates below 1.5 children per woman.

The United Nations Population Division (2009) projects that the population of the more-developed countries taken together will begin to decline between 2035 and 2040, but this outcome and its timing depend on the course that fertility rates take in the coming decades. Population aging is easier to predict because the future older population in 2050 is already alive today. Indicators of aging also are affected by fertility and the size of the younger population, but not as much as is overall population size.

The consequences of slowing growth or population decline for economic prosperity and national influence have been topics of research since at least the 1930s when, during the Great Depression, fertility declined below the replacement level in some countries (Espenshade & Serow, 1978; Hansen, 1937; Teitelbaum & Winter, 1985). More recently, although there is concern about the implications of and government interest in attempting to reverse decline or aging (as will be discussed in the section below), the predictions of negative consequences generally are not so dire. For example, Börsch-Supan and colleagues (2007) have argued that, in part, because aging is a gradual process, capital markets will anticipate the coming changes, and there will not be the feared "meltdown" of asset values when those born in the post-World War II baby boom years in Europe and the US reach retirement ages. The increased demand for capital as labor forces shrink plus economic globalization will help minimize the demographic consequences for capital returns. The bigger challenge will be to increase the productivity of a smaller labor force, especially through education and training. Another option is to supplement labor force size with more women, immigrants, or older people.

POLICY RESPONSES RELATED TO DEMOGRAPHIC FACTORS

Several countries in Asia and Europe have implemented policies to reverse or slow population aging. Such policies focus primarily on raising fertility, although there also has been considerable discussion of immigration policy. The other major policy response related to demographic factors involves accommodating population aging through increasing the ages of eligibility for age-based programs, such as public pensions.

Policies to Reverse or Slow Population Aging

Fertility

Although sometimes not explicitly couched in pronatalist terms, family-support policies and family-friendly work policies have been tried in Europe (Grant et al., 2004) and Asia (Straughan et al., 2008). Some of these policies have affected the timing of fertility, but the longer-term effects on the ultimate level of fertility have been minimal (Gauthier, 2007).

Some analysts have suggested that large amounts of money over extended periods of time would be necessary to have an effect on completed family size, whereas others have argued that fertility change is not amenable to public policy intervention (Balter, 2006).

Immigration

In 2001, a United Nations Population Division report raised the intriguing question of whether or not immigration could be used to slow or reverse population aging and decline (United Nations Population Division, 2001). The report presented different scenarios for the future, including ones in which immigration was increased to levels that would maintain then-current OADRs or maintain peak population sizes in the absence of immigration. The amounts of so-called "replacement migration" necessary to achieve these targets were enormous for most countries in comparison to current levels of immigration.

Modification of Ages of Eligibility for Age-Based Policies

Given limited resources and the heterogeneity of needs among older people, policies to accommodate population aging might be based ideally on need, rather than on age (Neugarten, 1982). However, for political and administrative reasons, program eligibility is frequently based on age. Given the changing meaning of age over time, as highlighted above, age-based programs might well incorporate automatic adjustments of eligibility age. The US made an ad hoc adjustment through its 1983 Social Security reform, which phased in a two-year increase in the eligibility age for full benefits from 2003 to 2025. Several European countries also are making such gradual adjustments (Organisation for Economic Co-operation and Development, 2007), although with less advanced warning. Countries now designing such programs for the first time might well build in flexibility from the start.

Another strategy would be to use as the eligibility criterion some sort of prospective age, as defined earlier, or a combination of chronological and prospective ages, as proposed by Sanderson and Scherbov (2008). Taking changes in life expectancy into account when defining ages of eligibility for public programs is receiving increasing attention (Shoven & Goda, 2008). For example, benefit levels are now linked to life expectancy in Germany, Finland, and Portugal (Organisation for Economic Co-operation and Development, 2007). In countries with relatively high life expectancies, such a strategy might save money at the macro level and could facilitate the targeting of those with the greatest potential need. In countries with lower life expectancies, it could embody recognition of the fact that a person may have considerable need long before he or she reaches an age such as 65, perhaps through a lifetime of poverty. However, in both types of countries, use of a fluctuating prospective age to determine eligibility may make it more difficult for individuals to plan their own futures.

DEMOGRAPHY IS NOT DESTINY

Demographic phenomena – changes in fertility and mortality – are the driving forces behind population aging, and population aging has important demographic and socioeconomic consequences. That said, demography is not destiny, and, as will be demonstrated in the other chapters in this handbook, much can be done to ameliorate the extent to which there are negative consequences of population aging. Nevertheless, for policy purposes, it will be important going forward to carefully track trends in fertility and mortality, so that more accurate forecasts of population aging can be made. Continuing data collection and research to enhance understanding of how the characteristics – both strengths and needs – of older people will likely change over time will also be essential.

REFERENCES

Albertini, M., Kohli, M., & Vogel, C. (2007). Intergenerational transfers of time and money in European families: Common patterns – different regimes? *Journal of European Social Policy, 17*(4), 319–334.

Balter, M. (2006). The baby deficit. *Science, 312,* 1894–1897.

Billari, F. (2005). Partnership, childbearing and parenting: Trend of the 1990s. In M. Macura, A. L. MacDonald & W. Haug (Eds.), *The new demographic regime: Population challenges and policy responses* (pp. 63–94). Geneva and New York: United Nations Economic Commission for Europe and United Nations Population Fund. http://www.unece.org/pau/_docs/pau/PAU_2005_Publ_NDRCh05.pdf, accessed July 31, 2009.

Bongaarts, J. (2001). Dependency burdens in the developing world. In N. Birdsall, A. C. Kelley & S. W. Sindig (Eds.), *Population matters: Demographic change, economic growth, and poverty in the developing world* (pp. 55–64). Oxford, UK: Oxford University Press.

Börsch-Supan, A., Ludwig, A., & Sommer, M. (2007). Aging and asset prices. *Mannheim Research Institute for the Economics of Aging Discussion Paper* (pp. 129–207), http://www.mea.uni-mannheim.de/publications/meadp_129-07.pdf, accessed August 7, 2009.

Bruno, R. R. (1987). Educational attainment in the United States: March 1982 to 1985. *Current Population Reports: Population Characteristics* (US Census Bureau). *P-20,* http://www.census.gov/population/socdemo/education/p20-415/tab-01.pdf, accessed July 30, 2009.

Chahnazarian, A. (1991). Determinants of the sex ratio at birth: Review of recent literature. *Social Biology, 35,* 214–235.

Chesnais, J. C. (1993). *The demographic transition: Stages, patterns, and economic implications.* Translated from the French by E. Kreager & P. Kreager. Oxford, UK: Clarendon Press.

Coale, A. J. (1956). The effects of changes in mortality and fertility on age composition. *The Milbank Memorial Fund Quarterly, 34*(1), 79–114.

Coale, A. J. (1987). Demographic transition. In J. Eatwell, M. Milgate & P. Newman (Eds.), *Social economics* (pp. 16–23). London: MacMillan Press.

Cowgill, D. O. (1974). The aging of populations and societies. *The ANNALS of the American Academy of Political and Social Science, 415*(1), 1–18.

Espenshade, T. J., & Serow, W. J. (Eds.), (1978). *Economic consequences of slowing population growth.* New York: Academic Press.

Finch, C. E., & Crimmins, E. M. (2004). Inflammatory exposure and historical changes in human lifespans. *Science, 305*(5691), 1736–1739.

Freedman, V. A., Martin, L. G., & Schoeni, R. F. (2002). Recent trends in disability and functioning among older US adults. *Journal of the American Medical Association, 288*(24), 3137–3146.

Gauthier, A. H. (2007). The impact of family polices on fertility in industrialized countries: A review of the literature. *Population Research and Policy Review, 26,* 323–346.

Grant, J., Hoorens, S., Sivadasan, S., van het Loo, M., DaVanzo, J., Hale, L., et al. (2004). *Low fertility and population ageing: Causes, consequences, and policy options.* Santa Monica, CA: RAND Corporation. (MG-206-EC)

Hansen, A. H. (1937). Economic progress and declining population growth. *American Economic Review, 29*(1), 1–15.

Hermalin, A. I. (2002). Capturing change: Transitions at older ages and cohort succession. In A. I. Hermalin (Ed.), *The well-being of the elderly in Asia* (pp. 519–541). Ann Arbor: University of Michigan Press.

Hill, K., & Choi, Y. (2004). *The adult mortality in developing countries project: Substantive findings.* Paper presented for the Adult Mortality in Developing Countries Workshop, Marin County, California, July. http://www.ceda.berkeley.edu/events/AMDC_Papers/Hill_Choi_Summary-amdc.pdf, accessed July 31, 2009.

Japan Statistics Bureau. (2009). *Japan Statistical Yearbook 2009*, http://www.stat.go.jp/data/nenkan/zuhyou/y0227000.xls, accessed July 21, 2009.

Jeune, B., & Vaupel, J. W. (Eds) (1999). *Validation of exceptional longevity*. Monograph on Population Aging, 6. Odense, Denmark: Odense University Press.

Kinsella, K., & He, W. (2009). *An aging world: 2008*. Washington, DC: US Bureau of the Census, Series P95/09-1.

Kinsella, K., & Phillips, D. R. (2005). Global aging: The challenge of success. *Population Bulletin, 60*(1), 1–40.

Kinsella, K., & Velkoff, V. (2001). *An aging world: 2001*. Washington, DC: US Bureau of the Census, Series P95/01-1.

Lee, R. D. (2003). The demographic transition: Three centuries of fundamental change. *Journal of Economic Perspectives, 17*(4), 167–190.

Leon, D. A., Saburova, L., Tomkins, S., Andreev, E., Kiryanov, N., McKee, M., et al. (2007). Hazardous alcohol drinking and premature mortality in Russia: A population based case-control study. *The Lancet, 369*(9578), 2001–2009.

Lutz, W., Sanderson, W., & Scherbov, S. (2008). The coming acceleration of global population ageing. *Nature, 451*, 716–719.

Manton, K. G., Corder, L. S., & Stallard, E. (1997). Chronic disability trends in elderly United States populations: 1982–1994. *Proceedings of the National Academy of Sciences, 94*, 2593–2598.

Martin, L. G. (1990). The status of South Asia's growing elderly population. *Journal of Cross-Cultural Gerontology, 5*, 93–117.

Meslé, F. (2004). Mortality in Central and Eastern Europe: Long-term trends and recent upturns. *Demographic Research*, Special Collection 2, Article 3, http://www.demographic-research.org/special/2/3/s2-3.pdf, accessed July 21, 2009.

Neugarten, B. L. (Ed.), (1982). *Age or need? Public policies for older people*. Beverly Hills, CA: Sage.

Notestein, F. W. (1945). Population: The long view. In T. W. Schultz (Ed.), *Food for the world* (pp. 36–57). Chicago, IL: University of Chicago Press.

Ofstedal, M. B., Zimmer, Z., Hermalin, A. I., Chan, A., Chuang, Y., Natividad, J., et al. (2007). Short-term trends in functional limitation among older Asians: A comparison of five Asian settings. *Journal of Cross-cultural Gerontology, 22*(1), 243–261.

Omran, A. R. (1971). The epidemiologic transition: A theory of the epidemiology of population change. *The Milbank Memorial Fund Quarterly, 49* (Part 1)(4), 509–538.

Organisation for Economic Co-operation and Development. (2007). Pension reform: The unfinished agenda. *OECD Policy Brief*. Paris: OECD, http://www.oecd.org/dataoecd/16/24/39310166.pdf, accessed August 7, 2009.

Population Reference Bureau (2008). *2008 world population data sheet*. Washington, DC: Population Reference Bureau.

Rosero-Bixby, L., Castro-Martin, T., & Martin-García, T. (2009). Is Latin America starting to retreat from early and universal childbearing? *Demographic Research, 20*(9), 169–194.

Samir, K. C., Barakat, B., Goujon, A., Shirbekk, V., & Lutz, W. (2009). *Projection of populations by level of educational attainment, age and sex for 120 countries for 2005–2050*. International Institute for Applied Systems Analysis and Vienna Institute of Demography. http://www.iiasa.ac.at/Research/POP/Edu07FP/index.html?sb=12, accessed March 17, 2009.

Sanderson, W., & Scherbov, S. (2005). Average remaining lifetimes can increase as human populations age. *Nature, 435*, 811–813.

Sanderson, W., & Scherbov, S. (2007). A new perspective on population aging. *Demographic Research, 16*(2), 27–58.

Sanderson, W., & Scherbov, S. (2008.) Rethinking age and aging. *Population Bulletin, 63*(4), 1–16. Supplemental table available at http://www.prb.org/excel08/age-aging_table.xls, accessed July 30, 2009.

Serow, W. J. (1987). Why the elderly move: Cross-national comparisons. *Research on Aging, 9*(4), 582–597.

Shoven, J. B., & Goda, G. S. (2008). Adjusting government policies for age inflation. *NBER Working Paper Series* (National Bureau of Economic Research), 14231, 1–29.

Straughan, P. T., Jones, G. W., & Chan, A. W. M. (Eds.), (2008). *Ultralow fertility in Pacific Asia: Trends, causes, and policy issues*. London: Routledge.

Stuckler, D., King, L., & McKee, M. (2009). Mass privatisation and the post-communist mortality crisis: A cross-national analysis. *The Lancet, 373*(9682), 399–407.

Suzman, R. M., Willis, D. P., & Manton, K. G. (Eds.), (1992). *The oldest old*. New York, NY: Oxford University Press.

Swicegood, C. G., Sobczak, M., & Ishizawa, H. (2006). *A new look at the recent fertility of American immigrants: Results for twenty-first century*. Paper presented at the annual meeting of the Population Association of America, Los Angeles, 1 April.

Taeuber, I. B. (1960). Japan's demographic transition re-examined. *Population Studies, 14*(1), 28–39.

Teitelbaum, M. J., & Winter, J. M. (1985). *The fear of population decline*. Orlando, FL: Academic Press.

Torrey, B. B., Kinsella, K., & Taeuber, C. M. (1987). *An Aging World*. Washington, DC: US Bureau of the Census, Series P95/78.

United Nations Division for the Advancement of Women. (2001). Widowhood: Invisible women, excluded or secluded. *Women 2000*, December, 1–19. http://www.un.org/womenwatch/daw/public/wom_Dec%2001%20single%20pg.pdf, accessed July 31, 2009.

United Nations Population Division (2001). *Replacement Migration: Is it a solution to declining and ageing populations?* New York: United Nations.

United Nations Population Division (2004). *World Population to 2300.* New York: United Nations.

United Nations Population Division. (2009). *World Population Prospects: The 2008 revision.* http://esa.un.org/unpp, accessed July 15, 2009.

US Census Bureau. (2005). *Current Population Survey, 2004 Annual Social and Economic Supplement.* Internet Release Date: February 22, 2005. http://www.census.gov/population/www/socdemo/foreign/ppl-176.html, accessed July 17, 2009.

US Census Bureau. (2006). *Current Population Survey, 2005 Annual Social and Economic Supplement.* Internet Release Date: October 26, 2006. http://www.census.gov/population/socdemo/education/cps2005/tab01-01.xls, accessed July 29, 2009.

US Census Bureau. (2009). *International data base, updated June 2009.* http://www.census.gov/ipc/www/idb/informationGateway.php, accessed July 21, 2009.

US National Institute of Aging (2007). *Growing older in America: The health and retirement study.* Bethesda, MD: National Institutes of Health.

University of California, Berkeley, & Max Planck Institute for Demographic Research (2009). *Human Mortality Database.* University of California, Berkeley (USA), and Max Planck Institute for Demographic Research (Germany). http://www.mortality.org, accessed July 30, 2009.

Zaridze, D., Brennan, P., Boreham, J., Boroda, A., Karpov, R., Lazarev, A., et al. (2009). Alcohol and cause-specific mortality in Russia: A retrospective case-control study of 48,557 adult deaths. *The Lancet, 373*(9682), 2201–2214.

Zick, C. D., & Holden, K. (2000). An assessment of the wealth holdings of recent widows. *Journal of Gerontology: Social Sciences, 55B*(2), S90–S97.

Zimmer, Z., Martin, L. G., & Chang, M. (2002). Changes in functional limitation and survival among older Taiwanese, 1993, 1996, and 1999. *Population Studies, 56,* 265–276.

Chapter | 4 |

Trends in Longevity and Prospects for the Future

S. Jay Olshansky

School of Public Health, University of Illinois in Chicago, Chicago, Illinois

INTRODUCTION

The modern rise in life expectancy is one of humanity's crowning achievements. After more than 200 000 years of stagnant or slow increases in the average duration of life, a new chapter in the book of human longevity began in the nineteenth century when the rise in life expectancy accelerated (McNeill, 1976). The extrinsic forces of death (e.g. infectious diseases and accidents) that precluded survival beyond the first few years of life for most people throughout history were dramatically reduced as advances in public health and medical technology began to insulate people from the normal hazards of the outside world. Our past was dominated by fluctuations in mortality caused by episodes of highly lethal, infectious disease outbreaks that were punctuated by intermittent periods of less volatile but still high mortality. For those who survived childhood even as far back as the Roman Empire, a more regular age pattern of death emerged in later life. People who lived during this transitional phase attained ages that would be considered old even by today's standards.

The thirty-year rise in life expectancy at birth during the twentieth century was a seminal moment in human history, but it was accompanied by an unwelcome, although not unexpected, trade-off. People who ordinarily would have died early in life, from what are considered today to be preventable causes, began to live long enough to experience aging-related diseases such as cancer, cardiovascular diseases, osteoporosis, and sensory impairments. This medical and epidemiologic transition did not lessen the inevitability of death, but it made its temporal nature far more predictable. The evidence for this transition is easily seen in developed nations today where the chances of a long life are so high that about 80–90% of all deaths occur after age 65 and anywhere from 30–50% of deaths now occur past age 85 (Human Mortality Database, 2009).

Although it has been suggested recently that dramatic increases in longevity are on the near horizon (Christensen et al., 2009; de Grey, 2008; Kurzweil & Grossman, 2004), such extreme views require that almost all current pressures on human mortality be eliminated, and the biological process of aging itself would have to be stopped. There is no empirical evidence to support the view that aging is just another disease that can be eliminated (Carnes et al., 2008), but there is reason to believe that life expectancy will rise by the middle of this century beyond official government projections due, in part, to decelerated aging

DOI: 10.1016/B978-0-12-380880-6.00004-6

(Olshansky et al., 2009). Scientists are now optimistic that such breakthroughs are forthcoming (Butler et al., 2008; Miller, 2009; Sierra et al., 2008).

EPIDEMIOLOGIC TRANSITION

The transition in developed nations from infectious diseases expressed early in life to chronic degenerative diseases that kill later in life – the phenomenon that led to the rapid increase in life expectancy in the last two hundred years – is known as the epidemiologic transition (Omran, 1971). The third and final stage in Omran's theory is referred to as the age of chronic degenerative diseases, supposedly the stage that most developed nations reside in today. However, scientists have since speculated that new trends in old-age mortality late in the twentieth century justify the presence of a new stage in this epidemiologic model. Rogers and Hackenberg (1987) suggested that individual behaviors have had unique competing effects on life expectancy – some reducing the risk of death and others increasing it – thus warranting what these authors referred to as a new "hybristic stage."

Olshansky and Ault (1986) contend that modern nations have entered a fourth stage of the epidemiologic transition, which is characterized primarily by the same causes of death that exist in the third stage, but delayed to later ages by medical technology and behavior modification, referred to as "the age of delayed degenerative diseases" (Figure 4.1). It has also been suggested that perhaps the entire epidemiologic transition model is misguided because

it is based on observations of human fertility and mortality over a very short time window, about 150 years (Olshansky et al., 2000). These authors suggest that the modern decline in mortality could resemble any one of a large number of other troughs or low points in mortality that existed periodically in the past, and that humanity never in fact left the first stage. In other words, it has been suggested that, just like in the past, the low death rates enjoyed in most developed nations today could be followed by the rise and re-emergence of infectious diseases, a cycle that humanity has faced repeatedly for thousands of years. There is evidence emerging that suggests that infectious diseases could rise again in this century (Olshansky et al., 1997). Alternatively, the same authors suggested that the combination of antibiotic resistance and the emergence of new communicable diseases could soon lead to rising death rates for reasons that are fundamentally different from our past, perhaps leading humanity toward a new, fifth stage of the epidemiologic transition. This author's personal view is that humanity is headed toward a new fifth stage characterized by accelerating declines in death rates for some subgroups of the population and rising death rates for others.

FROM VOLATILITY TO STABILITY IN OUTER REGIONS OF THE LIFESPAN

Evidence of the transformation toward a more stable and predictable pattern of mortality at middle

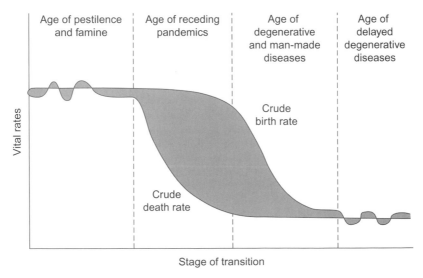

Figure 4.1   Stages of the epidemiologic transition.
Source: Olshansky & Ault, 1986.

and older ages can be observed in the vital records of those nations that have kept reliable vital statistics dating back to the middle of the eighteenth century. Consider the example of Sweden, where it is evident that the conditional probability of death [q(x)] at age 60 for both men and women has shifted from unpredictable patterns between 1751 and 1950 to a steady decline observed throughout the last half century (Figure 4.2). Although some of the instability in mortality rates observed in the Middle Ages was due to relatively small population size, overall, this more recent stable pattern of mortality at older ages for both men and women is real and has become commonplace throughout the developed nations of the world. More importantly, the amplitude of the annual absolute change in q(60) (Figure 4.3) has also experienced a consistent dampening across the centuries. Today, this trend in the movement of death rates for almost all older age-sex groups in low mortality populations has now become highly predictable, even over short time frames.

THE BIOLOGY OF LIFE AND DEATH

As countermeasures to early death from communicable diseases were discovered, the survivors who lived into increasingly older regions of the lifespan (past age 60) during the last 150 years were exposed with increasing frequency to the mortality risks associated with aging. Benjamin Gompertz (1825), a British actuary from the early nineteenth century, found such a remarkable regularity in the age pattern of death among people surviving beyond childhood that he referred to it is as a "law of mortality" – a discovery that he believed was on par with Newton's law of gravity. Today, death still harvests the living with "law-like" temporal regularity, and scientists are now uncovering the biological reasons for this mathematical regularity (Carnes et al., 1996). The significance of Gompertz's observation is the suggestion that regularity in human life tables arises from a highly predictable trajectory of biological decline that can be accurately referred to as an "intrinsic" pattern of death (Carnes & Olshansky, 1997). The concept of "intrinsic mortality" is not new; it has been part of the scientific literature for more than a century (Makeham, 1867; Pearl & Miner, 1935).

There was a time when scientists thought aging and the diseases that accompany the passage of time were direct products of natural selection. In fact, it is still a common misconception among many that evolution "designed" aging and death as mechanisms for enabling older generations to get out of the way in order to make room for the young. Under this perspective, the human genome was thought to contain genes whose primary role is to *cause* decrepitude, frailty, illness, and ultimately death – referred to as aging or death genes. Today, scientists recognize that the ultimate task of all genes is to transform a fertilized egg into a healthy adult capable of reproducing

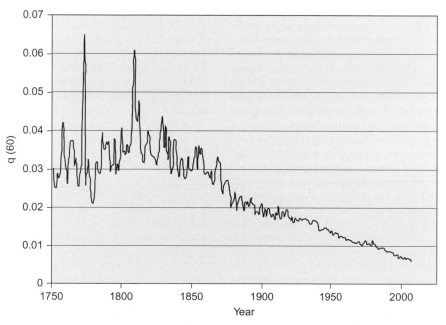

Figure 4.2 Conditional probability of death at age 60 for men and women combined (Sweden, 1751–2007).
Source: Human Mortality Database: http://www.mortality.org/

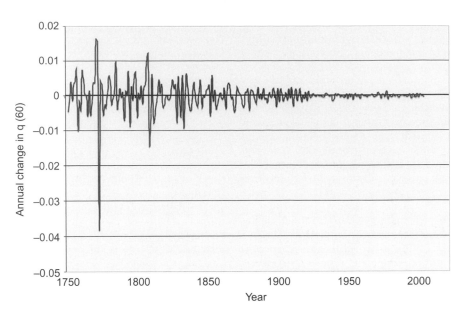

Figure 4.3 Absolute annual change in the conditional probability of death at age 60 for men and women combined (Sweden, 1751–2007).
Source: Human Mortality Database: http://www.mortality.org/

(Carnes & Olshansky, 1993). Neither aging nor death genes could arise under the direct force of natural selection in humans because their presence would have required for natural selection to operate in older regions of the lifespan among our earliest ancestors – a condition that could not have been possible because humans did not live to older ages with any degree of regularity until the nineteenth century. Aging is a product of evolutionary neglect, not evolutionary intent; it is what happens when genes themselves fall prey to the inevitable accumulation of detrimental changes over time. Thus, aging, disease, and death are most appropriately thought of as inadvertent or accidental byproducts of fixed genetic programs that operate deterministically, with clock-like precision, in other regions of the lifespan.

This view of aging has two important implications. First, aging and age-related diseases are a byproduct of predictable changes in the internal (intrinsic) workings of the body. Diseases of the cardiovascular and central nervous systems, cancers, and many other lethal and disabling conditions are "Achilles' heels" that emerge when the biology we inherited from our ancestors is pushed (by human ingenuity) beyond its normal operating time – the biological equivalent of a warranty period. These fundamental elements to the way in which our bodies operate exist in all of us; they are remnants of clock-like genetic programs that operate with remarkable precision early in life to regulate growth, development, and reproduction, but that later in life inadvertently lead to what all of us recognize as aging and disease (Hamilton, 1966;

Medawar, 1952; Williams, 1957). The passage of time that affects us all reveals the blueprint of a body that was not "designed" to fail, but that was also not intended for long-term use (Olshansky et al., 2001). This observation is important because it implies that most of what goes wrong with us as we grow older is not our fault.

It is fortunate that aging and death are not products of fixed genetic programs. If they were, the fate of our biological destiny would be outside of our control. Since aging and death are not hardwired into our biology, health and length of life are modifiable through such things as behavior modification, medical intervention, and biomedical technology. In fact, most of the gain in healthy lifespan in the latter part of the twentieth century has been manufactured by secular declines in smoking (Wang & Preston, 2009), healthier lifestyles, pharmaceuticals, and medical technology.

The downside of having some measure of control over our health is that we can also choose lifestyles that are harmful (e.g. smoking, obesity, excessive alcohol consumption, etc.), or, by misfortune of birth or socioeconomic status, we fall victim to harmful behavioral and environment conditions such as poverty, differential access to health care, lack of education, or pollution. Herein lies the dilemma currently faced by public health officials. There is now compelling evidence emerging to suggest that behavioral, environmental, and medical conditions for some subgroups of the population will lead them to higher levels of life expectancy than currently anticipated (Bongaarts & Feeney, 2002; Oeppen & Vaupel, 2002; Olshansky et al., 2009; Tuljapurkar et al., 2000; Wilmoth, 1998; Christensen et al., 2009). At the same time, equally compelling evidence suggests that other subgroups of the population are on the verge of the first significant decline in life expectancy in the modern era in developed nations (Olshansky et al., 2005; Olshansky & Persky, 2008; Wang et al., 2008). Uncertainty about the future of both short-term and long-term mortality has resurfaced because our biology is malleable enough to accommodate future *increases* and *decreases* in longevity.

FUTURISTS, OPTIMISTS, AND REALISTS

Scientific views of the future of human longevity have coalesced into three main schools of thought. One group claims that life expectancy will soon rise dramatically to hundreds or even thousands of years, physical immortality is on the horizon, and some people alive today will drink from the equivalent of a yet-to-be-discovered fountain of youth. The beneficiaries of these technological advances will be some people alive today and all future generations, and, according to the proponents of this view, people will either live indefinitely or at least for more than a billion years (de Grey, 2008; Kurzweil & Grossman, 2004). Here we will refer to the proponents of this view as *futurists*.

Futurist reasoning is based on the premise that information technology (IT) will increase at an exponential rate, eventually leading to dramatic new technological advances (such as nanobots) that will wipe out all diseases and aging itself (Kurzweil & Grossman, 2004, 2009); or, they rely on the premise that "regenerative medicine" will engineer new or refurbished body parts that will lead to increases in life expectancy that occur at a faster pace than the passage of time itself (de Grey et al., 2002). Under both of these futurist scenarios, physical immortality and eternal youth will be achieved for all of humanity in this century; people over age 85 will become indistinguishable (physically and mentally) from people at young and middle ages; old age as we know it today will literally cease to exist; and the world will become populated only by those who are physically healthy and mentally vibrant.

The futurist line of reasoning is extraordinarily appealing to the popular news media because it feeds on a deeply rooted fear of death and the long-held desire by every generation to believe that "our science" will lead us down the path toward immortality, or at least much longer and healthier lives. This is not an uncommon theme – Gruman (1961) documented this futurist view going back several thousand years,

noting that this vision of immortality and the belief that we could intervene in aging itself was previously known as prolongevity.

As appealing as the futurist argument may be, there are some underlying problems in defending it. For example, at the foundation of Kurzweil's view of bridges to immortality is the view that it will be IT that will drive future increases in longevity (Kurzweil & Grossman, 2009). Although there is no doubt that IT has been advancing exponentially in recent decades, there is no evidence provided by Kurzweil that links IT to how long people live. In fact, to the contrary, during the time when IT was rising exponentially in the latter part of the twentieth century, human longevity was increasing arithmetically in some parts of the world and actually declining in others (Olshansky, 2004; United Nations, 2003). The concept of regenerative medicine is also appealing, but so far there has been no science provided to support de Grey's (2008) assertions that such technological developments are forthcoming, nor is there any scientific evidence provided to defend assertions that the first billion-year-old person is already alive, or that there is a 50% chance of regenerative medicine yielding immortality by 2040 (de Grey, 2008). The futurist line of reasoning is totally dependent on something that does not currently exist – life-extending technologies that yield eternal life.

Optimists contend that observed declines in death rates observed during the last two centuries will continue throughout this century, leading to life expectancies as high as 100 years in some countries (Oeppen & Vaupel, 2002), with half of the babies born today expected to become centenarians (Christensen et al., 2009). The empirical method of choice among optimists is extrapolation, which is to say that they develop and use statistical methods of extending past trends in mortality and/or life expectancy into the future. Advocates of this approach have declared that there are no biological or demographic reasons why death rates cannot decline to zero (Wilmoth, 2001), and biological factors that influence how long individuals and populations can live (Carnes et al., 2003) are rejected (Wilmoth, 1998). Data offered to support the optimist position include unabated historical increases in the world record (also known as "best practice") life expectancy at birth (defined by one country annually; see Oeppen & Vaupel, 2002), largely unabated increases in the maximum age at death in Sweden (defined by one man and one woman annually in only one country; see Wilmoth et al., 2000), as well as steady declines in old-age mortality observed in G7 nations (nations whose finance ministers come together frequently to discuss global financial issues: they include Canada, France, Germany, Italy, Japan, the UK, and the US, see Tuljapurkar et al., 2000). Optimists do not base their arguments on any specific technological advances expected on the horizon; instead they rely entirely on the mathematical extrapolation of the past into the future without regard to the biological factors that influence duration of life or observed trends in behavioral risk factors (e.g. obesity) that have a negative effect on life expectancy (Olshansky & Carnes, 2010).

Realists contend that there are competing forces that will lead to simultaneous increases in life expectancy for some subgroups of a population and declines for others. On the one hand, scientists appear to be on the verge of a major breakthrough that will soon make it possible to slow the biological process of aging (Butler et al., 2008; Kenyon, 2005; Miller, 2002; Sierra et al., 2008). This intervention, along with other anticipated advances in the biomedical sciences, will lead to increasingly more effective treatments for diseases and their complications and continued downward pressure on death rates in the coming decades (Olshansky et al., 2009). On the other hand, there is equally compelling evidence documenting the presence of biological and environmental barriers to radical life extension (Carnes et al., 2003) and the deteriorating health of younger cohorts across the globe due to rising levels of obesity, diabetes, indications that coronary artery disease may be on the verge of rising (Nemetz et al., 2008), the emergence of antibiotic resistant microbes (Olshansky et al., 1997), and the adverse health impact of environmental pollution.

Regardless of which camp is eventually proven right, all of the scientists involved in this debate are in agreement that, in the short-term, progress against most major fatal diseases will continue at a pace that can be measured and modeled with a high degree of reliability. It is also worth emphasizing that optimists and realists are in agreement that the health and longevity benefits of biomedical progress will not be shared equally, at least not in the short-term. Poverty and other social inequities will continue to deny access to longer and healthier lives for the disadvantaged segments of the population (see also Chapter 9), but there is reason to be optimistic that many of these health disparities can be overcome (Olshansky et al., 2009).

LONGEVITY/MORTALITY "SHOCKS"

For public policymakers, pension fund managers, and insurance companies, of great interest now is the question of whether secular changes in death rates will be slow and predictable, as they have been during most of the last half century, or whether there is any prospect of returns to highly fluctuating death rates – referred to here as "shocks." The answer to this question is important as small slow changes are predictable, while large changes in either direction

can wreak havoc with age entitlement programs and pension funds.

According to Figures 4.1 and 4.2, historical shocks to mortality were common prior to the middle of the twentieth century due exclusively to the periodic but persistent presence of communicable diseases. Periods of high mortality were followed by notably lower death rates not only because the infectious agents completed their spread throughout the population, but also because the survivors represented a heartier subgroup. What are the potential shocks to longevity and mortality that could occur within the next few decades?

According to the historical record, the only dramatic shocks to mortality that yielded large changes in death rates over short time periods are negative – that is, they lead to rapidly increasing death rates. Notable examples in the twentieth century include the 1918 influenza pandemic that killed millions within an 18-month time span and the rise and spread of HIV/AIDS beginning in 1984. In both examples, neither of which could have been anticipated in advance, humanity experienced a global event that led to a short-term spike in the number of deaths and either a drop in life expectancy or a significant dampening of the rate of increase.

Given that influenza pandemics occur with an alarming regularity of about three times per century and that the H1N1 virus is spreading across the globe at an alarming pace, the obvious negative shock that is most evident today would be a strain of influenza that is far more deadly than seasonal flu. This is predictable in the sense that scientists can see it only after it has emerged, but before it wreaks havoc with death rates – giving scientists and public health workers only months, at best, to prepare.

What is particularly relevant with flu pandemics is the timing with which they occur, their lethality, and the age segments of the population most affected. The difficulty with influenza is that the virus can mutate rapidly, leaving large segments of the population largely unprotected from the new strain. The good news is that global alert systems are particularly effective in identifying the location and following the spread of the disease, and scientists now have the ability to isolate the genetic material from new viruses and create vaccines in relatively short time periods. In fact, that is exactly what happened with the H1N1 pandemic flu that emerged in Mexico early in 2009. By the end of the same year in which the pandemic first appeared, a vaccine that protected against this new strain had already become widely available. Thus, although negative shocks caused by communicable diseases cannot be eliminated, they can be dampened through human ingenuity.

Another negative shock that remains visible today is the rise and emergence of adult and childhood-onset obesity. Beginning around 1980, humanity witnessed what is nothing short of a dramatic change in the average weight of our population. The initial wave of obesity was expressed primarily among adults, and, within just the last three decades (from levels present in 1970), the prevalence of overweight and obesity has risen by two-thirds in most populations in the developed world (Fontaine et al., 2009). The link between obesity and mortality risk has been documented, so there is little doubt that we are already witnessing a dampening effect on the rise in life expectancy (Stewart et al., 2009), with possible declines on the horizon for some subgroups (Olshansky et al., 2005; Reither et al., 2009). The largest negative shock that is already visible is the dramatic increase in childhood obesity. Because these children will carry the health risks of extra weight with them for decades longer than the adults who are now obese, it is possible that we may witness declines in health status and notable increases in death rates among future cohorts of people reaching their third, fourth, and fifth decades of life.

The positive "shocks" to longevity and mortality that occurred in the twentieth century were dramatic in their impact, but they took place over much longer time periods. The most dramatic of all was the introduction of antibiotics in the middle of the century. However, scientific evidence suggests that advances in basic public health measures (e.g. sanitation, waste disposal, refrigeration, clean water, controlled indoor living and working environments) contributed to significant drops in mortality from the diseases that were brought under greater control with antibiotics, even before these medications were introduced and broadly disseminated (McKeown & Record, 1962). The combination of advances in diagnostic tools and surgical procedures, the development of new and more effective treatments for CVDs and cancer, and secular declines in smoking, led to significant reductions in death rates from these killer diseases, contributing to notable increases in life expectancy during the last quarter century. However, these improvements in longevity and mortality were gradual – not exactly shocks, but rather a persistent force that could be measured and predicted with some degree of reliability.

THE FUTURE OF HUMAN LONGEVITY

Do any future positive shocks lie ahead? Perhaps. The futurists provide an interesting set of sound bites claiming that immortality is on the horizon, and, if true, these would indeed represent a positive shock with no parallel in history. The absence of empirical evidence to support the futurist perspective leads this realist to be skeptical. The optimists have argued repeatedly that half of the babies born today in developed nations will live to 100 (Christensen et al., 2009; Oeppen & Vaupel, 2002), but these authors provide no specific projection scenarios for this assertion beyond a generic declaration that past trends would need to continue into the future. If past trends serve as the only basis upon which forecasts of life expectancy are made, then recent observed trends in obesity across the globe should lead the futurists to conclude that declines in life expectancy are forthcoming. The fact that negative trends in health and life expectancy are ignored by the optimists, who rely on extrapolation, indicates the presence of a bias (Olshansky & Carnes, 2010).

Because estimates of the future of life expectancy are important for addressing issues of public policy, governments are often responsible for making forecasts of longevity and population size as a method of determining tax rates and future outlays for age entitlement programs (such as Social Security and Medicare). In the US, the Social Security Administration (SSA) independently makes forecasts of the size and age structure of the population each year (Social Security Administration, 2008), and the US Census Bureau (CB) does so periodically (US Census Bureau, 2008). In its most recent forecasts of life expectancy, the SSA used national vital statistics data on age, sex, and underlying cause as the basis for choosing what they referred to as ultimate annual rates of improvement in age-sex-cause-specific death rates. From now until 2032, the SSA assumed that total mortality will decline annually by 0.86% at all ages (from 0 through 100+). From 2032 to 2082, the SSA assumed that, for those under age 65, total mortality will fall each year by 0.73% and that, at ages 65 and older, it will fall each year by 0.65%. The SSA therefore assumes that rates of mortality improvement will decelerate throughout this century because they are assuming constant percentage reductions in death rates (yielding smaller annual absolute declines), and because they explicitly assume a shift toward smaller percentage reductions in death rates after 2032. The CB's recent forecasts are somewhat more optimistic than those of the SSA, and they go further by declaring that, by 2075, the risk of death for all population subgroups would converge into the "non-Hispanic all other races" group that currently has the highest life expectancy in the US.

In November 2008 the MacArthur Foundation in Chicago funded a new Research Network on an Aging Society, consisting of twelve scientists who were charged over the next few years with identifying the magnitude of the effect of aging on individual- and population-level trends in function and longevity for our society and among subgroups. In addition, their goal is to facilitate public policy that enhances the opportunities and mitigates the challenges posed by the consequences of individual and population aging. As a baseline for the work, the Network decided to formulate a new set of population and mortality fore-casts for the US to the year 2050 to assess the effects of anticipated developments in the biomedical sciences. The rationale was that the SSA and CB both assume improvements in mortality will continue to occur over the next few decades, but underlying their projections is the presumption that the pace of improvement will decelerate. The Network contends that these projections may be too conservative.

The Network generated a new set of life expectancy forecasts for the US to 2030 and 2050 under two basic assumptions: (1) future declines in death rates will accelerate due to anticipated breakthroughs against major fatal diseases – referred to as the delayed disease model – and (2) the scientific means to delay biological aging will soon become a mainstream approach to extending healthy life – referred to as the delayed aging model. In both models it was assumed that the rate of improvement in mortality would accelerate in the coming decades and that progress would be made against current negative health trends (such as the rise of obesity). These forecasts represent the first-ever published demonstration of how a nation would be affected by successful efforts to slow aging – which the Network anticipates will be developed and disseminated in full force by mid-century. It was also acknowledged that the gains in life expectancy anticipated by the Network could be attenuated by persistent health disparities that are currently challenging the health and longevity of some subgroups of the population. Details of the methodology, assumptions, and conclusions based on a variety of projection scenarios are available at the Network website (http://agingsocietynetwork.org/demographic-forecasts). A summary of the initial results was published by Olshansky et al. (2009).

Results from the Network forecasts suggest that the SSA and CB may be underestimating the rise in life expectancy for US men and women combined by 3.1 to 7.9 years by the year 2050. Differences of this magnitude may seem small, but the Network demonstrated that each one-year underestimation in life expectancy at birth in 2050 would yield about 53 million more person-years-of-life (PYL) lived by people aged 65 and older between now and mid-century. When errors of this magnitude are added up between now and 2050, this means there could be as many as 419 million more PYL lived cumulatively over the next four decades. The effects of such an underestimation on the future cost of age entitlement programs are staggering – perhaps as high as US$8.3 trillion (Olshansky et al., 2009).

Although Network forecasts of life expectancy for the US do not even come close to the prediction of others that suggesting humanity is on the verge of achieving immortality (de Grey, 2008), or even 50 percent survival to age 100 for current birth cohorts (Christensen et al., 2009), the differences in future life expectancy between the Network and official government sources are sufficiently large to get the attention of public policymakers. The immediate shock on death rates from either of the Network's mortality projection scenarios will not be dramatic. Rather, they are expected to occur gradually in the coming decades as anticipated interventions slowly make their way into the standard of practice in medicine and public health. However, if the delayed aging model is shown to be efficacious by significantly reducing the risk of a broad range of fatal and non-fatal but disabling conditions, and also proven to be safe, then health care costs may be reduced as morbidity and disability become compressed near the end of life, leading to significant reductions in health care costs. In any case, the Network anticipates that people alive today may bear witness to the first major positive shock to mortality that is equivalent to the effects on longevity of public health interventions, vaccines, and medical technology developed throughout the twentieth century.

CONCLUSIONS

The future of human longevity has always been a topic of great interest to scientists and the lay population, and now public policymakers recognize the importance of efforts to gain some understanding of the future. Some have argued that our demography is our destiny (Peterson, 1999) and that we have little control over our future. If there is one thing we have learned in the last two centuries, it is that what separates us from all other species, who certainly face a demographic destiny that is outside of their control, is that humanity has already exercised so much control over the environment within which we live that it can now be said with confidence that we have gained some measure of control over important elements of our biological and evolutionary destiny. Humanity has the capacity to shape its future, not just let it unfold, so the question of how long we might live and how healthy we could be in the coming decades or centuries is still open to a broad range of interpretation and possibilities.

Research on aging is at a critical juncture. The focus of most of our attention on the biological and medical side has been to attack one disease at a time, as if they are independent of one another. Yet, evidence from animal models suggests that aging has common attributes across many forms of life, and that the diseases expressed at older ages are not solely byproducts of harmful lifestyles. Rather, diseases expressed in people that live to older regions of the lifespan are also influenced by biological processes of aging. This implies that the current medical model of attacking diseases independently of each other will eventually yield diminishing returns in terms of health and quality of life, and that a new model of health promotion for this century should include an accelerated research effort to slow aging. If we succeed in such an effort, even at a minor level of slowing aging by just a few years, the resulting extension of healthy life would reduce health care costs, enable people to remain in the labor force longer, compress morbidity and disability into a shorter duration of time before death, and economically benefit those who live longer and the countries in which they reside.

Regardless of which path human longevity takes in this century, global population aging resulting from life extension of any magnitude, combined with the inevitable upward shift in the age structure, will require a re-engineering of many of the social, economic, and physical infrastructures of our society. Key institutions such as education will need to be refashioned in order to help create new working opportunities for people reaching older ages. Current notions of retirement will have to be rethought to accommodate the shifting age structure. Population aging is going to occur so rapidly in some parts of the world that it will be difficult for social institutions to keep pace. The time has arrived for a new research agenda on human aging that addresses all facets of the changes in our society that are forthcoming.

REFERENCES

Bongaarts, J., & Feeney, G. (2002). How long do we live? *Population and Development Review, 24,* 271–291.

Butler, R. N., Miller, R. A., Perry, D., Carnes, B. A., Williams, T. F., Cassel, C., et al. (2008). New model of health promotion and disease prevention for the 21st century. *British Medical Journal, 337,* 149–150.

Carnes, B. A., & Olshansky, S. J. (1993). Evolutionary perspectives on human senescence. *Population and Development Review, 19,* 793–806.

Carnes, B. A., & Olshansky, S. J. (1997). A biologically motivated partitioning of mortality. *Experimental Gerontology, 32,* 615–631.

Carnes, B. A., Olshansky, S. J., & Grahn, D. (1996). Continuing the search for a law of mortality. *Population and Development Review, 22,* 231–264.

Carnes, B. A., Olshansky, S. J., & Grahn, D. (2003). Biological evidence for limits to the duration of life. *Biogerontology, 4,* 31–45.

Carnes, B. A., Staats, D. O., & Sonntag, W. E. (2008). Does senescence give rise to disease? *Mechanisms of Ageing and Development, 129,* 693–699.

Christensen, K., Doblhammer, G., Rau, R., & Vaupel, J. W. (2009). Ageing populations: The challenges ahead. *Lancet, 374,* 1196–1208.

de Grey, A. (2008). The singularity and the Methuselarity: Similarities and differences. In R. N. Bushko (Ed.), *Strategy for the Future of Health* (pp. 157–165). Amsterdam: IOS Press.

de Grey, A. D., Ames B. N., Andersen J. K., Bartke A., Campisi J., Heward C. B., et al. (2002). Time to talk SENS: Critiquing the immutability of human aging. *Annals of the New York Academy of Sciences. 959,* 452–462; discussion 463–455.

Fontaine, K. R., Greenberg, J. A., Olshansky, S. J., & Allison, D. B. (2009). Obesity's final toll: Influence on mortality rate, attributable deaths, years of life lost and population life expectancy. In V. R. Preedy & R. R. Watson (Eds.), *Handbook of Disease Burdens and Quality of Life Measures* (pp. 1085–1105). New York: Springer.

Gompertz, B. (1825). On the nature of the function expressive of the law of human mortality and on a new mode of determining life contingencies. *Philosophical Transactions of the Royal Society of London, 115,* 513–585.

Gruman, G. J. (1961). The rise and fall of prolongevity hygiene, 1558–1873. *Bulletin of the History of Medicine, 35,* 221–229.

Hamilton, W. D. (1966). The moulding of senescence by natural selection. *Journal of Theoretical Biology, 12,* 12–45.

Human Mortality Database. (2009). http://www.mortality.org/

Kenyon, C. (2005). The plasticity of aging: Insights from long-lived mutants. *Cell, 120,* 449–460.

Kurzweil, R., & Grossman, T. (2004). *Fantastic voyage: Live long enough to live forever.* Emmaus, PA: Rodale Press.

Kurzweil, R., & Grossman, T. (2009). *Transcend: Nine steps to living well forever.* Emmaus, PA: Rodale Press.

Makeham, W. M. (1867). On the law of mortality. *Journal of the Institute of Actuaries, 13,* 325–358.

McKeown, T., & Record, R. G. (1962). Reasons for the decline of mortality in England and Wales during the nineteenth century. *Population Studies, 16,* 94–122.

Medawar, H. (1952). *An Unsolved Problem of Biology.* London: Lewis.

McNeill, W. H. (1976). *Plagues and peoples.* Garden City: Anchor.

Miller, R. A. (2002). Extending life: Scientific prospects and political obstacles. *The Milbank Quarterly, 80*(1), 155–174.

Miller, R. A. (2009). "Dividends" from research on aging – can biogerontologists, at long last, find something useful to do? *Journal of Gerontology: Biological Sciences, 64,* 157–160.

Nemetz, P. N., Roger, V. L., Ransom, J. E., Bailey, K. R., Edwards, W. D., & Liebson, C. L. (2008). Recent trends in the prevalence of coronary disease: A population-based autopsy study of nonnatural deaths. *Archives of Internal Medicine, 168,* 264–270.

Oeppen, J., & Vaupel, J. W. (2002). Demography: Broken limits to life expectancy. *Science, 296,* 1029–1031.

Olshansky, S. J. (2004). The future of human life expectancy. In *World Population to 2300,* pp. 159–164. New York: United Nations.

Olshansky, S. J., & Ault, A. B. (1986). The fourth stage of the epidemiologic transition: The age of delayed degenerative diseases. *The Milbank Quarterly, 64,* 355–391.

Olshansky, S. J., & Carnes, B. A. (2010). Ageing and health. *Lancet, 375,* 25.

Olshansky, S. J., & Persky, V. (2008). The canary in the coal mine of coronary artery disease. *Archives of Internal Medicine, 168,* 261.

Olshansky, S. J., Carnes, B., Rogers, R. G., & Smith, L. (1997). Infectious diseases – New and ancient threats to world health. *Population Bulletin, 52,* 1–52.

Olshansky, S. J., Rogers, R. G., Carnes, B. A., & Smith, L. (2000). Emerging infectious diseases: The fifth stage of the epidemiologic transition? *World Health Statistics Quarterly, 51,* 207–217.

Olshansky, S. J., Carnes, B. A., & Butler, R. N. (2001). If humans were built to last. *Scientific American, 284,* 50–55.

Olshansky, S. J., Passaro, D. J., Hershow, R. C., Layden, J., Carnes, B. A., Brody, J., et al. (2005). A potential decline in life expectancy in the United States in the 21st century. *The New England Journal of Medicine, 352,* 1138–1145.

Olshansky, S. J., Goldman, D. P., Zheng, Y., & Rowe, J. W. (2009).

Aging in America in the twenty-first century: Demographic forecasts from the MacArthur research network on an aging society. *The Milbank Quarterly, 87,* 842–862.

Omran, A. R. (1971). The epidemiologic transition. A theory of the epidemiology of population change. *The Milbank Memorial Fund Quarterly, 49,* 509–538.

Pearl, R., & Miner, J. R. (1935). Experimental studies on the duration of life. XIV. The comparative mortality of certain lower organisms. *Quarterly Review of Biology, 10,* 60–79.

Peterson, P. (1999). *Gray dawn: How the coming age wave will transform America – and the world.* New York: Times Books.

Reither, E. N., Hauser, R. M., & Yang, Y. (2009). Do birth cohorts matter? Age-period-cohort analyses of the obesity epidemic in the United States. *Social Science & Medicine, 69,* 1439–1448.

Rogers, R. G., & Hackenberg, R. (1987). Extending epidemiologic transition theory: A new stage. *Social Biology, 34,* 234–243.

Sierra, F., Hadley, E., Suzman, R., & Hodes, R. (2008). Prospects for life span extension. *Annual Review of Medicine, 60,* 457–469.

Social Security Administration. (2008). Assumptions and methods underlying actuarial estimates. Retrieved September 22, 2009 from http://www.ssa.gov/OACT/TR/TR08/V_demographic.html#155199.

Stewart, S. T., Cutler, D. M., & Rosen, A. B. (2009). Forecasting the effects of obesity and smoking on U.S. life expectancy. *New England Journal of Medicine, 361,* 2252–2260.

Tuljapurkar, S., Li, N., & Boe, C. (2000). A universal pattern of mortality decline in the G7 countries. *Nature, 405,* 789–792.

United Nations. (2003). World population in 2300. Proceedings of the United Nations expert meeting on world population prospects (Working Paper No. ESA/WP 187). New York: United Nations.

US Census Bureau. (2008). 2008 National Population Projections. Retrieved September 22, 2009 from http://www.census.gov/population/www/projections.

Wang, H., & Preston, S. H. (2009). Forecasting United States mortality using cohort smoking histories. *Proceedings of the National Academy of Sciences of the United States of America, 106,* 393–398.

Wang, Y., Beydoun, M. A., Liang, L., Caballero, B., & Kumanyika, S. K. (2008). Will all Americans become overweight or obese? Estimating the progression and cost of the US obesity epidemic. *Obesity, 16,* 2323–2330.

Williams, G. C. (1957). Pleiotropy, natural selection, and the evolution of senescence. *Evolution, 11,* 298–311.

Wilmoth, J. R. (1998). The future of human longevity: A demographer's perspective. *Science, 280,* 395–397.

Wilmoth, J. R. (2001). How long can we live? A review essay. *Population and Development Review, 27,* 791–800.

Wilmoth, J. R., Deegan, L. J., Lundstrom, H., & Horiuchi, S. (2000). Increase of maximum life-span in Sweden, 1861–1999. *Science, 289,* 2366–2368.

Chapter | 5 |

Disability, Functioning, and Aging

Vicki A. Freedman

Institute for Social Research, University of Michigan, Ann Arbor, Michigan

CHAPTER CONTENTS

INTRODUCTION

The risks of disability – defined broadly as impairments in body functioning, limitations in activities, and restrictions in participation – increase dramatically with age. In the US, about 14 million adults aged 65 and older (40%) report a disability, and about 3 million (roughly 9%) report more severe limitations in self-care activities (Institute of Medicine [IOM], 2007). Estimates of severe late-life disability in other developed countries are of similar magnitude or higher, generally ranging from approximately 8%–20% (Lafortune et al., 2007). In more and less developed countries alike, the number of older adults living with disability is expected to increase (IOM, 2007; Jacobzone et al., 2000–2001; Kinsella & He, 2009). The consequences associated with loss of functioning can be far-reaching for individuals, families, and communities in terms of both economic costs and quality of life. As such, although not inevitable outcomes of aging, disability and functioning are central topics in the study of later life.

Over the past few decades, research has advanced our understanding of the critical components of disability in later life, its varied progression at later ages, and population-level changes in disability that occur as a consequence of population aging. This chapter covers both conceptual and empirical issues that intersect with the topics of disability and aging. The next section reviews emerging definitions of disability and corresponding advances in measurement. We then have an overview of the demography of disability, including a brief review of research on disability trajectories. A fourth section focuses on recent population-level trends. Concluding remarks, including future research directions, are provided in a final section.

DOI: 10.1016/B978-0-12-380880-6.00005-8

DEFINING AND MEASURING DISABILITY

Disability has been defined and operationalized in countless ways. In this chapter, the term "disability" is used broadly to include impairments in body functions and structures; reduction in person-level physical, cognitive, and sensory capacity; loss of ability to carry out daily self-care or household tasks independently and corresponding changes in how such tasks are performed; and limitations in the ability to participate in productive, social, and community life. However, as explained below, other interpretations persist in the gerontological literature and likely will remain in use for the near future, until new measures are implemented that reflect the latest conceptualizations. Indeed, in recent years there has been interest in developing new measures of late-life disability that go beyond activity limitations (Wunderlich, 2009) and recent advances in conceptualizing disability have provided an important backdrop for expanded efforts in this area.

The International Classification of Functioning, Disability, and Health (ICF)

The disability model now making its way into the gerontological literature is the International Classification of Functioning, Disability, and Health (ICF). This framework was put forth by the World Health Organization (WHO, 2002) nearly a decade ago and has been widely embraced by researchers in countries around the world and by disability researchers in the US, but has only recently and sporadically come into use in the US gerontological community (Jette, 2009). Developed through a global consensus process, the ICF provides a systematic coding scheme for classifying the consequences of health conditions and linking them to participation in society.

As shown in Figure 5.1, in the ICF, health conditions are distinguished from impairments in body functions or structures, which in turn are distinguished from person-level limitations in activities or restrictions in participation. Participation is defined as "involvement in life situations" and includes productive activities such as work or volunteering as well as more socially oriented activities such as being involved in community, social, and civic life. Personal and environmental factors influence the entire continuum.

The Institute of Medicine's Committee on the Future of Disability in America (IOM, 2007) has endorsed the use of the ICF in both research and policy for several reasons. The model offers the

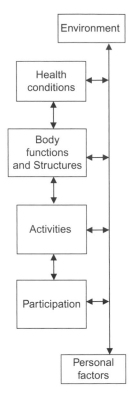

Figure 5.1 The language of the ICF framework.
Source: Adapted from WHO, 2002.

advantages of a commonly accepted, internationally agreed-upon language. In addition, it offers both "positive" and "negative" descriptors; for example, the positive analog to disability is functioning. The approach also recognizes that there are activities beyond self-care and maintenance that are of value to people with disabilities, a fact long-recognized in the gerontological literature but not explicit in current models. Unlike earlier models, the ICF explicitly recognizes the salient role of environmental factors, such as assistive technologies; home modifications; social supports and relationships; and services, systems, and policies, which may influence and shape whether an impairment in body function results in a participation restriction. Finally, the dual-headed arrows offer recognition that secondary health conditions may also emerge consequent to disability.

Despite these advantages, several barriers have slowed the use of the ICF by researchers interested in disability and aging (Freedman, 2009). First, the widely used measures of functional limitations, activities of daily living (ADLs), and instrumental activities of daily living (IADLs), which are included in most existing surveys and studies of older adults, do not map precisely into the ICF categories. Second, critical distinctions between the building blocks of activities – mobility, upper and lower body movements, sensory functions, and cognitive capabilities – and activities themselves are not readily apparent, although they can be easily incorporated by distinguishing *capacity for* from *performance of* activities. Third, the ICF is not a dynamic framework per se, so it remains an important task to elaborate process models based on the ICF language (IOM, 2007). Finally, as at the time of publication, measures of participation and the environment are not widely available, although work is underway to remedy this last limitation (Freedman, 2009; Noonan et al., 2009; Whiteneck & Dijkers, 2009). Consequently, the gerontological literature now offers a mixture of nomenclatures reflecting multiple conceptualizations.

Alternative Conceptualizations

Alternative perspectives on disability lead to fundamentally different ways of thinking about, measuring, and classifying the population. The medical conceptualization of disability, for instance, which is embedded in many US support programs for people with disabilities, emphasizes the underlying physiologic or mental cause of an individual's disability. In workers' compensation and disability insurance programs, for example, applicants are classified according to the condition causing their disability. However, this approach is limited for studying disability and aging because it does not explicitly recognize the social context of disability, and thus does not lead one to consider or foster environmental adaptations that might alleviate restrictions. In contrast, the disablement model developed by Nagi (1965) and advanced by Verbrugge and Jette (1994) and others distinguishes an individual's capacity for activities from socially defined limitations. Disablement is depicted as consisting of four stages (see Figure 5.2): compromised organ function because of chronic or acute conditions or injury ("pathology"); loss of system function ("impairment"); person-level limitations in physical or mental actions ("functional limitations"); and inability to carry out socially defined roles ("disability"). The Nagi model has been widely used in gerontological and geriatric research. As Guralnik and Ferrucci (2009) point out, there are well-developed measures for each stage of the process and there is an accumulated body of evidence of the predictive value of each stage for the next. Like the ICF, the Nagi model provides a framework for studying the role of environmental factors and compensatory strategies (Verbrugge & Jette, 1994).

Having alternative conceptualizations is not necessarily a detriment, and ultimately a blend of language and models could perhaps prove to be useful in moving research on disability and aging forward. In the meantime, to avoid confusion around core terms such as "disability," clarity around measures is especially important in bridging the language divide.

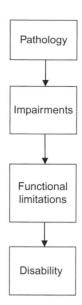

Figure 5.2   The Nagi Disablement Framework.
Source: Adapted from Institute of Medicine, 1991.

Measuring Capacity for Activities

Person-level capacity to carry out activities has been measured in surveys and clinical studies alike with both self-reported items and performance-based measures. Nagi (1965) first developed measures of functional limitation to explore rehabilitation potential for social security disability applicants. The items were administered by a team of medical evaluators. This evaluation along with a self-assessment by the applicant was used to score an applicant's maximum capacity and the physical requirements for the applicant's job (both using a numeric scale from 0 for "No Ability" to 7 for "No Restriction"). Wide variation is evident across national surveys in the implementation of functional limitation items, although studies generally include both upper (reaching up, reaching out, grasping) and lower (bending, lifting and carrying, climbing stairs) body movements. Most often respondents are asked about difficulty without help from another person or use of special equipment.

Performance measures involve individuals conducting movements or tasks according to a standardized protocol whilst trained observers make ratings using objective, predetermined criteria (Guralnik et al., 1989). Batteries have been developed to administer performance tests in the home setting that reflect the basic components of functioning (strength, balance, coordination, flexibility, endurance) as well as physical movements (e.g. walking). One of the most common performance-based measures is the Short Physical Performance Battery (SPPB) (Guralnik et al., 1995), which includes tests of gait speed, standing balance, and time to rise from a chair multiple times. Mobility disability has also been measured by longer timed walks, such as the 400-meter walk in the Health, Aging and Body Composition Study (Newman et al., 2006).

Cognition assessments also may be considered part of the family of performance tests, as participants are typically administered tasks (to tap, for example, memory, orientation, or executive functioning) using a standardized protocol, which is then scored using predetermined criteria. Some common cognition assessments incorporated into population-based studies include Folstein's Mini-Mental Status Exam (Folstein et al., 1975), the Telephone Interview for Cognitive Status (Brandt et al., 1988), and the Clinical Dementia Rating scale (Morris, 1993).

Measuring Activity Limitations

Activity limitations are most often measured in later life using two scales developed in the 1960s. The ADL scale was initially developed for an institutional setting to assess patients' ability to independently bathe, dress, to the toilet, transfer, control urination and bowel movements, and self-feed (Katz et al., 1963). Clinicians were asked to rate patients' independence on a three-category scale and detailed descriptions were provided for each category. Lawton and Brody's (1969) IADL scale was developed to facilitate communication about clients' everyday functional competence among different personnel and agencies involved in treatment plans. The authors proposed representative activities for consideration: women were to be evaluated by their ability to shop, cook, and do laundry whereas men were to be evaluated by their performance in transportation and handling money.

Although designed for clinical purposes, ADLs and IADLs have made their way onto most surveys of aging and health, with wide variation in both the number of activities considered and how items are worded. Most surveys ask about difficulty with ADLs and IADLs, and some but not all items explicitly refer to difficulty *without help or equipment* (in some cases a hypothetical situation). Also common are questions about *help* with ADLs and IADLs (often interpreted as "dependence" in daily activities), but items vary as to whether they elicit needing help or using help, as well as follow-up items that attempt to assess the reason for the difficulty/need for help (e.g. because of a health or memory problem, a health or physical problem, or a physical or mental health condition?). Historically, little information has been obtained on how the activity is carried out (e.g. is bathing taking a bath in a tub, showering, or washing up some other way? Is money management accomplished by going to the bank or checking balances online? Are adaptive or assistive technologies being used to facilitate performance?).

Measuring Participation

Although ADLs and IADLs have been used widely in research and policymaking, such items do not represent the full, rich array of meaningful experiences of older adults. Measures of participation in more societally oriented and other valued activities recently have been introduced into surveys and studies (Noonan et al., 2009). Whiteneck and Dijkers (2009) make the critical distinction between objective measures of participation, typified by frequencies of various types of engagement, and subjective measures that elicit the value of items to individuals and/or how satisfied they are with their level of participation. A third approach is illustrated by the National Health Interview Survey (NHIS), which asks about the amount of difficulty with leisure activities such as going out to things like shopping, movies, or sporting events; participating in social activities; and doing things to relax at home or for leisure.

More generally, information on how older adults spent their time (i.e. "time use") can help provide insight into participation in a range of activities in later life. Time use information is typically collected either with "stylized" questions about time spent doing a particular type of activity during a reference period (e.g. last week or last month) or using "diaries" that elicit all activities in a 24-hour period (typically yesterday). For the purposes of studying aging and disability, the former measures are available in the HRS whereas the latter are collected as part of the ongoing American Time Use Survey (ATUS) and are also available for older couples in the 2009 Panel Study of Income Dynamics.

Measuring the Environment and Accommodations

Over the last decade, awareness has grown that disability cannot be assessed outside of the physical, social, and technological environment in which individuals carry out activities. A number of instruments have been developed explicitly to measure the environments in which daily tasks are performed. Keysor (2006) summarizes three general approaches: respondent reports of their perceptions of how the environment influences participation; observation of study subjects as they avoid/encounter various features in the physical environment; and respondent assessment of the presence or absence of various features in the environment (rather than perceptions about their roles as barriers). The first approach is illustrated by the Craig Hospital Inventory of Environmental Factors (CHIEF) (Whiteneck et al., 2004), a 24-item self-report instrument that asks how often various barriers in the environment (related to attitudes and support, services and assistance, physical and architectural features, policies, work, and school) have been a problem in the past 12 months. An example of the second approach was developed by Shumway-Cook and colleagues (2003), who observed subjects' mobility patterns and assessed dimensions of the physical environment thought to influence mobility. The third approach is illustrated by the 36-item Home and Community Environment Instrument (Keysor et al., 2010) and the Pilot Study of Aging and Technology instrument (Freedman et al., 2005), both of which assess the presence of environmental features that may enhance (e.g. grab bar) or impede (e.g. steps with no railing) functioning.

With respect to accommodations, in addition to measures of dependence mentioned earlier, studies sometimes include measures of use of assistive technologies, and, less often, measures of other, more subtle, behavioral changes. Two general approaches have been taken to assistive technology use measurement (Cornman et al., 2005). Some surveys embed questions about assistive device use within activity limitation measures (i.e. asking only those who report difficulty with an activity about their device use). Other surveys, such as NHIS, use a single item (e.g. "Do you now have any health problem that requires you to use special equipment, such as a cane, a wheelchair, a special bed, or a special telephone?") Both approaches may lead to underestimates, since often individuals who do not report having difficulty with activities use devices and, in the case of a global item, estimates are likely sensitive to items that are named as examples. With respect to more subtle behavioral changes, Fried and colleagues (2001b) have advanced the notion of "preclinical" disability, defined as changes in how an activity is accomplished without frank difficulty or dependence.

Related Concepts

Several additional concepts, which are distinct from but related to disability, are found in the aging literature. Here we briefly discuss three common terms: frailty, health-related quality of life QOL, and healthy aging, and provide insight into how they differ from disability as defined above.

Frailty has been defined as "increased vulnerability to stressors due to impairments in multiple, interrelated systems that lead to decline in homeostatic reserve and resiliency" (Bergman et al., 2007). This concept has been operationalized in several different ways. Rockwood and Mitnitski (2007), for example, focus on frailty as an accumulation of deficits. Applying this approach to survey data, demographers have demonstrated that an index of accumulated deficits is an indicator of physiologic decline that is independent of age (Kulminski et al., 2007). An alternative conceptualization of frailty by Fried and colleagues (sometimes referred to as "geriatric frailty") is a distinct clinical syndrome manifested by at least three of the following five symptoms: exhaustion, weak grip strength, slow walking speed, low energy expenditure, and weight loss (Fried et al., 2004). This recognizable phenotype, whose prevalence increases steeply with age, predicts limitations in mobility, onset of activity limitations, and mortality in community-based studies (Bandeen-Roche et al., 2006; Fried et al., 2001a). Both approaches to frailty measurement include disability components: The former approach sums across different ICF domains whereas the latter includes measures of capacity along with symptoms that extend beyond disability into the realm of symptoms.

Disability is also distinct from, albeit closely related to, health-related QOL, defined as a measure of how changes in health influence a person's day-to-day life. Such measures have emerged from efforts to quantify disease impact. Common health-related QOL measures include self-rated physical and mental health, unhealthy days, activity limitations, mobility limitations, and symptoms such as pain or low energy levels. The Centers for Disease Control and Prevention's (CDC) measure of health-related QOL, for example, uses a set of four items (see Figure 5.3). The first three items are clearly focused on health, whereas the last item measures activity limitations. Other commonly used health-related QOL instruments include the

---

1. Would you say that in general your health is Excellent, Very good, Good, Fair, or Poor?

2. Now thinking about your physical health, which includes physical illness and injury, for how many days during the past 30 days was your physical health not good?

3. Now thinking about your mental health, which includes stress, depression, and problems with emotions, for how many days during the past 30 days was your mental health not good?

4. During the past 30 days, for about how many days did poor physical or mental health keep you from doing your usual activities, such as self-care, work, or recreation?

Figure 5.3   Center for Disease Control's Healthy Days Measures.
Source: http://www.cdc.gov/hrqol/methods.htm

SF-36 (Ware & Sherbourne, 1992) and EQ-5D (Kind et al., 2005).

How is disability related to healthy aging? As defined by the CDC, healthy aging is the development and maintenance of optimal physical, mental, and social well-being and function. Promotion of healthy aging is not merely a matter of preventing disease and disability. Instead, healthy aging focuses on the maximization of function at every level of ability. For individuals living without disease and disability, healthy aging emphasizes health promotion and disease prevention activities such as screenings, inoculations, and an active lifestyle. For those who have already developed impairments in function, healthy aging emphasizes maintenance of remaining functions and adaptations to remain engaged in activities that promote well-being. In other words, healthy aging is a central public health goal, particularly in societies that are experiencing population aging (Albert & Freedman, 2009).

THE DEMOGRAPHY OF LATE-LIFE DISABILITY

The lack of common language has made estimating the number of older adults living with disability a challenging task. The Institute of Medicine (2007), for instance, noted that the number of individuals (of all ages) in the US with impairments, activity limitations, or participation restrictions is at least 40 million, but may be as high as 50 million – a 25% range. Similarly, using four national surveys, Gregory (2004) found that estimates of activity limitations among older adults ranged from 13% to 20%.

Chief among the reasons for such variation is that each survey uses its own sequence of questions to identify older adults with limitations. One study (Freedman et al., 2004) found that variation across five national surveys narrowed when definition was taken into account. For example, estimates of difficulty with ADL ranged from 25%–30%, estimates of getting help or using equipment ranged from 15%–20%, and estimates of getting (or needing) help ranged from 7%–10%. The remaining variation can presumably be accounted for by other methodological factors such as mode of administration, nonresponse and proxy rates, coverage of population living in institutions and group quarters, and other content on the survey that may influence self-reports. Such sources of variation should be kept in mind when reviewing statistics on the demography of disability.

In this section, we present data from two ongoing sources of disability data in the US: the NHIS and the HRS, to illustrate basic features of the demography of disability. Both surveys are national in scope and offer complementary measures for understanding disability and functioning. The NHIS is an ongoing cross-section study of the noninstitutionalized population with an emphasis on health and functioning. The HRS is a panel study of the population aged 51 and older at baseline, with a focus on the intersection of health and economic issues. Both surveys have expanded their disability measures in recent years, and we highlight those innovations here.

Capacity to Carry Out Activities

According to the 2007 NHIS, 64% of adults aged 65 and older reported difficulty with an upper or lower body movement (Table 5.1). The prevalence was over 10 percentage points higher for women than men and increased with age from 55% among 65–74 year olds to nearly 83% among those aged 85 or older. Non-Hispanic blacks (hereafter blacks) had a higher prevalence than non-Hispanic whites (hereafter whites) and those of Hispanic origin. Percentages also varied by type of activity: twice as many older adults reported difficulty walking a distance of three blocks than did so for reaching up (40% vs 19%).

Not highlighted in the table is the important finding that adults aged 65 and older make up only about one-third of the population with difficulty in upper or lower body actions (Altman & Bernstein, 2008). In other words, at least two-thirds of those with limitations in such actions develop them before the age of 65. Indeed, in the NHIS nearly half (45.4%) of people aged 55–64 have a limitation in upper or lower body functioning. This finding suggests a massive opportunity for intervention well before late life begins.

Performance measures from the 2006 HRS are shown on the right-hand side of Table 5.1. In general, the two physical performance measures – walking speed and a series of balance tests – show variation similar to the self-reported lower body limitations. That is, a "low" score (in the case of walking speed, about 2.2 feet per second or more slowly; for balance, unable to hold for at least 10 seconds a stance with the heel of one foot touching the big toe of the other) is more prevalent among women and blacks and increases with age. The question of how to handle missing values is especially important when evaluating performance tests, because many older adults who do not attempt the test may have impaired capacity. In the HRS, approximately one in five eligible participants aged 65 and older did not have a walking or balance test score.

The percentage of older adults with cognitive impairment is shown in the last column. The tests included here are the TICS, immediate and delayed recall, and counting back by 7s from 100, and the scale ranges from 0 to 35 (Ofstedal et al., 2005). In about 6% of cases, a proxy's evaluation of the respondent's memory as poor is used in place of a

Table 5.1 Percentage of older Americans with impaired capacity to carry out activities.

	SELF-REPORTED			PERFORMANCE-BASED				
	UPPER OR LOWER BODY	WALKING 3 BLOCKS	REACHING UP	WALKING SPEED		BALANCE		COGNITION[1]
	% reporting difficulty	% reporting difficulty	% reporting difficulty	% low score[2]	% low or missing score[3]	% low score[4]	% low or missing score[3]	% low score[5]
Male	58.0	33.8	14.0	18.5	37.3	6.5	22.2	8.0
Female	68.7	45.5	22.0	28.5	49.3	10.3	28.1	6.6
65–74	55.4	33.0	15.6	16.9	34.3	4.3	17.4	5.6
75–84	71.7	45.4	19.9	29.5	49.0	11.1	28.7	8.0
85+	82.5	62.1	28.8	40.0	72.4	20.0	51.0	11.5
Non-Hispanic white	64.5	39.9	26.2	23.1	41.3	8.4	23.9	6.6
Hispanic	57.8	39.3	21.7	29.7	59.2	10.2	33.2	11.9
Non-Hispanic black	66.7	47.5	17.3	34.2	67.4	10.7	39.6	11.2
Total	64.1	40.4	18.6	24.2	44.2	8.7	25.6	7.2

Sources: 2007 National Health Interview Survey (N=4583) and 2006 Health and Retirement Study (N=5112 for walking speed and balance performance and N=5544 for cognition).
[1] Cognition is measured with items from the Telephone Interview Cognition Screen and the Mini Mental Status Exam or a proxy's rating of poor memory.
[2] %low score=Among those eligible and not by phone, percentage with 0.67 meters/second (2.2 feet/second) or more slowly (approximately the lowest quartile among those with non-missing scores) on the faster of two walks (2.5 meter course).
[3] % low or missing = Among those eligible and not by phone, percentage with low score or who were missing because they had an interview by proxy (2%), did not consent (about 7%), or consented but did not complete the test (11% for walking; 8% for balance). The latter group consists of individuals who felt (or whose interviewer felt) the test was not safe for them to perform and those who refused for other reasons.
[4] % low score=Among those eligible and not by phone, unable to hold semi-tandem stand for 10 seconds.
[5] % low score=8 or fewer out of 35.

poor score. Low cognitive scores (≤ 8 out of 35) show a different pattern from physical measures: women are *not* more likely to have poor cognition than men, and Hispanics and blacks both have nearly twice the rate of whites. Note that such tests are better considered "screening" tools and not diagnostic indicators per se. Estimates from the HRS' Aging, Demographics, and Memory Study, which draw upon more sensitive measurement tools, suggest that 22% of people aged 71 and older have cognitive impairment without dementia, and 14% meet the more stringent criteria for dementia (Plassman et al., 2007, 2008).

Activity Limitations and Social Participation Restrictions

Not all older adults with reduced physical or cognitive capacity report ADL or IADL limitations. In 2007, among adults aged 65 and older, 6.8% reported needing help with "personal care needs, such as eating, bathing, dressing, or getting around inside their home" and 12.7% reported needing help "handling routine needs, such as everyday household chores, doing necessary business, shopping, or getting around for other purposes" (see Table 5.2). Like self-reported capacity, however, the prevalence of ADL and IADL limitations is higher for women than for men and increases sharply with age. Racial variation differs from self-reported capacity: Blacks reported the highest prevalence but those of Hispanic origin fall between blacks and whites.

Turning to socially oriented activities, nearly 17% of older adults report difficulty going out to do things such as shopping and 12% report difficulty participating in social activities (visiting friends, attending clubs or meetings, or going to parties). Like measures of capacity and activity limitations, measures of participation restrictions rise with age in a

Table 5.2 Percentage of older americans with activity limitations and participation restrictions.

	ACTIVITY LIMITATIONS (2007)		PARTICIPATION RESTRICTIONS (2004–2007)	
	NEED HELP WITH ADL	NEED HELP WITH IADL	DIFFICULTY GOING OUT FOR SHOPPING AND LEISURE	DIFFICULTY SOCIALIZING
Male	4.9	8.4	12.6	9.9
Female	8.4	16.0	19.6	13.9
65–74	3.3	6.3	11.6	8.1
75–84	7.7	14.5	19.2	13.9
85+	21.5	38.0	34.1	27.6
Non-Hispanic white	6.3	12.0	16.1	11.5
Hispanic	8.2	13.6	19.0	14.7
Non-Hispanic black	10.6	18.9	21.0	17.5
Total	6.9	12.7	16.6	12.2

Sources: 2007 National Health Interview Survey (N=9439) and Schoenborn & Heyman (2009)'s analysis of the 2004–2007 National Health Interview Survey.

fashion comparable to the increase for needing help with IADLs. Racial disparities also exist, with blacks most likely to report difficulty; however, Hispanics and whites report very similar levels of difficulty.

Use of Assistive Devices and Modifications to the Home Environment

Assistive devices and physical attributes of the home environment are important because they can facilitate, or in some cases impede, the performance of daily activities. Estimates from six national surveys conducted from 1999 to 2002 suggest that approximately 14%–18% of the US population aged 65 or older uses assistive devices: most often, devices for mobility (canes, walkers) and bathing (grab bars, bath seats, railings) (Cornman et al., 2005).

In a 2006 module administered to a random subsample of HRS participants, information was collected not only about whether respondents used particular home features, but whether they had them and whether they or their families had added such features. Table 5.3 shows results for two common home modifications: a grab bar or seat for the shower or tub area and a grab bar around the toilet or raised toilet seat. The table also includes estimates of mobility device use in the last 30 days, also collected in the same module.

Like measures of capacity, use of modifications and mobility devices varies by sex, age, and race/ethnicity. Women are more likely to have, to have added, and to have used home modifications and mobility devices, and rates increase substantially with age. Racial and ethnic patterns for mobility device use follow patterns for self-reported and performance-based lower body limitations. That is, blacks appear to be using mobility devices in proportion to underlying need. However, despite their greater need, blacks are essentially equally as likely as whites, and Hispanics far less likely, to have a bathroom or toilet modification. This finding likely may reflect differences in housing ownership as well as other socioeconomic factors.

The Varied Course of Disablement

The course of disablement in later life varies and is inextricably linked to experiences much earlier in life (Mayer, 2009). As noted earlier, a large proportion of adults have already developed essentially permanent impairments in functioning by the time they reach age 65. For these individuals, factors earlier in life have already extended their influence on late-life functioning. Some of these influences may be genetic or programmed early in life; others may be the result of behaviors linked to social and economic resources in childhood or midlife. Other adults reach late life

Table 5.3 Percentage of older Americans with home modifications and mobility device use among the population 65 and older.

	BATH/SHOWER MODIFICATION			TOILET MODIFICATION			MOBILITY DEVICE USE[1]
	Have it	Added it	Used it[1]	Have it	Added it	Used it[1]	
Male	46.4	24.3	22.2	19.9	13.6	13.7	16.1
Female	55.9	32.4	35.2	30.6	19.8	24.1	21.6
65–74	44.4	21.8	19.6	20.5	13.3	14.3	12.8
75–84	57.7	32.7	39.2	26.7	16.7	20.7	21.5
85+	72.1	54.0	51.0	53.1	39.2	44.7	45.6
Non-Hispanic white	52.9	29.0	30.0	26.4	17.1	20.0	18.7
Hispanic	34.6	23.7	23.7	18.3	10.2	13.4	20.0
Non-Hispanic black	48.3	30.6	29.9	25.8	21.0	19.8	25.3
Total	51.2	28.9	29.7	26.1	17.2	19.7	19.3

Sources: 2006 Health and Retirement Study.
[1]Used in the last 30 days

without limitations, but then experience either a gradual or steep loss of ability to carry out daily activities (Ferrucci et al., 1996). Notably, a substantial proportion of older adults who experience functional decline also experience improvements (Crimmins & Saito, 1993).

A recent focus by investigators has been on identifying signature types of common trajectories experienced in later life, sometimes at the very end of life. Two distinct approaches have been undertaken. Lunney et al. (2003), for instance, have categorized decedents according to cause of death/condition and identified several characteristic trajectories: sudden death characterized by no activity limitations prior to death; a short period of decline, typical of many cancers; a longer period of limitations with multiple exacerbations, typical of organ system failure; and a slow, prolonged, and unrelenting decline typical of dementia, disabling stroke, and frailty. A second approach uses prospective data and advanced modeling methods to identify distinctive groupings. By estimating group-based mixture models, for example, Liang et al. (2010) and Dodge et al. (2006) both have identified three trajectories: consistently high functioning/no decline, a moderate decline, and a steep decline.

In order to maximize functioning and identify junctures for intervention, it is important to understand what factors increase the risks of onset of particular trajectories and progression along those pathways. Most studies of predictors of onset and progression have focused on simple transitions to and from activity limitations. Onset of activity limitations in later life is consistently higher for people with deficits in earlier stages of the disablement process – that is, those with multiple health conditions or with cognitive, sensory, or mobility impairment (Stuck et al., 1999), or preclinical disability (Fried et al., 2001b). Recently, the importance of the physical environment has been highlighted as well (Keysor, 2006). Less proximate risk factors that increase an older adult's risk of disability include infrequent social contacts, little physical activity, smoking, weight loss, and poor nutrition (Bartali et al., 2006; Stuck et al., 1999). House and colleagues (2005) have highlighted the contributions of socioeconomic status to the onset and progression of activity limitations, and found that education is linked to onset whereas income proves to be more salient in accounting for progression. Others have focused explicitly on factors linked to the risks of recovery. Hardy and Gill (2004, 2005), for instance, demonstrated that risks of recovery are higher for those who are cognitively intact, non-frail, have milder or fewer activity limitations, and have regular physical activity prior to the onset of limitations. More work is needed to understand what factors are associated with movements along particular trajectories and to develop interventions to maximize functioning within and across such groupings.

POPULATION TRENDS IN LATE-LIFE DISABILITY

A final central question related to disability and aging at the population level is whether declines in mortality have been accompanied by improvements in health and functioning. Typically, changes in population health and functioning are measured in one of two ways: by examining trends in the prevalence of disability (or other morbidity measures) or by comparing active life expectancy measures over time. In assessing the former, it is important to be clear about whether rates being compared are crude or adjusted for shifts in the proportion in each age group, since crude rates will underestimate declines (or overstate increases) if the population is aging. Because of reliance on age-specific rates, active life expectancy measures are by design age-adjusted. That is, the measure yields insight into how many years on average could be expected to be lived without activity limitations if age-specific rates of activity limitations and mortality here to hold over a hypothetical cohort's lifetime.

Several competing theories have been developed to explain how population health changes in the face of mortality declines. For example, Gruenberg (1977) asserted that medical advances (such as antibiotics and insulin) would lead to the increased survival of persons with chronic morbidity, which in turn would result in an expansion of the proportion of life spent with morbidity or disability, and concomitant increases in disability prevalence. This theory portends increases in life expectancy but no change in active life expectancy. In contrast, Fries' (1980, 1983) compression of morbidity theory asserts the opposite: because maximum life expectancy is fixed, as the onset of chronic disease is postponed into later ages, the period of morbidity and disability will be compressed into a smaller amount, and smaller proportion, of life expectancy. Consequently, one could expect disability prevalence to decline.

Two additional theories suggest more variable experience in the face of mortality declines. Manton's (1982) theory of dynamic equilibrium uniquely recognizes that interventions designed to reduce mortality also have an influence on morbidity, and vice versa. As such, years of life gained are assumed to be achieved through a combination of postponement of disease onset, reductions in severity of disease and disease progression, and improvements in clinical management. This theory predicts increases in life expectancy, active life expectancy, and years of life expected to be lived with disability; however, depending on the specific reasons for years of life gained, the ratio of active life expectancy to life expectancy could expand or contract, as could disability prevalence. Similarly, Robine and Michel (2004) suggest that populations may go through an ordered set of stages of expansion and compression as they age.

In practice, studying disability trends over time is challenging. Any change – whether in question wording; mode; response rates; rules about using proxies; or, for panel surveys, the extent of loss to follow-up over time – can introduce bias into trends. Nevertheless, a large and growing literature on late-life disability trends has emerged on this topic (for reviews, see Crimmins, 2004; Parker & Thorslund, 2007; Schoeni et al., 2008). Here we provide a brief overview of such trends, with an emphasis on the US experience.

Trends in the Prevalence of Activity Limitations

The evidence for activity limitation trends in the US during the 1980s and early 1990s was mixed, with Manton and colleagues reporting large declines in the age-adjusted prevalence of activity limitations (1997) and Crimmins and colleagues (1997a) concluding that there was no clear ongoing trend. During the 1990s, however, there was a convergence of evidence that suggested substantial decline in IADL limitations (Freedman et al., 2002) and that declines in three IADL activities – managing money, shopping for groceries, and doing laundry – were notably large from 1984 to 1999 (Spillman, 2004). Smaller declines in the use of help and difficulties with ADLs were also documented (Freedman et al., 2004). Not all groups have benefited equally; instead, improvements have been smaller for less advantaged groups – i.e. those with fewer years of education or lower income, and minorities (Schoeni et al., 2005). The trends observed in the US do not appear to be occurring in all low-mortality countries; for example, trends in ADL limitations vary across eight European countries (Jacobzone et al., 2000–2001).

Trends in Active Life Expectancy

In the US, trends in active life expectancy have differed across time periods and socioeconomic groups. From 1970 to 1980, for example, data for the entire US population were consistent with the expansion of the morbidity hypothesis (Crimmins et al., 1997b). That is, most of the increase in life expectancy consisted of years of life with activity limitations. Studies of the US in the 1980s and 1990s, three of which are summarized in Table 5.4, suggest a pattern consistent with the compression of morbidity (Cai & Lubitz, 2007; Crimmins et al., 2009; Manton et al., 2006a). The studies use different measures, methods, and time periods, and suggest different levels of active life expectancy, but all three show increases in the percentage of life expectancy to be spent without activity limitations. Findings by Crimmins and Saito (2001),

Table 5.4 Life expectancy, active life expectancy, and percentage of years expected to be lived without activity limitations.

	LONGITUDINAL STUDY OF AGING		NATIONAL LONG-TERM CARE SURVEY		MEDICARE CURRENT BENEFICIARY SURVEY	
	1984	**1994**	**1982**	**1999**	**1992**	**2003**
Active life expectancy	10.9	11.6	12.9	13.9	9.5	10.3
Life expectancy	13.7	14.3	17.5	17.7	16.8	17.3
% of life without activity limitations	80%	81%	74%	79%	57%	60%

Sources: Cai & Lubitz, 2007; Crimmins et al., 2009; Manton et al., 2006a.

however, suggest that such a compression may be concentrated among more educated groups.

Variation is also evident in other more developed countries. An analysis by Robine and colleagues (2008) of 14 countries in the European Union (EU) found a slight increase between 1995 and 2005 in the number of years lived without disability in Europe. However, no consistent pattern was evident across countries.

Reasons for Trends

The mechanisms by which population-level changes in activity limitations and active life expectancy occur are of great interest. In the US, where evidence of decline has been most robust, exploration into reasons for declines has revealed a combination of factors at work (Schoeni et al., 2008). Three salient reasons appear to be the shifting socioeconomic profile of older adults, changes in chronic disease severity, and changes in the way daily activities are carried out by older adults.

With respect to socioeconomic status (SES), older adults have greater educational attainment on average today than they did in the mid-1980s and such a change accounts for a substantial portion, but not all, of the decline in limitations (Freedman & Martin, 1999). The pathways from education to late-life functioning are complex and at times indirect. Education, along with other socioeconomic, demographic, and cultural factors, may be linked to the risk of developing health conditions and associated impairments, by influencing access to health care throughout life, preventive care, occupational history, social standing (and consequent stress and environmental exposures), and risk-taking behaviors. More educated people may have a greater ability to marshal resources to optimize their health outcomes and to accommodate impairments through changes to the physical environment and use of assistive technologies.

Evidence also suggests that some chronic conditions are less debilitating now than previously, despite increases in the prevalence of many chronic conditions (Freedman et al., 2007). In particular, arthritis, cardiovascular diseases (CVD), and vision limitations are less likely to be reported to cause activity limitations. It could be that earlier diagnosis and better management of such conditions has led to lower reported rates of disabilities. In the case of less debilitating vision limitations, cataract surgery has been implicated.

Finally, the nature of daily activities, particularly common household tasks such as shopping, preparing meals, and managing money, has changed over the last few decades. Moreover, many more seniors are living in supportive living environments, such as continuing-care retirement communities, assisted living facilities, and other retirement communities, which provide assistance with daily tasks and transportation. Other tasks are facilitated by the use of assistive technologies and environmental supports. One analysis suggests that shifts toward the use of assistive technologies by older adults with ADL limitations account for a sizeable share of the reduction in use of personal help (Freedman et al., 2006).

Future Late-Life Disability Trends: Tracking the Baby Boom Generation

Given the exceptionally large size of the cohorts born between 1946 and 1964, which are poised to enter late life, there is considerable interest in understanding whether declines in late-life disability trends will continue, slow, or reverse their course over the next few decades. Indeed, although published estimates from the National Long Term Care Survey suggest declines among the population aged 65 and older have continued (Manton et al., 2006b), the most recent evidence from the Medicare Current Beneficiary Survey suggests that declines may be leveling off (Federal Interagency Forum on Aging-Related Statistics, 2008).

Disagreement also exists about the health and functioning trends among the generations approaching late life and their implications for future late-life trends (see Martin et al., 2009; Seeman et al., 2010; Weir, 2007). Many measures suggest stable or improved health and functioning in the baby boom generations compared to prior cohorts. At the same time, troubling increases in limitations in ADLS have been identified, albeit rates remain at relatively low levels for adults under age 65.

What do such trends imply for the future? Some researchers have warned that trends in obesity and other potentially disabling conditions among working-age adults could offset future improvements in late-life functioning and that the beneficial effects of education will not be as large in the future. The most recent evidence available at publication concludes, however, that the increase in obesity has recently "paused," and that favorable trends in education and smoking are continuing (see Martin et al., 2010 for a review).

SUMMARY AND CONCLUSION

This chapter has offered a glimpse into both conceptual and empirical issues at the intersection of disability and aging. Concepts and nomenclatures continue to evolve, and new measures that will further our understanding of disability, functioning, and aging are being developed and implemented. Disparities by age, sex, and race/ethnicity persist in all spheres of disablement, in some cases linked to events and exposures much earlier in life. Disablement is a highly individualized experience, but work is underway to identify signature pathways that may be useful for tailoring interventions to maximize functioning.

Research has also attempted to characterize trends in limitations as mortality declines. Population aging does not necessarily mean greater prevalence of disability; to the contrary, in the US and in other more developed countries, the proportion of life expected to be lived without limitations has increased in recent years, as the prevalence of limitations in later life has declined. Like the individual disablement trajectories that characterize later life, the reasons for such trends are varied and complex. Recently, declines may have leveled off in the US, and disparities remain an important target for interventions in the future.

Further research is needed in several areas to ensure continued progress in maximizing functioning in later life. First, additional measurement work is needed to fully implement the ICF as a model for disablement in later life. Second, a better understanding of disparities in the disablement process in the US and around the world and predictors of entry into and progress along signature trajectories would be valuable. Understanding the relative importance of changes in capacity vs environmental components to such trajectories remains essentially unexplored territory. Third, continued vigilance in tracking population trends is needed for planning and intervention purposes and may also help settle theoretical disagreements about changes in health and functioning as populations age. Such trends are particularly important to monitor as the large baby boom cohorts enter later life.

Beyond basic description of disablement, further research is needed to identify cost-effective public health interventions that will extend years of life that are active and characterized by engagement. There are a number of promising approaches to disability interventions in later life, including comprehensive geriatric assessments; risk reduction programs; volunteer programs for older adults; multi-factorial fall prevention programs; depression screening and treatment; physical activity and fitness programs; and prehabilitation programs. In the coming years, additional attention needs to be given to the challenges of implementing cost-effective interventions to promote maximization of functioning at both individual and population levels.

ACKNOWLEDGMENTS

A special thanks to colleagues Linda Martin, Robert Schoeni, Emily Agree, Judy Kasper, Chris Seplaki, Jennifer Cornman, Patti Andreski, Douglas Wolf, and Steven Albert for allowing me to draw upon on collaborative efforts in preparing this chapter. Funding was provided in part through the National Institute of Aging (U01-AG032947).

REFERENCES

Albert, S. M., & Freedman, V. A. (2009). *Public health and aging: Maximizing functioning and wellbeing*. New York: Springer.

Altman, B., & Bernstein, A. (2008). *Disability and health in the United States, 2001–2005*. Hyattsville, MD: National Center for Health Statistics.

Bandeen-Roche, K., Xue, Q. L., Ferrucci, L., Walston, J., Guralnik, J. M., Chaves, P., et al. (2006). Phenotype of frailty: Characterization in the women's health and aging studies. *Journal of Gerontology: Medical Sciences,* 61A(3), M262–M266.

Bartali, B., Semba, R. D., Frongillo, E. A., Varadhan, R., Ricks, M. O., Blaum, C. S., et al. (2006). Low micronutrient levels as a predictor of incident disability in older women. *Archives of Internal Medicine,* 166(21), 2335–2340.

Bergman, H., Ferrucci, L., Guralnik, J., Hogan, D. B., Hummel, S., Karunananthan, S., et al. (2007). Frailty: An emerging research and clinical paradigm – Issues and controversies. *Journal of Gerontology: Medical Sciences,* 62A, 731–737.

Brandt, J., Spencer, M., & Folstein, M. (1988). The telephone interview for cognitive status. *Neuropsychiatry, Neuropsychology, and Behavioral Neurology,* 1, 111–117.

Cai, L., & Lubitz, J. (2007). Was there compression of disability for older Americans from 1992 to 2003. *Demography,* 44, 479–495.

Cornman, J. C., Freedman., V. A., & Agree, E. M. (2005). Measurement of assistive device use: Implications for estimates of device use and disability in late life. *The Gerontologist,* 45(3), 347–358.

Crimmins, E. M. (2004). Trends in the health of the elderly. *Annual Review of Public Health,* 25, 79–98.

Crimmins, E. M., & Saito, Y. (1993). Getting better and getting worse. *Journal of Aging and Health,* 5, 3–36.

Crimmins, E. M., & Saito, Y. (2001). Trends in healthy life expectancy in the United States, 1970–1990: Gender, racial, and educational differences. *Social Science & Medicine,* 52, 1629–1641.

Crimmins, E. M., Saito, Y., & Reynolds, S. L. (1997a). Further evidence on recent trends in the prevalence and incidence of disability among older Americans from two sources: the LSOA and the NHIS. *Journal of Gerontology: Social Sciences,* 52B(2), S59–S71.

Crimmins, E. M., Saito, Y., & Ingegneri, D. (1997b). Trends in disability-free life expectancy in the United States, 1970–1990. *Population and Development Review,* 23, 555–572.

Crimmins, E. M., Hayward, M. D., Hagedorn, A., Saito, Y., & Brouard, N. (2009). Change in disability-free life expectancy for Americans 70-years-old and older. *Demography,* 46(3), 627–646.

Dodge, H. H., Du, Y., Saxton, J. A., & Ganguli, M. (2006). Cognitive domains and trajectories of functional independence in nondemented elderly persons. *Journal of Gerontology: Medical Sciences,* 61, 1330–1337.

Federal Interagency Forum on Aging-Related Statistics. (2008). *Older Americans 2008: Key indicators of well-being.* Washington, DC: Government Printing Office.

Ferrucci, L., Guralnik, J. M., Simonsick, E., Salive, M. E., Corti, C., & Langlois, J., (1996). Progressive versus catastrophic disability: A longitudinal view of the disablement process. *Journal of Gerontology: Medical Sciences,* 51, M123–M130.

Folstein, M. F., Folstein, S. E., & McHugh, P. R. (1975). Mini-mental state: A practical method for grading the cognitive state of patients for the clinician. *Journal of Psychiatric Research,* 12(3), 189–198.

Freedman, V. A. (2009). Adopting the ICF language for studying late-life disability: A field of dreams? *Journal of Gerontology: Medical Sciences,* 64(11), 1172–1174.

Freedman, V. A., & Martin, L. G. (1999). The role of education in explaining and forecasting trends in functional limitations among older Americans. *Demography,* 36(4), 461–473.

Freedman, V. A., Martin, L. G., & Schoeni, R. F. (2002). Recent trends in disability and functioning among older adults in the United States: A systematic review. *Journal of the American Medical Association,* 288(24), 3137–3146.

Freedman, V. A., Crimmins, E., Schoeni, R. F., Spillman, B. C., Aykan, H., Kramarow, E., et al. (2004). Resolving inconsistencies in trends in old-age disability: Report from a technical working group. *Demography,* 41(3), 417–441.

Freedman, V. A., Agree, E., & Cornman, J. (2005). Development of an assistive technology and home environment assessment instrument for national surveys: Final report. Part I. Recommended modules and instrument development process. Report prepared for DHHS Office of the Assistant Secretary for Planning and Evaluation. Available at: http://aspe.hhs.gov/daltcp/reports/ATEAdevI.pdf

Freedman, V. A., Agree, E. M., Martin, L. G., & Cornman, J. C. (2006). Trends in the use of assistive technology and personal care for late-life disability, 1992–2001. *Gerontologist,* 46, 124–127.

Freedman, V. A., Schoeni, R. F., Martin, L. G., & Cornman, J. C. (2007). Chronic conditions and the decline in late-life disability. *Demography,* 44(3), 459–477.

Fried, L. P., Tangen, C. M., Walston, J., Newman, A. B., Hirsch, C., Gottdiener, J., et al. (2001a). Frailty in older adults: Evidence for a phenotype. *Journal of Gerontology: Medical Sciences,* 56(3), M146–M156.

Fried, L. P., Young, Y., Rubin, G., & Bandeen-Roche, K., for the WHAS II Collaborative Research Group (2001b). Self-reported preclinical disability identifies older women with early declines in performance and early disease. *Journal of Clinical Epidemiology,* 54, 889–901.

Fried, L. P., Ferrucci, L., Darer, J., Williamson, J. D., & Anderson, G. (2004). Untangling the concepts of disability, frailty, and comorbidity: Implications for improved targeting and care. *Journal of Gerontology Medical Sciences,* 59(3), M255–M263.

Fries, J. F. (1980). Aging, natural death and the compression of morbidity. *The New England Journal of Medicine,* 303, 130–135.

Fries, J. F. (1983). The compression of morbidity. *Milbank Memorial Fund Quarterly,* 61, 397–419.

Gregory, S. R. (2004). In Brief: Disability: Federal survey definitions, measurements, and estimates. Washington, DC: AARP.

Gruenberg, E. M. (1977). The failures of success. *Milbank Memorial Fund Quarterly,* 55(1), 3–24.

Guralnik, J. M., & Ferrucci, L. (2009). The challenge of understanding the disablement process in older persons: commentary responding to Jette AM. Toward a common language of disablement. *Journal of Gerontology: Medical Sciences, 64A*(11), 1169–1171.

Guralnik, J. M., Branch, L. G., Cummings, S. R., & Curb, J. D. (1989). Physical performance measures in aging research. *Journal of Gerontology: Medical Sciences, 44,* M141–M146.

Guralnik, J. M., Ferrucci, L., Simonsick, E. M., Salive, M. E., & Wallace, R. B. (1995). Lower-extremity function in persons over the age of 70 years as a predictor of subsequent disability. *New England Journal of Medicine, 332,* 556–561.

Hardy, S. E., & Gill, T. M. (2004). Recovery from disability among community-dwelling older persons. *Journal of the American Medical Association, 291*(13), 1596–1602.

Hardy, S. E., & Gill, T. M. (2005). Factors associated with recovery of independence among newly disabled older persons. *Archives of Internal Medicine, 165*(1), 106–112.

House, J. S., Lantz, P. M., & Herd, P. (2005). Continuity and change in the social stratification of aging and health over the life course: Evidence from a nationally representative longitudinal study from 1986 to 2001/2002. *Journal of Gerontology: Social Sciences, 60,* S15–S26.

Institute of Medicine, (1991). *Disability in America: Toward a national agenda for prevention.* Washington, DC: National Academy Press.

Institute of Medicine, (2007). *The future of disability in America.* Washington, DC: National Academy Press.

**Jacobzone, S., Cambois, E., & Robine, J. M. (2000–2001). *Is the health of older persons in OECD countries improving fast enough to compensate for population ageing? (Publication No. 30).* Paris: Organisation for Economic Co-operation and Development.

Jette, A. M. (2009). Toward a common language of disablement. *Journals of Gerontology: Medical Sciences, 64,* 1165–1168.

Katz, S., Ford, A. B., Moskowitz, R. W., Jackson, B. A., & Jaffee, M. W.

(1963). Studies of illness in the aged. The Index of ADL, a standardized measure of biological and psychosocial function. *Journal of the American Medical Association, 185,* 914–919.

Keysor, J. J. (2006). How does the environment influence disability? Examining the evidence. In M. J. Field, A. M. Jette & L. Martin (Eds.), *Appendix D in Workshop on Disability in America: A New Look: Summary and Background Papers* (pp. 88–100). Washington, DC: National Academies Press.

Keysor, J. J., Jette, A. M., Lavalley, M. P., Lewis, C. E., Torner, J. C., Nevitt, M. C., et al. (2010). Community environmental factors are associated with disability in older adults with functional limitations: The MOST Study. *Journal of Gerontology: Medical Sciences, 65,* 393–399.

Kind, P., Brooks, R., & Rabin, R. (Eds.), (2005). *EQ-5D concepts and methods: A developmental history.* New York: Springer.

Kinsella, K., & He, W. (2009). *An Aging World 2008.* Washington, DC: Government Printing Office.

Kulminski, A. M., Ukraintseva, S. V., Akushevich, I. V., Arbeev, K. G., & Yashin, A. I. (2007). Cumulative index of health deficiencies as a characteristic of long life. *Journal of the American Geriatrics Society, 55*(6), 935–940.

Lafortune, G., & Balestat, G., & the Disability Study Expert Group Members. (2007). *Trends in severe disability among elderly people: Assessing the evidence in 12 OECD countries and the future implications.* Paris: Organisation for Economic Co-operation and Development.

Lawton, M. P., & Brody, E. M. (1969). Assessment of older people: Self-maintaining and instrumental activities of daily living. *The Gerontologist, 9,* 179–186.

Liang, J., Xu, X., Bennett, J. M., Ye, W., & Quiñones, A. R. (2010). Ethnicity and changing functional health in middle and late life: A person-centered approach. *Journal of Gerontology: Social Sciences, 65*(4), 470–4.

Lunney, J. R., Lynn, J., Foley, D. J., Lipson, S., & Guralnik, J. M. (2003). Patterns of functional decline at the end of life. *Journal*

of the American Medical Association, 289(18), 2387–2392.

Manton, K. G. (1982). Changing concepts of morbidity and mortality in the elderly population. *Milbank Memorial Fund Quarterly: Health and Society, 60,* 183–244.

Manton, K. G., Corder, L., & Stallard, E. (1997). Chronic disability trends in elderly United States populations: 1982–1994. *Proceedings of the National Academy of Sciences USA, 94*(6), 2593–2598.

Manton, K. G., Gu, X., & Lamb, V. L. (2006a). Long-term trends in life expectancy and active life expectancy in the United States. *Population and Development Review, 32*(1), 81–106.

Manton, K. G., Gu, X., & Lamb, V. L. (2006b). Changes in chronic disability from 1982 to 2004/2005 as measured by long-term changes in function and health in the U.S. elderly population. *Proceedings of the National Academy of Sciences USA, 103*(48), 18374–18379.

Martin, L. G., Freedman, V. A., Schoeni, R. F., & Andreski, P. (2009). Baby boom health and functioning approaching 60. *Journal of Gerontology: Social Sciences, 64*(3), S369–S377.

Martin, L. G., Schoeni, R. F., & Andreski, P. M. (2010). Trends in health of older adults in the United States: Past, present, future. *Demography, 47.*

Mayer, K. U. (2009). New directions in life course research. *Annual Review of Sociology, 35,* 413–433.

Morris, J. C. (1993). The Clinical Dementia Rating (CDR): Current version and scoring rules. *Neurology, 43,* 2412–2414.

Nagi, S. Z. (1965). Some conceptual issues in disability and rehabilitation. In M. B. Sussman (Ed.), *Sociology and Rehabilitation* (pp. 100–113). Washington, DC: American Sociological Association.

Newman, A. B., Simonsick, E. M., Naydeck, B. L., Boudreau, R. M., Kritchevsky, S. B., Nevitt, M. C., et al. (2006). Association of long-distance corridor walk performance with mortality, cardiovascular disease, mobility limitation, and disability. *Journal* of the American Medical Association, 295, 2018–2026.

Noonan, V. K., Kopec, J. A., Noreau, L., Singer, J., Chan, A., Mâsse, L. C., et al. (2009). Comparing the content of participation instruments using the international classification of functioning, disability and health. Health Quality Life Outcomes, 7, 93.

Ofstedal, M. B., Fisher, G. G., & Herzog, A. R. (2005). HRS/ AHEAD Documentation of cognitive functioning measures in the health and retirement study. HRS Documentation Report DR-006. Ann Arbor, MI: University of Michigan.

Parker, M. G., & Thorslund, M. (2007). Health trends in the elderly population: Getting better and getting worse. The Gerontologist, 47, 150–158.

Plassman, B. L., Langa, K. M., Fisher, G. G., Heeringa, S. G., Weir, D. R., Ofstedal, M. B., et al. (2007). Prevalence of dementia in the United States: The aging, demographics, and memory study. Neuroepidemiology, 29(1–2), 125–132.

Plassman, B. L., Langa, K. M., Fisher, G. G., Heeringa, S. G., Weir, D. R., Ofstedal, M. B., et al. (2008). Prevalence of cognitive impairment without dementia in the United States. Annals of Internal Medicine, 148(6), 427–434.

Robine, J. M., & Michel, P. J. (2004). Looking forward to a general theory on population aging. Journal of Gerontology: Medical Sciences, 59, M590–M597.

Robine, J. M., Jagger, C., Van Oyen, H., & Cambois, E. (2008). Increasing healthy life expectancy and reducing longevity gaps between European countries. European

Health Report. Brussels: European Commission.

Rockwood., K., & Mitnitski, A. (2007). Frailty in relation to the accumulation of deficits. Journal of Gerontology: Medical Sciences, 62, 722–727.

Schoenborn, C. A., & Heyman, K. M. (2009). Health characteristics of adults aged 55 years and over: United States, 2004–2007. National Health Statistics Reports; no. 16. Hyattsville, MD: National Center for Health Statistics.

Schoeni, R. F., Martin, L. G., Andreski, P., & Freedman, V. A. (2005). Persistent and growing socioeconomic disparities in disability among the elderly: 1982–2002. American Journal of Public Health, 95(11), 2065–2070.

Schoeni, R. F., Freedman, V. A., & Martin, L. G. (2008). Why is late-life disability declining? Milbank Memorial Quarterly, 86(1), 47–89.

Seeman, T. E., Merkin, S. S., Crimmins, E. M., & Karlamangla, A. S. (2010). Disability trends among older Americans: National Health and Nutrition Examination Surveys, 1988–1994 and 1999–2004. American Journal of Public Health, 100(1), 100–107.

Shumway-Cook, A., Patla, A. E., Stewart, A., Ferrucci, L., Ciol, M.A., & Guralnik, J., (2003). Environmental components of mobility disability in community-living older persons. Journal of the American Geriatrics Society, 51(3), 393–398.

Spillman, B. C. (2004). Changes in elderly disability rates and the implications for health care utilization and cost. Milbank Memorial Fund Quarterly, 82(1), 157–194.

Stuck, A. E., Walthert, J. M., Nikolaus, T., Büla, C. J., Hohmann, C., &

Beck, J. C. (1999). Risk factors for functional status decline in community-living elderly people: A systematic literature review. Social Science and Medicine, 48, 445–469.

Verbrugge, L. M., & Jette, A. M. (1994). The disablement process. Social Science & Medicine, 38, 1–14.

Ware, J. E., & Sherbourne, C. D. (1992). The MOS 36-Item Short-Form Health Survey (SF-36®): I. Conceptual framework and item selection. Medical Care, 30(6), 473–483.

Weir, D. (2007). Are Baby Boomers living well longer? In B. Madrian, O. S. Mitchell & B. J. Soldo (Eds.), Redefining retirement: How will Boomers fare? (pp. 95–111). New York: Oxford University Press.

Whiteneck, G., & Dijkers, M. P. (2009). Difficult to measure constructs: Conceptual and methodological issues concerning participation and environmental factors. Archives of Physical Medicine & Rehabilitation, 90 (11 Suppl.), S22–S35.

Whiteneck, G. G., Harrison-Felix, C. L., Mellick, D. C., Brooks, C. A., Charlifue, S. B., & Gerhart, K. A., (2004). Quantifying environmental factors: A measure of physical, attitudinal, service, productivity, and policy barriers. Archives of Physical Medicine & Rehabilitation, 85(8), 1324–1335.

World Health Organization. (WHO) (2002). Towards a common language for functioning, disability, and health, ICF. Geneva: WHO.

Wunderlich, G. S. (2009). Improving the measurement of late-life disability in population surveys. Washington, DC: National Academies Press.

Chapter | 6 |

Global Aging

Elizabeth Frankenberg[1], Duncan Thomas[2]

[1]Sanford School of Public Policy, Duke University, Durham, North Carolina [2]Department of Economics, Duke University, Durham, North Carolina

INTRODUCTION

The globe is graying. Among the greatest achievements and greatest challenges that society faces today is that people across the world are living to unprecedented ages. During the second half of the twentieth century, the combination of increased life expectancy and reduced fertility resulted in sharp increases in the share of the population at older ages in the developed world. Middle-income countries have begun this transition and the rest of the world is catching up at an unprecedented pace.

These late-comers account for a large and increasing share of the world's population. The fraction aged 60 and older is projected to double in the next two decades – a dramatic increase. Yet only a handful of developing countries have policies and institutions in place to serve older adults.

Social research on global aging is a rapidly growing field. The questions are important and the data infrastructure is fast improving as more high-quality population-based surveys from developing countries become available. Exciting opportunities for scientific research abound.

The goal of this chapter is to provide an overview of what is known, highlight emerging lines of inquiry that are likely to have an important impact on science, and discuss challenges that have hindered progress. Linda Martin described the demography of aging in Chapter 3. We briefly review the aggregate demographic features that drive global aging. We focus on current patterns and future trends in low-income countries with respect to three dimensions of aging: health; work and retirement; and living arrangements and transfers. Low- and middle- income countries provide most of the evidence but we draw contrasts with more developed countries where informative.

As noted in Chapter 3, between 1950 and 2000, the proportion of the population aged 60 or older almost doubled to 15% in more developed countries (MDCs) while it increased by about a quarter to 5% in less developed countries (LDCs). These changes were largely driven by increases in life expectancy and declines in fertility. Between 1950 and 2000, life expectancy rose by 10 years (to 76) in

DOI: 10.1016/B978-0-12-380880-6.00006-X

MDCs, but rose by more than 20 years in LDCs (to 65 years). The total fertility rate (TFR), the number of children per reproductive age woman at current age-specific levels of childbearing, fell from 2.8 to 1.6 in MDCs and declined from 6.2 to 2.7 in LDCs. In these dimensions, LDCs in 2000 look much like the MDCs did fifty years earlier. Between 2000 and 2050, life expectancy is projected to increase by 10 years in LDCs (and by about half that in MDCs) and fertility is expected to fall to about replacement level.

Enormous gains in longevity have occurred since 1900, with life expectancy more than doubling in some countries. In developed countries improvements were most rapid during the first half of the century. Between 1950 and 2000, life expectancy in developing countries rose by more than 20 years, and the gap in life expectancy at birth between more- and less-developed countries was reduced by a decade, to about 12 years. By 2050, life expectancy is projected to rise by six years in MDCs and ten years in LDCs. In 2050, the life expectancy gap between the regions will be only eight years. For those who survive to age 60, individuals in MDCs can expect to live another 21 years, vs 18 for those from LDCs.

The implications of these changes are illustrated by population pyramids, which summarize the distribution of the population by age and sex. Pyramids for MDCS, presented in Figure 3.3 of Chapter 3, illustrate the gradual shift from a triangle in 1950 to a rectangle in 2050. Pyramids for LDCs are presented in Figure 6.1. Whereas the shape changed little over the last half of the twentieth century, projecting forward to 2050, the rectangularization of the pyramid reflects the rapid rate of graying of LDC populations. This unprecedented tempo will carry with it new challenges and new opportunities. Between 2006 and 2030, the number of older people in LDCs is projected to increase by 140%, vs 51% in MDCs (US NIA, 2007).

Although contrasting the population structures of LDCs and MDCs in aggregate is useful, enormous heterogeneity exists within these groups, as shown in Table 6.1. Consider Uganda and China, for example. In 2005, they stood at different ends of the distribution of median population age for LDCs, with median ages of 15 and 33, respectively.

Figure 6.2 displays the population pyramids for Uganda and China in 1950, 2000, and 2050. In 1950, Uganda and China both resemble the overall pattern for LDCs at that time (Figure 6.1), reflecting similar demographic profiles, with life expectancies around 40 and TFRs over 6.

By the year 2000, the population compositions had diverged. In Uganda life expectancy rose by about a decade, but fertility rates remained high (>7), resulting in a low median age and a pyramid with an exceptionally wide base. Over the same period, China's aggressive family planning program sharply curtailed fertility, while life expectancy rose by some three decades. By 2000 the base of China's pyramid had compressed and the middle and the top had widened.

The third column of Figure 6.2 depicts the expected pyramids in 2050, based on United Nations population projections (medium variant). By 2050 Uganda's projected life expectancy is 70 and its TFR is 3.4. The growth of Uganda's population will have slowed, but the population will remain young for decades to come. China, meanwhile, is projected to have a life expectancy of 80 and a TFR of 1.9. By 2050 the people who made up the young cohorts in 2000 will be middle-aged and older and China's pyramid will be much more rectangular.

Uganda and China exemplify the variation in developing countries. Table 6.1 provides summary statistics for Uganda, China, Bangladesh, South Africa, Mexico, and Indonesia. We highlight these countries both because their key demographic indicators fall at various points along the distributions for all LDCs and because good household data exist to highlight the implications of population aging.

The second and third rows present life expectancy and TFR for each country in 1950. Fertility and mortality are high everywhere. By 2005–10 major differences emerge. Life expectancy in South Africa has dropped a point, but is a full 76 years in Mexico. The TFR also exhibits tremendous variation, ranging from only 1.7 in China to 7.1 in Uganda.

The phenomena of declines in life expectancy (South Africa) and stubbornly high fertility (Uganda) are observed in other countries. A number of countries in sub-Saharan Africa have seen an erosion of progress in life expectancy as a result of HIV/AIDS, and parts of the former Soviet Union have also lost ground (Varnik et al., 2001). TFRs are above 6 in six countries other than Uganda.

The projection-generated statistics for 2045–2050 suggest that cross-LDC heterogeneity in demographic rates will diminish. For this period, life expectancy is between 76 and 80 for four of the six countries, and the TFR is 1.9 for all countries but Uganda. Whether these patterns materialize depends on how closely reality follows the projection assumptions. The most uncertain parameters are the timing and pace of decline in fertility in high-fertility countries and whether fertility will rise slightly in very low-fertility countries. Nevertheless, shifts to lower rates of fertility and mortality in developing countries will produce populations with much higher proportions of older people than is the case today, and at a far more rapid pace than in the developed world.

These fundamental shifts have powerful implications for society as services will focus more on the needs of older adults. Already, noncommunicable diseases (NCDs) are major causes of death in LDCs. As their prevalence rises, pressures on the health care

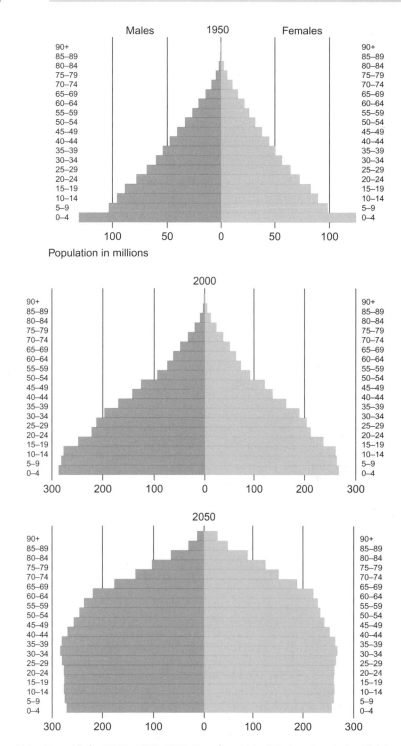

Figure 6.1 Population Pyramids for LDCS, 1950–2050. Data from United Nations Population Division, 2009, medium variant.

system will increase and health care costs will rocket. More generally, the public finance implications of an older population are daunting. Pensions and social security will absorb increasing fractions of global resources while the ratio of workers to dependents will decline. These pressures will be greatest where the number of older people increases while the total population shrinks. Other changes in society will occur

Table 6.1 Aging indicators for selected developing countries.

	UGANDA	BANGLADESH	SOUTH AFRICA	MEXICO	INDONESIA	CHINA
Median Age in 2005	15	22	24	25	27	33
1950–55						
Life expectancy	40	38	45	51	38	41
TFR	6.9	6.7	6.5	6.9	5.5	6.2
2005–10						
Life expectancy	52.1	65	44	76	69	73
TFR	7.1	3.0	2.6	2.1	2.2	1.7
2045–50						
Life expectancy	70	76	59	81	77	80
TFR	3.4	1.9	1.9	1.9	1.9	1.9
Total dependency ratio 2007	112	114	58	55	50	40
Total dependency ratio 2050	70	62	49	61	54	65

Source: United Nations, 2007a

as well. New options in elder care will emerge. Social safety nets will be developed to backstop the care that adult children typically provide and to support elderly individuals who have exhausted their own resources. Changes in age structures will have important implications for education and work opportunities, taxation of earnings and wealth, savings and insurance vehicles, and how earnings are taxed.

GLOBAL AGING AND HEALTH

Aging is a relative concept, with a meaning that differs across societies with different life expectancies. This complexity raises a host of issues, many of which are apparent in the literature on aging, health, and healthy aging.

Life expectancy is largely driven by deaths at early ages and so increases in life expectancy have presaged major shifts in the global burden of disease. Omran (1971) characterized change in causes of death as the epidemiologic transition, summarized as a shift of the major killers from infectious and acute diseases that primarily affect children, to chronic and degenerative NCDs. A hallmark of movement along the epidemiologic transition is that deaths associated with metabolic dysfunction and malignant neoplasms account for the majority of deaths. In Singapore, for example, over a 30-year period, life expectancy at birth rose by the same number of years, and the share of deaths from cardiovascular diseases rose from 5% to 32%, while the share from infectious diseases fell from 40% to 12% (Kinsella & He, 2009).

Causes of Death and the Epidemiologic Transition

Imperfect at best, cause-of-death data are weakest where health services are most stretched and death registers are absent. Major differences in the cause-of-death structure remain between developed and developing countries. A widely used scheme for classifying cause of death relies on three broad groups: communicable, perinatal, maternal, and nutritional conditions comprise Group I causes; NCDs comprise Group II causes; and injuries and accidents comprise Group III causes. In both MDCs and LDCs, deaths from injuries and accidents account for just under 10% of all deaths. In MDCs most other deaths (86% of the total) are from noncommunicable (Group II) diseases; in LDCs a full 40% of deaths are from Group I causes. Our example countries illustrate the continuum along which countries fall with respect to the importance of Group II vs Group I causes (Table 6.2). In China most deaths are from Group II causes, in South Africa the reverse is true, and in Bangladesh Groups I and II account for similar percentages of deaths.

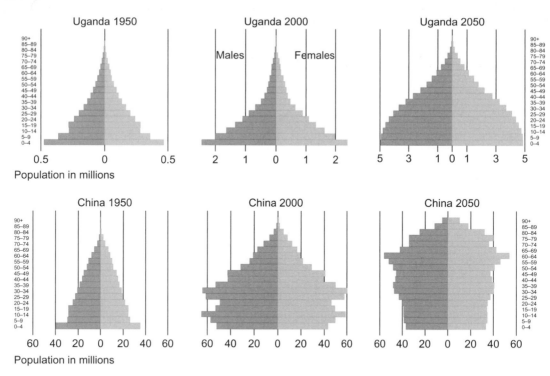

Figure 6.2 Evolution of population pyramids for Uganda and China. Data from United Nations Population Division, 2009, medium variant.

Table 6.2 Selected indicators: Health status, labor force participation, and living arrangements.

	BANGLADESH	SOUTH AFRICA	MEXICO	INDONESIA	CHINA
Health Indicators					
% deaths from Group I	46	65	16	29	12
% deaths from Group II	44	28	72	61	77
% deaths from Group III	10	7	11	10	11
% of male adults who smoke	47	28	37	66	60
Labor Force Participation					
Males aged 65+	66	26	46	69	34
Males aged 25-44	99	83	96	99	95
Females aged 65+	9	15	10	37	17
Females aged 25-44 yrs	27	65	53	54	84
Living Arrangements					
% males married at 60+	49	78	77	84	50
% females married at 60+	43	47	45	36	
Men per 100 women, 80+ years	88	41	72	70	58
% men living alone at age 60	1.8	8	7.2	2.4	8.1
% women living alone at age 60	3.3	8.2	9.6	11.9	8.1
Sources: United Nations, 2007a; Kinsella & He, 2009					

Delving into more detailed causes of death based on the Global Burden of Disease project, in both low-income and high-income countries, about one third of all deaths are caused by lower respiratory tract infections, ischaemic heart disease, cerebrovascular disease, or chronic obstructive pulmonary disease (WHO, 2006). In low-income countries, other big killers include diarrhoeal diseases, HIV/AIDS, tuberculosis, malaria, and prematurity and low birthweight, vs cancers, diabetes, and Alzheimer's disease (AD) in high-income countries. Based on projections to 2030, this partial overlap in top killers will remain relatively stable through to 2030, although for both low- and high-income countries diabetes will play a more important role by the end of the period (Mathers & Loncar, 2006).

Nutrition Transition and Global Epidemic of Obesity

For many years the nutritional difference between LDCs and MDCs that has received the most attention is the prevalence of malnutrition in poor countries. In contrast, one of the greatest public health achievements of the twentieth century in the developed world has been the eradication of nutrition deficiencies as the relative price of calories collapsed and foods were fortified with essential micro-nutrients. In recent years, attention has turned to the global epidemic of obesity.

Body mass index (BMI), which is weight (in kg) divided by height (in m) squared, has proved to be a very convenient summary, particularly for adults. Extreme values of BMI (underweight = BMI < 18.5 and overweight = BMI > 25) have been shown to be associated with elevated morbidity and mortality (Fogel, 2004; Waaler, 1984). Overweight adults, and particularly obese adults (BMI > 30), are at elevated risk of *inter alia* heart disease, dislipidemia, type II diabetes, stroke, and some types of cancers. Many of these are the NCDs prevalent among older adults in high-income countries, suggesting that the epidemiologic transition is likely to be accompanied by a nutrition transition (Popkin, 1994, 2002).

Figure 6.3 displays the distribution of BMI for adult males and females (aged 22 through 75) using survey data from six countries: Bangladesh, Indonesia, China, South Africa, Mexico, and the US. The countries are arrayed from poorest (at the top) to richest (at the bottom). Figure 6.3 presents non-parametric estimates of the shapes of the BMI distributions. Stark differences distinguish the three poorest countries in the upper half from the three richest in the lower half of the figure. In general, the distribution of BMI shifts to the right as development proceeds.

In Bangladesh, over half the adult population is underweight and less than 5% are overweight. Moving up the GDP distribution to China, only about 10% of the population is underweight whereas about 15% is overweight. Generally, women are more likely to be overweight than men, but differences are particularly dramatic in South Africa. The co-existence of under-nutrition and over-nutrition is a hallmark of many LDCs as they move through the nutrition transition.

Continuing up the GDP ladder, in Mexico, under-nutrition is rare but almost three-quarters of the population is overweight or obese. The Mexican and US distributions are very similar, although income per capita is about four times higher in the US than in Mexico. In terms of BMI, the developing world is catching up or surpassing the developed world, although incomes lag far behind.

The rate of increase in BMI in LDCs is far faster than it was in MDCs. In the US, the fraction of adults who were overweight doubled between 1960 and 2005. In Indonesia, the fraction doubled in the last 10 years. The drama of this transition is evident in Figure 6.4, which displays the fraction of the population that is overweight by birth cohort for the same respondents measured 10 years apart. Growth in the likelihood of being overweight is concentrated among younger adults. An Indonesian born in 1970 is around four times more likely to be overweight in 2007 relative to 1997. As the younger cohorts age, the prevalence of elevated BMI in Indonesia will increase dramatically, as will the health problems that are likely sequelae.

The availability of cheap calories high in fat and sugar, coupled with declines in energy output, are proximate contributors to the global epidemic of obesity, but they are not the whole story. In the poorest countries, older adults are more likely to be underweight than prime-age adults. In contrast, in richer countries, older adults are more likely to be overweight than prime-age adults. At the aggregate level, BMI and GDP are positively correlated. Within a population the association is more complex. BMI and SES tend to be positively associated in societies characterized by undernutrition and negatively correlated in societies characterized by overnutrition. As a population moves through the nutrition transition, the nutrition of the most educated (and highest income) improves first. This group is also the first to adjust diet and physical activity to avoid being overweight, suggesting that behavioral changes have important impacts on health outcomes. Across the globe, better-educated women tend to be on the vanguard of this transition. The relative importance of information, resources, technology, and other factors in these processes has not been established (see Monteiro et al., 2004 and Popkin, 1993 for excellent discussions of these issues).

Overweight and obesity are multisystem conditions that are associated with elevated mortality. Obesity has been implicated as a risk factor for type 2 diabetes, coronary heart disease, cancer, and other complications. While the costs of overweight and obesity

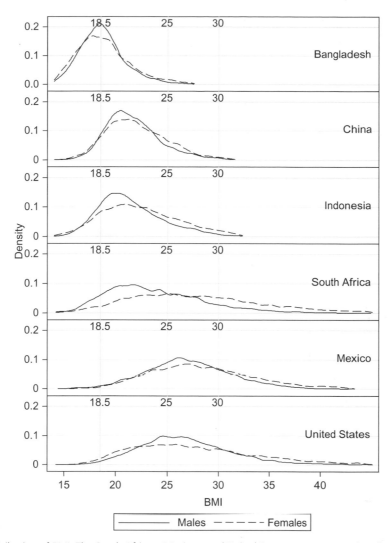

Figure 6.3 Distribution of BMI. The South African, Mexican, and United States surveys are nationally representative; the Indonesian survey is representative of about 80% of the Indonesian population; the Chinese survey is representative of nine provinces; and the Bangladesh survey is representative of one district.

are hard to estimate, they do include costs on the health care system and on economic output (such as treatment costs, reduced lifespan, and possibly direct costs). Olshansky et al. (2005) estimate that obesity reduces life expectancy by between one-third and three-quarters of a year in the US, and Preston (2005) discusses the merits of major campaigns for behavioral change akin to efforts waged on smoking and drunk driving. A case study of the direct and indirect costs of obesity in China concludes that the costs of obesity and related dietary and physical activity patterns account for between 3.6% and 8.7% of gross national product (GNP) in 2000 and 2025, respectively (Popkin et al., 2006).

The meaning and significance of BMI varies spatially and temporally. Optimal BMI (as measured by its association with mortality) has shifted up in developed countries over the last 30 years (Fogel, 2004). Moreover, BMI does not distinguish between lean tissue weight and weight due to body fat but the implications for health differ. For example, stress causes fat deposits around the abdomen, which in turn is a risk factor for some health conditions linked to obesity.

Elevated blood pressure is associated with stress and predicts CVD. In the US, about one-third of the population is either hypertensive (systolic blood pressure ≥140 mmHg or diastolic blood pressure ≥90 mmHg) or controlling hypertension with drugs. Figure 6.5 displays hypertension rates in Indonesia. The patterns and levels are very similar to those in the US, except that in the US around one-half of those who suffer from hypertension are controlling it with drugs. In Indonesia, less than one in twenty with hypertension

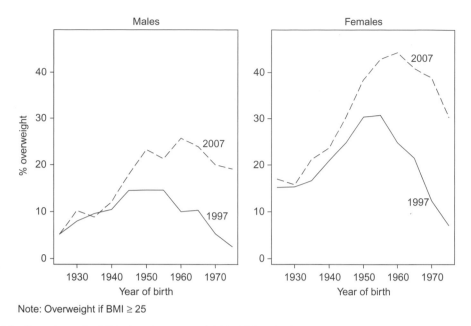

Note: Overweight if BMI ≥ 25

Figure 6.4 Percentage of adult Indonesians overweight by birth cohort.

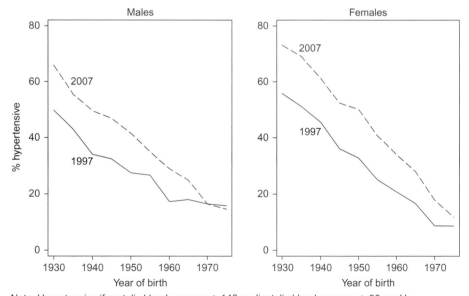

Note: Hypertensive if systolic blood pressure ≥ 140 or diastolic blood pressure ≥ 90 mmHg

Figure 6.5 Percentage of adult Indonesians hypertensive, by birth cohort.
Source: Panel respondents measured in 1997 and 2007 waves of Indonesia Family Life Survey.

are treated. High levels of undiagnosed hypertension are common in LDCs and will exact a toll as populations age.

The patterns reviewed above are important because research suggests that metabolic-related risk factors for CVD and diabetes may not be additive. Risks of CVD and diabetes are greatest among those who suffer from the so-called metabolic syndrome (a combination of elevated BMI, adiposity, elevated blood pressure, dyslipidemia, and inflammation).

The other side of the nutritional status coin in LDCs is micronutrient adequacy. Recent work hypothesizes that micronutrient deficiencies may cause mitochondrial damage that leads to late onset of degenerative diseases, including cancer (Ames, 2006). Mild-to-moderate deficiencies in iodine, Vitamin A, and zinc are common throughout the developing world, but the micronutrient that has received the most attention is iron. In low- and middle-income countries, iron deficiency anemia ranks 10th amongst causes of years lost to disability (WHO, 2008a). Rates of anemia among reproductive-age women are much higher than among same-age men, and iron deficiency contributes to more disabilities for women than men. Among older adults in developing countries, rates rise with advancing age (Patel, 2008). In Indonesia, rates of anemia in the late 1990s exceeded 25% for men 65 and older and more than 45% for women in that age range (Thomas et al., 2004).

Nutrition and disease insults during the fetal period and in early childhood are associated with poor health outcomes in mid- and later life, including elevated risks of obesity, dyslipidemia, glucose intolerance, and CVD (Barker, 2006; Finch & Crimmins, 2004). Health insults in early life may induce organs, metabolism, or gene expressions to adapt to the environment to ensure survival, with deleterious consequences for adult health. The consequences may be exacerbated if a child adapts to a nutritionally restricted environment in utero but enters a calorie-abundant environment at birth, in which the "thrifty gene" is maladaptive. This literature suggests an important contributing factor to the rapid increases in obesity and CVD in LDCs. Moreover, investments in improved reproductive and child health in developing countries today are likely to yield returns well into the future, given links between early- and later-life health.

Health-Related Behaviors

Obesity and smoking partially explain lower life expectancy in the US relative to other wealthy countries (Preston & Ho, 2009). The costs of smoking and obesity cumulate over the life course, emerging many years after onset. Ezzati and Lopez estimate that in 2000, nearly five million premature deaths were attributable to smoking worldwide, with deaths roughly equally divided between developed and developing countries. Nearly 80% of those who died were men, and over two million deaths were of individuals aged 70 and older (Ezzati & Lopez, 2004).

The implications for global aging are troubling. About one half of the world's smokers live in China, India, and Indonesia. In China and Indonesia, six or seven out of every ten men smoke, as do four or five out of every ten men in Mexico and Bangladesh (Table 6.2). Whereas developed countries have succeeded in reducing smoking, progress is more elusive in developing countries.

Use of alcohol is also relatively high in many developing countries. In Russia, for example, life expectancy has declined in recent years and the explanation is thought to lie with alcohol consumption and psychosocial stress (Brainerd & Cutler, 2005).

Other Measures of Population Health

Biological markers of health status have revolutionized research on population health, but relying exclusively on those markers and health-related behaviors limits progress on understanding global aging. Efforts to conduct population-based studies that measure other dimensions of health in the developing world have increased knowledge of health conditions, particularly for children and women of reproductive age. The evidence on the health of men and older adults is more fragmented.

Disability

Over the past 15 years a framework has been developed for quantifying how various health problems and diseases affect quality of life. The Global Burden of Disease project computes disability-adjusted life years, which measure the number of years of healthy life lost as a function of both premature death *and* disability from various conditions. More years of healthy living are lost in LDCs from both premature death and from disabilities than is the case in high-income countries.

If one restricts attention to the disability component, psychological conditions are an important source of poor health. Across the globe, depressive disorders account for the largest share of years lost to disability, in part because such a small fraction is treated. Very little research has explored the impact of traumatic events – such as an earthquake, tsunami, war, or even a financial crisis – on the well-being of the elderly. More generally, little is known about whether older adults are at greater risk than others of suffering from mental health problems in LDCs. Results from a recent round of surveys in 11 low- and middle-income countries do reveal that dementia is the foremost contribution to disability for the elderly (Sousa et al., 2009).

Putting aside the level of severity and considering adults more generally, poor vision and hearing account for a substantial portion of disabilities worldwide. These conditions are often untreated. The policy response to aging in developing countries will need to include increasing access to technologies that reduce the impact of these disabilities, as has happened in developed countries.

After age 40, the prevalence of moderate and severe disability rises sharply with age but evidence on disabilities is limited because of the complexities associated with measurement in population-based studies

(WHO, 2004a). Particularly in developing countries, this problem limits the scope for a precise understanding of how individuals cope with and adjust to disabilities.

Gender Differences in Health and Mortality

Apart from a few sub-Saharan African countries, life expectancy is higher for women than men. Women live some seven years longer in much of the developed world, whereas, in LDCs, the gap is closer to three years. The smaller gap in the developing world reflects, in part, higher rates of maternal mortality (450 vs 11 per 100 000). Over time the gender gap in life expectancy is expected to diminish in developed countries but increase somewhat in developing countries.

The reasons for women's systematic survival advantage are not entirely clear. Men use and abuse alcohol and tobacco at greater rates than women, and men also face greater occupational exposure to hazards. Injury and suicide rates are higher for men than for women. Women, on the other hand, typically experience higher rates of disability overall (Kinsella & He, 2009).

With respect to gender differences in mental health, men and women experience about the same burden from neuro-psychiatric disorders but causes are different. Depression is the leading cause for both men and women but the burden is about 50% higher for women. Women also suffer more from anxiety disorders, AD, and migraines (WHO, 2004a).

Health Services for Older Adults in Developing Countries

Public health services in developing countries typically do not reflect the needs of an aging population because they were originally designed with the goal of reducing infant and child mortality from infectious diseases. Improved child health likely yields benefits over the entire life course, but the health sector will increasingly face pressure to provide services geared towards NCDs and the needs of older adults.

As populations age and the most important causes of poor health shift towards NCDs, pressure will mount to change health sector priorities, particularly as health conditions increasingly reflect lifestyle choices such as smoking, poor diet, or inadequate exercise. Development of broad-based health policies that reduce risks for NCDs, in combination with effective and affordable primary care interventions for those with chronic NCDs, is essential (WHO, 2008b).

Other issues with the health care sector in many developing countries are that it is inefficient, and quality is low on average but highly variable. As the costs of treating an aging population increase, these problems must be addressed. The financing of health care services raises a multitude of challenges because public health services are typically heavily subsidized.

Worldwide, the distribution of the health work forces does not reflect the global burden of disease. The Americas Region (as defined by WHO, and including Canada and the US) accounts for 10% of the global burden of disease but claims as residents almost 37% of the world's health workers and more than 50% of health care expenditures (WHO, 2006). Indeed, a significant fraction of the health personnel trained in developing countries are working in the developed world where wages and working conditions are relatively better.

WORK, RETIREMENT, AND WEALTH ACCUMULATION IN AN AGING WORLD

The shape of a country's population pyramid provides a visual image of how the ratio of prime-age adults to younger and older individuals will change as time passes and individuals age. The pace of change of a country's working-age population has important implications for the economic resources on which the country can draw. Countries that can look forward to years of steady growth in the working-age population have the potential for sustained economic growth, a phenomenon called the "demographic dividend." But, in much of the developed world, growth of the working age population will slow or turn negative in the coming decades. In Japan, for example, population is projected to decline by 17% over the next 25 years. By 2050, there will be only 1.4 workers for every retiree in Japan (as opposed to a ratio of 3.4 today)

The adjustments that economies will make to changes in population age composition are unclear. If productivity of the existing workforce can be increased, reductions in workforce growth will be absorbed. Other responses that focus more explicitly on the size of the workforce include encouraging more immigration, increased labor force participation, and higher fertility.

Over the next 25 years a number of countries, including Japan, Russia, Spain, Germany, and South Korea, will experience a contraction in the size of the work force. China, Australia, and the US can expect moderate labor force growth (0%–25%). Growth of the labor force will range from 25% to 50% in countries such as Brazil, India, and Indonesia, but will exceed 50% in the Middle East and much of sub-Saharan Africa. These trends drive changes in the dependency ratio. While steady growth of the working-age population is generally an advantage with respect to economic performance, it is important to note that countries with very rapid growth in the working-age population face the challenge of finding employment for all those who want it and averting discontent among the un- and underemployed (Hayutin, 2007).

Age-Specific Rates of Work

Although a population's age composition roughly delineates the size of the groups likely to be working, whether one works is an individual choice and the fraction working varies dramatically both by age and sex. Among prime-age men (25–44), participation rates are universally high, typically 85% or more. In developed countries labor force participation rates drop off sharply with age, so that, at ages above 65, rates for men are below 10% in most European countries and between 10% and 20% in North America and Oceania (Kinsella & He, 2009).

Participation rates among older adults are markedly higher in many developing countries. In our illustrative countries (Table 6.2), male labor force participation at age 65 and above varies from 26% in South Africa to 69% in China. Differences in the decline in participation rates by age are correlated with differences in GNP (United Nations, 2007b). In countries that have social security and pension programs, these mechanisms can provide some measure of financial security in older age.

Female labor force participation is lower than male participation at all ages. Among prime-age women in developed countries, rates are 75% to 85%. In developing countries rates vary tremendously, for example from 27% in Bangladesh to 84% in China. At 65 and above, rates are much lower: ranging from 9% in Bangladesh to 17% in China.

In Europe and the US, labor force participation of older adults has risen markedly since the 1980s (Kinsella & He, 2009). The fraction of working men aged 65–69 increased from a quarter to a third between 1985 and 2005 (Rix, 2009). For women, the growth was even more dramatic. These changes are likely driven by a number of factors interrelated in complex ways: rising education levels that may affect motivation to work; decline in physically demanding work; changes in Social Security so that work past retirement age is rewarded rather than penalized; shifts from defined benefit (DB) pensions to defined contribution (DC) pensions; and economic downturn.

Less information is available on change over time in participation rates of older people in developing countries, but data from some more advanced LDCs suggest that, for men 65 and older, participation rates declined between the early 1970s and the late 1990s (Kinsella & Velkoff, 2001).

Retirement and the Lifecycle Model of Savings

The term "retirement" suggests an abrupt switch from full-time work to full-time leisure. In reality, for most of the world's population the process of moving out of the labor force is far more gradual, even in developed countries. In industrialized countries the term "bridge employment" is used to describe a myriad of work arrangements that serve as stepping stones out of the labor force, such as reduced hours at the same job, performing a different job for the same employer, or changing jobs and employer to one with fewer demands.

In developing countries work is far less regulated and so age-related shifts in the nature of work are more fluid. That said, shifts toward reduced hours or into different tasks may begin at earlier ages in developing countries because many jobs are based on manual labor and so are more physically demanding. In addition, health declines in LDCs tend to begin at earlier ages.

The lifecycle model of savings posits that people save during their prime working years in order to finance consumption during retirement. In Thailand and Taiwan, however, increased rates of savings have been documented at all ages (Deaton, 1992; Deaton & Paxson, 1994, 2000).

As life expectancy has risen, an obvious question is whether individuals anticipate living longer and plan for that by working longer, saving more, or both. Analyses of data from Taiwan suggest that the rise in saving rates there closely tracks the increases in life expectancy and that in many cases the savings are passed on as bequests to the next generation (Tsai et al., 2000). Bloom and colleagues (2007) analyzed this issue for the US, using data on subjective probabilities of survival provided by respondents to the HRS. They found that people who expect to live longer accrue higher levels of wealth, but do not actually work longer. It is not entirely clear how to interpret this association.

Institutional Regulation of Employment and Old-Age Support

The notion of "working one day, retired the next" was perhaps most apt for developed countries in the 1950s and earlier when pension receipts were tightly tied to age. Over time, governments in developed countries have tried various policy levers to influence employment by age. Whether these policies aim to ease older workers out of employment to clear the way for younger workers, or to keep older workers employed because of a need for labor, depends on a country's age structure and economic situation.

One policy that strongly affects employment rates is the extent of benefits for workers in poor health. Other important policies are the age at which retired workers become eligible for full benefits, and the extent to which retiring at a later age is rewarded or penalized. Gruber and Wise (2007) analyzed cross-country data on the relationship between social security policies and labor force participation, concluding that a three-year increase in the retirement age could cut the costs of old-age security programs by over one-quarter.

Over the past several decades the number of countries with old-age, disability, and survivor programs has increased five-fold, from 33 in 1940 to 167 in 2004 (Kinsella & He, 2009). All of the developing countries we consider in this chapter have some type of program in place and many of the programs have been reformed several times. (South Africa's first law took effect in 1928. Mexico and China introduced legislation in 1943 and 1951, respectively. Uganda, Indonesia, and Bangladesh were relative latecomers, adopting laws in 1967, 1977, and 1998, respectively.) The majority of programs are geared towards workers in the public sector or the formal private sector. Benefits for the self-employed and those who are employed informally are less well-developed. Some countries have instituted programs to support all older adults, or the least well-off, placing a large burden on public finances and subsequent generations.

The Old Age Pension program in South Africa illustrates some of the complexities associated with designing, implementing, and evaluating the impact of these programs. The noncontributory program in South Africa provides income to adults aged 60 (or 61) and older who satisfy an income and asset means test. When instituted in 1993, the benefit was extremely generous: beneficiaries received about twice the median per capita income of households in rural South Africa and most older blacks in the country were eligible for the benefit. The program absorbed around 1.4% of GDP. Since then, the value of the benefit has declined by over a third in real terms. Evidence suggests that the program has benefited not only the elderly but also others in their extended families either directly or indirectly through reduced demands on the resources of younger generations. A major challenge for research lies in understanding how public and private support interact in societies where living arrangements are fluid and family obligations particularly across generations are strong.

Macroeconomics and the Age Structure

A large body of literature discusses the potential for a demographic dividend arising because of the macroeconomic consequences of changes in age structure of populations (Bloom & Canning, 2001; Lee et al., 2001). The dividend is thought to have two components. First, over the course of the demographic transition, an opportunity for sustained economic growth emerges because of increased shares of the population in working ages. Whereas some countries, particularly Taiwan, Korea, and Singapore, have realized this first dividend, others countries have not (Clark et al., 2007), suggesting an important role for institutions and policies to harvest such benefits.

A second dividend may arise as a consequence of increases in wealth that also arise from changes in age structure. Within a population, the elderly are often the wealthiest, so, as their share of the population rises, so do average wealth holdings (Mason & Lee, 2007). These assets support the elderly, reducing the extent to which they rely on those currently in the labor force for support. Mason & Lee (2007) developed a model of these processes, concluding that, if policies focus solely on providing for the elderly through the transfer of resources from the working-age population to the elderly, the opportunity that asset accumulation provides for sustaining permanently higher standards of living will not be realized. Fully understanding the costs and benefits of the "demographic dividend" remains an important challenge for research.

FAMILIES, LIVING ARRANGEMENTS, AND INTERGENERATIONAL TRANSFERS

Worldwide, family members are the most important providers of support and care for older people. Because declines in fertility rates are relatively recent phenomena in LDCs, the current generation of older people typically has surviving siblings and children that form an important support network. The density of these networks will diminish as lower-fertility cohorts begin to age and family structures evolve toward the "beanpole" families (decreased numbers of members within each generation and an increase in the number of living generations) that characterize MDCs.

The survival advantage of women has important implications for living arrangements at older years. The older population is dominated by women. In Russia, for every 100 women above age 65 there are only 45 men. Ratios are low in other Eastern European countries as well, reflecting both heavy male mortality during World War II and higher male mortality at the adult ages (Brainerd, 2001; Mesle & Vallin, 2002). In most developed countries women predominate at older ages.

In LDCs, the ratios of men to women are much higher (about 90 for the 65–79 age range and around 67 for age 80 and above). These aggregate figures mask tremendous cross-country variation. Drawing on our illustration countries, at 80 years and above the number of men per 100 women is only 41 in South Africa but is 88 in Bangladesh (Table 6.2). The larger ratio in Bangladesh arises in part because women's survival advantage is smaller there than in many other parts of the world.

A related phenomenon of old age is that many more women than men are unmarried. The sex ratio at older ages contributes to this. So do the facts that women tend to marry older men (which compounds the effect of men's survival disadvantage) and that men are more likely than women to remarry after the death of a spouse. In developed and developing countries, at ages over 75, some 70% of men are married vs only about 20% of women (Kinsella & He, 2009).

In our sample countries, the fraction of men married at age 60 and older ranges from 49% in South Africa to 84% in Indonesia. For women in this age group the variation is much smaller, from 36% in Indonesia to 47% in South Africa. While establishing a causal relationship is far from straightforward, the descriptive evidence indicates that, at older ages, marriage is associated with physical and mental health benefits (see Manzoli et al., 2007). This suggests that being single at older ages, and living arrangements more generally, may have important implications for the QOL of older people.

A number of factors shape the choices older people make about living arrangements as well as patterns in living arrangements across countries. These include marital status, kin availability, wealth, health, preferences, and cultural and institutional contexts. Norms regarding children's responsibilities to older parents are important aspects of culture in many regions, and in China have even been adopted into law (Frankenberg & Kuhn, 2004; Zeng & George, 2010). Moreover, few developing countries have any institutional capacity to provide long-term residential care for aging citizens, although the need for such capacity will increase dramatically over the next 50 years.

For older adults who are married, the most common arrangement is to live with one's spouse. In developed countries older women who are widowed tend to live alone, whereas in developing countries this group more typically lives with kin. Worldwide the fraction of individuals age 60 and above who live alone is estimated at about 14%, but the rate is more than twice as high for women as for men (United Nations, 2005).

There is considerable regional variation in the fraction of older people living alone. The United Nations data put rates of solo living below 10% in most African and Asian countries and between 10% and 20% in Latin America and the Caribbean. In contrast, in the more developed countries between one-fifth and one-third of those aged 60 and above live alone (United Nations, 2005).

The availability of kin, most notably offspring, is important in determining living arrangements. In developing countries, opportunities to live with kin are relatively widespread, and living with or near kin is very common. Data from the United Nations confirm that, in most countries in Africa, Asia, Latin America, and the Caribbean, more than 60% of older individuals co-reside with children or grandchildren (United Nations, 2005). Analysis of Demographic and Health Survey (DHS) data on living arrangements across 43 countries confirms these general patterns (Bongaarts & Zimmer, 2002). Bongaarts and Zimmer show that, in countries where educational levels are higher, older adults are more likely to live alone or in smaller households with fewer children. This relationship does not extend to other dimensions of SES and well-being, such as per capita GNP and life expectancy.

Some work has drawn on panel data to examine transitions in living arrangements. In Indonesia, Singapore, and Taiwan, not only do most older people share a residence with kin at a point in time, but they also tend to stay in this pattern for many years (Frankenberg et al., 2002).

In some countries intergenerational co-residence is declining. In Japan, adult children used to pre-empt the inevitable by sharing a residence with older parents before the needs of those parents necessitated it; now the pattern has shifted towards delaying co-residence until necessity intervenes (Takagi et al., 2007). A trend towards lower levels of intergenerational co-residence has also been observed in many European countries (Kinsella & He, 2009).

It is important to note that intergenerational co-residence reflects needs and preferences of both generations, not just one or the other. In some developed countries, older people share residences with children, but these children are still relatively young and may simply not yet have left home, or older children have returned to the homes that their parents own with the idea that they will one day inherit the residence (Frankenberg et al., 1999; United Nations, 2005). In countries where agriculture and small-scale family enterprise are important components of the economy, the older generation may control key economic assets such as land and equipment. Moreover, older people can provide labor for both home production and businesses, with the former of perhaps particular importance as the labor force participation of women with children rises.

In Africa, HIV/AIDS has shifted the picture of intergenerational relations to some degree. When prime-age individuals become ill, it is often their older parents who assume responsibility first for their care and then for the care of any grandchildren (Merli & Palloni, 2006). Skipped-generation households, in which young children live with their grandparents because their parents have died, are increasingly common.

Using DHS data from counties in sub-Saharan Africa, Zimmer (2007) shows that about 14% of older people live in a skipped-generation household. How long these arrangements will endure, and who will provide for the eventual needs of aging grandparents as the grandchildren get older, is unclear.

Institutional living is an important component of the living arrangements landscape in more developed countries, particularly for the oldest old and for women. Limited data are available on the proportion of older people in institutions, but, in developed countries in the late 1990s, rates ranged from 4% to 12% (Gibson et al., 2003). Few such institutions even exist in developing countries. Reviewing census data from China in 2000, Zeng & George (2010) report that in urban areas 5% and 3% of women and men aged 65+ lived in nursing homes for the elderly, vs 2% and 1% for rural older men and women.

A decline in kinship support through co-residence seems inevitable in China, because the ratio of older adults to eligible prime-age kin will increase. Eventually, couples who are each from "one child" families will have up to four parents and eight grandparents for whom to provide support.

Two other phenomena have the potential to further erode patterns of adult child–older parent co-residence. One is childlessness. Considerable cross-country variation exists in the proportion of individuals who are childless, but rates of childlessness have increased among middle-aged women in the developed world, and will likely rise eventually in the developing world as well. A second factor is migration. As young and prime-age adults move out of rural to urban areas or international destinations, older parents may find themselves left behind and alone in rural areas.

But adult children may substitute financial help for shared living. A number of studies have explored the occurrence and correlates (and in some cases the magnitudes) of intergenerational exchange in contexts in which industrialization is well under way (for example, Agree et al., 2005; Biddlecom et al., 2002; Chan, 1999; Knodel et al., 1992; Lee et al., 1994). The preponderance of evidence from Asia suggests that, although co-residence has declined in some East Asian countries, the majority of parents receive financial support from their children, despite the potentially centrifugal forces of industrialization and modernization.

Frankenberg and Kuhn (2005) compared parent–child transfers in Indonesia and Bangladesh, countries whose development has proceeded at different paces and with very different norms regarding the responsibilities of sons and daughters for parental support. They found strong evidence that traditional patterns of family organization leave an enduring imprint on transfer patterns, based on cross-country differences in the relative roles of adult sons and daughters in providing for their parents. Studies of intergenerational transfer flows in other historically patriarchal and patrilineally oriented societies (Taiwan and South Korea) suggest that sons play a more important role than daughters in providing financial support to elders, particularly following marriage (Lee et al., 1994). In Vietnam, also a relatively patriarchal society, the relative roles of sons and daughters in the provision of financial assistance to elderly parents are less pronounced (Knodel et al., 2000). Biddlecom et al. (2002) presented results regarding the roles of sons and daughters with respect to financial support for parents in Thailand, the Philippines, and Taiwan. In the Philippines and Thailand (where kinship is reckoned bilaterally), parents are slightly more likely to receive financial support from daughters than from sons. In Taiwan parents are much more likely to receive support in the form of money from sons than from daughters, but the reverse is true for support in the forms of goods.

As with co-residence, transfers do not flow unilaterally from children to older parents. The data from Bangladesh and Indonesia show that parents both give and receive transfers with non-co-resident children, although the latter is more common (Frankenberg & Kuhn, 2004). On the other hand, data from the US and Europe show that most older parents are more likely to provide assistance to children than to receive it (US National Institute of Aging, 2007). These differences likely reflect in part the greater availability of institutional mechanisms that support saving for old age in developed countries.

GLOBAL AGING, POPULATION WELL-BEING, AND FUTURE RESEARCH

Global aging represents one of the most remarkable triumphs of mankind and, at the same time, poses one of the greatest challenges for society. Within a few years, for the first time in recorded history, older adults (age >65) will outnumber children (age <5). The developed world made the transition over the last two or three generations. Developing countries will do it within the space of a single generation. Not only is the tempo faster but the scale is greater given the size of the population in the developing world.

The impact of global aging on the well-being of the elderly and the generations behind them is not well understood. Much can be learned from the experience of the developed world. But much remains to be learned in developing countries. This is an exciting area for innovative research that has the potential to contribute to a better understanding of the meaning of aging and how it varies over contexts; the factors that influence healthy aging; and the consequences of aging for well-being across the generations.

Recent advances in the availability and quality of population-based data from LDCs will have a major impact on the field. Many of these surveys have been designed to assure comparability with studies in other developed and developing countries. These publicly accessible data afford unique opportunities to exploit the social, economic, health, demographic, and genetic heterogeneity that exists across the globe to better understand the behavioral choices of individuals and their families along with shedding new light on the drivers that underlie human health and well-being.

The field of global aging is in its infancy. An exciting area for innovative research, it provides unparalleled opportunities for making major contributions to both policy and science.

ACKNOWLEDGMENTS

We are very grateful to Linda George and Steve Cutler, whose comments substantially improved this work. Some of the research reported here has been conducted with financial support from the National Institutes on Aging (R01AG031266, R01AG030668, and R01AG20276).

REFERENCES

Agree, E. M., Biddlecom, A. E., & Valente, T. W. (2005). Intergenerational transfers of resources between older persons and extended kin in Taiwan and the Philippines. *Population Studies, 59*, 181–195.

Ames, B. (2006). Low micronutrient intake may accelerate the degenerative diseases of aging through allocation of scarce micronutrients by triage. *PNAS, 103*(47), 17589–17594.

Barker, D. J. P. (2006). Esther and Isadore Kesten Memorial Lecture, Leonard David School of Gerontology *California: University of Southern California*

Biddlecom, A., Chayovan, N., & Ofstedal, M. B. (2002). Intergenerational support and transfers. In A. I. Hermalin (Ed.), *The Well-being of the Elderly in Asia. A four-country comparative study* (pp. 185–207). Ann Arbor: University of Michigan Press.

Bloom, D. E., & Canning, D. (2001). Cumulative casualty, economic growth, and the demographic transition. In N. Birdsall, A. C. Kelley & S. W. Sinding (Eds.), *Population Matters: Demographic change, economic growth, and poverty in the developing world* (pp. 165–200). Oxford: Oxford University Press.

Bloom, D. E., Canning, D., Mansfield, R. K., & Moore, M. (2007). Demographic change, social security systems, and

savings. *Journal of Monetary Economics, 54*, 92–114.

Bongaarts, J., & Zimmer, Z. (2002). Living arrangements of older adults in the developing world: An analysis of demographic and health survey household surveys. *Journal of Gerontology: Social Sciences, 57*, S145–S157.

Brainerd, E. (2001). Economic reform and mortality in the former Soviet Union: A study of the suicide epidemic in the 1990s. *European Economic Review, 45*, 1007–1019.

Brainerd, E., & Cutler, D. M. (2005). *Autopsy on an Empire: Understanding mortality in Russia and the former Soviet Union.* William Davidson Institute Working Paper, Number 740.

Chan, A. (1999). The role of formal versus informal support of the elderly in Singapore: Is there substitution? *Southeast Asian Journal of Social Science, 27*(2), 87–110.

Clark, R., Ogawa, N., & Mason, A. (2007). *Population aging, intergenerational transfers and the macroeconomy.* Northampton, MA: Edward Elgar Publishing Inc.

Deaton, A. (1992). *Understanding consumption.* Oxford: Oxford University Press.

Deaton, A., & Paxson, C. (1994). Intertemporal choice and inequality. *Journal of Political Economy, 102*, 437–467.

Deaton, A., & Paxson, C. (2000). Growth, demographic structure,

and national saving in Taiwan. *Population and Development Review, 26*, 141–173.

Ezzati, M., & Lopez, A. D. (2004). Regional, disease specific patterns of smoking-attributable mortality in 2000. *Tobacco Control, 13*, 388–395.

Finch, C. E., & Crimmins, E. M. (2004). Inflammatory exposure and historical changes in human life-spans. *Science, 305*, 1736–1739.

Fogel, R. W. (2004). *The escape from hunger and premature death, 1700–2100.* Cambridge: Cambridge University Press.

Frankenberg, E., & Kuhn, R. S. (2004). The role of social context in shaping intergenerational relations in Indonesia and Bangladesh. *Annual Review of Gerontology and Geriatrics, 24*(1), 177–199.

Frankenberg, E., & Kuhn, R. S. (2005). The implications of family systems and economic context for intergenerational transfers in Indonesia and Bangladesh. CCPR Working Paper, 027-04, UCLA.

Frankenberg, E., Beard, V., & Saputra, M. (1999). The kindred spirit: The ties that bind Indonesian children and their parents. *Southeast Asian Journal of Social Science, 27*, 65.

Frankenberg, E., Chan, A., & Ofstedal, M. B. (2002). Stability and change in living arrangements in Indonesia, Singapore, and

Taiwan, 1993-99. *Population Studies, 56*, 201–213.

Gibson, M., Gregory, S., & Pandya, S. (2003). *Long-term care in developed nations: A brief overview.* AARP Policy and Research Report, 2003-13. Washington, DC.

Gruber, J., & Wise, D. A. (2007). *Social security programs and retirement around the world.* Chicago: University of Chicago Press.

Hayutin, A. M. (2007). How population aging differs across countries: A briefing on global demographics. Palo Alto, CA: Stanford University.

Kinsella, K., & He, W. (2009). *An aging world: 2008.* In US Census Bureau (Ed.), *International Population Reports* P95/09-1. Washington, DC: US Government Printing Office.

Kinsella, K., & Velkoff, V. A. (2001). *An aging world: 2001.* US Census Bureau (Ed.), *International Population Report* P95/01-1. Washington, DC: US Government Printing Office.

Knodel, J., Napaporn, C., & Siriwan, S. (1992). The impact of fertility decline on familial support for the elderly. *Population and Development Review, 18*, 79–103.

Knodel, J., Friedman, J., Anh, T., & Cuong, B. (2000). Inter-generational exchanges in Vietnam: Family size, sex composition, and the location of children. *Population Studies, 54*, 89–104.

Lee, R. D., Mason, A., & Miller, T. (2001). Saving, wealth, and population. In N. Birdsall, A. C. Kelley & S. W. Sinding (Eds.), *Population matters: Demographic change, economic growth, and poverty in the developing world* (pp. 137–164). Oxford: Oxford University Press.

Lee, Y. J., Parish, W. L., & Willis, R. J. (1994). Sons, daughters, and intergenerational support in Taiwan. *American Journal of Sociology, 99*, 1010–1041.

Manzoli, L., Villari, P., Pirone, G. M., & Bocciab, A. (2007). Marital status and mortality in the elderly: A systematic review and meta-analysis. *Social Science & Medicine, 60*, 77–94.

Mason, L., & Lee, R. (2007). Transfers, capital and consumption over the demographic transition. *Population Aging, Intergenerational Transfers and the Macroeconomy*, 128–162.

Mathers, C., & Loncar, D. (2006). Projections of mortality and global burden of disease from 2002–2030. *PLoS Medicine, 3*(11), 2011–2030.

Merli, M. G., & Palloni, A. P. (2006). The HIV/AIDS epidemic, kin relations, living arrangements and the African elderly in South Africa. In B. Cohen & J. Menken (Eds.), *Aging in sub-Saharan Africa: Recommendations for furthering research* (pp. 117–165). Washington, DC: National Academies Press.

Mesle, F., & Vallin, J. (2002). Mortality in Europe: The divergence between east and west. *Population, 57*, 171–212.

Monteiro, C., Moura, E., Wolney, L., & Popkin, B. (2004). Socioeconomic status and obesity in adult populations of developing countries: A review. *Bulletin of the World Health Organization, 82*(12), 940–946.

Olshansky, S. J., Passaro, D. J., Hershow, R. C., Layden, J., Carnes, B. A., Brody, J., et al. (2005). A potential decline in life expectancy in the United States in the 21st century. *New England Journal of Medicine, 352*, 1138–1145.

Omran, A. R. (1971). Epidemiological transition: A theory of the epidemiology of population change. *Milbank Quarterly, 49*, 509–538.

Patel, K. V. (2008). Epidemiology of anemia in older adults. *Seminars in Hematology, 45*, 210–217.

Popkin, B. M. (1993). Nutritional patterns and transitions. *Population and Development Review, 19*, 138–157.

Popkin, B. M. (1994). The nutrition transition in low-income countries – An emerging crisis. *Nutrition Reviews, 52*, 285–298.

Popkin, B. M. (2002). The shift in stages of the nutrition transition in the developing world differs from past experiences! *Public Health Nutrition, 2002*(5), 205–214.

Popkin, B. M., Kim, S., Rusev, E. R., Du., S., & Zizza, C. (2006). Measuring the full economic costs of diet, physical activity and obesity-related chronic diseases. *Obesity Reviews, 7*, 271–293.

Preston, S. H. (2005). Deadweight? – The influence of obesity on longevity. *New England Journal of Medicine, 352*, 1135–1137.

Preston, S. H., & Ho, J. Y. (2009). *Low life expectancy in the United States: Is the health care system at fault?* Cambridge, MA: National Bureau of Economic Research.

Rix, S. E. (2009). Employment at older ages. In P. Uhlenberg (Ed.), *International handbook of population aging* (pp. 445–470). Dordrecht: Springer-Verlag.

Sousa, R. M., Ferri, C. P., Acosta, D., Albanese, E., Guerra, M., Huang, Y., et al. (2009). Contribution of chronic diseases to disability in elderly people in countries with low and middle incomes: A 10/66 Dementia Research Group population-based survey. *The Lancet, 374*(9704), 1821–1830.

Takagi, E., Silverstein, M., & Crimmins, E. (2007). Inter-generational coresidence of older adults in Japan: Conditions for cultural plasticity. *Journal of Gerontology: Social Sciences, 62*, S330–S339.

Thomas, D., Frankenberg, E., Friedman, J., Habicht, J. P., McKelvey, C., Pelto, G., et al. (2004). *Causal effect of health on labor market outcomes.* CCPR Working Paper 022-04, UCLA.

Tsai, I. J., Chu, C. Y. C., & Chung, C. F. (2000). Demographic transition and household saving in Taiwan. *Population and Development Review, 26*, 174–193.

United Nations (2005). *Living arrangements of older persons around the world.* New York, NY: United Nations.

United Nations (2007a). *World population ageing 2007.* New York, NY: United Nations.

United Nations (2007b). *World economic and social survey 2007: Development in an ageing world.* New York, NY: United Nations.

US National Institute of Aging (2007). *Why population aging matters: A global perspective.*

Washington, DC: US Department of State.

Varnik, A., Wasserman, D., Palo, E., & Tooding, L. (2001). Registration of external causes of death in the Baltic States 1970–1997. *European Journal of Public Health, 11*, 84–88.

Waaler, H. T. (1984). Height, weight, and mortality: The Norwegian experience. *Acta Medica Scand suppl., 679*, 1–51.

World Health Organization. (2004a). *Healthy life expectancy (HALE) at birth and age 60, by sex, WHO Member States, 2002*. The World health report 2004: Changing history. Geneva: World Health Organization.

World Health Organization (2004b). *Regional overview of social health insurance in South-East Asia.* New Delhi: World Health Organization, Regional Office for South-East Asia.

World Health Organization. (2006). *Working together for health.* The World Health Report 2006. Geneva: WHO.

World Health Organization. (2008a). *Global burden of disease: 2004 update.* The World Health Report 2008. Geneva: WHO.

World Health Organization. (2008b). *Primary health care: Now more than ever.* The World Health Report 2008. Geneva: WHO.

Zeng, Y., & George, L. K. (2010). Population aging and old age insurance in China. In W. D. Dannefer & C. Phillipson (Eds.), *Handbook of social gerontology.* Thousand Oaks, CA: Sage.

Zimmer, Z. (2007). *HIV/AIDS and the living arrangements of older persons across the sub-Saharan African Region.* University of Utah Institute of Public and Internal Affairs Working Paper, 21 November.

Chapter | 7 |

Racial and Ethnic Influences Over the Life Course

James S. Jackson[1], Ishtar O. Govia[2], Sherrill L. Sellers[3]

[1]*University of Michigan, Ann Arbor, Michigan,* [2]*University of the West Indies, Mona, Jamaica and University of Michigan, Ann Arbor, Michigan,* [3]*Miami University, Oxford, Ohio*

CHAPTER CONTENTS

INTRODUCTION

This chapter presents a framework for how age-, period-, and cohort-related phenomena might intersect with identities and other status characteristics to influence the health of racial and ethnic group members across the life course in the US. We propose that life course models of the aging of racial and ethnic minority persons in the US must attend to historical, cohort, age, and other social status factors, including generation, socioeconomic position (SEP), and gender, to be fully reflective of the complex realities of life among ethnic and racial minorities. Nuanced life course models are particularly imperative now in comparison to prior eras in US history, because of the unprecedented number of aging persons who are projected for the world and the US by 2050. Age distributions across the globe are being fundamentally reshaped by increased individual longevity, reduced population fertility, and low levels of immigration (Christensen et al., 2009), such that there soon will be more individuals over 60 than there are under 15 years of age in the US (Rowe & Berkman, 2009). We suggest a framework of aging among racial and ethnic groups that addresses the dynamic intersections of age-, period-, and cohort-related phenomena, social identities, and other social and psychological statuses.

Longevity gains are a significant achievement of the twentieth and early twenty-first centuries; over this period advanced industrial nations have reduced death by childbirth and infectious diseases, reduced rates of infant mortality, and controlled chronic illnesses more effectively. In spite of longevity boosts in many industrialized countries, however, these countries differ in how quickly changes in their aging pyramids have, or will, transition. For example, the coming of the aging society in the US is delayed when compared to many parts of Europe, but it is inevitable (Olshansky et al., 2009).

In the US, racial and ethnic minority persons contribute in multiple ways to the enormous diversity

DOI: 10.1016/B978-0-12-380880-6.00007-1

that will characterize the reshaped aging pyramid. First, increased longevity is quite prevalent among several racial and ethnic groups (e.g. Chinese, Japanese, Cuban, and Mexican Americans). Second, the younger native populations of these groups typically have higher fertility rates than non-Hispanic whites (e.g. Mexican Americans). Third, a large proportion of the populations in these groups, particularly Hispanics, are foreign-born (US Census Bureau, 2008). By 2030, all of these trends will produce a society in which the non-Hispanic white population will be the numerical minority in the US population. In addition, the population of ethnic minority elderly is increasing at a faster rate than their majority counterparts and by 2050 will constitute 42% of the population aged over 65. Non-Hispanic whites have declined from being 80% of the total elderly population in 1980 to 74% in 2008 and are expected to constitute only 58% of the total elderly population by 2050 (US Census Bureau, 2008).

Second, implicit in these demographic transitions is that there will also be increased diversity in countries and cultures containing significant numbers of ethnic and racial minority groups. These group members possess histories and life course experiences that unfortunately are often associated with early disadvantages culminating in health inequalities in later life (Adler et al., 2010; Jackson & Govia, 2009). These changes are generating new challenges for individuals and governments (Robinson et al., 2007).

Considering social, economic, health, and psychological disparities among social groups over the life course demands that we consider how such disparities arise, how they are maintained, and how they are reproduced across generations. Most theoretical formulations are either silent about the sources of such disparities or static in their notions of fundamental social causes (Phelan et al., 2004). In this chapter we conceptualize disparities as a complex, dynamic intersectional function of intergenerational positioning, historical time, period events, and compositional differences among cohorts. While this conceptualization increases the complexity of the notion of fundamental social causes, we think it is appropriate and necessary. It will aid in understanding at any given point in time, space, and individual age how group memberships shape socioeconomic statuses, life chances, and health statuses.

People arrive at specific points in their life course at particular ages; in particular spaces; with particular liabilities because of an intricate web of genetics, epigenetic influences, parental opportunities, and early life experiences; their family, friends, and institutional memberships; and their own unique life trajectories. Equally important: because group memberships produce very complex, interweaving experiences dictated by genetic endowments; historical family experiences and opportunities; environmental circumstances; and

individual and group life experiences; any individual sharing a particular social attribute (gender, race, ethnicity, etc.) may become enmeshed with the life experiences of others who share their race, ethnicity, gender, or geographical location. Thus, the individual intergenerational and life course experiences become interwoven with those of other, non-familial, members of their social groups, for whom their contact may only be imagined over vast geographical (and historical) distances (Anderson, 1989).

These intersections produce contemporary social, economic, psychological, and health disparities at differing points in the individual life course when the racial, ethnic, or socioeconomic group membership(s) of one person is compared to the group membership(s) of another. What produces these differences is an inevitable intersection of genetic and epigenetic influences; congenital and early life circumstances; life exposures; and life experiences that eventuate in late-life inequalities among groups and individuals by social, economic, racial, and ethnic statuses (Jackson, 2004).

In this chapter we focus on the age, gender, socioeconomic, cultural, racial, and ethnic graded influences on life course development and material and health outcomes among different groups. Because of space limitations we will give illustrative examples. Even with this limitation, we hope that the intersectional examination we present will reveal the appropriateness and utility of the basic life course framework, encompassing the intersection of genetic influences, socialization, cumulative life experiences, and risk exposures on the fundamental nature of individual development.

DEFINING RACIAL AND ETHNIC DIFFERENCES IN SOCIOECONOMIC AND HEALTH STATUSES: UNEQUAL TREATMENT AND UNEQUAL OUTCOMES

Across the life course, SES as well as racial and ethnic statuses are intricately related to health and health disparities (Adler & Rehkopf, 2008; Crimmins et al., 2004; George, 2005). Often the complexity of SES, however, is not explored in health disparities research. An examination of 2008/2009 data from the US CB's CPS helps illustrate this concern. There is considerable racial and gender variation among older individuals in terms of years of formal education and poverty, two widely used measures of SES. For example, 23% of all elders have not completed high school. Among black elders, 40% have less than 12 years of formal education. In 2008, over 60% of blacks aged 65 and older had finished high school, compared with 1970, when only 9% of elderly blacks were high school graduates. Also in 2008, over 12% of blacks aged 65 and older had a bachelor's degree or higher. In 2008, about 46% of the Hispanic population aged 65 and older had finished high school, compared with 77% of the total older population. Also in 2008, 9% of Hispanic older Americans held a bachelor's degree or higher, compared with 21% of all older persons (Administration on Aging, 2009).

Poverty status, another important indicator of SES, varies by race and ethnicity, education, and gender among elders in the US. Census data indicate that 11.2% of white elders reside in households that fall below the poverty line. Nearly one out of four black (24.7%) and Hispanic (23.2%) elders lives in poverty. The level of poverty among Asian elders is comparable to that of white elders (11.8%) (Administration on Aging, 2009). Although the poverty rate in 2008 for black elderly (65 and older) was more than twice the rate for all elderly, this figure represents a significant decline (from 48% in 1968) in the poverty rate for black elderly over the last five-decade period.

Women, across all racial and ethnic minority groups in the US, are much more likely to live in households that fall below the federal poverty line. Black and Hispanic women are particularly vulnerable. Forty percent of elderly black women who have not completed high school are poor; 33% of Hispanic elderly women with less than 12 years of education live in poverty. Slightly over 12% of elderly white women with less than 12 years of education fall below the poverty line. These data highlight unequal opportunities across race, ethnicity, and gender that inevitably affect health across the life course, but that are often not attended to in life course health disparities research.

On the other hand, the independent contributions of SES and racial and ethnic statuses have been explored in several theoretical and empirical chapters and articles. For example, research suggests that lower SES is positively associated with poor health outcomes (Hayward et al., 2000), restricted access to health care (Huguet et al., 2008; Weitzman & Berry, 1992), and poorer treatment in the health services industry (Spencer & Chen, 2004). Cutting-edge biological research reveals that persons with lower social statuses, including poorer persons, may age biologically earlier in life (Cherkas et al., 2006; Crimmins et al., 2009).

After establishing statistically significant and practically meaningful connections between SES and health, research in this area has been moving in the direction of exploring possible biological (Szanton et al., 2005; Zajacova et al., 2009), psychological (Taylor & Seeman, 1999), chronic stressors exposure-related (Adler & Rehkopf, 2008; Baum et al., 1999; Kahn & Fazio, 2005), and economic mechanisms through which SES likely affects health outcomes. Although this shift in focus is indicative of the widespread acceptance of the compelling effect that SES

has on health, there has also been parallel research on the ways in which racial and ethnic group statuses may independently affect health (Chatters & Jackson, 1989; Turnbull & Mui, 1995).

An extensive body of research has developed over the past several decades to examine the relationship between membership of specific racial and ethnic groups and health outcomes. Mortality is often used as a general indicator of health and tends to show racial gaps in survival for blacks and whites. Examination of mortality data from the CDC highlight these gaps. Life expectancy in the US has risen over the last 40 years across all groups; however, race and gender variations are also apparent. In 1976, life expectancy was 69.9 years for white men and 77.5 years for white women. By 2006, life expectancy was 75.7 years for white men and 80.6 years for white women. In 1976, life expectancy was 62.9 years for black men and 71.6 years for black women. By 2006, the life expectancy for black men had increased by nearly 7 years to 69.7 years; for black women the increase was more modest, to 76.5 years. Although there has been considerable improvement, the life expectancy of black men in 2006 is still below that of white men 40 years ago (Administration on Aging, 2009). The data suggest different mechanisms may be at work in the mortality rates, and, by extension, in the health outcomes of different racial and ethnic groups. For example, black men are less like to survive to age 65 than white men. Although the difference is smaller, a similar pattern is evident for black and white women. By age 85, however, there appears to be a race-related mortality crossover, perhaps more prominent among women, revealing that blacks have longer life expectancies than whites.

Empirical studies suggest that some risk factors are culturally specific and that risk and resource factors are unevenly distributed among racial and ethnic groups. For example, comparisons between non-Hispanic whites and racial and ethnic minority groups suggest that health services are underutilized (Neighbors et al., 2007) among racial and ethnic minorities. In addition, research on racial and ethnic health disparities suggests that risks for severe mental illness and specific physical diseases are greater among certain ethnic groups than others. Further, rates differ depending on factors such as nativity and, among immigrants, time in the country to which they have relocated (e.g. Alegría et al., 2007; Zsembik & Fennell, 2005). In addition, research suggests that racial and ethnic minorities may engage in poor health behaviors as forms of self-regulation to cope with differential exposure to chronic stressors (Jackson & Knight, 2006). For example, a recent study (Jackson et al., 2010) found that poor health behaviors among African Americans, but not among white Americans, were protective of risk for major depression, but contributed independently to poor physical health outcomes among blacks but not among whites. Researchers in this area, however, tread carefully because of the risk of seeming to engage in race-based biological determinism. In recent years attention has increasingly focused on understanding whether and how racial and ethnic status as distinct concepts become embodied in the differential health outcomes among racial and ethnic groups (Gravlee, 2009; Krieger, 2005; Lee, 2009).

In spite of the progress of research that has investigated the independent effects that SES, race, and ethnicity demonstrate in health outcomes over the life course, research that examines the joint effects of SES, race, and ethnicity is still in nascent stages (Williams et al., 2010). Yet, this joint effect is highly likely given evidence that SES provides the context for understanding within racial and ethnic group differences in health (Schoenbaum & Waidmann, 1997). One example of this type of effect is that racial differences in poor health outcomes are most apparent at lower SES levels (Lillie-Blanton et al., 1996). Further, applying the lens of race and ethnicity helps to nuance SES-specific findings. For example, despite the health disadvantages that racial and ethnic minority group members face across the life course, the number of oldest old in these groups is substantial. It is likely that those who survive to these ages have the advantage of hardiness accrued throughout their life experiences (Antonucci & Jackson, 2009).

In short, SES and racial and ethnic statuses have been, and promise to be, dimensions of analyses that shed enormous light on the mechanisms of health disparities across the life course. Examining their joint contributions to health outcomes provides a deeper understanding of the myriad ways in which cumulative advantage and disadvantage manifest in physical and psychological health. An exciting area for future research will be the development of methodological and statistical techniques that can appropriately examine the ways in which these multiple locations, such as SES, race, and ethnicity, contribute to health and health disparities across the life course, particularly among racial and ethnic minorities.

OBSERVED DIFFERENCES IN AGING AMONG RACE AND ETHNIC GROUPS: MULTIPLE AND INTERSECTING CAUSATION

Ethnicity and racial status are complex social, psychological, and religious constructs. In addition, there is a complex interplay among genes and environmental factors, especially as people age. On the one hand, there exist some bases for genetic groupings of population groups, but this classification is hardly definitive for observed complex morbidity and mortality differences. On the other hand, the notion of race as "merely" a social construction is probably too simplistic. Racial categorizations are most likely social manifestations based upon genetically caused phonotypical differences, and the genes responsible for observed and commonly used racial markers may be the most unstable and under the most selective pressures (Jackson, 2004). In parsing causal factors, environmental and GE interaction are probably most important in any health and disease risk assessment. Skin tone is the most often used marker of racial differences (Jablonski & Chaplin, 2002). But skin tone, like most physical difference attributes, can be explained by environmental adaptation. Its instability may make it the least likely external marker for evolutionary relations among human groups (Jablonski & Chapin, 2002).

BIOLOGICAL AND SOCIAL PERSPECTIVES ON RACE CATEGORIZATION

Self-reported (or other-reported) race and ethnicity is the most frequent categorization in both social and biological research. A question not often posed is: why should we observe in the US such large and both consistent (African Americans) and often inconsistent (Caribbeans, Latinos, Asians, etc.) morbidity and mortality disparities among racial and ethnic groups, especially as they age? In the construal of race (and ethnicity) there are at least two processes operative in group categorization. The first is biologically based in the genetic underpinnings for observed phonotypical differences among individuals and groups. The second, however, is social and represents both self and the attributions of others to the meanings that these observed individual and observable markers come to possess. As noted elsewhere (Jackson, 2004), it is unlikely that biological processes alone in a heavily genetically admixed population like the US could account solely for the large observed racial and ethnic group differences in morbidity and mortality (Cooper, 2004). The categorization of racial groups within any country requires a complex interplay between those categorized and those being categorized. For example, the one-drop rule of hypo descent in the US stated that, regardless of phenotype, traceable African ancestry constitutes the categorization "black." Although the one-drop rule is based in the specific historical context of slavery and different forms of racial segregation, within the US today, many persons and institutions still subscribe to the belief that persons with any trace of African ancestry are black. For example, the debate surrounding

President Obama's racial background (as well as Tiger Woods' early racial claims) is recent evidence.

The largest and most consistent disparities are found between those who are categorized (by self and other) as black and white. Thus, self-described race in the US is related to large, observed differences in physical health morbidity and mortality, perhaps having little to do with the genetic differences between groups and more to do with socially produced systems of inequality (Braun, 2002).

One possible pathway for observer perceptions of race could be the effects of systematic discrimination. Several scholars (e.g. Williams, 1997; Williams et al., 2010) have noted that, while the exact mechanisms are unknown, racism and discrimination are ingrained in US culture and institutions. Further, internalization and other potential adaptation strategies and race-specific stressors, stress mediators, and stress outcomes may be operative, contributing even more to observed physical health differences. What is clear is that discrimination is not randomly distributed. In fact, discrimination is related to broader life contexts such as poverty. There are also differences within and among ethnic groups in exposure and risk. Racism itself can give rise to discrimination (Williams, 1997; Williams et al., 2010). Discrimination in turn can lead to differences in life-chances, which in turn affect health. Experiences of specific incidents of racism may have direct effects on health, and, as we have noted elsewhere (e.g. Jackson et al., 1996), coping strategies in the face of discrimination may be harmful to physical health.

Overall, discrimination and racism have health effects (William et al., 2010). Growing evidence argues against simplistic genetic determinism in complex disease differences among race and ethnic groups (e.g. Cooper, 2004; Jackson, 2004). Discrimination probably plays a role in health and services processes, but the role is complex. More research is needed on how discrimination and racism are similar to, and the same as, other mundane life stressors, and how the stress process itself may be implicated in the nature of gene expression. More broadly, while it is clear that experiences of unequal outcomes are easily observed among race groups, what is still unknown is exactly how discrimination operates in the context of social, political, economic, and cultural influences that change during historical time and affect individual experiences over the life course.

THE LAW OF SMALL EFFECTS

We have proposed (Jackson, 2004) the "Law of Small Effects," suggesting that there is no one single factor that produces observed race and ethnic group disparities. Most likely, there are a group of small differences that accumulate over the life course to produce observed differences in morbidity and mortality in adulthood and older ages among different racial and ethnic groups. These could include genetic effects, gene–gene interactions, GE interactions, epigenetic effects, discrimination, and life course selection effects. While none of these effects by themselves are large enough to produce the health disparities observed between blacks and whites in older ages, when taken together, and in interactions, they produce the type of consistent differences observed between groups such as blacks and whites in this society.

Disparities are not reducible to simple SES or genetic explanations. These observed differences are complex, multi-faceted, and life course-influenced. For example, why are race and ethnic disparities so significantly influenced, but not eliminated, by other factors, such as social and economic status, gender, and living arrangements? Finally, it is unclear why self-reported race should be related to morbidity and mortality outcomes at all, if genes play such a powerful role in these observed differences. We suggest that the pathways for how "self" and "other" conceptions of race affect health outcomes are potentially explicable. New studies are needed that take a more complex view, and greater attention needs to be paid to understanding the meaning of "environment" in any evolutionary and genetic perspective on complex human behaviors and diseases.

AGE, PERIOD, AND COHORT INFLUENCES ON RACE AND ETHNIC DIFFERENCES IN AGING: DEFINING THE SOCIAL GROUP

One of the most concrete ways in which to appreciate cohort – and, by extension, period and age effects – is to examine population trends and projections. Table 7.1 shows how the demographic distribution of the US is projected to shift from 2000 to 2030 and then to 2050. Some of these data are to be expected. As we move from 2000 to 2050, across race and ethnicity, the aging pyramid is anticipated to reflect greater numbers in the middle and older age groups, with the numbers of the oldest old expected to be greater than in prior decades. For the most part, the total number of women will continue to surpass the total number of men. And, as noted earlier, by 2030 Hispanics will clearly be the largest ethnic minority in the US.

The projections, however, also present data that are striking. One of the most notable trends concerns shifts in the sex ratios from 2000 to 2030 to 2050. Although the number of white women is expected

Table 7.1 Population projections by race, selected age groups, and sex: 2000, 2030, and 2050.

	BLACKS			HISPANICS			WHITES*		
	BOTH	MALE	FEMALE	BOTH	MALE	FEMALE	BOTH	MALE	FEMALE
2000 (N = 282 194 309)									
<20	12 406 914	6 295 812	6 111 102	13 758 998	7 096 353	6 662 645	54 379 773	27 893 823	26 485 950
20–24	2 678 048	1 304 479	1 373 569	3 444 737	1 897 691	1 547 046	13 004 820	6 576 973	6 427 847
25–44	10 749 565	5 070 754	5 678 811	11 767 707	6 221 525	5 546 182	62 513 584	31 285 165	31 228 419
45–64	6 532 963	2 980 710	3 552 253	4 918 705	2 391 883	2 526 822	50 960 873	24 999 513	25 961 360
65–84	2 526 980	996 390	1 530 590	1 604 689	686 957	917 732	26 659 893	11 525 628	15 134 265
85–99	308 859	84 544	224 315	151 636	50 163	101 473	3 761 036	1 100 343	2 660 693
100 +	8656	1631	7025	2512	674	1838	53 361	8828	44 533
TOTAL	35 211 985	16 734 320	18 477 665	35 648 984	18 345 246	17 303 738	211 383 340	103 390 273	107 943 067
2030 (N = 363 759 709)									
<20	12 997 217	6 639 831	6 357 386	18 573 529	9 489 750	9 083 779	59 109 619	30 196 188	28 913 431
20–24	3 117 217	1 583 223	1 533 994	4 349 446	2 205 940	2 143 506	14 910 459	7 577 147	7 333 312
25–44	12 676 530	6 306 234	6 370 296	19 072 859	9 365 836	9 707 023	57 855 379	29 039 951	28 815 428
45–64	10 407 502	4 847 990	5 559 512	17 805 862	8 891 692	8 914 170	56 374 536	27 573 180	28 801 356
55–84	6 491 248	2 682 087	3 809 161	8 561 558	3 975 440	4 586 118	50 710 821	23 494 680	27 216 141
85–99	732 328	223 330	508 998	1 034 561	376 976	657 585	8 522 952	3 200 855	5 322 097
100 +	26 000	4222	21 778	37 466	8349	29 117	392 623	85 838	306 785
TOTAL	46 448 042	22 286 917	24 161 125	69 435 281	34 313 983	35 121 298	247 876 386	121 167 839	126 708 550
2050 (N = 410 004 059)									
<20	13 364 175	6 827 476	6 536 699	21 807 416	11 144 877	10 662 539	62 811 847	32 090 838	30 721 009
20–24	3 239 603	1 645 409	1 594 194	5 373 589	2 728 616	2 644 973	15 253 191	7 752 683	7 500 508
25–44	13 189 082	6 595 015	6 594 067	22 143 451	10 919 562	11 223 889	61 696 641	30 913 399	30 783 242
45–64	12 185 763	5 901 623	6 284 140	21 506 013	10 265 787	11 240 226	58 291 053	28 692 270	29 598 783
65–84	7 906 001	3 415 432	4 490 569	16 208 301	7 689 579	8 518 722	47 925 534	22 437 029	25 488 505
85–99	2 103 209	693 884	1 409 325	3 972 548	1 620 114	2 352 434	19 054 402	7 587 220	11 467 182
100 +	126 061	25 761	100 300	243 107	65 474	177 633	1 603 072	434 976	1 168 096
TOTAL	52 113 894	25 104 600	27 009 294	91 254 425	44 434 009	46 820 416	266 635 740	129 908 415	136 727 325

Source: Demographic forecasts from the MacArthur Foundation Research Network on an Aging Society.
*Included in this group are Asians and Native Americans. Their numbers were so small that they were collapsed with the non-Hispanic whites.

to be consistently larger than the number of white men in 2030 and 2050, the other race groups highlighted show different trends. Female blacks outnumbered male blacks in 2000 and are anticipated to do so again in 2030. They are not expected, however, to outnumber them in 2050; projections indicate approximately four million more black men than women. Male Hispanics outnumbered female Hispanics in 2000 by approximately one million. However, projections suggest that Hispanic females will surpass the number of Hispanic males by about two million in 2050.

Another striking trend is the projections for increases in the numbers of centenarians. For blacks, in 2030 the number of these persons will increase three-fold compared to 2000, and, in 2050, will be 14 times greater than the 2000 numbers. For Hispanics, the number of centenarians will be 14 times greater in 2030 than in 2000. In 2050, the number of centenarians among Hispanics is expected to be six times more than in 2030; this number is an astounding 97 times more than in 2000. The 2030 projected number of whites is seven times the 2000 number. The number for this race group's centenarian population in 2050 is 30 times more than that in 2000.

Succinctly, projected changes in the numbers of centenarians indicate the inevitability of people on average living to older ages compared to earlier cohorts. Compared to cohort groups that lived in earlier eras there will undoubtedly be exponential growth (based upon prior advances) in biomedical technologies in the coming decades that may decrease in almost revolutionary fashion the illnesses and diseases that accompany aging. These later cohorts, however, must also contend with challenges that accompany their extended lives. One of the areas in which such challenges are likely to exist, given the demographic projections, is intergenerational relationships. With the expected shifts in sex ratios described earlier, intergenerational family patterns are likely to experience changed dynamics. The health implications of these shifted dynamics are likely to be a thriving area of research in coming years.

One of the most dramatic pictures that demographic projections paint is how the aging pyramid shifts dramatically from 2000 to 2030 to 2050 for the Hispanic population. In 2000 the most numerous age groups were those younger than 20. In 2030 and 2050, however, the most populous group will be the 25–44-year-olds. The 65–84-year-olds will increase from 1.6 million in 2000 to 8.5 million in 2030 and 16.2 million in 2050. These shifts portend changes in the ways in which families normatively choose to interact with and care for aging relatives. The demographic shifts in centenarians in the Hispanic population provide a concrete example of the different ways in which age, period, and cohort effects may influence familial norms and thus health outcomes

among older cohorts over the life course in decades to come. Specifically, for earlier cohorts of Hispanics, the population of the elderly that had to be cared for was much smaller than the numbers that will be present in coming cohorts.

In addition, these trends will be affected by period-specific effects, such as shifts in immigration policies related to family reunification. These likely changes in intergenerational relations must also be considered in the context of possible changes in age-specific norms and expectations for behaviors within multigenerational family contexts. Demographic comparisons are also useful for understanding how age, period, and cohort changes can have intersecting influences on health over the life course. Table 6.1 shows, for example, that, in comparing blacks and Hispanics, one of the most striking features is that, despite both groups beginning with population sizes of over 35 million in 2000, by 2030, the 69.4 million projected Hispanics far surpasses the projected 46.4 million for blacks. What may be contributing to these group differences? The data speak to the crucial role immigration likely plays in the shifting race, sex, and aging populations, given that, in 2000, more than 42% of the Hispanics in the US were foreign-born (Ramirez, 2004). Immigration, in turn, suggests period and cohort effects that can affect the aging process for all racial and ethnic group members. Specifically, if the majority of persons within a particular cohort must contend with limited or no access to health services because of their non-US citizenship status, this limited access will have direct and indirect repercussions on their health outcomes over their life course.

Another example in the population projections of the variance among different ethnic minority groups is how age, period, and cohort effects might be related to health outcomes. In 2000, among Hispanic persons aged 44 and younger, men outnumbered women. That this atypical sex ratio remains only for Hispanics aged 24 and younger in 2030 and 2050 suggests that distinct dynamics will contribute to health care and health status outcomes in these years more than in the 2000s because different sex-specific issues will be prominent. In short, population projections suggest how age-period-cohort conditions become crucial to understanding race and ethnic differences in health over the life course. Although different definitions of age-period-cohort effects have been used in different disciplines, and thus produce different findings regarding the relevance of these three linearly dependent factors (Keyes et al., 2010), one consistent finding in studies that examine health outcomes using these lenses is that the health of racial and ethnic group members across the life course must be understood in their particular periods. For instance, considering the health implications of the atypical sex ratios among Hispanics in the US, different historical periods have had distinct social norms regarding women's work outside the home as well as men being stay-at-home fathers. These period-specific norms play direct and indirect roles in health outcomes. Yet, little research to date has examined these APC effects and their intersections with gender in depth for specific ethnic groups. One of the main reasons for this dearth in the literature is that statistical tools and methodologies are only now becoming sufficiently sophisticated to disaggregate the effects of age, period, and cohort from one another (Harding, 2009; O'Brien et al., 2008; Osmond & Gardner, 1989; Smith, 2008; Yang & Land, 2008). Future methodological advances will thus need to explore how to address further intersections, such as gender, while attending to the age, period, and cohort effects that affect aging processes and outcomes.

LIFE COURSE, COHORT, AND PERIOD PERSPECTIVES ON RACE AND ETHNIC GROUP DIFFERENCES: THINKING ABOUT THE RACE AND ETHNIC GROUP LIFE COURSE

A core premise of the life course perspective is that current and aging cohorts of racial and ethnic minority groups have been, and are being, exposed to conditions that will influence significantly their material, social, psychological, and health statuses as they reach older ages in the years and decades to come (e.g. Baltes, 1987). Riley and her colleagues (e.g. Riley, 1994a, 1994b; Riley & Riley, 1994) proposed that changes in social structures that provide role opportunities and norms do not keep pace with the alterations in people's lives caused by cohort succession. This "structural lag" must be considered in models of aging and human development. Their main argument has been that, as people age, they encounter changing role opportunities and circumstances in society. This intersection between individual lives and role opportunities and structures for individuals can never be fully synchronized.

Clearly, the future is difficult to predict; but what is clear is that structural change will continue to be asynchronous with the course of people's lives. Flexible structures and processes for changes in opportunity and norms responsive to structural lags and the course of individual lives must be developed. For many ethnic and racial minorities in this country, and, in fact, many countries around the world, age integration is accomplished not so much by individuals directly in their relationship to complex social structures, but instead through family systems that provide productive relationships and connections across the age span (Jackson et al., 2004).

Some of the structural changes that may accompany the coming aging society may place these formal and informal familial arrangements at risk. These changes may weaken important buffers and facilitators in the lives of individual ethnic minority families. The family may be unable to shield these groups from the full brunt of structural changes that Riley discusses and that will occur with the coming aging society. Specifically, the continuing effects of discrimination may interact with structural changes and make it more challenging for families to adapt. For example, systematic barriers to education exist now for racial and ethnic minorities, barriers that affect not only the aging cohort members but also their offspring.

ELIMINATING RACE AND ETHNIC-BASED AGING DISPARITIES OVER THE LIFE COURSE: ARE THERE CRITICAL POINTS OF INTERVENTION?

There is a compelling need to develop better health interventions and policies directed to the growing US ethnic and racial minority populations (Antonucci & Jackson, 2009; Miles, 2009; Sellers et al., 2009). If we are to improve the health of underrepresented minority populations, especially blacks and Latinos, these policies must be responsive to life course considerations and the realities of family life. Research on discriminated-against minorities has focused on three major themes: heterogeneity, vulnerabilities due to societal maltreatment, and family strengths (e.g. Williams et al., 2010). A life course framework is needed to explore how sociohistorical context influences and interacts with individual and group resources to both impede and facilitate the quality of life and health of successive cohorts of discriminated-against minorities over the life course and in their individual human development experiences (Adler & Stewart, 2010; Antonucci & Jackson, 2009). For example, relationships between socioecologic factors, such as high crime rates, family dysfunction, high noise levels and social isolation, and negative health factors (e.g. hypertension) can affect all members of families and communities, thus possibly initiating poorer health among younger, as well as older, ethnic and racial groups (Glymour et al., 2009; Sellers et al., 2009).

Continuing gender imbalances, segregated geographic distributions, and disproportionate numbers in poverty, among other factors, will have profound effects on family structure, health status, and the well-being of many of these groups over the twenty-first century. As we noted earlier, ethnic and racial categories derive their interpretations from: (1) the sociohistorical and current circumstances that face the different groups with well-defined physical characteristics and (2) the self- and other-group attitudes and behaviors toward members who belong to these categories (Jackson, 2004; Sellers et al., 2009). While some genetic and biological factors may vary with race and ethnic categorization (Taylor, 2009), we suggest that the fundamental nature of inequality derives from discrimination and maltreatment (Sellers et al., 2009). While it is not yet clear how race and ethnic group categorizations fit exactly in biopsychosocial models of health, human development, and life course development (Jackson et al., 2004), it is vital that we integrate into the models of health, health promotion, and disease prevention, conditions under which race, ethnicity, sociocultural, and socioeconomic factors may serve as important resources in coping processes and adaptation to environmentally disadvantaged circumstances (Antonucci & Jackson, 2009).

Compared to Americans of European descent, at every point of their life course African Americans (and many Latino and Native American groups) have greater morbidity and mortality rates (Anderson et al., 2004). Among African Americans, as with most racial-ethnic groups in the US, cancer and cardiovascular disease are the two leading causes of death (Sellers et al., 2009). Hypertension is particularly deadly and affects one out of every three African Americans; blacks, for example, have a 60% greater risk of death and disability from stroke and coronary disease than whites (Taylor, 2009). Black women have three times the rate of high blood pressure compared to white women and are twice as likely as white women to die of hypertensive CVD (Mezuk, 2009). Similarly, cancer incidence rates for blacks are 6% to 10% higher than for whites (Sellers et al., 2009).

In sum, many race and ethnic groups, especially blacks, are at disproportionate risk for negative health outcomes when compared to white Americans (Anderson et al., 2004) and face significant challenges as they age. A number of factors may contribute to these disparities, ranging from biological dispositions (Adler & Stewart, 2010) to dietary habits (Taylor, 2009) to failure to receive adequate health care (Williams et al., 2010). The specific mechanisms, however, that produce these differential outcomes are less clear (Anderson et al., 2004). Given complex sociohistorical contexts, it may be more helpful in determining exact mechanisms to compare within specific race and ethnic groups. For example, black/white comparisons may be less illuminating than the examination of various intragroup social and cultural factors as possible sources of risk and resilience for African American men, women, and children (Sellers et al., 2009). It may be that we learn much more about how SES conditions life chances and morbidity and mortality differences by examining the influence of SES differences within ethnic and racial minority populations, rather than by examining racial and ethnic differences in SES.

It is important to develop frameworks within which the nature of the economic, social, and health circumstances of racial and ethnic groups can be explained and understood in the context of historical and current structural disadvantages and blocked mobility opportunities (Jackson, 1991). Such frameworks would contextualize individual and group experiences by birth cohort, period events, and individual aging processes (Sellers et al., 2009). It is clear, however, that blacks and other racial and ethnic minorities have, and do, arrive in adulthood and older ages with extensive histories of disease and ill health, and varied individual adaptive reactions to their poor health (Anderson et al., 2004). The available cohort data for cause-specific mortality and morbidity across the life course over the last few decades indicates that there are accumulated deficits that place black, Latino, and Native American middle-aged and older people at greater risk than comparable chronologically aged whites (Jackson, 1991). Similarly, the fact that blacks may actually outlive their white counterparts, the well-known and commonly described age cross-over effect in the very older ages, suggests possible selection factors at work that may result in hardier older blacks (Antonucci & Jackson, 2009). These selection factors may act on successive cohorts of blacks as they age in a "sandwich-like" manner, culling out the weaker members of a given cohort, leaving alternating groups of middle-aged and older blacks of relative wellness and good functional ability. The cohort experiences of blacks, and other racial and ethnic minority groups, undoubtedly play a major role in the nature of their health experiences over the life course in terms of the quality of health care from birth, exposure to risk factors, and the presence of exogenous environmental factors. Another contributing factor is the stressor role of prejudice and discrimination across the life course, even though it may differ in form and intensity as a function of birth cohort, period, and age (Anderson et al., 2004; Williams et al., 2010).

CONCLUSIONS: HOW SOCIAL GROUP DESIGNATIONS OF RACE AND ETHNICITY BECOME PHYSICAL REALITIES – A BIO-PSYCHOSOCIAL-ENVIRONMENTAL FRAMEWORK

Cooper (2004) and others (e.g. Jackson, 2004) have suggested that biological perspectives may be less relevant than social definitions and the consequences of racial and ethnic statuses. These social definitions provide important clues for understanding environmental causes of observed differences in material, social, and health statuses among ethnic and race groups. Other work notes the independent role of cultural and lifestyle differences among racial and ethnic groups in accounting for behavioral and health outcomes (e.g. Sellers et al., 2009). The assumption that race and ethnicity constitute just one of many sociocultural factors, rather than distinct cultural and social environment indicators, has precluded the types of research and analyses that examine the intersectional role of sociocultural factors in material, social, and health outcomes among racial and ethnic groups. Many researchers have even questioned the appropriateness and validity of SES and other sociocultural measures (e.g. occupation, coping resources, lifestyle factors) when making comparisons across race and ethnic groups (e.g. Hayward et al., 2000; Jackson et al., 2004).

Human development, aging, and the life course are critical constructs in understanding ostensible racial and ethnic group differences. We assume that different ethnic and racial groups have divergent life experiences because of sociostructural, socioeconomic, and cultural reasons (Sellers et al., 2009). These different experiences will have significant influences, both positive and negative, on individual, family, and group well-being at all stages of the life course, ultimately influencing adjustment to major life transitions (e.g. loss of spouse, retirement, and disability) in older ages. Race and ethnicity are summary, predisposing constructs that represent myriad other social, psychological, and possibly biological factors (Jackson, 2004; Jackson et al., 2004).

We need a coherent life course framework within which the nature of the material, social, and psychological lives of ethnic and racial minorities can be understood in the context of historical and current structural disadvantage and blocked mobility opportunities (Riley, 1994a). We need to understand how structural disadvantages in the environment are translated at different points in the individual and group life course into physical, social, and psychological aspects of group and self. It is clear that the age cohort into which group members are born; the social, political, and economic events that these cohorts experience; and the individual aging process at different points in a person's life course influence the adaptation and QOL of individuals, families, and larger ethnic and race groups in the US. The last half century has witnessed new knowledge about aging of biological, sensory, behavioral, physiological, and cognitive systems related to aging (Antonucci & Jackson, 2009). For example, people do not age in the same way; individuals differ greatly in age-related declines (and increments) in physical, behavioral, and cognitive functioning. Research clearly suggests that some aging processes are modifiable (Glynmour et al., 2009). Cognitive declines are not universal with age; some intellectual abilities are actually maintained or improve with age. In addition,

observed functional differences across individuals are greatly influenced by societal, environmental, and health-related statuses, and the background and makeup of the individual.

In this chapter we have speculated on the possibility of extending the life course framework to encompass an integrated, intersectional conceptualization of development and aging that includes historical, cohort, immigration, and cultural influences on successful social and psychological aging among racial and ethnic elders as part of a biopsychosocial model (Jackson et al., 2004). Intergenerational models of aging and human development are of critical importance in understanding individual aging trajectories. Period events and cohort membership play a determining role in aging processes, and, it is necessary to conceptualize age-related change and processes within an individual, family, and societal life course framework (Antonucci & Jackson, 2009).

On average, older race and ethnic minority adults show a relatively poorer status than comparable non-minority populations. Nonetheless, based upon current estimates of mortality and life expectancies, older minority populations have grown and will continue to do so (Jackson & Sellers, 2001). Some data indicate that some minority populations of advanced ages, for example blacks, may be more robust in comparison to whites, perhaps reflecting different aging processes and selection over time for hardier individuals. At every point earlier in the life course, however, most members of racial and ethnic groups are at greater mortality and morbidity risk than whites (Sellers et al., 2009).

Some studies have shown how recognition and inclusion of cultural and racial considerations in service delivery programs can increase the effectiveness and reduce the cost of delivering services to racial and ethnic minority populations (Miles, 2009). It is also our belief that the infusion of racial minority and ethnic content contributes to our understanding of the health status and health needs of the nation's elderly more generally, regardless of whether the direct focus of that work is on racial and ethnic groups (Sellers et al., 2009).

Although there is some convergence toward a risk and resources life course model of ethnicity that utilizes modern biopsychosocial theories of culture and acculturation (Jackson et al., 2004), the empirical literature has not kept pace. The work that we have briefly reviewed suggests directions that new health, behavioral, and social science research might take in this area. Theoretical frameworks of ethnicity and culture are beginning to emerge (Jackson & Govia, 2009; Sellers et al., 2009) that will lead to more and better empirical studies. Race, ethnicity, and cultural effects on biological and social functioning over the life course are not readily accounted for by current theories of aging (Adler & Stewart, 2010; Glynmour et al., 2009). A biopsychosocial life course framework encompassing the important contextual and intersecting factors of race, culture, ethnicity, gender, immigration, and social and economic statuses, which intersect over the life course and influence material, psychological, health, and social well-being, is needed to understand and ameliorate the needs of an increasingly diverse and heterogeneous older US population (Antonucci & Jackson, 2009; Jackson et al., 2004).

social identities, and other social and psychological statuses to influence the health of racial and ethnic group members across the life course.

SUMMARY

Age distributions across the globe are being fundamentally reshaped by increasing individual longevity, reduced population fertility, and shifting migration patterns. We propose a framework which addresses the dynamic intersections of age, period, and cohort,

ACKNOWLEDGMENTS

The preparation of this chapter was aided by grant support from the National Institute of Mental Health, National Institute of Aging, and National Center on Minority Health Disparities. The growing aging society is very much highlighted by the Jack Rowe lead MacArthur Foundation Network on the Aging Society. We would especially like to thank Dr. Jay S. Olshansky of the group for sharing their data with us. It was greatly appreciated. Finally we would like to thank the Program for Research on Black Americans for their continuing support.

REFERENCES

Adler, N. E., & Rehkopf, D. H. (2008). U.S. disparities in health: Descriptions, causes, and mechanisms. *Annual Review of Public Health, 29,* 235–252.

Adler, N. E., & Stewart, J. (2010). *Reaching for a healthier life. Facts on socioeconomic status and health in the U.S.* Chicago, IL: MacArthur Foundation.

Administration on Aging (2009). Retrieved February 2, 2010, from AoA website: http://www.aoa. gov/AoARoot/Aging_Statistics/ minority_aging.

Alegría, M., Sribney, W., Woo, M., Torres, M., & Guarnaccia, P. (2007). Looking beyond nativity: The relation of age of immigration, length of residence, and birth cohorts to the risk of onset of psychiatric disorders for Latinos. *Research in Human Development, 4,* 19–47.

Anderson, B. (1989). *Imagined communities: Reflections on the origins and spread of nationalism.* London and New York: Verso.

Anderson, N. B., Bulatao, R. B., & Cohen, B. (Eds.), (2004). *Critical perspectives on racial and ethnic differences in health in later life.* Washington, DC: The National Academies Press.

Antonucci, T. C., & Jackson, J. S. (Eds.), (2009). *Life-course perspectives on late life health inequalities.* New York: Springer.

Baltes, P. B. (1987). Theoretical propositions of life-span developmental psychology: On the dynamics between growth and decline. *Developmental Psychology, 23,* 611–626.

Baum, A., Garofalo, J. P., & Yali, A. M. (1999). Socioeconomic status and chronic stress: Does stress account for SES effects on health? *Annals of the New York Academy of Sciences, 896,* 131–144.

Braun, L. (2002). Race, ethnicity, and health: Can genetics explain disparities? *Perspectives in Biology and Medicine, 45,* 159–174.

Chatters, L. M., & Jackson, J. S. (1989). Quality of life and subjective well-being among Black Americans. In R. L. Jones (Ed.), *Black adult development and aging* (pp. 191–213). Berkeley, CA: Cobb & Henry Publishers.

Cherkas, L. F., Aviv, A., Valdes, A. M., Hunkin, J. L., Gardner, J. P., Surdulescu, G. L., et al. (2006). The effects of social status on biological aging as measured by white-blood-cell telomere length. *Aging Cell, 5,* 361–365.

Christensen, K., Doblhammer, G., Rau, R., & Vaupel, J. W. (2009). Ageing populations: The challenges ahead. *Lancet, 374,* 1196–1208.

Cooper, R. S. (2004). Genetic factors in ethnic disparities in health. In N. B. Anderson, R. A. Bulatao & B. Cohen (Eds.), *Critical perspectives on racial and ethnic differences in health in later life* (pp. 269–309). Washington, DC: National Research Council.

Crimmins, E. M., Hayward, M. D., & Seeman, T. (2004). Race/ethnicity, socioeconomic status and health. In N. B. Anderson, R. A. Bulatao & B. Cohen (Eds.), *Critical perspectives on racial and ethnic differences in health in later life* (pp. 310–352). Washington, DC: The National Academies Press.

Crimmins, E. M., Kim, J., & Seeman, T. (2009). Poverty and biological risk: The earlier "aging" of the poor. *Journal of Gerontology: Medical Sciences, 64A,* 286–292.

George, L. K. (2005). Socioeconomic status and health across the life course: Progress and prospects. *Journal of Gerontology: Social Sciences, 60*(Special Issue 2), S135–S139.

Glymour, M. M., Ertel, K. A., & Berkman, L. A. (2009). What can life-course epidemiology tell us about health inequalities in old age? In T. C. Antonucci & J. S. Jackson (Eds.), *Life-course perspectives on late life health inequalities* (pp. 27–56). New York, NY: Springer.

Gravlee, C. C. (2009). How race becomes biology: Embodiment of social inequality. *American Journal of Physical Anthropology, 139,* 47–57.

Harding, D. J. (2009). Recent advances in age-period-cohort analysis. A commentary on Dregan and Armstrong, and on Reither, Hauser and Yang. *Social Science & Medicine, 69,* 1449–1451.

Hayward, M. D., Crimmins, E. M., Miles, T. P., & Yang, Y. (2000). The significance of socioeconomic status in explaining the racial gap in chronic health conditions. *American Sociological Review, 65,* 910–930.

Huguet, N., Kaplan, M. S., & Feeny, D. (2008). Socioeconomic status and health-related quality of life among elderly people: Results from the Joint Canada/United States Survey of Health. *Social Science & Medicine, 66,* 803–810.

Jablonski, N. G., & Chaplin, G. (2002). Skin deep. *Scientific American, 288,* 74–81.

Jackson, J. S. (1991). Introduction. In J. S. Jackson (Ed.), *Life in Black America* (pp. 1–12). Newbury Park, CA: Sage Publications.

Jackson, J. S. (2004). Discussion: Genetic explanation for health disparities: What is at stake? In E. Singer & T. C. Antonucci (Eds.), *Proceedings of the Conference on Genetics and Health Disparities,* March (pp. 20–21). Ann Arbor, MI: Institute for Social Research, University of Michigan.

Jackson, J. S., & Govia, I. O. (2009). Quality of life for ethnic and racial minority elders in the 21st century: Setting a research agenda. In G. Cavanaugh & P. Sanford (Eds.), *Diversity and aging* (pp. 148–169). Washington, DC: AARP.

Jackson, J. S., & Knight, K. M. (2006). Race and self-regulatory health behaviors: The role of the stress response and the HPA axis in physical and mental health disparities. In K. W. Schaie & L. L. Carstensen (Eds.), *Social structures, aging, and self-regulation in the elderly* (pp. 189–239). New York, NY: Springer Publishing Co.

Jackson, J. S., & Sellers, S. L. (2001). Health and the elderly. In R. Braithwaite & S. E. Taylor (Eds.), *Health in Black communities* (pp. 81–96) (2nd ed.). San Francisco, CA: Jossey Bass.

Jackson, J. S., Brown, T. N., Williams, D. R., Torres, M., Sellers, S. L., & Brown, K. (1996). Racism and the physical and mental health status of African Americans: A thirteen year national panel study. *Ethnicity & Disease, 6,* 132–147.

Jackson, J. S., Antonucci, T. C., & Brown, E. (2004). A cultural lens on biopsychosocial models of aging. In P. T. Costa, Jr. & I. C. Siegler (Eds.), *Recent advances in psychology and aging* (pp. 221–241). Amsterdam: Elsevier.

Jackson, J. S., Knight, K. M., & Rafferty, J. A. (2010). Race and unhealthy behaviors: Chronic stress, the HPA axis, and physical and mental health disparities over the life-course. *American Journal of Public Health, 99,* 1–7.

Kahn, J. R., & Fazio, E. M. (2005). Economic status over the life course and racial disparities in health. *Journal of Gerontology: Social Sciences, 60B*(Suppl. Special Issue 2), S76–S84.

Keyes, K. M., Utz, R. L., Robinson, W., & Li, G. (2010). What is a cohort effect? Comparison of three statistical methods for modeling cohort effects in obesity prevalence in the United States, 1971–2006. *Social Science & Medicine, 70,* 1100–1108.

Krieger, N. (2005). Stormy weather: Race, gene expression, and the science of health disparities. *American Journal of Public Health, 95,* 2155–2160.

Lee, C. (2009). "Race" and "ethnicity" in biomedical research: How do scientists construct and explain differences in health? *Social Science & Medicine, 68,* 1183–1190.

Lillie-Blanton, M., Parsons, P. E., Gayle, H., & Dievler, A. (1996). Racial differences in health: Not just black and white, but shades of gray. *Annual Review of Public Health, 17,* 411–448.

Mezuk, B. (2009). Epidemiology of diabetes and cardiovascular disease: The emergence of health disparities over the life span. In T. C. Antonucci & J. S. Jackson (Eds.), *Life-course perspectives on late life health inequalities* (pp. 77–98). New York, NY: Springer.

Miles, T. P. (2009). Health care reform and health disparities: Reasons for hope? In T. C. Antonucci & J. S. Jackson (Eds.), *Life-course perspectives on late life health inequalities* (pp. 275–292). New York: Springer.

Neighbors, H. W., Caldwell, C., Williams, D. R., Nesse, R., Taylor, R. J., Bullard, K. M., et al. (2007). Race, ethnicity, and the use of services for mental disorders: Results from the National Survey of American Life. *Archives of General Psychiatry, 64,* 485–494.

O'Brien, R. M., Hudson, K., & Stockard, J. (2008). A mixed model estimation of age, period, and cohort effects. *Sociological Methods & Research, 36,* 402–428.

Olshansky, S. J., Goldman, D. P., Zheng, Y., & Rowe, J. W. (2009). Aging in America in the twenty-first century: Demographic forecasts from the MacArthur Foundation Research Network on an Aging Society. *The Milbank Quarterly, 87,* 842–862.

Osmond, C., & Gardner, M. J. (1989). Age, period, and cohort models: Non-overlapping cohorts don't resolve the identification problem. *American Journal of Epidemiology, 129,* 31–35.

Phelan, J. C., Link, B. G., Diez-Roux, A., Kawachi, I., & Levin, B. (2004). "Fundamental causes" of social inequalities in mortality: A test of the theory. *Journal of Health and Social Behavior, 45,* 265–285.

Ramirez, R. R. (2004). We the people: Hispanics in the United States. Census 2000 special reports (December), 1–18. Washington, DC: U.S. Census Bureau.

Riley, M. W. (1994a). Changing lives and changing social structures: Common concerns of social science and public health. *American Journal of Public Health, 84,* 1214–1217.

Riley, M. W. (1994b). Aging and society: Past, present, and future. *The Gerontologist, 34*, 436–446.

Riley, M. W., & Riley, J. W., Jr. (1994). Age integration and the lives of older people. *The Gerontologist, 34*, 110–115.

Robinson, M., Novelli, W., Pearson, C., & Norris, L. (2007). *Global health and global aging.* New York: John Wiley & Sons.

Rowe, J. & Berkman, L. (2009). *Investing over the life-course: A winning strategy.* The Huffington Post (www.huffingtonpost.com/ john-rowe/investing-over-the-life-c_b_210391.html), June 23, 2009.

Schoenbaum, M., & Waidmann, T. (1997). Race, socioeconomic status, and health: Accounting for race differences in health. *Journal of Gerontology: Social Sciences, 52B*, 61–73.

Sellers, S. L., Govia, I. O., & Jackson, J. S. (2009). Health and black older adults: Insights from a life-course perspective. In R. Braithwaite, S. E. Taylor & H. M. Treadwell (Eds.), *Health issues in the black communities* (pp. 95–116) (3rd ed.). San Francisco, CA: Jossey Bass.

Smith, H. L. (2008). Advances in age-period-cohort analysis. *Sociological Methods & Research, 36*, 287–296.

Spencer, M. S., & Chen, J. (2004). Effect of discrimination on mental health service utilization among Chinese Americans. *American Journal of Public Health, 94*, 809–814.

Szanton, S. L., Gill, J. M., & Allen, J. K. (2005). Allostatic load: A mechanism of socioeconomic health disparities? *Biological Research for Nursing, 7*, 7–15.

Taylor, J. Y. (2009). Genetic influences on disparities in hypertension and obesity in late life. In T. C. Antonucci & J. S. Jackson (Eds.), *Life-course perspectives on late life health Inequalities* (pp. 99–114). New York, NY: Springer.

Taylor, S. E., & Seeman, T. E. (1999). Psychosocial resources and the SES–health relationship. *Annals of the New York Academy of Sciences, 896*, 210–225.

Turnbull, J. F., & Mui, A. C. (1995). Mental health status and needs of black and white elderly: Differences in depression. In D. K. Padgett (Ed.), *Handbook on ethnicity, aging, and mental health* (pp. 73–98). Westport, CT: Greenwood Press/Greenwood Publishing Group.

US Census Bureau (2008). Projections of the population by age and sex for the United States: 2010 to 2050 (NP2008-T12/ NP2008-T14). (http://www. census.gov/population/www/ projections/2008projections. html) Washington, DC: Population Division, US Census Bureau.

Weitzman, B. C., & Berry, C. A. (1992). Health status and health care utilization among New York City home attendants: An illustration of the needs of working poor, immigrant women. *Women & Health, 19*, 87–105.

Williams, D. R. (1997). Race and health: The added effects of racism and discrimination. *Annals of Epidemiology, 7*, 322–333.

Williams, D. R., Mohammed, S. A., Leavell, J., & Collins, C. (2010). Race, socioeconomic status, and health: Complexities, ongoing challenges, and research opportunities. In N. E. Adler & J. Stewart (Eds.), *The biology of disadvantage* (pp. 69–101). New York: Annals of the New York Academy of Science.

Yang, Y., & Land, K. C. (2008). Age-period-cohort analysis of repeated cross-section surveys: Fixed or random effects? *Sociological Methods & Research, 36*, 297–326.

Zajacova, A., Dowd, J., & Aiello, A. (2009). Socioeconomic and race/ethnic patterns in persistent infection burden among U.S. adults. *The Journals of Gerontology: Medical Sciences, 64A(2)*, 272–279.

Zsembik, B. A., & Fennell, D. (2005). Ethnic variation in health and the determinants of health among Latinos. *Social Science & Medicine, 61*, 53–63.

Chapter | 8 |

Stratification and Inequality Over the Life Course

Scott M. Lynch[1], J. Scott Brown[2]

[1]Department of Sociology and Office of Population Research, Princeton University, Princeton, New Jersey, [2]Department of Sociology and Gerontology and Scripps Gerontology Center, Miami University, Oxford, Ohio

CHAPTER CONTENTS

INTRODUCTION

Stratification is the "layering" of individuals and larger social units in society, and inequality is both the antecedent and consequence of stratification. Social scientists have long been concerned with stratification and inequality in human societies, especially socioeconomic inequalities, where "socioeconomic" refers to educational attainment, occupational status, earnings, and wealth. A comprehensive understanding of stratification and inequality, given that they are processes, implicitly requires a life course approach, and much of the historical research on inequality has implicitly adopted a life course view, albeit a narrow one. Yet, over the history of stratification and inequality research, there have been major changes both within the field of stratification and outside this domain that have ultimately led to a more explicit and broader life course focus. These changes include:

(1) a shift from broad theoretical and historical discussions of stratification and inequality with little empirical investigation to full-fledged empirical studies with a narrower focus;

(2) an expansion of empirical investigation into stratification mechanisms, including sex and race;

(3) an expansion of empirical investigation into additional inequalities (outcomes of stratification), including, predominantly, health;

(4) the development of an explicit life course theory coupled with the collection of longitudinal data and the development of statistical methods that make life course research in stratification possible; and

(5) growing sophistication in conceptualizing and modeling stratification and inequality as processes that unfold across the individual life course and change across sociohistorical time.

This last development includes the recognition that inequalities in health, educational attainment, earnings, and wealth are simultaneously the causes and consequences of stratification both within and between generations.

In this chapter, we discuss each of these major changes in the field. First, we provide a brief overview of the history of theory and research in stratification and inequality from the late 1800s through the 1960s. We then discuss the expansion of stratification research in the 1960s and 1970s to include sex and race as predictors of socioeconomic differences.

DOI: 10.1016/B978-0-12-380880-6.00008-3

Next, we discuss the simultaneous growth in interest of health inequality as a key outcome of stratification in the 1970s. Then we discuss the emergence of a life course perspective in the 1980s and its explicit integration into stratification research coupled with the acquisition of longitudinal data that make life course research possible. In this discussion, we provide a conceptual diagram that illustrates the complexities of researching stratification from a life course perspective, and we highlight the breadth of contemporary research investigating various components of this diagram. Finally, we provide an in-depth discussion of data, methods, and challenges therein that have emerged and continue to evolve in inequality research as a result of the life course focus.

Our goal is not to provide an exhaustive account of research on stratification and inequality. Instead, our goal is to show that stratification and inequality research has evolved to provide a deeper understanding of inequality at both the within-individual level and the between-individual level both within and between birth cohorts. Specifically, research has expanded to include additional important sources and outcomes of inequality, namely health, as well as to view the production of inequality as an interactive one that unfolds across the life course of individuals, and unfolds differentially across time.

There are a number of topics in stratification and health research that we do not cover. First, we focus on stratification and inequality in the US; we do not discuss international or comparative research. Second, we do not discuss aggregate studies of inequality in earnings, wealth, and health (e.g. Kawachi et al., 1997). Third, we do not address health research that does not involve investigation of socioeconomic inequality. Finally, we do not discuss research on sex and race inequalities that do not have socioeconomic outcomes as the key focus. For example, we do not discuss gender role stratification or changes in racial prejudice and discrimination that are not the focus of stratification and inequality research. Along these same lines, we do not discuss research on crime as a predictor of socioeconomic inequality, despite some evidence that incarceration may play a significant role in affecting stratification, especially among blacks and other racial minorities (e.g. Pager, 2007; Western, 2006).

A BRIEF HISTORY OF INEQUALITY STUDIES

Identifying and understanding inequality is a cornerstone of research in the social sciences, especially in sociology. In sociology, interest in stratification and inequality began with Durkheim, Marx, and Weber. Durkheim's work, *The Division of Labor in Society* ([1893] 1997), initiated interest in inequality by highlighting that agricultural surpluses led to a division of labor and ultimately the unequal distribution of resources in society (see Davis & Moore, 1945 for a detailed presentation of the functionalist approach that derived from Durkheim's work for the first half of the twentieth century; see also Massey, 2007; Tumin, 1953). Marx's work focused more directly on inequality, but he focused on earnings only, and, ultimately, the distinction between two economic classes: those who possessed capital (the bourgeoisie) and those who were exploited by capital (the proletariat) (Marx, [1894] 1972). Implicit in his work is the recognition that inequality maintains itself within generations and is reproduced across generations. Within a generation, there is no room for advancement; i.e. capital and labor are fixed, caste-like positions. Across generations, inequality between capital and labor grows as capital continually seeks to squeeze more profit from labor. Marx argued that such a system is unsustainable, because the product of labor must be purchased for profit to be realized (one of the earliest "demand side" economic views), and the masses of labor would be increasingly unable to purchase the fruits of their labor with below-subsistence wages.

Of course, capitalism has survived – and perhaps succeeded – in the US for more than two centuries, leading to revisions of Marx's original thesis. One early revision can be found in Weber's work ([1922] 1948). Weber argued that the class system in capitalistic societies is more complex than the dichotomous, earnings-based system laid out by Marx. Instead, Weber argued, consumption patterns and prestige systems also play a role in the stratification system. Subsequent theorists, both Marxist and non-Marxist, have argued that the evolution of a credit system enabled the survival of capitalism by allowing consumption patterns of rich and poor to blur actual income/class differences (see Bourdieu & Passeron, 1977; Sobel, 1983; Veblen, 1973). These theoretical debates continue today, but quantitative research on inequality did not begin in earnest until the 1950s.

In the late 1950s, following the drastic expansion of the middle class after World War II, sociologists became interested in both intragenerational and intergenerational mobility. Early work focused on intergenerational status attainment (Blau & Duncan, 1967; Duncan & Hodge, 1963). This early work focused on occupational mobility and whether and to what extent (white) fathers transmit status to their (white) sons. This research implicitly adopted (or anticipated) a life course perspective, given its focus on *transmission* of status across generations, but the temporal focus was limited. Such studies focused on status transmission only across two generations, did not generally consider historical change in status transmission processes, and provided little explicit discussion of the life course. Subsequent status attainment work focused on the mechanisms linking social origins to schooling and earnings outcomes, including the intertwined effects of race, gender, and social-psychological forces, though this work met with mixed success (see Bielby, 1981, for an overview).

In the late 1960s and 1970s, stratification and inequality research began focusing on race and sex inequalities, following the Civil Rights Movement and the push for gender equality (e.g. with the "sexual revolution" and the proposed equal rights amendment; see for example Firestone, 1972; Reich, 1977). An example of this is the Double Jeopardy Hypothesis on racial inequality in health, which originated in civil rights debates in the 1960s and which focused on the joint effects of gender and race. Later this was expanded to "triple jeopardy," which added old age and (less frequently) poverty status (Brown & Lynch, 2004).

In the 1970s, research began to investigate health inequality as a consequence of socioeconomic stratification/inequality. One of the earliest works in this area was Kitagawa and Hauser's (1973) seminal research on educational differences in mortality. Their work was primarily demographic, focusing on the three key demographic variables of age, sex, and race, and showed that (1) mortality was inversely related to socioeconomic status (SES), defined both by educational attainment and income and (2) the socioeconomic differential in mortality varies across age, sex, and race. Beyond noting age differences in the socioeconomic differential (largest at midlife and smallest at young and old ages), however, the life course was ignored.

Research in the stratification of health has continued since the 1970s (e.g. House et al., 1994; Sorlie et al., 1995), but it exploded in the 1990s approximately at the same time as interest emerged, within both the political sphere and the general population, in changing health care policy to make access – and presumably health – more equitable. From 1990, the stratification of health has been a major area of investigation, much of which has centered on determining the mediating mechanisms through which SES operates to affect health (e.g. Mirowsky & Ross, 2003; Ross & Wu, 1995).

In sum, the study of inequality has a long history in social research, and, although early research often had an implicit life course focus, much of it did not adopt an explicit life course perspective until later. The movement toward a life course perspective on stratification had to wait until the development of an integrated life course framework, beginning in earnest in the 1980s. Further, while health inequalities became a central area of study for health scholars between 1970 and 1990, its integration with stratification research waited until the 1990s and continues today.

THE LIFE COURSE PERSPECTIVE AND INEQUALITY

Stratification and resulting inequality are processes and not static phenomena. An explicit life course focus has emerged in inequality research over the last two decades. Recent research focuses on differentiating within-individual change across the individual life course from between-individual differences both within the life course and across birth cohorts and/or periods. Two developments largely account for this shift in focus: the development of an explicit theoretical life course paradigm and an explosion in the availability of data and methods that allow us to disentangle within-individual aging processes from between-cohort sociohistorical change.

The key insight – or defining characteristic – of the life course perspective is the recognition that the passage of time has implications for both individual- and societal-level outcomes. These outcomes evolve over time and the processes that account for them also are an important component of life course research.

Both Mills (1959) and Ryder (1965) laid early groundwork for the life course perspective. Mills' discussion of the intersection of history and biography in his development of the concept of the "sociological imagination" laid the basis for understanding that individual lives are embedded within the social context in which they exist. Thus, individual lives do not play out in a sociohistorical vacuum but instead are heavily influenced by a larger social and historical context. Ryder's discussion of the birth "cohort" facilitated understanding how society changes: that the birth cohort is a vehicle for social change. Matilda White Riley (1987) integrated these two views to form an enduring life course perspective: individual development unfolds within a social context that is defined and shaped largely by the succession of birth cohorts.

This life course view informs contemporary thinking about stratification and inequality. Individuals are born into a society that is already stratified – that is, differentiated – along key dimensions, including sex, race, and SES, and these dimensions are interrelated. Put another way, inequality exists at the outset for individuals. Individuals' lives then unfold across age within this initially stratified system, and inequality may expand or contract as social conditions change (or do not). Life course research on stratification and inequality, therefore, must attend to both within-individual change over age ("aging") and broader sociohistorical history ("social change").

Figure 8.1 demonstrates some of the complexity involved in a life course perspective on inequality. We use this figure as a heuristic device to structure our discussion of both substantive and methodological issues in contemporary inequality research. At the

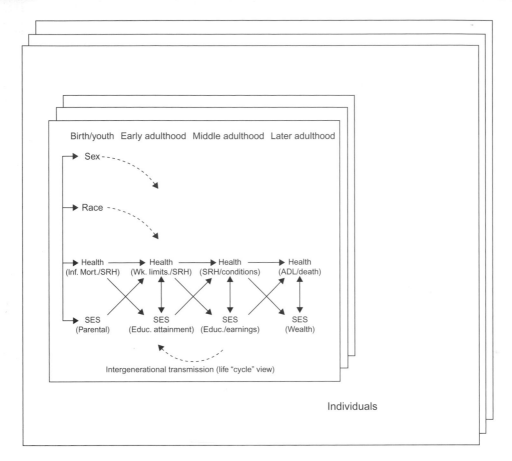

Birth cohorts

Figure 8.1 Depiction of life course stratification processes.

lowest level, that is, the individual level, the figure shows a relatively complex within-individual process in which stratification plays out across the life course of individuals. Via layered boxes – and to some extent via characteristics that differentiate individuals such as sex, race, early life SES, and early life health – the figure shows that the individual life course is differentiated across individuals. That is, individuals are differentiated at birth, and throughout life, by their acquired statuses (e.g. sex, race, parental SES, and health at birth), and these early life statuses partially shape subsequent health and socioeconomic inequality. Finally, via larger layered boxes, the figure shows that the process of stratification that unfolds across age, and that is differentiated across individuals, plays out across a broader historical context, with the cohorts within which individuals are born acting as the vehicles of change.

No research to date has investigated the entire model in Figure 8.1 (although some work does engage large portions; see Elder, 1974). However, all

stratification research to date can be placed within the diagram, and recent research captures larger portions of this diagram than earlier studies did. Research has evolved in several directions within the bounds of this figure. As noted previously, early theory focused primarily on the evolution of the stratification system (e.g. Durkheim, Marx, and Weber; represented loosely in the figure via the larger layered boxes). Research in the middle of the last century moved from broad, theoretical discussions to between-cohort (or short-term intergenerational) transmission of SES. We represent this focus as the dashed, curved path from middle adulthood back to early adulthood (which is admittedly misplaced; i.e. the dashed line should link the middle adulthood of an individual in the earlier generation with the early adulthood of a younger generation individual). Contemporary demographic research on health inequalities has focused on the larger boxes in examining change in socioeconomic inequalities, especially in mortality (Elo & Preston, 1996; Pappas et al., 1993). In general, this research has shown that income and wealth inequality, as well as health inequality, have generally expanded over the last century (see Massey, 2007 for in-depth discussion of the growth in earnings and wealth inequality over the last quarter century).

Research focusing on socioeconomic and health inequality across birth cohorts (or time) has tended to ignore within-individual aging and the role of SES at that level. Nonetheless, another body of research, largely in social epidemiology, social psychology, and sociology more broadly, has simultaneously evolved to focus on between-individual differences in health, wealth, and SES that unfold across the life course (e.g. Farkas & O'Rand, 1998; House et al., 1994; O'Rand, 1996; Ross & Wu, 1996).

Research has generally found that inequality widens across the life course: From unequal beginnings emerge even more unequal endings. Merton (1968, 1988) provided an early theoretical and empirical basis for this "Matthew Effect" in studying scientific careers, finding that the publication gap between scientists at high vs low status colleges and universities that existed in early careers widened over time. In both the stratification and health inequality literature, this pattern has been referred to as the "cumulative dis/advantage" perspective (see Crystal & Shea, 1990; Dannefer, 1991; Dannefer & Sell, 1988). The basic tenet of this theory is that initially modest social distinctions become amplified over the life course as minor social advantages lead to additional social opportunities for individuals with higher status relative to their less-well-off peers such that these differences become quite substantial by mid- and late life. Applying this theory to economic inequalities is straightforward. Socioeconomic advantage is passed to children; educational attainment is strongly predicted by parental attainment and status. Early adult educational attainment translates into differential occupations to which differential earnings are attached. Differential earnings then translate into differential rates of salary progression and wealth accumulation. Therefore, at the end of the life course, what began as a modest differential has become a substantial differential at retirement and beyond (for an extended discussion, see O'Rand & Henretta, 1999).

Cumulative dis/advantage theory also has been applied to health inequalities, although the pathways to health inequalities are somewhat more complex. To be brief, although health disparities exist at birth, contemporary youth in the US are predominantly healthy. However, socioeconomic inequalities tend to lead to differences in exposure to risk factors for poor health (e.g. smoking, alcohol consumption, lack of exercise, and less nutritious diets), as well as differences in health care access and social psychological skills that may buffer the effects of stress. After long-term exposure to risk factors and the inability to mitigate stressors, a health differential emerges across age (Dannefer, 2003; Ross & Wu, 1996).

A competing theory emerged as the result of empirical findings that health gaps between socioeconomic groups widen across early and middle adulthood, but then narrow in later life. Kitagawa and Hauser first observed this pattern in 1973, but paid little attention to it. Subsequent research, based on a life course perspective, found a similar pattern and developed a theoretical explanation. House et al. (1994) argued that, although social factors have strong effects on health early in the life course, biological processes begin to dominate in later life (see also House, 2002). In brief, as biological organisms age, they experience increased susceptibility to chronic diseases, declines in functioning, and an increase in mortality risk, and these come to overpower social factors in later life, making SES differences less important. Crystal and Shea (1990) make a similar argument regarding the narrowing of economic gaps in old age due to the attenuation of economic inequality by progressive social programs such as public pensions that redistribute income and offset market forces.

Contemporary research on life course and cohort differences in health has integrated these two temporal dimensions. Lauderdale (2001), for example, showed that mortality differentials persist across age, even when cohort differences in mortality are taken into account. Her research showed, specifically, that, when widening mortality differentials across time (cohort) are considered, the within-cohort age pattern of mortality widened. Lynch (2003) expanded this view and showed that, if cohort differences in self-rated health were controlled, the observed narrowing of socioeconomic health differentials disappeared and was consistent with the widening health differentials observed by Ross and Wu (1996); that is, consistent with cumulative dis/advantage theory.

Other research in stratification and health inequalities has become more refined in its focus on within-individual change over the life course. In our figure, this corresponds to the interrelationship of health and SES across the life course; in particular, the diagonal arrows from SES and health at one stage of the life course to another.

Recent research on inequality and health over the life course has progressed in two complementary directions. Research over the last decade, especially in economics, has focused on the role that health during childhood and adolescence plays in producing inequality in socioeconomic outcomes later in life. At its extreme, such research has found (or at least argued) that the entirety of the SES–health relationship is explained by selection; that is, that later-life health and SES are purely the function of early life health (e.g. Smith & Kingston, 1997).

Additionally, sociological and epidemiologic research has focused on the effects of early life health on later socioeconomic attainment/status. Barker's research (1990, 1992, 1995; see also Joseph & Kramer, 1996) is among the earliest work in this area. Barker showed that early life conditions, including in utero conditions, influence later-life health and longevity. Although Barker's focus was not on the role of stratification/inequality in producing early-life health inequality, his research spearheaded a focus on the persistence of health inequality as a major factor in later-life health inequality in sociology. Specifically, sociologists have been focused on the role that SES, especially early in life (e.g. particularly educational attainment; see Lauderdale, 2001; Lynch, 2003) plays in the production of health inequalities later in life. Since publication of Barker's study, research on the effects of early life course conditions on adult and late-life health inequality has blossomed and become a major area of investigation (see Gunnell et al., 1998; Hayward & Gorman, 2004; McLeod & Almazan, 2003; Shanahan & Mortimer, 1996; Wheaton & Clarke, 2003).

Barker's work dovetailed nicely with one additional development in the life course study of socioeconomic and health inequality: the role of biomarkers and genetics in the production of later-life health. This area of investigation mainly falls outside the domain of stratification and inequality research, but there has been growing interest within sociology in researching the role of genetics and biomarkers in producing later-life health disparities (see National Research Council, 2000).

In inequality research focused on non-health outcomes, contemporary work on within-individual life course differences has developed in areas such as educational attainment, social mobility, and work, and often includes a focus on associated race and/ or gender inequalities. For example, Johnson (2002) links early life course experiences and social origins to the development of work value trajectories as adolescents transition from schooling to employment in young adulthood, noting the particularly strong effects of race and gender as they interact with life course development and occupational opportunity structures. Some social mobility work has begun to combine the well-established findings regarding the role of "weak-ties" in social networks in obtaining employment with a greater focus on the longitudinal nature of employment trajectories. Wegener (1991), for example, notes the importance of the social status/prestige of earlier employment in determining whether such ties are effective in gaining subsequent employment. His findings show that individuals from low status employment pathways gain no benefit from the weak ties established in their prior jobs. Likewise, work in educational attainment continues to explore the mechanisms that produce the now well-established inequalities noted in the early status attainment models. For example, Cameron and Heckman (2001) investigated the sources of race-ethnic disparities in college attendance in the US. While prevailing wisdom among scholars had suggested that the strong negative impact of lower parental income among minority students was a matter of credit constraints faced by families with college-aged children – a fundamentally economic argument – their results demonstrated that parental background and family environment accounted for most of the differential in college attendance a strongly life course finding (i.e.: the linked lives of parent and child rather than immediate economic circumstances was most important in explaining differences in educational attainment).

In sum, incorporating a life course perspective in stratification research and health research has increased our understanding of how time, especially as measured by cohort differences, influences the relationship between SES and health. In addition, the life course perspective has led to a deeper understanding of the interrelationship between SES and health across the lives of individuals. What remains to be discussed is the role that data and methodological developments play in the study of stratification and inequality.

METHODOLOGICAL ISSUES IN THE LIFE COURSE STUDY OF INEQUALITY

The widespread emergence/acquisition of data that facilitate life course investigations into inequality began in the mid-to-late 1970s in conjunction with the development of life course theory. Prior to this, most studies of inequality used single-year cross-sectional data sets. To be sure, some long-term longitudinal data collection efforts began prior to the 1970s. For example, the Terman Study began in the 1920s (see Elder and Johnson, 2003) and the Wisconsin Longitudinal Study began in 1957 (see Sewell et al., 2004). However, such efforts were limited prior to the 1970s, and samples were often not nationally representative. The explosion in availability of nationally representative repeated cross-sections and panels began in the 1970s and facilitated richer investigations. An explicit life course approach to studying inequality, however, brings with it a host of methodological issues that must be addressed to reach valid conclusions.

It is true that a purely cross-sectional, or static, approach to studying inequality also raises numerous methodological issues, but these problems become more apparent when one takes a life course view. In part, these problems become more apparent because of the nature of the data used in life course research. For example, missing data due to attrition and mortality in panel studies is a larger – or at least more recognizable – concern for data collected over time than for "snap-shot" studies.

Part of the reason that life course research using repeated cross-sectional or panel data brings such issues to the forefront is that longitudinal data potentialize the ability to address and resolve some of the problems that simple cross-sectional data do not. For example, without sophisticated methods and/or assumptions, little can be done about mortality prior to recruitment into a single cross-sectional study. In this section, we highlight some key methodological issues that challenge life course research in general and life course research on inequality specifically.

Age-Period-Cohort Issues

Perhaps the greatest contribution that the life course perspective has made to research on inequality is recognition that the meaning of age, as a variable, is multifaceted. In a single cross-sectional study, age is often incorporated as a control variable in regression models, and the meaning of its coefficient (i.e. its "effect") is uncertain, permitting multiple interpretations. In early aging research, investigators often interpreted coefficients for age as genuine aging effects; that is, as the consequence to the outcome variable (i.e. earnings) of an individual growing older. This interpretation may be sensible for outcomes such as chronic illness or mortality risk, which increase with age. This kind of interpretation makes less sense, however, for variables such as educational attainment, which cannot decrease with age. In cross-sectional data, education is, in fact, negatively related to age: Education has a mean of about 13 years at age 30 and a mean of less than 11 years at age 89+ in the GSS (see Riley, 1987 for an early discussion of this result). In contrast, when education is regressed on age and birth cohort using repeated cross-sectional data, the effect of both cohort and age is positive. That is, mean educational attainment has increased across birth cohorts, and it increases slightly across age within birth cohorts (Riley, 1987).

The life course perspective can explain these seemingly disparate results. Simply put, age represents the influence of three different components of time: age, cohort, and period. Education is largely fixed, at the individual level, by age 30. Educational attainment has increased across the last century, however, as the result of policies such as compulsory education laws and the creation of the GI Bill for veterans. The result is that successive birth cohorts have obtained higher average levels of education by age 30.

Within birth cohorts, mean educational attainment increases across age for two reasons. First, returning to school after age 30 has become popular among baby boomers, for retraining, personal, or other reasons (see Elman & O'Rand, 1998, 2004). Second, selective mortality – that is, greater mortality among less-educated members of a birth cohort across age – reduces a birth cohort to its more educated members, thereby increasing the mean (see Lleras-Muney, 2005).

A single cross-sectional study does not allow the disentangling of these processes, but repeated cross-sectional studies and panel studies do. The evolution of data sources from simple, one-shot cross-sectional studies to repeated cross-sections and panels has enabled us to separate the effect of different dimensions of time in contemporary research. However, life course research seeking to disentangle age, cohort, and period effects confronts two limitations.

First, the APC "dilemma" is well-known. Put succinctly, regardless of data availability, only two dimensions of time can be modeled at once without strong assumptions, because the third dimension is determined by the first two. If we know, for example, the year of a study and the ages of the respondents in it, we know their birth cohort(s) as well. This problem has been well-recognized for decades (see Smith, 2008 for a review of its history), but recent methodological work (as described in Chapter 2) suggests that age, period, and cohort effects can be differentiated. Although the proponents of new methods recognize the limitations of their new approaches, it is important to note that simply understanding that age can represent at least two different dimensions of time is important given that, with appropriate data, we can at least differentiate between-individual differences from within-individual change over time.

Second, the very structure of extant studies limits our ability to fully disentangle temporal patterns. Panel studies are generally implemented without replenishment to compensate for attrition and/or to recruit new cohorts in the desired age range. Thus, the birth cohorts that begin a longitudinal study are the only ones studied. As a result, the portion of the total "lexis" surface (i.e. a two-dimensional grid created by intersecting age in years with period in years) covered by most panel studies constitutes only a set of diagonal bands of the full surface. With most panel studies (e.g. the ACL survey, the National Health Epidemiologic Follow-up surveys, and the National Longitudinal surveys), data are restricted to an initial set of cohorts that were studied at baseline. Thus, there is relatively little overlapping of the age-range coverage of birth cohorts that is needed to facilitate a full life course disentanglement of age and cohort (let alone period) patterns (see Lynch & Lin, 2008). Additionally, the few panel studies that do replenish portions of their samples by adding more recent cohorts, such as the National Long-Term Care Survey or the HRS, are limited, because they are typically restricted to narrow age ranges (e.g. over age 65 in the NLTCS and over age 51 in the HRS).

Repeated cross-sectional studies are not a panacea either, although they cover a larger portion of the lexis surface. A major problem with repeated cross-sectional studies is that they do not permit investigation of endogeneity and selection, including selective survival.

Endogeneity and Selection

Endogeneity and selection are key problems for research on inequality. Technically, endogeneity occurs when a predictor variable (x) in a regression model is correlated with the error term (e) in the model. This can occur under a variety of conditions, but two cases are especially common in inequality research: (1) when important variables are omitted from the model (called "omitted variable bias") and (2) when the outcome variable is a predictor of x and not simply a response to x (called "simultaneity bias"). At least part of the latter problem is often called "selection."

The former problem is well-known in social research, and, indeed, many studies use this bias to an advantage. One of the most common approaches to investigating mediators of a social process is to estimate a regression model first with only the key x variable of interest predicting the outcome and then estimate a second model that includes hypothesized mediators of the relationship. The researcher can then compute the proportion of the total effect of x that is "explained" by the mediators (the "indirect effect") and the proportion that remains attributable to x (the "direct effect"). The change in the coefficient of x is a result of omitted variable bias: In the first model, the omission of mediators led to an overestimate of the direct effect of x.

Omitted variable bias has been the point of departure for countless studies of inequality. For example, explanations of sex and race differences in earnings and wealth are often considered to be a function of (i.e. to be mediated by) differences in educational attainment between groups. This research has consistently found that a large proportion of sex and race differences is attributable to educational attainment differences between groups (see Corcoran & Duncan, 1979; Jacobs, 1996).

A more insidious and difficult type of endogeneity occurs when the outcome variable of interest is, in fact, a predictor of the x variable(s) in a model. Ignoring this simultaneity produces biased coefficients that generally lead to overestimation of the effect size of x in regression models. In inequality research, simultaneity has been especially problematic when the outcome of interest is health because it is possible – indeed probable – that health has reciprocal effects on educational attainment, occupational status (including employment status), and earnings.

Historically, with simple cross-sectional data sets, it was difficult to resolve endogeneity problems. First, early cross-sectional studies tended to have small samples and few variables. Such studies made handling omitted variable bias difficult because there were few variables beyond those of interest that could be included to rule out spurious threats to validity. Further, a common method for dealing with endogeneity in economic research was, and still is, the use of instrumental variables methods involving two- and three-stage least squares estimation. In brief, the most basic instrumental variables methods involve (1) finding "replacement" variables ("instruments") that are correlated with an endogenous x variable but are uncorrelated with the error term, (2) regressing the original x variable on these instruments and forming predicted values from this result to replace the original endogenous x, and (3) regressing the outcome on the exogenous x variables and the predicted values formed in step (2).

Yet, finding appropriate instruments is difficult if not impossible in studies with few variables. Further still, handling endogeneity due to simultaneity is virtually impossible with cross-sectional data because all variables are measured simultaneously. Ultimately, results of analyses using such data rested on theoretical arguments about the temporal priority of variables and the theoretical plausibility of reciprocal effects.

The growth in the availability of repeated cross-sectional and, especially, panel data sets enabled the development of better approaches to handling endogeneity in the study of inequality. In health research, for example, a rapidly growing area of investigation is in the role that early-life health inequality plays in later-life health inequality (e.g. Hayward & Gorman, 2004). This research has attempted to determine the role that early-life health and SES play in affecting later-life health, corresponding to the bottom half of Figure 8.1.

Selective Mortality/Survival

Selective mortality (or selective survival) is also a problem in the study of inequality but has only been explicitly discussed in research on health inequality. Selective mortality is the process by which a cohort of individuals becomes less heterogeneous as a result of differential survival of its members. The result of selective mortality is that the explanatory power of predictors (like education) weakens as a cohort of individuals becomes more homogeneous across age (see Lynch, 2003 for discussion; selective mortality may mask cumulative disadvantage).

Some of the earliest contemporary work on selective survival was done by Vaupel and Yashin (1985), who found that the age pattern of mortality risk itself was affected by differential mortality rates within a cohort. For example, if two subpopulations within a single birth cohort each have exponential (Gompertz) mortality hazards across age, but one subpopulation has substantially lower mortality than the other, the aggregate mortality pattern for the entire cohort will not be exponential over age.

Indeed, Horiuchi and Wilmoth (1998) showed that, if a cohort is comprised of multiple subpopulations, each having its own exponential mortality hazard across age (with the range of variation ["frailty"] in these hazards following a particular probability distribution [gamma] in the population), the resulting hazard for the entire cohort follows a logistic pattern, such that the aggregate rate of mortality increase begins to taper beyond midlife and becomes flat at the oldest ages.

In the case of mortality, then, selective survival produces a weakening effect of age on the mortality hazard across age. Although this problem may seem relevant only to the study of mortality, others have shown that such (potentially unobserved) subpopulation heterogeneity has far-reaching implications on understanding health inequalities across the life course. As discussed above, there is an ongoing debate in the literature on the effect of education (and income) on health across age. The cumulative disadvantage hypothesis argues that health disparities between SES groups widen across age (e.g. Lynch, 2003; Ross & Wu, 1996), while the age-as-leveler hypothesis contends that SES-based health disparities decline post midlife (Beckett, 2000; House et al., 1994).

A corresponding argument appears in the literature on race and mortality. On the one hand, the "double jeopardy hypothesis" proposes that health gaps between whites and blacks should widen across age as a function of the "double" threat to health that aging and racial minority status pose (Ferraro & Farmer, 1996). On the other hand, empirical findings indicate that the health and mortality risk gap between blacks and whites narrows across age. Indeed, a mortality "crossover" occurs beyond age 75 in which whites are more likely to die than blacks. Some have argued that this finding is the result of unreliable age reporting among blacks; others have argued that selective survival accounts for the crossover (see Lynch et al., 2003 for discussion; Markides & Black, 1996). A mortality crossover or convergence in the effect of SES on health *could* be purely an artifact of strong mortality selection, but extant data sets provide little opportunity to verify this conclusion.

Beyond health, selective survival may be important for understanding life course processes that do not (at least directly) bear on health. For example, we can find no investigation in the literature on differences in earnings or differences in wealth accumulation that consider – or even mention – the role of selective survival in earnings and wealth accumulation at advanced ages. Yet, to the extent that earnings and wealth accumulation predict health earlier in life, and to the extent that health predicts survival, it is surely the case that observed earnings and wealth differentials in later adulthood may be larger than have been estimated with models that fail to compensate for selective survival.

Missing Data

Data in simple, one-shot cross-sectional studies that address inequality are often missing. While it is rare for data to be missing on key life course stratification variables such as age, sex, race, and education, it is quite common for data to be missing on earnings, wealth, occupation, and health variables. Indeed, it is common for 15% or more of respondents to refuse to report earnings and wealth. In studies of the effects of SES on health, it is also common for similarly substantial percentages of health data to be missing as well (or, to be measured via proxy respondents and therefore discounted). Thus, missing data pose a significant problem for the study of inequality, and the problem is often accentuated in repeated cross-sectional and, especially, panel studies. At the root of missing data problems is the failure of many studies to consider the many ways that "missingness" may occur in life course research.

The key issue with missing data is that ignoring it may produce biased results. The "trick" is to determine when missing data are problematic. Since the late 1980s, scholars have attempted to develop schema that document and explain the consequences of missing data. To date, the most important schema that has emerged comes from Little and Rubin (2002), who classify missing data as (1) missing completely at random (MCAR), (2) missing at random (MAR), and (3) observed at random (OAR). To avoid the use of double negatives, we can reduce this typology to the following. If the propensity for missingness on a variable y is not predicted by any variable x nor y itself, then the data that are missing on y are MCAR. If the propensity for missingness on y is a function of x, but not y, then the missing data are not OAR. Finally, if the propensity for missingness on y is a function of y itself, then the missing data are not MAR. For example, consider earnings as the outcome of interest. If a person's education (or some other variable, but not earnings) predicts whether s/he answers the earnings question in a survey, then missingness on earnings is not OAR. In contrast, if the value of the person's earnings itself predicts whether s/he answers the earnings item (e.g. persons with high earnings do not answer the earnings question), then missingness on earnings is not MAR.

As Little and Rubin (and others) have shown, when missing data are either MCAR or MAR, the missing data mechanism is "ignorable," meaning that we may proceed with any variety of methods that have emerged over the last decade or so to deal with it. In the past, list-wise deletion (or "complete case analysis") was the usual method of dealing with missing data. The only problem with this strategy when the data are at least MAR is that it can produce a significant loss of sample size (statistical power). More recently, other, increasingly popular, methods for handling missing data have emerged that help preserve statistical power, including methods that involve altering the model itself (e.g. full information maximum likelihood [FIML] analysis), methods that involve altering the parameter estimation strategy (e.g. expectation-maximization [EM] algorithms), and methods that involve augmenting the data (e.g. multiple imputation) (see Little & Rubin, 2002 for in-depth technical discussion of these methods).

All of these "solutions" for missing data are particularly problematic for inequality research because they all assume that the missing data are MAR. There are a number of common sources of missingness in life course research on inequality, and many, if not most, of them do not justify the MAR assumption. Missingness in panel data is the easiest to consider. Individuals may be missing on key variables in panel data because of unit or item nonresponse. Unit nonresponse means that an individual (or family) did not participate in a wave of a study because of (1) mortality, (2) movement/unlocatability, or (3) refusal or inability (e.g. onset of dementia) to participate. In these cases, the entire record for an individual (or family) will be missing, and missingness may be related to the outcome of interest. For example, if one is interested in a socioeconomic outcome, individuals with lower SES will have a greater propensity to die between waves of a study. Lower SES individuals may also have a greater propensity to become institutionalized, making them more difficult to locate or more likely to be unable to participate in an interview. At the other end of the SES spectrum, those with higher SES are more likely to move. Even if we know that the individual died, the fact that the unobserved socioeconomic outcome is related to mortality makes the missingness not MAR. And, if the individual did not die (and/or we cannot confirm it), we cannot simply assume that missingness is MAR. Knowing that the individual refused (or was unable) to participate is not necessarily good news, either: refusal may be predicated on the outcome of interest, much as we know high income earners are often less likely to report their income, and those with the poorest health may be unable to report their health.

Item nonresponse may be less problematic because we may be able to use contemporaneous measures to predict who refuses to answer particular items (e.g. wealth). Unless we are certain that observed covariates explain entirely (e.g. pseudo-R-squared = 1) why a respondent refuses to respond to an item, however, we cannot conclude that the missingness is MAR. In brief, we simply cannot know how (or why) nonrespondents differ from respondents in panel studies because the data required to determine this are missing.

In repeated cross-sectional data, as opposed to panel data, missingness may appear to be less of a problem. That is, a few percent missing at each wave on particular items may seem to be offset by the fact that we ultimately have more observed data points. However, a subtle type of missingness in such studies is selective mortality prior to inclusion in the cross-section. For example, in studies of mid-adulthood earnings, selective mortality reduces the pool of potential respondents from a given birth cohort to the highest-earning subset, thereby reducing earnings gaps in mid-to late adulthood.

There are procedures for handling selective mortality and other forms of attrition in panel studies, but to date few studies in inequality research have addressed this issue. Failing to address this issue may influence (i.e. bias) studies' findings, especially with regard to wealth inequalities in late adulthood. Given the dearth of research addressing this issue, however, we can only speculate about the implications of selective survival on substantive findings.

CONCLUSIONS

The study of stratification and inequality has a long history in social science research, dating back to the late 1800s. While the earliest research was primarily theoretical and driven by macro-historical and political views of political economies, empirical research on stratification and inequality began in earnest in the middle of the last century. A few decades later, sex and race began to be studied as central mechanisms in the production of socioeconomic inequality, and health inequality began to be studied as an important outcome of stratification by sex, race, and SES. Late in the century, the emergence of long-term longitudinal data – both repeated cross-sections and panel studies – as well as the development of more sophisticated statistical methods for analyzing such data facilitated an expansion of research following a life course perspective. Contemporary research has therefore expanded in two directions: toward a broader understanding of the inter-linkage of life course processes within sociohistorical (cohort) change and toward a more in-depth understanding of the process of stratification over the life course of individuals. From our view, with the ever-expanding wealth of longitudinal data, the ever-expanding ability of statistical methodology to address the problems that such data present, and the increasing permanence and refinement of the life course paradigm, future research will become less piecemeal and more integrative to provide a richer understanding of inequality.

We see several directions, both substantive and methodological, in which the study of inequality should expand. Substantively, first, future research on inequality should continue to expand its focus on the production of inequality over the life course of individuals. We are only beginning to understand how early life events and conditions shape inequality across adulthood and later life. Future research should pay particular attention to the potential role of biology and health in both producing inequality and responding to it. Second, as the US becomes more diverse, future research on inequality needs to broaden its focus on racial and ethnic differences in stratification. Specifically, the typical racial categories of "white" and "nonwhite," (or even "black" and "other"), and the simple ethnic categories of "Hispanic" and "non-Hispanic" are simply insufficient for understanding inequality in a society in which a large and growing proportion are of mixed racial and ethnic ancestry.

In order to obtain a richer understanding of inequality along these lines, studies of inequality must continue to use and develop advanced statistical techniques designed to address life course research questions using longitudinal data. Traditional methods for the analysis of cross-sectional contingency table data, and even some more advanced regression modeling methods, are simply insufficient tools for modeling life course processes that are inherently replete with endogeneity problems. At the same time, future research needs to approach new techniques with a healthy level of skepticism. For example, while some innovative new statistical approaches to the APC problem now provide new capabilities for addressing this issue (see Chapter 3) and new applications of latent growth curve modeling claim capabilities that match more directly with fundamental life course inequality research questions (Mirowsky & Kim, 2007), such techniques rely on very strong assumptions that may frequently be incompatible with theorized life course and/or inequality patterns.

Indeed, these fundamental issues/questions may ultimately be unaddressable by any techniques, instead requiring data that are more compatible with the notion of inequality processes that unfold over the entire life course. That is, to understand inequality across the life course, one may need data that capture the full life courses of individuals from birth to death, and this should be a long-term goal for inequality researchers. Collection of such data will require scientists and the organizations that fund and organize data collection to rethink the processes surrounding collection given that this type of study is unobtainable within the lifetime of any single investigator. Indeed, we might learn a great deal about how such data can be collected by looking back at the handful of studies, like the Terman Study, that in a limited way have already succeeded in doing so.

REFERENCES

Barker, D. J. P. (1990). The fetal and infant origins of adult disease. *British Medical Journal*, 301, 1111.

Barker, D. J. P. (Ed.), (1992). *Fetal and infant origins of adult disease*. London: BMJ Publishing.

Barker, D. J. P. (1995). Fetal origins of coronary heart disease. *British Medical Journal*, 311, 171–174.

Beckett, M. (2000). Converging health inequalities in later life – An artifact of mortality selection? *Journal of Health and Social Behavior*, 41, 106–119.

Bielby, W. T. (1981). Models of status attainment. In D. J. Treiman & R. V. Robinson (Eds.), *Research in social stratification and mobility* (Vol. 1, pp. 3–26). Greenwich, CT: JAI Press.

Blau, P. M., & Duncan, O. D. (1967). *The American occupational structure*. New York: Wiley.

Bourdieu, P., & Passeron, J. C. (1977). *Reproduction in education, society, and culture*. Beverly Hills: Sage.

Brown, J. S., & Lynch, S. M. (2004). Race, aging, and health: The history and future of the double jeopardy hypothesis. *Contemporary Gerontology*, 10, 105–109.

Cameron, S. V., & Heckman, J. J. (2001). The dynamics of educational attainment for black, Hispanic, and white males. *Journal of Political Economy*, 109, 673–748.

Corcoran, M., & Duncan, G. J. (1979). Work history, labor force attachment, and earnings differences between the races and sexes. *The Journal of Human Resources*, 14, 3–20.

Crystal, S., & Shea, D. (1990). Cumulative advantage, cumulative disadvantage, and inequality among elderly people. *Gerontologist*, 30, 437–443.

Dannefer, D. (1991). Differential gerontology and the stratified life course: Conceptual and methodological issues. *Annual Review of Gerontology and Geriatrics*, 8, 3–36.

Dannefer, D. (2003). Cumulative advantage/disadvantage and the life course: Cross-fertilizing age and social science theory. *Journal of Gerontology: Social Sciences*, 58B, S327–S337.

Dannefer, D., & Sell, R. (1988). Age structure, the life course, and "aged heterogeneity": Prospects for research and theory. *Comprehensive Gerontology*, B2, 1–10.

Davis, K., & Moore, W. E. (1945). Some principles of stratification. *American Sociological Review*, 10, 242–249.

Duncan, O. D., & Hodge, R. W. (1963). Education and occupational mobility: A regression analysis. *American Journal of Sociology*, 68, 629–644.

Durkheim, É. ([1893] 1997). *The division of labour in society*. New York: The Free Press.

Elder, G. H., Jr. (1974). *Children of the great depression*. Chicago: University of Chicago Press.

Elder, G. H., Jr., & Johnson, M. K. (2003). The life course and aging: Challenges, lessons, and new directions. In R. A. Settersten Jr. (Ed.), *Invitation to the life course: Toward new understandings of later life* (pp. 49–81). Amityville, NY: Baywood Publishing.

Elman, C., & O'Rand, A. M. (1998). Midlife work pathways and educational entry. *Research on Aging, 20,* 475–505.

Elman, C., & O'Rand, A. M. (2004). The race is to the swift: Socioeconomic origins, adult education, and wage attainment. *American Journal of Sociology, 110,* 123–160.

Elo, I. T., & Preston, S. H. (1996). Educational differentials in mortality: United States, 1979–85. *Social Science and Medicine, 42,* 47–57.

Farkas, J. I., & O'Rand, A. M. (1998). The pension mix for women in middle and late life: The changing employment relationship. *Social Forces, 76,* 1007–1032.

Ferraro, K. F., & Farmer, M. M. (1996). Double jeopardy to health hypothesis for African Americans: Analysis and critique. *Journal of Health and Social Behavior, 37,* 27–43.

Firestone, S. (1972). *The dialectic of sex.* New York: Bantam.

Gunnell, D., Smith, G. D., Frankel, S., Nanchahal, K., Braddon, F. E. M., Pemberton, J., et al. (1998). Childhood leg length and adult mortality – Follow-up of the Carnegie survey of diet and growth in pre-war Britain. *Journal of Epidemiology and Community Health, 52,* 142–152.

Hayward, M. D., & Gorman, B. K. (2004). The long arm of childhood: The influence of early-life social conditions on men's mortality. *Demography, 41,* 87–107.

Horiuchi, S., & Wilmoth, J. R. (1998). Deceleration in the age pattern of mortality at older ages. *Demography, 35,* 391–412.

House, J. S. (2002). Understanding social factors and inequalities in health: 20th century progress and 21st century prospects. *Journal of Health and Social Behavior, 43,* 125–142.

House, J. S., Lepkowski, J. M., Kinney, A. M., Mero, R. P., Kessler, R. C., & Herzog, A. R. (1994). The social stratification of aging and health. *Journal of Health and Social Behavior, 35,* 213–234.

Jacobs, J. A. (1996). Gender inequality and higher education. *Annual Review of Sociology, 22,* 153–185.

Johnson, M. K. (2002). Social origins, adolescent experiences, and work value trajectories during the transition to adulthood. *Social Forces, 80,* 1307–1341.

Joseph, K. S., & Kramer, M. S. (1996). Review of the evidence on fetal and early childhood antecedents of adult chronic disease. *Epidemiological Review, 18,* 158–174.

Kawachi, I., Kennedy, B. P., Lochner, K., & Prothrow-Stith, D. (1997). Social capital, income inequality, and mortality. *American Journal of Public Health, 87,* 1491–1498.

Kitagawa, E. M., & Hauser, P. M. (1973). *Differential mortality in the United States: A study in socioeconomic epidemiology.* Cambridge, MA: Harvard University Press.

Lauderdale, D. S. (2001). Education and survival: Birth cohort, period, and age effects. *Demography, 38,* 551–562.

Little, R. J. A., & Rubin, D. B. (2002). *Statistical analysis with missing data* (2nd ed.). Hoboken, NJ: John Wiley & Sons.

Lleras-Muney, A. (2005). The relationship between education and adult mortality in the United States. *Review of Economic Studies, 72,* 189–221.

Lynch, S. M. (2003). Cohort and life-course patterns in the relationship between education and health: A hierarchical approach. *Demography, 40,* 309–331.

Lynch, S. M., & Lin, T. (2008). Growth curve modeling and disentangling age and cohort patterns. Paper presented at the annual meeting of the American Sociological Association, Boston, MA, August.

Lynch, S. M., Brown, J. S., & Harmsen, K. G. (2003). Black-white differences in mortality deceleration and compression and the mortality crossover reconsidered. *Research on Aging, 25,* 456–483.

Markides, K. S., & Black, S. A. (1996). Race, ethnicity, and aging: The impact of inequality. In R. H. Binstock & L. K. George (Eds.), *Handbook of aging in the social sciences* (pp. 153–170) (4th ed.). San Diego, CA: Academic Press.

Marx, K. ([1894] 1972). *Capital* (3 vols.). London: Lawrence and Wishart.

Massey, D. S. (2007). *Categorically unequal: The American stratification system.* New York: Russell Sage Foundation.

McLeod, J. D., & Almazan, E. P. (2003). Connections between childhood and adulthood. In J. T. Mortimer & M. J. Shanahan (Eds.), *Handbook of the life course* (pp. 391–411). New York: Kluwer Academic/Plenum Publishers.

Merton, R. K. (1968). The Matthew effect in science: Theoretical and empirical investigations. *Science, 199,* 55–63.

Merton, R. K. (1988). The Matthew effect in science, II: Cumulative advantage and the symbolism of intellectual property. *ISIS, 79,* 606–623.

Mills, C. W. (1959). *The sociological imagination.* Oxford, UK: Oxford University Press.

Mirowsky, J., & Kim, J. (2007). Graphing age trajectories: Vector graphs, synthetic and virtual cohort projections, and virtual cohort projections, and cross-sectional profiles of depression. *Sociological Methods & Research, 35,* 497–541.

Mirowsky, J., & Ross, C. E. (2003). *Education, social status, and health.* New York: Aldine de Gruyter.

National Research Council. (2000). *Cells and surveys: Should biological measures be included in social science research?* Committee on population: C. E. Finch, J. W. Vaupel, & K. Kinsella (Eds.), *Commission on behavioral and social sciences and education.* Washington, DC: National Academy Press.

O'Rand, A. M. (1996). The precious and the precocious: Understanding cumulative disadvantage and cumulative advantage over the life course. *Gerontologist, 36,* 230–238.

O'Rand, A. M., & Henretta, J. C. (1999). *Age and inequality:*

Diverse pathways through later life. Boulder, CO: Westview Press.

Pager, D. (2007). *Marked: Race, crime, and finding work in an era of mass incarceration.* Chicago: University of Chicago Press.

Pappas, G., Queen, S., Hadden, W., & Fisher, G. (1993). The increasing disparity in mortality between socioeconomic groups in the U.S., 1960 and 1986. *The New England Journal of Medicine, 329,* 103–109.

Reich, M. (1977). The economics of racism. In D. M. Gordon (Ed.), *Problems in political economy: An urban perspective* (pp. 184–188). Lexington, MA: D.C. Health.

Riley, M. W. (1987). On the significance of age in sociology. *American Sociological Review, 52,* 1–14.

Ross, C. E., & Wu, C. (1995). The links between education and health. *American Sociological Review, 60,* 719–745.

Ross, C. E., & Wu, C. (1996). Education, age, and the cumulative advantage in health. *Journal of Health and Social Behavior, 37,* 104–120.

Ryder, N. (1965). The cohort as a concept in the study of social change. *American Sociological Review, 30,* 843–861.

Sewell, W. H., Hauser, R. M., Springer, K. W., & Hauser, T. S. (2004). As we age: A review of the Wisconsin Longitudinal study, 1957–2001. In K. T. Leicht (Ed.), *Research in social stratification and mobility* (Vol. 20, pp. 3–111). London: Elsevier.

Shanahan, M. J., & Mortimer, J. T. (1996). Understanding the positive consequences of psychosocial stressors. *Advances in Group Processes, 13,* 189–209.

Smith, H. (2008). Advances in age-period-cohort analysis. *Sociological Methods and Research, 36,* 287–296.

Smith, J. P., & Kington, R. S. (1997). Race, socioeconomic status, and health in late life. In L. G. Martin & B. J. Soldo (Eds.), *Racial and ethnic differences in the health of older Americans* (pp. 105–162). Washington, DC: National Academy Press.

Sobel, M. E. (1983). Lifestyle differentiation and stratification in contemporary U.S. society. In D. J. Treiman & R. V. Robinson (Eds.), *Research in social stratification and mobility* (Vol. 2, pp. 115–144). Greenwich, CT: JAI Press.

Sorlie, P. D., Backlund, E., & Keller, J. B. (1995). U.S. mortality by economic, demographic, and social characteristics: The national longitudinal mortality study. *American Journal of Public Health, 85,* 949–956.

Tumin, M. M. (1953). Some principles of stratification: A critical analysis. *American Sociological Review, 18,* 378–394.

Vaupel, J., & Yashin, A. I. (1985). Heterogeneity's ruses: Some surprising effects of selection on population dynamics. *The American Statistician, 39,* 176–185.

Veblen, T. (1973). *The theory of the leisure class.* Boston: Houghton Mifflin.

Weber, M. ([1922] 1948). *Economy and society.* Berkeley: University of California Press.

Wegener, B. (1991). Job mobility and social ties: Social resources, prior job, and status attainment. *American Sociological Review, 56,* 60–71.

Western, B. (2006). *Punishment and inequality in America.* New York: Russell Sage Foundation.

Wheaton, B., & Clarke, P. (2003). Space meets time: Integrating temporal and contextual influences on mental health in early adulthood. *American Sociological Review, 68,* 680–706.

Part | 3 |

Social Factors and Social Institutions

Chapter | 9 |

Health Disparities Among Older Adults: Life Course Influences and Policy Solutions

Pamela Herd[1], Stephanie A. Robert[2], James S. House[3]

[1]*Department of Sociology, University of Wisconsin, Madison, Wisconsin,* [2]*School of Social Work, University of Wisconsin, Madison, Wisconsin,* [3]*Department of Sociology and Gerald R. Ford School of Public Policy, University of Michigan, Ann Arbor, Michigan*

CHAPTER CONTENTS

INTRODUCTION

In the US, as in all countries, the health of the population is distributed unevenly: there are disparities in health by education, income, race and ethnicity, neighborhood, and other social factors. We refer to health "disparities" as the unequal distribution of health between groups. Many disparities are also "inequities," differences in health that are unfair because they are socially produced and therefore modifiable. There has been growing attention to this issue in the US, although most of the attention has focused on children and working-age adults. In this chapter, we focus on older adults. We apply a life course approach, highlighting how health disparities arise and accumulate over the life course and into old age.

Attention to health disparities in the US has focused primarily on racial and ethnic differences in health, highlighting the disadvantaged health status of most racial/ethnic minorities, and the unequal access to and quality of care received by many racial/ethnic minorities (IOM, 2002). Racial differences in health are largely, although not exclusively, explained by the lower socioeconomic position (e.g. by education, income, occupation) of racial and ethnic minority groups in the US (Williams & Collins, 1995).

This chapter focuses on SEP: health disparities by education, income, and occupation, and their importance over the life course. We also highlight how disadvantages across multiple social statuses, particularly by SEP, race, and gender, combine to produce large health disparities among older adults. Further, we emphasize that policy solutions to address them must be rooted in a fundamental cause perspective. In short, a key assumption embedded in this perspective is that the route to ameliorating, or even weakening, health disparities is through the distribution of resources (income and educational attainment), what fundamental cause theorists label "upstream" factors, rather than through tackling intermediary factors, such as obesity and smoking, that fundamental cause theorists label "downstream" factors (House et al., 1990; Link & Phelan, 1995, 2002).

We first summarize research on SEP and racial/ethnic disparities in health at older ages, while also emphasizing the need to understand them in the context of a life course perspective. We then explore what has been learned about how to address health disparities at older ages by focusing on social and economic policies for older adults. In particular, we emphasize the importance of focusing on "upstream" factors, such as SEP, as opposed to "downstream" solutions, such as access to medical care or behavioral interventions. We conclude by highlighting some priority research areas that need attention in order to best improve health and reduce health disparities across the life course and at older ages.

HEALTH DISPARITIES AMONG OLDER ADULTS

Over the last few decades in the US, rates of disability among older adults have declined significantly (Freedman et al., 2002; Manton & Gu, 2001; Spillman, 2004; Wolf et al., 2005) and there have been improvements in elders' overall health as well (Martin et al., 2007; Soldo et al., 2006). People are living longer and their lives are, on average, characterized by more years of good physical functioning. Overall trends in improved functional status among older adults partly result from the fact that the average SEP of older adults has improved in recent decades, reflected in higher education, income, and wealth levels (Schoeni et al., 2008).

However, these *average* improvements in both SEP and health among the current cohort of older adults mask the fact that there are still great and ever-growing *disparities* in both SEP and health among older adults (Schoeni et al., 2005). Not surprisingly, inequities in SEP among older adults are associated with disparities in health status. This has stark implications for the health of women and racial minorities, who are much more likely to have lower SEP (Harrington Meyer & Herd, 2007).

SEP Disparities in Health at Older Ages

Although some measures of health have improved among current cohorts of older adults in the US, large disparities in health among older adults by SEP remain. Indeed, evidence suggests that educational differences in disability-free life expectancy in the US have actually widened over the last few decades (House et al., 2005; Schoeni et al., 2005; Singh & Siahpush, 2006). On average, older adults with lower income, less wealth, less education, and lower occupational status have worse health, greater disability, lower health-related quality of life, worse mental health, and earlier mortality than their higher SEP peers (House et al., 1994; Luo & Waite, 2005; Robert et al., 2009).

For example, Schoeni et al. (2005) used data from the NHIS from 1982 to 2002 to examine how changes in morbidity over time were patterned by educational attainment and income among older adults. Although all socioeconomic groups experienced improvements in physical function over time, the rate of improvement in function was much higher and more consistent among those older adults with higher income and educational attainment than, among those with lower SEP. Chaudhry et al. (2004) demonstrate that, among those aged 70 and older, those with low educational attainment (less than 8 years) compared to those with more education (at least 12 years) were 1.4 times more likely to have more functional limitations six months after, as compared to the month before, hospitalization.

The body of research on SEP and health highlights how various dimensions of SEP are each independently associated with health outcomes at older ages. Older adults with lower occupational status (from their longest or last occupation) have worse health and greater disability than those in higher occupational categories (Chandola et al., 2007; Gueorguieva et al., 2009; Guilley & Lalive d'Epinay, 2008). Income is strongly related to mortality among older adults (Feinglass et al., 2007), and predicts the progression of disease and disability over the life course (Herd et al., 2007; Zimmer & House, 2003). Although each greater increment of income is associated with better health, the relationship is curvilinear, such that having low income or being in poverty is most strongly related to poor health at older ages (Backlund et al., 1996; Luo & Waite, 2005; McDonough et al., 1997). Education is also strongly related to the onset of disease and disability, independent of income and occupation (Herd et al., 2007; Zimmer & House, 2003). It is hypothesized that education provides a set of psychological and cognitive skills that facilitate better health (Ross & Wu, 1995). Finally, subjective social status, or how one rates one's social status compared to one's peers, is associated with multiple health outcomes among older men (for self-rated health, depression, and long-standing illness) and older women (for self-rated health, depression, long-standing illness, diabetes, and high-density lipoprotein cholesterol), after adjusting for many covariates, including wealth, education, and occupational class (Demakakos et al., 2008).

Beyond personal SEP, studies show that the socioeconomic context of one's neighborhood contributes to the physical, psychological, and cognitive health of older adults, over and above their own SEP (Diez-Roux et al., 1997; Lawlor et al., 2005a; Morenoff et al., 2007; Robert & Ruel, 2006; Sheffield & Peek, 2009). The hypothesized links between poor neighborhoods and health range from the stress and limited social networks produced by violent neighborhoods (psychosocial pathways) to the lack of accessible grocery stores and restaurants with fresh fruits and vegetables (material pathways).

Racial/Ethnic Disparities in Health at Older Ages

Health status among older adults is also significantly stratified by race and ethnicity in the US. African American older adults have worse health than white older adults on virtually all measures of physical and mental health function (Bulatao & Anderson, 2004). However, Asian older adults in the US have better health and functioning, on average, than non-Hispanic white older adults (Mutchler et al., 2007). American Indian older adults have much higher rates of morbidity and earlier mortality than whites (Harrington et al., 2007). Although Hispanic older adults have greater functional disability and poorer self-rated health than non-Hispanic white older adults (Schoeni et al., 2005), they have comparable mortality rates (Hummer et al., 2004). This latter finding is often referred to as the "Hispanic Paradox," wherein some Hispanic groups have better health than would be expected given their average lower SEP in comparison to non-Hispanic whites. A recent study by Turra and Goldman (2007) suggests that this Hispanic health advantage at older ages is found only among the lowest SEP groups. Hispanic older adults with low income or education have better mortality in middle and older ages than their non-Hispanic white peers. The paradox also appears to reflect nativity. US-born Hispanics with high education levels have worse mortality than their highly educated non-Hispanic white peers at middle and older ages. Finally, it is important to keep in mind that the health of Hispanics varies by country of origin. Some Hispanic groups, such as Cubans, have substantially better health outcomes when compared to other groups, such as Mexicans.

Because most racial and ethnic minority groups have lower SEP in the US, and because SEP is so strongly associated with health, racial disparities in health are substantially explained by individual SEP at older ages (e.g. Hayward et al., 2000; Williams & Oh, 2009). This suggests that addressing SES differences by race in the US would improve population health and reduce racial disparities in health across the life course. This includes addressing the racial and socioeconomic residential segregation of people in the US, which contributes to racial disparities in health (Cagney et al., 2005; Robert & Ruel, 2006; Subramanian et al., 2005; Yao & Robert, 2008).

Despite this important role of SEP in understanding the reasons for racial disparities in health, once SEP is controlled for, some racial disparities persist in both physical health (Crimmins et al., 2004; Farmer & Ferraro, 2005; Kahn & Fazio, 2005; Robert & Lee, 2002; Williams & Collins, 1995) and mental health (Skarupski et al., 2005). Research finds that, despite Medicare, racial differences in access to, and quality of, care contribute to poor health outcomes among racial and ethnic minorities (Voelker, 2008). However, health care does not account for all of these disparities, and a growing research agenda is exploring how racial differences in stress, discrimination, sense of control, social support, and other psychosocial factors may contribute to the additional burden of illness among racial/ethnic minorities (Williams & Mohammed, 2009; Williams & Oh, 2009).

One area of limited research is the interaction between race, SEP, and gender. For example, among those born in 1970, white women will outlive African American women by seven years (Hayward & Heron, 1999). But we know little about what might explain these differences and the extent to which SEP mediates and moderates these associations. Since low SEP is disproportionately concentrated among women and minority older adults, the combination of these lower statuses at older ages and their relation to health outcomes need to be understood.

LIFE COURSE APPROACH TO UNDERSTANDING HEALTH DISPARITIES AT OLDER AGES

A life course approach is critical to understanding health disparities at older ages. A life course approach, as discussed in Chapter 10, focuses on how processes of stratification work over the lifespan of individuals, groups, and cohorts to produce health outcomes in later life (Mortimer & Shanahan, 2004). Life course perspectives highlight that social status can affect health at any point in one's life, and that the timing of exposures and experiences linked to inequity may matter more at some ages in the lifespan. Alwin and Wray (2005) highlight that "the structure, sequence, and dynamics of events, transitions, and trajectories (social pathways) that take place within life-stage phases over the lifespan have consequences on health" (p. 10).

A life course approach looks at how SEP is related to health at older ages, but also how SEP and health affect each other in complex ways over the life course to produce health disparities at older ages. From this perspective, SEP in older adulthood may affect health at older ages, but a lifetime of dynamic and cumulative exposures and experiences also contributes to health at older ages. SEP and health have reciprocal relationships across the life course, contributing to chains of risk and accumulation of risk that individuals face as they age (Haas, 2008; Hayward & Gorman, 2004; Robert et al., in press).

In early life, evidence demonstrates that having parents with limited socioeconomic resources, both education and income, leads to accumulating health disadvantages across the life course (Case et al., 2002; Luo & Waite, 2005). Children who grow up poor or with parents with limited education and occupational attainment, have worse health outcomes throughout childhood and into adulthood (Guralnik et al., 2006; Lawlor et al., 2005b; Power et al., 2005; Singh-Manoux et al., 2004) and old age (Blackwell et al., 2001; Holland et al., 2000). The literature, however, is inconsistent regarding how these effects vary by gender and race. For example, Hamil-Luker and O'Rand (2007) found that adverse socioeconomic conditions in childhood were predictive of heart attack in adulthood for women but not for men.

There is less agreement regarding the extent to which adults' SEP weakens the health effect of childhood SEP. The Barker hypothesis suggests that most sources of later-life health disparities can be found in fetal and infant life (Barker, 1992; Barker et al., 1993). Poor maternal health, which itself is often a product of poverty, leads to an in-utero environment that stagnates infant development. These childhood antecedents of ill health may not emerge until later in life. In essence, this unhealthy in-utero environment leads to biological programming of ill health. Indeed, one explanatory factor for why the infant mortality rate for African American mothers with college degrees is the same as white mothers without a high school degree is that African American women's childhood deprivation leads to health problems during their pregnancies (Lu & Halfon, 2003). However, some studies that have more effectively adjusted for adult SEP contradict the Barker hypothesis. These studies find that adult SEP is a better predictor of health outcomes than childhood SEP (Pensola & Martikainen, 2003; Wamala et al., 2001)

Poor health also affects socioeconomic trajectories across the life course. A growing body of literature documents how childhood health affects educational attainment and adult income (Case et al., 2005; Haas, 2006; Palloni, 2006). But even if poor childhood health negatively affects educational attainment, the root source of health disparities remains growing up in a household with limited socioeconomic resources. In order to understand the relationship between SEP and health in old age, we must look earlier in the life course to sort out the underlying dynamics that drive these relationships.

Cumulative Effects and Double Jeopardy vs "Age as Leveler"

There are competing theories about whether health disparities by SEP and race/ethnicity should widen or decline across the life course. One life course theoretical approach, "cumulative advantage/disadvantage" theory, suggests that racial and socioeconomic disparities in health widen over time as disadvantages or advantages compound or accumulate over the life course (Dannefer, 2003; Kahn & Fazio, 2005; O'Rand, 1996; O'Rand & Hamil-Luker, 2005). Consistent with this theory, a "double jeopardy" hypothesis suggests that older age itself is a disadvantage that amplifies the effects of race/ethnicity and/or SEP on health among older adults (e.g. Ferraro & Farmer, 1996). Similarly, some gerontological literature suggests that neighborhood context may be particularly salient to the health and functioning of people who have already experienced health challenges (Lawton, 1998; Wen et al., 2005). More generally, those experiencing health or other challenges at older ages may be particularly susceptible to the effects of neighborhood context and other stressors on changes in physical and mental health.

Cumulative disadvantage theory highlights how early disadvantage or advantage affects how cohorts differentiate in health over time (Ferraro & Kelley-Moore, 2003). Some evidence from Russia supports a cumulative disadvantage model where each additional life course socioeconomic risk factor was associated with a greater likelihood of poor self-rated health at older ages (Nicholson et al., 2005). Lawlor and colleagues (2005b) found that there was cumulative risk for heart disease among older women: the more socioeconomic risk factors they had, the more likely they were to develop coronary heart disease.

Results from other studies suggest that SEP disparities in physical health (Ferrie et al., 2002; Gueorguieva et al., 2009) and mental health (Miech et al., 2005) are set during early or middle adulthood, and just persist or perpetuate after that without either declining or increasing. For example, Miech et al. (2005) found that education disparities in psychopathology arise and are set in early adulthood, and then persist as individuals and cohorts age. At older ages, personal and financial resources are not enough to make up for some of the SEP disadvantages in health set earlier in adulthood.

In contrast to cumulative disadvantage theory, the age-as-leveler theory suggests that social factors may not be as strongly associated with changes in health at older ages as they are at younger and middle ages. This theory views human development as a multidimensional process of growth involving gains, losses, and adjustments across the lifespan (Alwin & Wray, 2005; Baltes et al., 1998). It suggests that social factors that affected health at earlier ages may not continue to affect health change as strongly later in life, as people learn to adapt to life changes. Or, social factors may be less crucial than biological factors at older ages.

Indeed, much research has found that individual SEP is more weakly associated with health and health-related QOL at older ages than at middle and early old age (Herd, 2006; House et al., 1994; Robert & House, 1996; Robert et al., 2009). The relationship between SEP, other risk factors, and health may be buffered by either biological robustness (in early adulthood) or biological frailty (in later old age). Research suggests that a cumulative index of biological risk is negatively associated with SEP (Kubzansky et al., 1999; Seeman et al., 2004). However, Seeman and colleagues (2008) found that, although education and income were each independently associated with cumulative biological risks among adults, these associations were weaker at older ages. Similarly, the associations between neighborhood SEP and cumulative biological risks are smaller among older adults (Bird et al., in press). Looking at biological frailty in old age by race, Crimmins et al. (2003) found racial differences in biological risk, although they were not as strong for those aged 70 and older.

Another explanation for stagnating or declining health disparities in old age, as opposed to being a product of biological, psychological, or interpersonal factors, is a changed structural context (Herd, 2006; House et al., 1994). Economic policies, such as Social Security and SSI, may affect the health of older adults, particularly those at the lowest income levels. Moreover, Medicare and other social policies available to older adults may buffer the effects of lower SEP at older ages. The health effects of social policy at older ages will be discussed in more detail in the next section.

It is also the case, however, that some of this weaker association between SEP and health at older ages may be due to the fact that the lowest SEP and sickest people select out of the population; i.e. they do not survive to older ages (Mirowsky & Ross, 2008). This results in a hardier group of older adults who survive to older ages, particularly the hardiest of the low SEP group. Dupre (2007) provides evidence that a cumulative disadvantage perspective applied to individuals may end up looking like an "age-as-leveler" phenomenon when applied to aggregate-level data at older ages. He finds strong effects of education on the onset of disease and mortality. Then, Dupre demonstrates how the selection of less-educated people out of the population through mortality contributes to the apparent weaker association between education and health at later ages. More work is needed to examine the size of the effect of selective mortality on SEP disparities in health across the life course.

THE LIFE COURSE, FUNDAMENTAL CAUSES, AND POLICY SOLUTIONS

But what do the research findings demonstrate about policy solutions to health disparities? The fact that health disparities grow across much of the life course, with some evidence of decline at (increasingly) older ages, implies two things. First, early-life interventions may play a significant role in reducing disparities in health throughout the entire life course. But life course theory also implies that interventions at any point in the life course may reduce existing disparities. Indeed, evidence suggests that African American women who were poor in early to mid-adulthood had equal health outcomes to African American women who had higher income at these ages, if the former group of women subsequently escaped poverty. Other studies reinforce this finding and suggest an additional compensatory effect of education on earlier-life socioeconomic disadvantage in predicting health outcomes (McDonough et al., 2005).

But while a life course perspective can guide us towards thinking about the differing effects policy choices may have at various points in the life course, fundamental cause theory provides more specific guidance about policy design. In short, it is premised on the fact that SEP is not simply a determinant of health status, but a fundamental cause of health status (House et al., 1990; Link & Phelan, 1995). Over the past 30 years, sociologists and epidemiologists documenting the consistent and inverse relationship between SEP and measures of both morbidity and mortality across the life course, across countries and across time, began to challenge the notion that SEP was simply a proxy for other factors that negatively affect health, such as access to health care, sedentary lifestyles, smoking, and obesity (Adler et al., 1994; House et al., 1994; Lantz et al., 1998).

Key evidence supporting fundamental cause theory shows that, while the intervening links between SEP and health have changed across time, the link between low SEP and poor health has not changed. For example, while the diseases responsible for and reflecting socioeconomic disparities in morbidity and mortality changed over the course of the twentieth century from infectious disease to chronic conditions, socioeconomic disparities in health either persisted or increased (Link & Phelan, 1995; Pappas et al., 1993). Further, the strong link between SEP and health persists across countries with vastly different social, political, and economic institutions (WHO, 2006). Finally, these differences also persist across the life course, even as risk factors for disease and mortality change (House et al., 1990). For example, even as old age is increasingly characterized by increased life expectancy and declining disability, these advantages have not been randomly distributed across socioeconomic groups (Goesling, 2006; House et al., 2005; Schoeni et al., 2005).

POLICY APPROACHES TO ADDRESSING HEALTH DISPARITIES

Medical Care and Insurance

The most common policy approaches to addressing socioeconomic and racial health disparities emphasize downstream solutions. They focus on changing health behaviors and improving access to health care via health insurance. Lack of health insurance adversely affects access to, and quality of, health care. Indeed, there is evidence that those who had been uninsured prior to age 65 face a lower likelihood for mortality once they transition onto Medicare (McWilliams et al., 2004). But, health insurance and health care probably account for only 10–20% of the relationship between SEP and health (McGinnis et al., 2002; Ross & Mirowsky, 2000). In part, this is because socioeconomic disparities in health are largely due to the differences in the onset, rather than progression, of poor health (Herd et al., 2007). Medical care does little to prevent the onset of poor health; it largely offsets health decline once individuals get sick. Access to health insurance is also not probable as a primary explanation for socioeconomic disparities among the elderly given nearly universal access to health insurance via Medicare.

However, despite near-universal access to health insurance at older ages, disparities in the quality of care contribute to disparities in health outcomes. First, there is evidence that African American Medicare beneficiaries do not receive the same care that white beneficiaries receive. Gornick et al. (1996) found that, among Medicare beneficiaries, African Americans are at least 50% less likely than whites to have bypass surgery, angioplasty, or hip replacement. African Americans also go to the doctor less and receive fewer mammograms and flu shots. But they are more likely than whites to go to the hospital and to die earlier. African Americans are three times more likely than whites to have a lower limb amputation due to

diabetes whereas whites are significantly more likely to have vein-stripping procedures that save the limb. Geiger (1996) reviewed 10 years of studies on the effect of race and class on medical treatment in the US and found that African Americans are consistently less likely to receive angioplasty, catheterization, bypass surgery, vein stripping, mammograms, less invasive vaginal hysterectomies, renal transplants, hip and knee replacements, and flu shots (IOM, 2002).

Another issue is the cost of health care for older Americans. Medicare beneficiaries currently devote 20% of their income to out-of-pocket health care costs. Further, out-of-pocket health care costs are particularly high among those with the fewest resources. Those without high school degrees have out-of-pocket health care costs that are almost twice those of college graduates. Those in the bottom income quartile have out-of-pocket costs that consume 30% of their income compared to 8% for the wealthiest individuals in the top income quartile (Crystal et al., 2000). By 2025, beneficiaries' average out-of-pocket health care costs could rise to 30%, and vulnerable groups will face the harshest repercussions. Those in poor health and with no supplemental insurance outside of Medicare are projected to devote as much as 63% of their income to health care (Maxwell et al., 2001).

Behavioral Approaches to Intervention

Another oft-cited solution to addressing socioeconomic and racial disparities in health involves getting individuals to "behave" better. In short, obesity, inactivity, tobacco use, and alcohol and other substance use or abuse all exert negative impacts on health. Indeed, those with low SEP are more likely to smoke, be underweight or overweight, exercise less, and drink immoderately. Although there is enormous public, media, and, increasingly, policy attention focused on these behavioral factors, they too account for just a minority portion of the relationship between race, SEP, and health. Studies find they account for just 10–20% of the relationship between SEP and heath and essentially none of the relationship between race and health, once SEP has been accounted for (Lantz et al., 1998).

Other Mediators of the Effect of SEP and Race/Ethnicity on Health

SEP affects health by structuring exposures to a range of material and psychosocial health risk and protective factors beyond access to medical care and health behaviors. Low SEP affects health through its effects on physical environment exposures, stress, healthy food availability, sense of control, social support, access to social services, and a range of other material and psychosocial factors that combine to affect health (House et al., 2005). But, again, any one or small set of these factors (e.g. chronic and acute stress) accounts for only 10–20% of socioeconomic, racial, or ethnic disparities. In essence, the powerful effects of SEP on health refer to the degree to which SEP structures peoples' exposure to or experience of almost all risk factors for health – biomedical, behavioral, psychosocial, social, and environmental.

A Fundamental Cause Perspective

From a fundamental cause perspective, however, focusing policy too heavily on any of these proximate or "downstream" biomedical, behavioral, or psychosocial risk factors is not the most effective strategy to reduce disparities in health (Link & Phelan, 1995), for a number of reasons. First, focusing on changing risky behaviors ignores the context in which they emerge. Attempting to reduce health disparities primarily by improving risky health behaviors ignores that such behaviors may sometimes be adaptive in the face of the conditions in which they arise, and/or that addressing behavior change may not be successful without improving the underlying conditions (such as low income, high crime neighborhoods) that give rise to the behaviors and/or sustain them. For example, stress may induce coping mechanisms that are bad for people's health. There is evidence that high levels of stress induce smoking, drinking, and drug use (Ng & Jeffrey, 2003) and consumption of high levels of starchy, high-caloric foods (Dallman et al., 2003). Such adaptive behaviors may be hard to change without changing the stressful situations.

Moreover, the context of individual or neighborhood material disadvantage can affect behavioral choices. Healthy foods, fresh fruits, vegetables, and whole grains cost more than processed foods with little nutritional value, and healthy foods are less available in some poor, urban neighborhoods (Dubowitz et al., 2008). In terms of exercise, meeting federal guidelines of an hour a day may be particularly challenging for those with low SEP. For example, one's neighborhood may preclude taking walks or running due to violence or crime and gym memberships may prove unaffordable (Lenthe et al., 2005).

Finally, fundamental cause theory suggests that new behavioral risk factors emerge just as old risky behaviors are eliminated or improved. For example, malnutrition drove many socioeconomic disparities in health throughout much of the twentieth century, but currently obesity poses a much greater risk. The recent preponderance of processed, highly caloric, and cheap food with little nutritional value has, in part, driven obesity trends. Thus, there is a certain irony in the fact that the War on Poverty in the 1960s,

which focused on malnutrition, is gradually being replaced by a war on obesity. The broader link to both malnutrition and obesity is SEP, just at different time periods (Herd, 2009).

SOCIAL AND ECONOMIC POLICIES

While downstream policy solutions have received considerable analysis and study, focusing primarily on interventions designed to improve smoking, drinking, exercise, and diet, there is less research examining whether "upstream" policy solutions impact health. In short, if education and income were improved or even redistributed, would health be affected? Although both medical care and health behaviors are the major focus of policy interventions and evaluations aimed at improving population health, the US spends nearly 600 billion dollars annually on social and economic policies for the elderly, aside from health care. As this chapter has described, there is reason to believe these "upstream" policies may impact the health of older adults.

Examining the health effects of social and economic policies targeted at the elderly is especially useful given that there are no other points in the life course when incomes are so extensively supplemented by income support policies. Indeed, in 2008, the US delivered $516 billion in Social Security benefits. On average, Social Security comprises 40% of annual incomes among those aged 65 and over. Moreover, it comprises 80% of incomes for one-fifth of those aged 65 and over (SSA, 2004). Further, for those that fall below eligibility guidelines for Social Security or those whose incomes fall well below the poverty threshold, there is another safety net to offset extreme poverty. Supplemental security income (SSI) subsidizes incomes for about 6% of elderly Americans.

Social Security and SSI have offset the most severe forms of economic deprivation among the elderly. This is critical from a health perspective because almost all prior evidence shows that the largest reductions in health are associated with changes in income among those with the lowest incomes (e.g. Backlund et al., 1996). Social Security has been effective at reducing poverty rates among the elderly. Between 1960 and 2005 the elderly poverty rate dropped from almost 30% to 10%. Almost all of this decline can be attributed to rising Social Security benefits (Engelhardt & Gruber, 2004). SSI further protects the very poor. At age 65, one would expect that the combination of eligibility for full Social Security benefits and SSI would further reduce poverty. Indeed, the percentage of those aged 65 to 69 falling below 75% of the poverty level fell to 4.4% (compared to 6.6% among those aged 61).

Income Support Policies and Health

So what is the evidence regarding the effects of income support policies on health? There have been only a handful of studies estimating the causal effects of income transfer policies on the health of the elderly. Indeed, some of the most promising studies have been in developing countries, though the extent of their applicability to the developed world is unclear. Most notably, under an income support experiment, titled PROGRESSA, the Mexican government has been providing about $800 million in aid to almost one-third of all rural families since 1997. Families must meet certain conditions to obtain aid. Families must seek preventative health care, children up to age five must have their growth monitored in clinic visits, those over age 50 must participate in a yearly preventative check up, and mothers must receive prenatal care and receive health education counseling. Additional family income supplements are also available if school-age children attend school. Finally, the income is distributed directly to mothers, an important distinction in a patriarchal culture (Gertler, 2000).

The results showed striking improvements in health for children, adults, and those over age 50. Those over age 50 had significant reductions in activity limitations due to illness, fewer days bedridden due to sickness, and more generally an increase in energy levels as measured by their ability to walk distances without significant fatigue. It is unlikely that all these improvements were due to the required yearly preventative check up, and much more likely that the improved family income contributed to such outcomes. Children and adults also showed improved outcomes. But it could not be initially proven that income had an independent effect on the children's health, due to the medical care requirements for children linked to the receipt of income benefits. However, subsequent research has demonstrated this in Mexico (Fernald et al., 2009) and Ecuador (Paxson et al., 2007) and the program is now being generalized to urban Mexico and adopted by Argentina, Columbia, Honduras, and Nicaragua.

There also is evidence about the impact of Social Security and the SSI program in the US on health outcomes. Social Security is an obvious program to examine, given its magnitude, its effect on elderly people's incomes, and its impact on poverty among elderly Americans. But it is difficult to estimate whether Social Security affects health. Simply examining whether those with higher Social Security benefits have better health will not indicate whether Social Security benefits caused the higher levels of health. Social Security benefits are based on individuals' prior earnings, which may have been negatively affected by their health over the life course. Thus, lower Social Security benefits may result from poor health, cause poor health, or both.

One approach to examining the effects of Social Security on health is to focus on the impact of Social Security on population health over time. Ongoing work by Peter Arno and his colleagues has examined this question by focusing on the mortality experience of different adult age groups over the twentieth century. The hypothesis is that two large positive exogenous shocks from Social Security to the income of the elderly occurred over this period, first at its inception in the late 1930s and early 1940s and second when it was indexed to inflation during the 1960s and early 1970s. These changes should have produced discontinuous acceleration of rates of mortality decline in the health of the elderly (aged 65–74 and 75–84), but not adult age groups below age 65, in the 10–15 years following these changes. Their preliminary data are consistent with a potential positive impact on health for the older population. This work suggests the utility of further research, which might yield clearer causal inferences about the relationship between Social Security and health outcomes.

Another strategy is to examine health impacts of an unanticipated change in income. Snyder and Evans (2006) used this type of design to examine the impact of Social Security benefits on mortality. New Social Security legislation led to a "notch," with individuals with the exact same work histories born just before January 1, 1917 receiving higher Social Security benefits in old age than those born just after this date. The experimental group (receiving the higher benefit), despite receiving about 7% higher Social Security benefits than the control group, had *higher* mortality rates after age 65 than the control group. While highly cited, this paper has two significant problems that highlight some of the nuance and difficulty of conducting such analyses. First, the poorest beneficiaries, who are most likely to have health effects from income increases, had negligible income increases. For example, a notch beneficiary retiring at age 62 without a high school degree had just a 1% higher benefit or a $5 higher monthly benefit. Second, dissertation research by Handwerker (2007) found mortality differences between the experimental and control groups previous to when these cohorts began collecting Social Security benefits. Thus, it would appear that the higher mortality rates of the "notch" group likely had little or nothing to do with the Social Security benefits, but rather the fact that they were sicker previous to receiving Social Security benefits.

Although Social Security may have had an important impact on health among older adults, it is difficult to design a study that can appropriately estimate its effect today because of its universality and the way in which individuals' health affects their choice to receive Social Security. Those in poor health receive Social Security benefits at earlier ages because poor health forces their labor force exit. SSI, though more limited in the population affected and its total effects on income, has some advantages for testing the effects of income supports on health. In particular, SSI is targeted at the poorest elderly Americans (although the blind and disabled under age 65 are also eligible), and past research suggests that income supports that raise the incomes of the very poorest should have the largest health effects (Backlund et al., 1996).

The first study that examined the health effects of SSI looked at whether the implementation of the program had any effect on health. Taubman and Sickles (1983) used the Retirement History Survey to examine how the health of elderly recipients changed after they started receiving SSI. Individuals reported how their health compared to those of similar age. They found that SSI had a positive impact on the reported health of elderly beneficiaries. Specifically, while the health of individuals eligible for SSI previous to implementation was statistically significantly worse than the health of those not eligible, this difference in health was no longer significant after SSI was implemented. There are two limitations of this study, however. First, declining differences in health may have been due to mortality selection: SSI recipients may have reflected a more robust group of survivors. Second, SSI eligibility also guaranteed access to Medicaid as a supplement to Medicare. Thus, improved health may have been due to Medicaid, not SSI.

Recent work by Herd and colleagues (2008) sought to build on both the promise and problems in Taubman and Sickle's work, with an alternative empirical design to estimate the impact of SSI on the health of the elderly. Instead of testing whether the implementation of SSI affected health, they tested whether variation in SSI maximum benefits over time within states predicts changes in health. Though there is a federal maximum SSI benefit, states can supplement the federal benefit. The federal minimum is set at 75% of the poverty line. As with Social Security, SSI is adjusted to account for inflation. In 2000, the federal monthly income minimum was $532 for single individuals and $789 for married couples. In 1990 and 2000, 25 and 27 states, respectively, supplemented this federal benefit. Thus, Herd and colleagues examined whether within-state changes in maximum SSI benefits over time correlated with within-state changes in disability. They found that increases in the maximum state SSI benefit were correlated with reductions in disability rates among the elderly, net of state and year fixed effects and other controls.

Other Social Policy Supports: Older Americans Act and Food Stamps

The other two significant social welfare policy supports targeted at older Americans include the Older Americans Act (OAA) ($2 billion) and food stamps ($3.5 billion). While Social Security dwarfs spending on these programs ($516 billion), they do provide some important benefits. Nearly half of OAA spending is on nutritional programs such as Meals on Wheels, which delivers hot food to older Americans confined to their homes. Although existing evidence on program outcomes is limited, it demonstrates a positive impact on nutritional outcomes among the elderly (Gollub & Weddle, 2004; Mathematica Policy Research, 1996).

Spending on food stamps for older Americans is another important social welfare policy support. However, relative to younger Americans, participation among the elderly is low. Only about 30% of eligible older adults are actually receiving benefits. There is some evidence, however, that those eligible and not receiving these supports may not need them (Haider et al., 2003). In part, this is because older people qualify for food stamps at higher income levels. Further, these individuals may be drawing on food banks or nutrition services under OAA instead (Nord, 2002). Generally, evaluations of food stamps indicate that they reduce food insecurity (Hoynes et al., 2007).

CONCLUSION: NEW PATHWAYS FOR RESEARCH

Although there has been growing attention to the existence and persistence of health disparities in the US, much remains unknown about what generates these disparities and how policies can intervene to reduce them. When thinking about how to improve health disparities at older ages, a life course approach suggests that we think about both prevention, via policies that improve outcomes early in the life course, and treatment, via policies that buffer or even reverse previous or accumulated health-detrimental exposures. Fundamental cause theory suggests that in both cases we attend to policies that address SEP directly: attending to the socioeconomic conditions of life that lead to a variety of risk and protective factors that produce health. Providing for economic security for families and children may be a precondition for setting babies and children on positive health trajectories. However, later interventions in education and income security may be important as well. Although SEP across the life course appears to accumulate to affect health, improvements in SEP in middle and older adulthood may buffer, or even override in some cases, the effects of early life disadvantage.

While research on policy interventions early in the life course and midlife is also needed, there are important reasons for focusing on later life. From a public policy perspective, enormous resources are devoted to extending the length and QOL among older adults. We spend nearly a half a trillion dollars annually on Medicare, the primary source of health insurance for those aged 65 and older, and a large fraction of overall health care spending is devoted to the elderly. Mortality rates rise substantially as people age and the most expensive year of life, in terms of medical expenditures, is the year before death. Yet, the later in old age that one dies, the smaller the amount of medical expenditures in that last year of life (Lubitz et al., 1995). Thus, postponement of mortality in old age, if due to better health, could lead to substantial savings in medical care. And given the fact that the fastest increases in medical spending have occurred among the elderly over the last 40 years, any reduction in medical spending on this group would help reduce rapidly rising health care costs (Meara et al., 2004).

From a fundamental cause perspective, there may be other ways to extend and improve life in old age beyond spending on medical care. We also spend over a half a trillion dollars annually to improve the economic well-being of older Americans via Social Security, SSI, and other programs discussed above. But we know relatively little about how these policies may be affecting health. If there is evidence that this spending affects health, this provides a powerful additional set of motivations and considerations for maintaining and strengthening existing income support policies, in addition to creating new ones. Currently, when policy analysts consider the ramifications of changes to income support policies such as Social Security, they do not consider the potential health implications when cutting or expanding these benefits. This additional outcome could profoundly impact cost–benefit analyses of policy formulation and reform.

Social and economic policies could be among the most important policies affecting health, even rivaling or exceeding the effects of health care policies, such as Medicare, and consequently may help resolve America's paradoxical crisis of paying more for health care than other developed countries but getting less in terms of levels of population health (Schoeni et al., 2008). The US spends about twice as much per capita on health care as other OECD Organisation for Economic Co-operation and Development countries. Yet, our population health measures frequently lag well behind these same countries. We consistently rank at the bottom of comparable countries in infant mortality and life expectancy (Starfield, 2000). At the same time, the US also has the highest poverty rates (calculated as the percentage of individuals living below half of median income) in the industrialized world (Smeeding et al., 2002). These high poverty rates are largely due to limited social welfare spending in the US compared to other countries (Smeeding et al., 2002). A large part of the explanation for lagging population health in the US may be economic deprivation.

Clearly, further research on the effects of social welfare supports on the health of elderly Americans could advance both the public policy agenda and our basic scientific understanding of the relationship between SEP and health. This evidence could fundamentally reframe how policymakers think about health policy by pushing policymakers to think beyond downstream solutions, such as expanding access to health insurance and expanding funding for health behavior change, to upstream solutions as an avenue for improving population health (Schoeni et al., 2008).

REFERENCES

Adler, N. E., Boyce, T., Chesney, M. A., Cohen, S., Folkman, S., Kahn, R. L., et al. (1994). Socioeconomic status and health: The challenge of the gradient. *American Psychologist, 49*, 15–24.

Alwin, D. F., & Wray, L. A. (2005). A life-span development perspective on social status and health. *Journal of Gerontology: Social Sciences, 60B*, 7–14.

Backlund, E., Sorlie, P., & Johnson, N. J. (1996). The shape of the relationship between income and mortality in the United States: Evidence from the National Longitudinal Mortality Study. *Annals of Epidemiology, 6*, 12–23.

Baltes, P. B., Lindenberger, U., & Staudinger, U. M. (1998). Lifespan theory in developmental psychology. *Handbook of Child Psychology, 1*, 1029–1143.

Barker, D. J. P. (Ed.), (1992). *Fetal and infant origins of adult disease.* London: British Medical Journal Books.

Barker, D. J., Gluckman, P. D., Godfrey, K. M., Harding, J. E., Owens, J. A., & Robinson, J. S. (1993). Fetal nutrition and cardiovascular disease in adult life. *Lancet, 10*, 938–941.

Bird, C. E., Seeman, T. E., Escarce, J. J., Basurto-Davila, R., Finch, B. K., Dubowitz, T., et al. (in press). Neighborhood socioeconomic status and biological "wear & tear" in a nationally representative sample of US adults. *Journal of Epidemiology and Community Health.*

Blackwell, D. L., Hayward, M. D., & Crimmins, E. M. (2001). Does childhood health affect chronic morbidity in later life? *Social Science & Medicine, 52*, 1269–1284.

Bulatao, R. A., & Anderson, N. B. (2004). *Understanding racial and ethnic differences in health in late life: A research agenda.* Washington, DC: National Academies Press.

Cagney, K. A., Browning, C. R., & Wen, M. (2005). Racial disparities in self-rated health at older ages: What difference does the neighborhood make? *Journal of Gerontology: Social Sciences, 60B*, 181–190.

Case, A., Lubotsky, D., & Paxson, C. (2002). Economic status and health in childhood: The origins of the gradient. *The American Economic Review, 92*, 1308–1334.

Case, A., Fertig, A., & Paxson, C. (2005). The lasting impact of childhood health and circumstance. *Journal of Health Economics, 24*, 365–389.

Chandola, T., Ferrie, J., Sacker, A., & Marmot, M. (2007). Social inequalities in self reported health in early old age: Follow-up of prospective cohort study. *British Medical Journal, 334*, 963–964.

Chaudhry, S., Friedkin, R., Horwitz, R., & Inouye, S. K. (2004). Educational disadvantage impairs functional recovery after hospitalization in older persons. *American Journal of Medicine, 117*, 650–656.

Crimmins, E. M., Johnston, M., Hayward, M., & Seeman, T. (2003). Age differences in allostatic load: An index of physiological dysregulation. *Experimental Gerontology, 38*, 731–734.

Crimmins, E. M., Hayward, M., & Seeman, T. E. (2004). Race/ethnicity, socioeconomic status, and health. In N. B. Anderson, R. A. Bulatao & B. Cohen (Eds.), *Critical perspectives on racial and ethnic differences in health in late life* (pp. 310–352). Washington, DC: National Academies Press.

Crystal, S., Johnson, R. W., Harman, J., Sambamoorthi, U., & Kumar, R. (2000). Out-of-pocket health care costs among older Americans. *Journal of Gerontology: Social Sciences, 55B*, 51–62.

Dallman, M., Pecoraro, N., Akana, S., la Fleur, S., Gomez, F., Houshyar, H., et al. (2003). Chronic stress and obesity: A new view of "comfort food". *Proceedings of the National Academy of Sciences, 100*, 116–196.

Dannefer, D. (2003). Cumulative advantage/disadvantage the life course: Cross-fertilizing age and social science theory. *Journal of Gerontology: Social Sciences, 58*, 327–S337.

Demakakos, P., Nazroo, J., Breeze, E., & Marmot, M. (2008). Socioeconomic status and health: The role of subjective social status. *Social Science & Medicine, 67*, 330–340.

Diez-Roux, A. F., Nieto, J., Muntaner, C., Tyroler, H., Comstock, G., Shahar, E., et al. (1997). Neighborhood environments and coronary heart disease: A multilevel analysis. *American Journal of Epidemiology, 146*, 48–63.

Dubowitz, T., Heron, M., Bird, CE., Lurie, N., Finch, BK, Basurto-Davila, R., et al. (2008). Neighborhood socioeconomic status and fruit and vegetable intake among whites, blacks, and Mexican Americans in the United States. *American Journal of Clinical Nutrition, 87*, 1883.

Dupre, M. E. (2007). Educational differences in age-related patterns of disease: Reconsidering the cumulative disadvantage and age-as-leveler hypothesis. *Journal of Health and Social Behavior, 48*, 1–15.

Engelhardt, G., & Gruber, J. (2004). Social Security and the evolution of elderly poverty. *NBER Working Paper No. 10466.* Cambridge, MA: NBER.

Farmer, M. M., & Ferraro, K. F. (2005). Are racial disparities in health conditional on socioeconomic status? *Social Science & Medicine, 60*, 191–204.

Feinglass, J., Lin, S., Thompson, J., Sudano, J., Dunlop, D., Song, J., et al. (2007). Baseline health, socioeconomic status, and 10-year mortality among older middle-aged Americans: Findings from the Health and Retirement Study, 1992–2002. *Journal of Gerontology: Social Sciences, 62*, S209–S217.

Fernald, L. C., & Gunnar, M. R. (2009). Poverty-alleviation program participation and salivary cortisol in very low income children. *Social Science & Medicine, 68*(12), 2180–2189.

Ferraro, K. F., & Farmer, M. M. (1996). Double jeopardy, aging as leveler, or persistent health inequality? A longitudinal analysis of white and black Americans. *Journal of Gerontology: Social Sciences, 51*, 319–328.

Ferraro, K. F., & Kelley-Moore, J. A. (2003). Cumulative disadvantage and health: Long-term consequences of obesity? *American Sociological Review, 68*, 707–729.

Ferrie, J. E., Shipley, M. J., Smith, G. D., Stansfeld, S. A., & Marmot, M. G. (2002). Change in health inequalities among British civil servants: The Whitehall II study. *Journal of Epidemiology and Community Health, 56*, 922–926.

Freedman, V. A., Martin, L. G., & Schoeni, R. F. (2002). Recent trends in disability and functioning among older adults in the United States: A systematic review. *Journal of the American Medical Association, 288*, 3137–3146.

Geiger, H. J. (1996). Race and health care – an American dilemma? *New England Journal of Medicine, 335*, 815–816.

Gertler, P. (2000). *Final report: The impact of PROGRESA on health.* Washington, DC: International Food Policy Research Institute.

Goesling, B. (2006). The rising significance of education for health. *Social Forces, 85*, 1621–1644.

Gollub, E. A., & Weddle, D. O. (2004). Improvements in nutritional intake and quality of life among frail homebound older adults receiving home-delivered breakfast and lunch. *Journal of the American Dietetic Association, 104*, 1227–1235.

Gornick, M. E., Eggers, P. W., Reilly, T. W., Mentnech, R. M., Fitterman, L. K., Kucken, L. E., et al. (1996). Effects of race and income on mortality and use of services among Medicare beneficiaries. *New England Journal of Medicine, 335*, 791–799.

Gueorguieva, R., Sindelar, J. L., Falba, T. A., Fletcher, J. M., Keenan, P., Wu, R., et al. (2009). The impact of occupation on self-rated health: Cross-sectional and longitudinal evidence from the Health and Retirement Survey. *The Journal of Gerontology: Social Sciences, 64*, 118–124.

Guilley, E., & Lalive d'Epinay, C. J. (2008). Social status and mortality with activity of daily living disability in later life. *Journals of Gerontology: Social Sciences, 63*, S192–S196.

131

Guralnik, J. M., Butterworth, S., Wadsworth, M. E. J., & Kuh, D. (2006). Childhood socioeconomic status predicts physical functioning a half century later. *Journal of Gerontology: Medical Sciences, 61*, 694–701.

Haas, S. A. (2006). Health selection and the process of social stratification: The effect of childhood health on socioeconomic attainment. *Journal of Health and Social Behavior, 47*, 339–354.

Haas, S. A. (2008). Trajectories of functional health: The 'long arm' of childhood health and socioeconomic factors. *Social Science & Medicine, 66*, 849–861.

Haider, S. J., Jacknowitz, A., & Schoeni, R. F. (2003). Food stamps and the elderly: Why is participation so low? *The Journal of Human Resources, 38*, 1080–1111.

Hamil-Luker, J., & O'Rand, A. M. (2007). Gender differences in the link between childhood socioeconomic conditions and heart attack risk in adulthood. *Demography, 44*, 137–158.

Handwerker, E. A. W. (2007). Empirical essays in the economics of aging, Doctoral dissertation, University of California, Berkeley. Proquest Dissertations and Theses, 3275438.

Harrington Meyer, M., & Herd, P. (2007). *Market friendly or family friendly? The state and gender inequality in old age.* New York: Russell Sage.

Hayward, M. D., & Gorman, B. (2004). The long arm of childhood: The influence of early life conditions on men's mortality. *Demography, 41*, 87–108.

Hayward, M. D., & Heron, M. (1999). Racial inequality in active life expectancy among adult Americans. *Demography, 36*, 77–91.

Hayward, M. D., Crimmins, E. M., Miles, T. P., & Yang, Y. (2000). The significance of socioeconomic status in explaining the racial gap in chronic health conditions. *American Sociological Review, 65*, 910–930.

Herd, P. (2006). Do functional health inequalities decrease in old age? Educational status and functional decline among the 1931–1941 birth cohort. *Research on Aging, 28*, 375–392.

Herd, P. (2009). Social class, health, and longevity. In P. Uhlenberg (Ed.), *International Handbook of Population Aging* (pp. 583–604). New York: Springer.

Herd, P., Goesling, B., & House, J. S. (2007). Unpacking the relationship between socioeconomic position and health. *Journal of Health and Social Behavior, 48*, 223–238.

Herd, P., Schoeni, R. F., & House, J. S. (2008). Upstream solutions: Does the Supplemental Security Income program reduce disability in the elderly? *Milbank Quarterly, 86*, 5–45.

Holland, P., Berney, L., Blane, D., Davey Smith, G., Gunnell, D. J., & Montgomery, S. M. (2000). Life course accumulation of disadvantage: Childhood health and hazard exposure during adulthood. *Social Science & Medicine, 50*, 1285–1295.

House, J. S., Kessler, R., & Herzog, A. (1990). Age, socioeconomic status and health. *Milbank Quarterly, 68*, 383–411.

House, J. S., Lepkowski, J. M., Kinney, A. M., Mero, R. P., Kessler, R. C., & Herzog, A. R. (1994). The social stratification of aging and health. *Journal of Health and Social Behavior, 35*, 213–234.

House, J. S., Lantz, P. M., & Herd, P. (2005). Continuity and change in the social stratification of aging and health over the life course: Evidence from a nationally representative longitudinal study from 1986 to 2001/2002 (the Americans' Changing Lives Study). *Journal of Gerontology: Social Sciences, 60*, S15–S26.

Hoynes, H. W., Schanzenbach, D., & Drive, O. S. (2007). Consumption responses to in-kind transfers: Evidence from the introduction of the food stamp program. NBER Working Paper No. W13025. Cambridge, MA: NBER.

Hummer, R. A., Benjamins, M. R., & Rogers, R. G. (2004). Racial and ethnic disparities in health and mortality among the U.S. elderly population. In N. B. Anderson, R. A. Bulatao & B. Cohen (Eds.), *Critical perspectives on racial and ethnic differences in health in later life* (pp. 53–94). Washington, DC: National Academies Press.

Institute of Medicine. (2002). *Committee on understanding and eliminating racial and ethnic disparities in health care.* Washington, DC: National Academies Press.

Kahn, J. R., & Fazio, E. M. (2005). Economic status over the life course and racial disparities in health. *Journal of Gerontology: Social Sciences, 60*, 76–84.

Kubzansky, L., Kawachi, I., & Sparrow, D. (1999). Socioeconomic status and risk factor clustering in the normative aging study: Any help from the concept of allostatic load? *Annals of Behavioral Medicine, 21*, 330–338.

Lantz, P., House, J. S., Lepowski, J. M., Williams, D., Mero, R., & Chen, J. (1998). Socioeconomic factors, health behaviors, and mortality. *Journal of the American Medical Association, 279*, 1703–1708.

Lawlor, D. A., Davey Smith, G., Patel, R., & Ebrahim, S. (2005a). Life-course socioeconomic position, area deprivation, and coronary heart disease: Findings from the British Women's Heart and Health Study. *American Journal of Public Health, 95*, 91–97.

Lawlor, D. A., Ebrahim, S., & Davey Smith, G. (2005b). Adverse socioeconomic position across the life course increases coronary heart disease risk cumulatively. *Journal of Epidemiology and Community Health, 59*, 785–793.

Lawton, J. (1998). Contemporary hospice care: The sequestration of the unbounded body and 'dirty dying.' *Sociology of Health & Illness, 20*, 121–143.

Lenthe, FJ., Brug, J., & Mackenbach, J. P. (2005). Neighborhood inequalities in physical inactivity: The role of neighborhood attractiveness, proximity to local facilities and safety in the Netherlands. *Social Science & Medicine, 60*, 763–765.

Link, B. G., & Phelan, J. (1995). Social conditions as fundamental causes of disease. *Journal of Health and Social Behavior (Extra Issue)*, 80–94.

Link, B. G., & Phelan, J. C. (2002). McKeown and the idea that social conditions are fundamental causes of disease. *American Journal of Public Health, 92*(5), 730–732.

Lu, M. C., & Halfon, N. (2003). Racial and ethnic disparities in birth outcomes: A life-course perspective. *Maternal and Child Health Journal, 7*, 13–30.

Lubitz, J., Beebe, J., & Baker, C. (1995). Longevity and Medicare expenditures. *New England Journal of Medicine, 332*, 999–1003.

Luo, Y., & Waite, L. J. (2005). The impact of childhood and adult SEP on physical, mental and cognitive well-being. *The Journal of Gerontology: Social Sciences, 60*, 93–101.

Manton, K. G., & Gu, X. L. (2001). Changes in the prevalence of chronic disability in the United States black and nonblack population above age 65 from 1982 to 1999. *Proceedings of the National Academy of Sciences of the United States of America, 98*, 6354.

Martin, L. G., Schoeni, R. F., Freedman, V. A., & Andreski, P. (2007). Feeling better? Trends in general health status. *Journal of Gerontology: Social Sciences, 62*, S11.

Mathematica Policy Research (1996). *Serving elders at risk, the Older Americans Act nutrition program*. Washington, DC: US Department of Health and Human Services.

Maxwell, S., Moon, M., & Segal, M. (2001). Growth in Medicare and out-of-pocket spending: Impact on vulnerable beneficiaries. *New England Journal of Medicine, 344*, 928–931.

McDonough, P., Duncan, G. J., Williams, D., & House, J. S. (1997). Income dynamics and adult mortality in the United States, 1972 through 1989. *American Journal of Public Health, 87*, 1476–1483.

McDonough, P., Sacker, A., & Wiggins, R. D. (2005). Time on my side? Life course trajectories of poverty and health. *Social Science & Medicine, 61*, 1795–1808.

McGinnis, M. J., Williams-Russo, P., & Knickman, J. (2002). The case for more active policy attention to health promotion. *Health Affairs, 21*, 78–93.

McWilliams, J. M., Zaslavsky, A. M., Meara, E., & Ayanian, J. Z. (2004). Health insurance coverage and mortality among the near-elderly. *Health Affairs, 23*, 223–233.

Meara, E., White, C., & Cutler, D. (2004). Trends in medical spending by age, 1963–2004. *Health Affairs, 23*, 176–183.

Miech, R., Eaton, W., & Brennan, K. (2005). Mental health disparities across education and sex: A prospective analysis examining how they persist over the life course. *Journal of Gerontology: Social Sciences, 60*, 93–98.

Mirowsky, J., & Ross, C. E. (2008). Education and self-rated health – Cumulative advantage and its rising importance. *Research on Aging, 30*, 93–122.

Morenoff, J., House, J., Hansen, B., Williams, D., Kaplan, G., & Hunte, H. (2007). Understanding social disparities in hypertension prevalence, awareness, treatment, and control: The role of neighborhood context. *Social Science & Medicine, 65*, 1853–1866.

Mortimer, J. T., & Shanahan, M. J. (Eds.), (2004). *Handbook of the life course*. New York: Springer.

Mutchler, J. E., Prakash, A., & Burr, J. A. (2007). The demography of disability and the effects of immigrant history: Older Asians in the United States. *Demography, 44*, 251–263.

Ng, D., & Jeffrey, R. (2003). Relationships between perceived stress and health behaviors in a sample of working adults. *Health Psychology, 22*, 638–642.

Nicholson, A., Bobak, M., Murphy, M., Rose, R., & Marmot, M. (2005). Socio-economic influences on self-rated health in Russian men and women – A life course approach. *Social Science & Medicine, 61*, 2345–2354.

Nord, M. (2002). Rates of food insecurity and hunger unchanged in rural households. *Rural America, 16*, 42–47.

O'Rand, A. M. (1996). The precious and the precocious: Understanding cumulative disadvantage and cumulative advantage over the life course. *The Gerontologist, 36*, 230–238.

O'Rand, A. M., & Hamil-Luker, J. (2005). Processes of cumulative adversity: Childhood disadvantage and increased risk of heart attack across the life course. *Journal of Gerontology: Social Sciences, 60*, 117–124.

Palloni, A. (2006). Reproducing inequalities: Luck, wallets, and the enduring effects of childhood health. *Demography, 43*, 587–615.

Pappas, G., Queen, S., Hadden, W., & Fisher, G. (1993). The increasing disparity in mortality between socioeconomic groups in the United States, 1960 and 1986. *New England Journal of Medicine, 329*, 103–109.

Paxson, C., & Schady, N. (2007). Cognitive development among young children in Ecuador. *Journal of Human Resources, XLII*(1), 49–84.

Pensola, T. H., & Martikainen, P. (2003). Cumulative social class and mortality from various causes of adult men. *Journal of Epidemiology and Community Health Services, 57*, 745–751.

Power, C., Hypponen, E., & Davey Smith, G. (2005). Socioeconomic position in childhood and early adult life and risk of mortality: A prospective study of the mothers of the 1958 British birth cohort. *American Journal of Public Health, 95*, 1396–1402.

Robert, S. A., Cagney, K. A., & Weden, M. M. (in press). A life-course approach to the study of neighborhoods and health. In C. Bird, P. Conrad, A. Fremont, & S. Timmermans (Eds), *The handbook of medical sociology*. Nashville, TN: Vanderbilt University Press.

Robert, S., & House, J. (1996). SEP differentials in health by age and alternative indicators of SEP. *Journal of Aging and Health, 8*, 359–388.

Robert, S. A., & Lee, K. Y. (2002). Explaining race differences in health among older adults: The contribution of community socioeconomic context. *Research on Aging, 24*, 654.

Robert, S. A., & Ruel, E. (2006). Racial segregation and health disparities between black and white older adults. *Journal of*

Gerontology: Social Sciences, 61, 203–211.

Robert, S. A., Cherepanov, D., Palta, M., Dunham, N. C., Feeny, D., & Fryback, D. G. (2009). Socioeconomic status and age variations in health-related quality of life: Results from the National Health Measurement Study. *Journal of Gerontology: Social Sciences, 64,* 378–389.

Ross, C., & Wu, L. (1996). Education, age, and the cumulative advantage in health. *Journal of Health and Social Behavior, 37*(1), 104–120.

Ross, C. E., & Mirowsky, J. (2000). Does medical insurance contribute to socioeconomic differentials in health? *The Milbank Quarterly, 78,* 291–321.

Schoeni, R. F., Martin, L. G., Andreski, P., & Freedman, V. (2005). Persistent and growing socioeconomic disparities in disability among the elderly: 1982–2002. *American Journal of Public Health, 95,* 2065–2070.

Schoeni, R. F., Freedman, V. A., Martin, L. G. (2008). Why is late-life disability declining?. *Milbank Quarterly, 86,* 47–89.

Seeman, T. E., Crimmins, E., Huang, M. H., Singer, B., Buceur, A., Gruenwald, T., et al. (2004). Cumulative biological risk and socio-economic differences in mortality. *Social Science & Medicine, 58,* 1985–1997.

Seeman, T. E., Merkin, S. S., Crimmins, E., Koretz, B., Charette, S., & Karlamangla, A. (2008). Education, income and ethnic differences in cumulative biological risk profiles in a national sample of US adults: NHANES III (1988–1994). *Social Science & Medicine, 66,* 72–87.

Sheffield, K. M., & Peek, K. (2009). Neighborhood context and cognitive decline in older Mexican Americans: Results from the hispanic established populations for epidemiologic studies of the elderly. *American Journal of Epidemiology, 169,* 1092–1101.

Singh, G. K., & Siahpush, M. (2006). Widening socioeconomic inequalities in U.S. life expectancy, 1980–2000. *International Journal of Epidemiology, 35,* 969–979.

Singh-Manoux, A., Ferrie, J., Chandola, T., Marmot, M. (2004). Socioeconomic trajectories across the life course and health outcomes in midlife: Evidence for the accumulation hypothesis? *International Journal of Epidemiology, 33,* 1072–1079.

Skarupski, K. A., Mendes de Leon, C. F., Bienias, J. L., Barnes, L. L., Everson-Rose, S. A., Wilson, R. S., et al. (2005). Black-white differences in depressive symptoms among older adults over time. *Journal of Gerontology: Psychological Sciences, 60,* 136–142.

Smeeding, T., Rainwater, L., & Burtless, G. (2002). United States poverty in a cross-national context. In S. Danziger. & H. Haveman (Eds.), *Understanding poverty* (pp. 162–189). New York: Russell Sage Foundation.

Snyder, S. E., & Evans, W. N. (2006). The effect of income on mortality: Evidence from the social security notch. *The review of economics and statistics, 88,* 482–495.

Soldo, B., Mitchell, O. S., Tfaily, R., & McCabe, J. F. (2006). Cross-cohort differences in health on the verge of retirement. *NBER Working Paper* No.12762. Cambridge, MA: NBER.

Spillman, B. C. (2004). Changes in elderly disability rates and the implications for health care utilization and cost. *Milbank Quarterly, 82,* 157–194.

Social Security Administration (2004). *Income of the aged chartbook.* Baltimore, MD: Social Security Administration.

Starfield, B. (2000). Is U.S. health really the best in the world? *Journal of the American Medical Association, 284,* 483.

Subramanian, S. V., Acevedo-Garcia, D., & Osypuk, T. L. (2005). Racial residential segregation and geographic heterogeneity in black/white disparity in poor self-rated health in the U.S.: A multilevel statistical analysis. *Social Science & Medicine, 60,* 1667–1679.

Taubman, P. J., & Sickles, R. C. (1983). Supplemental social insurance and the health of the poor. *NBER Working Paper No. 1062.* Cambridge, MA: NBER.

Turra, C. M., & Goldman, N. (2007). Socioeconomic differences in mortality among US adults:

Insights into the hispanic paradox. *Journal of Gerontology: Social Sciences, 62,* S184.

Voelker, R. (2008). Decades of work to reduce disparities in health care produce limited success. *Journal of the American Medical Association, 299,* 1411–1413.

Wamala, S., Lynch, J., & Kaplan, G. (2001). Women's exposure to early and later life socioeconomic disadvantage and coronary heart disease risk: The Stockholm female coronary risk study. *International Journal of Epidemiology, 30,* 275–284.

Wen, M., Cagney, K. A., & Christakis, N. A. (2005). Effect of specific aspects of community social environment on the mortality of individuals diagnosed with serious illness. *Social Science & Medicine, 61,* 1119–1134.

Williams, D. R., & Collins, C. (1995). U.S. socioeconomic and racial differences in health: Patterns and explanations. *Annual Review of Sociology, 21,* 349–386.

Williams, D. R., & Mohammed, S. A. (2009). Discrimination and racial disparities in health: Evidence and needed research. *Journal of Behavioral Medicine, 32,* 20–47.

Williams, D. R., & Oh, H. J. (2009). The contribution of race and SEP to the health of the Black elderly. In J. S. Jackson (Ed.), *African American Elderly: Current research on biological, social and psychological aging* (pp. 152–178). New York: Springer Publishing.

Wolf, D. A., Hunt, K., & Knickman, J. (2005). Perspectives on the recent decline in disability at older ages. *Milbank Quarterly, 83,* 365–395.

World Health Organization (2006). Commission on the social determinants of health. New York: The United Nations.

Yao, L., & Robert, S. A. (2008). The contributions of race, individual socioeconomic status, and neighborhood socioeconomic context on the self-rated health trajectories and mortality of older adults. *Research on Aging, 30,* 251.

Zimmer, Z., & House, J. (2003). Education, income, and functional limitation transitions among American adults: Contrasting onset and progression. *International Journal of Epidemiology, 32,* 1089–1097.

Chapter | 10 |

Molecular Genetics, Aging, and Well-being: Sensitive Period, Accumulation, and Pathway Models

Michael J. Shanahan[1], Scott M. Hofer[2]

[1]*Department of Sociology and Center for Developmental Science, University of North Carolina at Chapel Hill, Chapel Hill, North Carolina,* [2]*Department of Psychology, University of Victoria, Victoria, British Columbia, Canada*

INTRODUCTION

Aging reflects ongoing transactions between context and person across many decades of life. Life course sociology is now central to investigations focused on the dynamic social context of aging, with its distinctive emphasis on long-term patterns in people's statuses, roles, and relationships. At the same time, reflecting many decades of research, the genetic study of behavior is a well-established vantage point from which to view individual development. Indeed, recent advances in the understanding of the genome and its measurement have created new and exciting possibilities for studying the genetic basis of aging-related outcomes. In turn, the integration of life course sociology and the genetically

informed study of behavior represents an emerging, highly promising – and yet highly challenging – avenue for research focused on the mechanisms of aging and well-being.

Such an integration is facilitated by two considerations. First, genetic factors by themselves do not cause complex behaviors. Rather, the influence of genetic factors depends on, among other things, gene–environment processes, which refer to a family of mechanisms by which genetic and environmental factors jointly influence the likelihood of behaviors (Johnson, 2007; McClearn et al., 2001; Rutter, 2007; Shanahan & Hofer, 2005). Far from being a static set of instructions that dictate biological processes, the expression of the genome is dynamic and changes in response to socially situated experience (Kendler et al., in press). Further, the relationship between context and genetic factors may often be transactional, with influences extending reciprocally among environmental factors and genetic processes (e.g. Tollefsbol, 2009). (The interdisciplinary field of behavioral genetics uses the term "environment" to refer to social context – which may be defined as enduring patterns of interaction among people and shared ways of making sense of reality – but also to physical features of one's setting such as toxins, pollutants, nutrition, and even the intrauterine environment and infectious agents. To the extent that these physical characteristics are distributed in societies according to socioeconomic status and other social variables, however, both the social and physical aspects of the "environment" may be of interest to social and behavioral scientists.)

Second, many behaviors of interest to aging research have been productively studied with genetically informed data, including dimensions of cognitive

DOI: 10.1016/B978-0-12-380880-6.00010-1

aging (e.g. Houlihan et al., 2009), physical and mental health (e.g. Kendler et al., 2009), and the stress process (e.g. Charles & Almeida, 2007). Additionally, genetically informed studies have focused on life-long behaviors that are thought to be related to these outcomes, including attainment processes, interpersonal relationships, health-related behaviors, and deviance (Shostak & Freese, 2009). Genetic and social factors are thus central to characterizing life-long experiences of the person. Indeed, extant research is highly suggestive of links between social status and stress processes and how these classic concerns of life course sociology intersect with human biology from the intrauterine environment (and perhaps extending back to the experiences of prior generations; see Heijmans et al., 2008) to death.

Our chapter selectively reviews studies that suggest links between social and molecular processes extending across the phases of life. Very few empirical studies of aging draw upon both the life course and molecular genetics, but there is a rapidly growing number of studies from each perspective that suggest points of intersection. We emphasize studies of health, broadly defined as "a state of complete physical, mental and social well-being and not merely the absence of disease or infirmity" (WHO, 1948), because many gene–environment studies focus on indicators of physical and mental well-being.

What aspects of molecular genetics have been used to study human behavior and have implications for behavioral patterns and health over long periods of time? We discuss three classes of mechanisms: (1) genetic candidates; and genetic expression by way of (2) transcription and (3) epigenetics. For each, we briefly introduce the genetic mechanism and then discuss studies that suggest links with the life course and aging. We begin, however, by highlighting the potential for mutually beneficial exchanges between molecular genetics and the life course paradigm. Our chapter does not consider the social, legal, and ethical issues that sometimes attend to genetically informed studies of behavior. Also, a more detailed consideration of gene–environment interactions and correlations in the life course may be found in Shanahan and Boardman (2009).

To anticipate the broad message that emerges from our review: several molecular genetic mechanisms clearly interact with social experiences in the prediction of health and these processes extend over many decades of life. However, the features of social context that are decisive to these processes are poorly understood. Life course sociology has scarcely considered the issue of "environmental specificity" – whether specific contextual experiences are necessary precursors to a specific behavior or, in contrast, whether numerous contextual experiences would be substitutable precursors – but genetically informed studies of behavior highlight its importance. Further, the temporal properties of these gene–environment

processes are not well understood. There is presently a great deal of interest in the sensitive period model, according to which genes and social experiences coalesce during a delimited window of development to durably alter, for example, the person's reactivity to stress. However, accumulation and pathway models will likely also provide leverage in linking these gene–environment processes to health. This area of research is progressing rapidly and the present situation may be characterized as one of great opportunity for emerging biological models of disease that are informed by life course studies of social context.

CROSS-FERTILIZING MOLECULAR GENETICS AND THE LIFE COURSE PARADIGM

To date, research suggests several genetic mechanisms that are related to health and that may be studied productively with life course principles in mind. Clearly, a thorough explanation and review of these mechanisms is not possible in this chapter, but even a brief overview will highlight reasons why these mechanisms are relevant to social scientists.

In many instances, genetic processes provide causal mechanisms that link social experience with health. As has long been recognized, causal accounts must, at a minimum, satisfy the requirements of association and temporal ordering between the hypothesized independent and dependent variables and plausible linking mechanisms. In many cases, genetic processes provide a critical – yet presently underappreciated – part of linking accounts of how a social factor (e.g. SES, social isolation) could conceivably be related to indicators of health. Particularly given the non-experimental nature of most social research and the recognized history of false positives in studies of social context and health, future research can productively move forward by specifying chains of causal mechanisms that connect social and molecular genetic processes with health.

A related point: ideally, these linking mechanisms in turn suggest ways to refine the conceptualization and measurement of social experience. Specific biological mechanisms often suggest aspects of social experiences that apparently matter and likely bear on the issue of environmental specificity. Such genetic mechanisms can also help understand temporal dynamics – how social experiences and disease may be related over time. Genetic mechanisms are now known to extend from intergenerational patterns to relatively immediate processes, and temporal distinctions at the molecular level will help to elucidate issues of timing at the level of social context. It is now abundantly clear that static snapshots of molecular and social processes can

Table 10.1 Individual- and context-based perspectives on life course models of health.

	INDIVIDUAL-BASED PERSPECTIVE	CONTEXT-BASED PERSPECTIVE
Sensitive period	Biological system open to durable programming during delimited period	"Initial" context strongly bears on subsequent contexts (i.e. strong path dependence in social experiences originating from initial social circumstance)
Accumulation	Biological program endures; is reinforced by internal feedback	Stability of social contextual experiences in terms of risks and capital
Pathway	Biological program disrupted by internal correction, exhaustion, biological, or aging process	Contextual discontinuities disrupting largely stable pattern of advantageous or disadvantageous social experiences

be highly misleading when attempting to characterize a person's experiences (see papers in Kendler et al., in press).

Indeed, sensitive period, accumulation, and pathway models are helpful in situating gene–environment processes in a life course framework. Two perspectives on these models provide interesting contrast and complementarity (see Table 10.1, where the two perspectives shown are heuristic, intended to highlight different ways of thinking about life course models of health). First, an individual-based perspective highlights the person as a biological organism. Accordingly, the sensitive period model – sometimes referred to as a critical period or latency model – posits that specific biological systems are highly plastic (i.e. subject to change, also referred to as "programming") at specific points in development; that the resulting biological change takes place in response to the environment; and that the biological change is durable, potentially creating stable behavioral tendencies. From the individual-based perspective, the accumulation model posits that the stability of the programmed reactivity is maintained. Finally, a pathway model emphasizes the developmental properties of biological systems and the possibility for self-correction or a distinct worsening of programmed response patterns. Such a model recognizes that biological systems are dynamic and highly complex, possibly disrupting continuities that emerged in earlier phases of development.

Second, a context-based perspective highlights the social embeddedness of the individual. O'Rand (2006) has proposed a cumulative disadvantage model according to which early disadvantages initiate strongly path-dependent exposure to risks: a "chain of insults" (Hayward & Gorman, 2004) that extends across the phases of life. In contrast, people with advantageous early circumstances encounter a strongly path-dependent sequence of enriched environments marked by high levels of social capital, which may be defined as interpersonal relationships that facilitate the attainment of goals and positive development. From this

vantage point, a sensitive period model refers to social circumstances at a specific point in the life course that greatly influence subsequent social experiences. In keeping with a large empirical literature, O'Rand emphasizes the importance of the SES of the family-of-origin, which is highly influential with respect to life-long patterns of social capital and social risks. From the context-based perspective, the accumulation model then refers to the "chain of insults" (in the case of cumulative disadvantage) and the continuity of diverse forms of capital (in the case of cumulative advantage) across phases of life (see also Hertzman & Power, 2003; Lynch & Smith, 2005). The tendency toward diverging pathways suggested by this contrast (between early disadvantage and early advantage) may be complicated, however, by the possibility of randomly occurring insults. Although early disadvantage initiates strongly path-dependent exposures to subsequent social disadvantages, O'Rand (2006) suggests that early advantage is associated with comparatively greater variability in life course patterns because of randomly occurring stressors and challenges. Thus, the accumulation model suggests a tendency toward divergence of social experiences, and thus health, between people born into advantageous vs disadvantageous backgrounds, but notable variability among the former.

The third model, the "pathway model," directs attention to the highly contingent and varied life course patterns that people experience, marked by complex sequences and combinations of challenges and insults and forms of capital (Kuh, 2007; Kuh et al., 2003; Power & Hertzman, 1997). Such a view allows for social processes of resilience by which people encountering adversity adapt so as to avoid distressful outcomes, consistent with Elder's program of research on resilience in the life course (Elder & Shanahan, 2006). Accordingly, some people experience potentially debilitating combinations of stressors and genetic risks, yet avoid or delay serious decrements in well-being because of their social, psychological, and human capital. Such models are potentially quite pro-bative given that many people who experience early adversity and possess a genetic risk do not show symptoms of specific psychopathologies in later life.

The individual- and context-based perspectives are distinct but also complementary. As will be seen, each informs the other and neither perspective, alone, is capable of explaining behavioral development and aging. Given that genetic and social processes may thus be mutually informative, what genetic processes are relevant to life course research? We suggest three broad categories of such processes. Our discussion of molecular processes is highly simplified and abbreviated, intended only to provide sufficient background to then consider relevant empirical research.

MOLECULAR GENETIC PROCESSES IN THE LIFE COURSE

Candidate Genes in the Life Course

The term "gene" refers to a circumscribed chain of nucleotide bases that comprise coding and non-coding regions. The coding regions lead, by way of transcription, to specific proteins and the non-coding regions, or promoters, regulate transcription. A very large body of research focuses on associations between specific alleles (or variants of a gene) and specific behaviors (called "phenotypes"). Many such studies examine single nucleotide polymorphisms (or SNPs, which refer to variation in a single nucleotide base pair) or copy number variants (which describe differences in the number of times a gene or set of contiguous genes appear between genomes). The premise of such research is that a candidate gene is functional, reliably producing a discrete set of proteins that, in turn, are associated with cascades of biological, psychological, and social processes that result with regularity in a specific phenotype.

Within this framework, several issues deserve consideration. First, how should genetic variation be assessed? Advances in genotyping (the assessment of an individual's genome, the sum total genetic information) increasingly allow for genome-wide association studies (GWASs), which characterize genetic variation across an individual's entire genome. A difficult challenge of the GWAS approach is how best to use the exceptionally large body of resulting data. In any event, candidate genes are complicated by how fine-grained characterizations of the genetic variation should be (called "resolution"). For example, some studies focus on haplotypes – combinations of genes that tend to be transmitted together (forming a haplotype block) – which are thought to summarize all of the variation in the region where the block is located.

Second, how do we know when phenotypes are being measured appropriately? Many scholars advocate the use of endophenotypes (or intermediate phenotypes), which refer to behaviors that, in terms of chains of causal mechanisms, are very proximal to genetic processes. For example, variability in genes associated with dopamine receptors (alleles associated with DRD1 and DRD2) may be related to how efficiently a person can learn from rewarding and aversive experiences (Frank et al., 2007). In both instances, the candidate genes are associated with the within-person range of the availability in dopamine (which could be considered the endophenotype), which is related to how rewarding or aversive stimuli are actually experienced by the individual. Phenotypes that are further removed from these genetic variants might then result from differences in learning or impulsivity.

Third, how can we know when observed associations between candidates and phenotypes actually reflect causal mechanisms? The chief threat to internal validity is the possibility that observed associations are spurious, reflecting other genes, phenotypes, and unmodeled gene–environment associations. Spuriousness is a distinct possibility given that (1) random assignment to an allelic status is not possible (but see Davey Smith & Ebrahim, 2003, 2004), (2) many health-related outcomes are highly co-morbid (e.g. indicators of cardiovascular disease or internalizing psychopathologies), and (3) given the common understanding that one specific gene will have a small, additive effect on a phenotype. When randomization is impossible, such a threat to internal validity can be addressed, to some degree, by the strength of the conceptual model.

Compelling models are often made possible by drawing on non-human animal studies (typically involving rodents or primates) in which a candidate is silenced (either by physically knocking the locus out or by interfering with its expression) and then assigning animals to different environmental conditions. By way of such non-human animal studies, the functionality of a specific candidate can be assessed with randomization and the results can inform conceptual models that may then be generalized to humans. This strategy depends on several assumptions concerning the applicability of a specific non-human animal model to humans. But the premise is that a fairly small set of candidates can indeed be identified that, if altered, have a marked impact on genetic processes. (By analogy, thousands of parts are necessary for complex machines such as jet airplanes to work but only a few well-chosen parts need to be disrupted to create a shut-down.)

Of critical importance, candidate gene studies are ideally informed by strong conceptual models positing causal mechanisms that link the candidates to specific biological, psychological, and social processes that predictably result in specific phenotypes. Absent such conceptual models, usually based on previous empirical associations, studies of candidate genes and their associations with phenotypes, at best, provide suggestive evidence for future research and may well contribute to the well-known problem of false positive findings and non-replication (Rutter, 2008).

Journals devoted to aging have devoted considerable attention to candidates related to a multitude of diseases and forms of psychopathology, cognitive abilities, and motor and perceptual skills in old age, as well as longevity. One of the most investigated candidates is the APOE ε4 allele. The APOE gene is associated with apolipoprotein E, a lipoprotein that plays a critical role in the mobilization and distribution of cholesterol, phospholipids, and other fatty acids and is implicated in neuronal development, brain plasticity, and repair functions. The ε4 allele has been related to CVD, Alzheimer's disease, and impaired cognitive aging. While most research focuses on associations between ε4 and such phenotypes in late adulthood and old age, there is growing recognition that such associations may begin to form decades before the appearance of clinical signs of disease (e.g. Filippini et al., 2009, on cognitive differences in ε4 carriers and noncarriers in their late twenties).

The effects of candidate genes such as APOE are thought to be complicated by gene–environment interactions (GxE) and correlations (rGE). GxEs refer to processes by which a genetic effect on a phenotype is conditioned by an environmental factor, or vice versa. For example, Yaffe and colleagues (2000) report lower rates of cognitive decline associated with estrogen use in ε4-negative women but no reduced risk of decline in ε4-positive women (compared with never-users of estrogen).

A growing number of studies suggest that substantial adversities in early childhood may activate or trigger genetic propensities for psychopathologies that manifest in adulthood. Three studies are illustrative. Caspi and his colleagues (2002) were among the first to propose and test such a model with humans, finding that the MAOA gene – which metabolizes neurotransmitters – interacts with child maltreatment before the age of five to predict antisocial disorders in the early twenties. In turn, antisocial disorders in young adulthood are often followed by many psychosocial disadvantages throughout adulthood, including lowered socioeconomic attainments, social isolation, and other forms of psychopathology, and diminished health.

Gatt et al. (2009) report an interaction between early life stress and BDNF (a gene implicated in stress reactivity) in the prediction of adult depression, and Bet and his colleagues (2009) also examined early life stressors and their interaction with GR (a gene also related to stress reactivity). They observed that early-life stressors coupled with a risk variant of GR predicted depression in a random sample of adults aged 55 to 85. The Gatt and Bet studies are especially noteworthy because they examine mechanisms that link GxE and depression. Indeed, Gatt details two distinct brain arousal pathways by which the early stress–BDNF combination has a significant effect on depression and anxiety.

Studies such as those of Caspi, Gatt, and Bet have all been interpreted as examples of the individual-based sensitive period model, with the three-fold combination of a genetic risk, an environmental adversity, and the timing of the adversity in the person's life all combining to create a persistent vulnerability. A number of major questions remain to be studied, however. First, how delimited are the windows of biological sensitivity to the environment? Caspi's results are noteworthy because they reflect environmental risk in a relatively narrow time frame, before the age of five. More typical, however, are the Gatt and Bet studies, which rely on retrospective recall of several risks before the age of 18. As Casey and her colleagues (2009) note in the context of BDNF, defining the widow of sensitivity requires a detailed understanding of the gene and its influences on the organism in developmental terms. (Indeed, her research suggests that BDNF alleles can be risk factors at one point in development and protective factors at another point.)

A second, related, question is whether these windows of sensitivity typically occur in childhood or, as many studies suggest, even in utero. There is very little evidence for sensitive periods involving gene–environment interactions after adolescence. However, this may be a due to greater homogeneity in age-graded developmental processes early in life, increasing heterogeneity in terms of exposure and timing of events in middle adulthood, and the fact that early developmental periods have been more studied than periods in early and middle adulthood.

Third, what actually must occur within the window of biological sensitivity? The Caspi study is based on a multi-item scale of indicators of maltreatment ranging from parents raising their voices to sexual abuse, a wide range of behaviors. Among the successful replications of this study, many different measures of maltreatment have been used. Moreover, whatever indicators of maltreatment are used, this environmental risk frequently co-occurs with other significant risks, including poverty, family conflict, neighborhood disorganization, parental substance abuse, sibling hostility and lack of warmth, geographic mobility, income instability, and parental psychopathology (Shanahan & Hofer, 2005). Significantly, all of these factors are related to externalizing symptoms and antisocial behaviors in children.

Given networks of associations among environmental risks, it may be difficult to establish the unique, additive, and interactive roles of maltreatment per se. Put differently, is maltreatment necessary and sufficient during the window of sensitivity (i.e. the sole causal factor implicated in the main and interactive effects predicting antisocial behavior), unnecessary but sufficient (meaning that one or more of these other correlated candidates may substitute for maltreatment as a causal factor), or unnecessary and insufficient (meaning that one or more correlated candidates may substitute and maltreatment may or may not be part of the causal process)?

To be sure, childhood maltreatment is one example of this potential complexity but others can be identified, including health risks (e.g. Alamian & Paradis, 2009; Schuit et al., 2002), risks associated with poverty (e.g. McLeod & Almazan, 2003), environmental risks involving exposures to toxins and social indicators of poor living conditions (e.g. deFur et al., 2007; Evans, 2006), and psychosocial risks for psychopathology (e.g. Copeland et al., 2009). In these and other instances, specific environmental candidates do not occur in isolation but rather tend to coalesce with other factors to comprise the individual's social context. Thus, it may be very difficult to specify the range of environmental risks that must or could occur in the sensitive period to create a lasting vulnerability.

Fourth, is the sensitive period model, by itself, an etiological explanation of a later disease state? This possibility seems unlikely (if for no other reason than such models typically have modest explanatory power). In turn, what types of subsequent social experiences are necessary or sufficient? The context-based accumulation model emphasizes prolonged exposure to stressors, and the context-based pathway model raises the possibility of resilience because of sequences or configurations of diverse forms of capital. Accordingly, is maltreatment before age five actually a marker for a chain of stressors extending throughout the early life course? In this case the results do not correspond to the sensitive period model. At present, no studies examine the causal pathways that link the GxEs occurring in the early life course with disease states in adulthood. However, psychosocial research clearly shows that such pathways are highly informative (e.g. in the case of antisocial behaviors, the subject of the Caspi paper and its numerous replications; see papers in Laub, 2003; Robins & Rutter, 1992). A reasonable supposition is that individual- and context-based models of sensitive periods and accumulation coalesce to link early experiences with adult health.

A second form of gene–environment interplay involving candidate genes is the gene–environment correlation (rGE), which refers to processes by which genetic factors are associated with environmental features, perhaps strengthening the association between the genetic variance and the phenotype. For example, genetic susceptibility for depression could lead to social isolation, which in turn could increase depressive symptoms, particularly later in life.

Perhaps the most consistent theme in extant research is that rGEs have been observed for many facets of interpersonal relationships extending from childhood into adulthood. A recent review reported gene–environment correlations involving several aspects of parent–child relationships, including warmth, conflict, and rejection and also propensity to marry, marital quality, spousal conflict, likelihood of divorce, and social support (Jaffee & Price, 2007). More recently, twin and genome-wide association studies both suggest that family chaos reflects genetic factors (Price & Jaffee, 2008 and Butcher & Plomin, 2008, respectively); a biometric study suggests a genetic basis for exposure to a best friend with heavy substance use (independent of the genetic variance associated with one's own substance use) (Harden et al., 2008); and some aspects of social networks may be heritable (Fowler et al., 2009). The possibility that genetic factors are associated with interpersonal relationships makes intuitive sense, since relatively stable behavioral dispositions could elicit consistent reactions from other people (called an "evocative gene–environment correlation") and also influence the initial choice of interactional partners (the "active gene–environment correlation").

Thus far, studies of rGE have not been informed by sensitive periods, accumulation, or pathways models, although they are likely relevant. As noted, specific alleles may contribute to a biological sensitivity at circumscribed phases of life (e.g. BDNF in Casey et al., 2009), suggesting that rGEs will be more readily observed during such windows. Once such correlations form, however, they may continue through subsequent phases of life because of the person's behavioral continuities (i.e. individual-based accumulation) and also because of continuity in how others react (consistent with context-based accumulation). Despite the tendency toward behavioral continuity implied by genetic risks, the pathway model suggests the possibility for change. In terms of interpersonal relationships, this is vividly illustrated by Sampson and Laub's (1993) studies of criminal careers: many youth who were heavily engaged in delinquent behaviors did not engage in criminal acts in young adulthood because they married, became parents, and disengaged from antisocial peer groups.

Epigenetic Processes and Life Course Sociology

The sequence of nucleotides that make up each person's genes do not change from the moment of conception to death, but patterns of gene expression are likely dynamic across the life course. Gene expression refers to a range of mechanisms by which the connection between genes and their products (typically proteins) are modified. Gene expression is of critical importance because there is rarely a one-to-one correspondence between specific base pairs and specific phenotypes. Rather, the "genetic program" associated with the base pairs is modified by the person's experiences, resulting in changes in the rate of expression of genes.

Although there are many mechanisms of gene expression, only a few have been applied to the study of human behavior thus far. Epigenetic processes (tellingly, "above the gene") typically refer to alterations in the DNA that do not involve the base pairs themselves and that are relatively stable and may be heritable and reversible. Epigenetic mechanisms reflect changes to the genome that do not involve the DNA sequence but that activate or silence a part of that sequence. Such mechanisms are likely to be of keen interest to life course studies because they occur in response to the person's experiences and thus to their environment, including social context. There is presently a great deal of interest in epigenetic processes because they hold the potential to explain at least some gene–environment interactions (e.g. Foley et al., 2009; Waterland, 2009).

Two epigenetic mechanisms have been especially prominent in studies of well-being thus far. First, DNA methylation occurs when a methyl group is added to a component of the DNA (a CpG nucleotide) that is often associated with promoter regions of genes. (Methylation is also involved in two other forms of epigenetic modifications, imprinting and X-chromosome inactivation). Generally, the more a sequence is methylated, the less that sequence is expressed. Second, the genomic DNA is intricately wrapped around histones, which are proteins that serve as spools around which the DNA is wound. There are several molecular processes (e.g. acetylation) by which histones can be modified, and thus the "exposure" of a region of DNA changed such that a sequence of DNA is more or less expressed.

To date, epigenetic processes have been well-studied with respect to several types of cancers and they are believed to play roles in, for example, asthma, type 2 diabetes, and coronary heart disease (Jirtle & Skinner, 2007), as well as in some psychiatric disorders, including autism spectrum disorder, Rett's syndrome, drug addiction, and depressive disorders (Jiang et al., 2008). Prominent "environmental factors" include diet, endocrine disruptors, pollutants and environmental toxins, and infectious agents (Foley et al., 2009). To the extent that exposure to such factors depends on SES and other sociological variables, such associations provide mechanisms that link social inequalities with diseases.

Evidence also suggests that epigenetic processes may reflect "environmental factors" more akin to proximal social context. Three lines of research thus far are especially suggestive. First, Fischer and his colleagues (2007) report that environmental enrichments (e.g. the provision of toys and complex housing structures) boost memory in rats and mice and that these enhancements occur by way of histone modifications in the hippocampus. Such research may well intersect with a long line of studies suggesting that stimulating household environments (e.g. traditionally gauged by the number of books in the living room) are linked to children's cognitive development (Levenson et al.,

2004). Perhaps such processes may also explain why "enriched environments" across the life course are thought to correlate with enhancements in and the maintenance of brain functions. Generally, the enriched environments being studied with rodents are thought to be homologous to cognitively stimulating environments of people.

Second, Meaney and Szyf (2005) have examined the enduring effects of stressors in early life. Specifically, they have compared rat pups raised by nurturing and non-nurturing mothers, finding that the former are less anxious and less reactive to stressors experienced later in life. These differences reflect methylation patterns that interfere with the expression of the GR (glucocorticoid receptor) gene, which plays a role in stress reactivity. This much-discussed line of research is intriguing because it suggests a linking mechanism for studies of parent–child relationships and internalizing symptoms. Third, Tsankova and her colleagues (2006) studied chronic stress in mice, which induces depressive behaviors and is associated with several histone modifications that ultimately down-regulate BDNF. This line of research suggests linking mechanisms for models of learned helplessness and depression.

As Calvanese and his colleagues (2009) note, an epigenetic explanation of aging must detail specific epigenetic changes during development and then link such changes to the aging phenotype. There presently are no studies that satisfy these conditions although some plausible hypotheses have been formulated.

First, consistent with the sensitive period model, it may be that epigenetic processes explain the developmental origins of health and disease hypothesis (DOHaD), which posits that early environmental experiences – including the intrauterine environment – are the origins of CVD (Barker et al., 1990). This hypothesis was later extended to include cancers, type 2 diabetes, and obesity in adulthood and, significantly for our purposes, the DOHaD is thought by many to reflect epigenetic processes (e.g. Dolinoy & Jirtle, 2008). According to this perspective, epigenetic changes early in life represent a type of genetic "programming" whereby an experience during a critical period has long-term effects. Waterland and Michels (2007) suggest different molecular mechanisms by which this "durable programming" takes place during sensitive periods. (In Meany's rodent studies, for example, the methylation process specific to the GR receptors is complete by the sixth postnatal day.)

Thus, epigenetic mechanisms could provide insight into vulnerable windows very early in life that then have long-term implications for health and well-being. Fischer's studies, discussed above, raise the possibility that cognitively stimulating homes very early in development enhance the capacity for memory, an enhancement that may endure beyond early childhood. Similarly, the Meany and Tsankova programs of research suggest that early environments are capable of altering an individual's reactivity to stress, alterations that then persist. These possibilities raise a number of research questions in the human context. The threshold question is whether humans are subject to the same epigenetic mechanisms involving proximal environments and hippocampal methylation (Fischer), and changes in GR (Meany) and BDNF (Tsankova).

If so – and there is widely held belief that these studies offer major insights into human processes – what are the human analogues to the rodent's enriched environments, nurturing maternal care, and chronic social defeat? For example, what is the range of variability in households capable of inducing the epigenetic changes observed by Fischer and his colleagues and what are the salient features of such settings? These issues were similarly raised with respect to the candidate gene studies; i.e. what types of environmental features are necessary during the sensitive period?

Likewise, once again, the identification of the individual-based sensitive period is clearly of interest but, from a life course perspective, the persistence of epigenetic changes is especially intriguing and has wide-ranging implications. Stable cognitive deficiencies and heightened stress reactivity and anxiety may well contribute to social-based accumulation of more stressful experiences across the life course. That is, epigenetic mechanisms taking place during a sensitive period could then give rise to stressors throughout life and eventuate in disease states.

This possibility is dramatically suggested by a study that compared epigenetic modification of the promoter of the GR receptor in the hippocampus of suicide victims who were positive for child abuse vs suicide victims negative for abuse and controls (McGowan et al., 2009). The average ages of the suicide completers and controls were about 34 and 35, respectively. Results showed increased methylation, and hence lowered expression, of the GR promoter among suicide victims with a history of abuse when compared to controls. No differences were observed among suicide victims without a history of abuse when compared to controls. The findings have been interpreted to suggest that childhood adversity alters the development of the stress response system by way of methylation, enhancing the effects of stressors and the likelihood of mood disorders throughout life.

It is also possible that sensitive periods are not always necessary to link epigenetic patterns with disease. Rather, it may be that life-long experiences are associated with epigenetic processes that then explain decline and disease in later life consistent with the accumulation model. Bjornsson et al. (2008) assessed global methylation patterns in 100 adults at two occasions separated by 10 years. They observed a decrease in methylation levels with aging, which is thought to be associated with cancers, AD, and type 2 diabetes. Fraga and his colleagues (2005) compared epigenetic markers in a small number of identical twins, finding that older twins who lived apart and had numerous phenotypic differences showed greater epigenetic differences than younger identical twins who lived together. As noted, epigenetic processes reflect environment exposures (involving diet, endocrine disruptors, pollutants, and infectious agents) and psychosocial processes (maternal care, chronic stressors). Thus, a major research question requiring further study is whether life-long patterns of such exposures and experiences accumulate, at the cellular level, in terms of global and site-specific (e.g. promoter regions) epigenetic changes (e.g. demethylation), leading to different trajectories of morbidity and mortality in later life (an accumulation model).

Taken together, these two models – reflecting DOHaD and accumulation processes – suggest that the life course may be marked by both individual- and context-based sensitive periods during which salient experiences influence behavior for many years and/or wear-and-tear processes that accumulate over many decades. For example, perhaps children raised in settings lacking enrichment and parental nurturing then experience more stressors throughout their lives (owing to their actions, continuity in their environments, and their heightened reactivity), resulting in accelerated aging as indicated by patterns of morbidity and mortality. In contrast, children raised in enriched, nurturing settings may experience less stress and more rewarding experiences over many decades.

The pathway models are also likely relevant to epigenetic processes. Much-discussed research by Weaver and his colleagues (2004, 2006) suggests that the methylation changes in GR that Meany observed can be reversed (consistent with the pathway model). To what extent are early epigenetic processes reversible? Weaver and his colleagues relied upon an invasive pharmacological intervention. Can psychosocial experiences reverse methylation patterns as well? To what extent are subsequent experiences necessary for the maintenance of the changes? It seems implausible that proximal settings beyond the sensitive period are irrelevant but most discussions of DOHaD do not discuss this possibility and non-human animal studies have not investigated this complication.

Whatever the life course complexities relevant to epigenetic processes, it is presently thought that epigenetic differences will explain, in part, racial disparities in health, which are known to be pervasive and sometimes quite marked (Kuzawa & Sweet, 2009). Accordingly, African American mothers experience more stressors during pregnancy and the resulting intrauterine environment leads to epigenetic changes with life-long implications for metabolic patterns and stress reactivity. In turn, these differences translate into adult health disparities between whites and African Americans.

In principle, the process is especially invidious because these epigenetic changes are heritable, such that, for example, the methylation pattern of GR in the mother is transmitted to the child by way of heritability and also by way of a more distressed mother. This "double line" of transmission introduces the possibility for substantial continuity across generations in the stressfulness of intrauterine and early childhood environments. Consistent with this line of reasoning, Diorio and Meaney (2007) observed that nurturing mothers, by way of GR methylation, raised less anxious and stress-reactive pups, who then became more nurturing mothers themselves. Kuzawa and Sweet suggest that epigenetic mechanisms may likewise explain why children of Holocaust survivors and women who were pregnant during the 9/11 attacks showed evidence of changes in stress reactivity.

Transcriptional Processes in the Life Course

Roughly 10% of the variability in gene expression is thought to reflect epigenetic mechanisms, with most expression likely reflecting transcription regulation, the rate at which DNA is copied by way of RNA polymerase into messenger RNA and then proteins. Transcription factors attach to sequences of DNA near the genes that they regulate and then promote or block the RNA polymerase. By establishing links between rate of transcriptional activity and social experiences, scientists can begin to understand mechanisms by which environmental factors affect physical health. Although transcription itself is a vigorous area of research in molecular genetics, only recently have insights into these processes been applied to socially informed studies of human health. Nevertheless, several studies suggest that this is a most promising avenue for future research.

Miller and his colleagues (2008) studied links between chronic stress and transcription by conducting a genome-wide expression study (using microarray technology) on family caregivers of brain cancer patients and matched controls. The study clearly has implications for adult caregivers of aging parents and relatives. They hypothesized that chronic stress elevates cortisol, which in turn leads to (1) an eventual, compensatory down-regulation of glucorticoid receptors in monocytes (a type of white blood cell that is integral to immune response) but also (2) an enhancement of pro-inflammatory pathways. (Jointly, these processes are referred to as the glucocorticoid resistance hypothesis.) Caregivers reported higher levels of perceived stress and decreased satisfaction with their lives.

The authors then measured the transcription factor-binding motifs (TFBMs) in the promoter regions of differentially expressed genes. As expected, TFBMs occurred about 23% less frequently in genes associated with glucocorticoid receptors and they occurred more frequently in genes associated with pro-inflammation

in caregivers, compared to controls. The net result is that social stress has a "transcriptional fingerprint" involving resistance to glucocorticoids and mild systemic inflammation. A similar pattern was observed by Cole and his colleagues (2007; see also Cole, 2008) in their comparison of adults with high or low perceived loneliness (isolated vs integrated people, respectively).

The path-breaking work of Miller and Cole suggests the relevance of the accumulation model for transcriptional processes with their studies' emphases on chronic stress and social isolation (which is presumably fairly stable). As with gene candidates and epigenetic processes, these studies likewise raise the issues of environmental specificity and temporality. Are specific experiences necessary to alter the rate of a specific transcription process or are there many "functionally equivalent" environments that can produce the same effect? And how long must a stressful environment endure before the rate of transcription is altered?

One study is especially interesting from the life course perspective. Miller and his colleagues (2009) examined why children's SES affects health outcomes (such as indicators of CVD) in adulthood. The question is especially intriguing because low SES in childhood predicts coronary heart disease throughout adulthood even among people who attain high levels of SES later in life. Miller et al. suggest that early adversity increases the likelihood of a "defensive phenotype" characterized by exaggerated biological response to stress, including inflammatory response. As stressors accumulate in the life course, individuals with this defensive phenotype will be more prone to inflammatory diseases, including some types of cardiovascular and respiratory diseases and cancers.

Consistent with this model, the authors observe that, controlling present SES, children from low-SES households (as indicated by parents' occupations during the first five years of life) showed several transcriptional changes consistent with a defensive phenotype at about age 34. These findings imply that early socioeconomic experiences result in durable programming of the stress response system. Although the use of occupational prestige to indicate "adversity" deserves further consideration, the empirical findings raise the possibility that early experiences are capable of enduring biological programming (by way of transcription) in response to social circumstances. As Cole and his colleagues (2007, see also Cole, 2008) concluded, such studies call for greater nuance with respect to life course patterns of social settings. What types of early experiences are actually capable of enduring programming (i.e. individual-based sensitive period model) of the defensive phenotype? What roles do mediating experiences (i.e. the context-based accumulation model) play? And how are pathways of experiences related to continuities and discontinuities in programming into old age?

LOOKING FORWARD

Although three genetically informed approaches to health and well-being have been reviewed, there is a surprising degree of convergence among them both in terms of the relevance of life course models and the issues that call for further study. The predominant, cross-cutting theme is presently that genetic and social factors combine (typically in childhood) to create vulnerabilities in the form of behavioral tendencies (or propensities) that are then associated with disease states well into adulthood, consistent with combinations of the individual- and context-based sensitive period, accumulation, and pathway models shown in Table 10.1. And this model in turn opens two major new avenues for future research.

First, what social experiences need to happen during a sensitive period? Human studies thus far have studied SES, social isolation, and "early adversity," which are relatively general descriptors of proximal settings. Non-human animal studies have examined licking and grooming (in the case of rodents) and the removal of the mother (in the case of primates), which do not generalize neatly to specific features of human social contexts. Moreover, all of the studied environmental features to date are highly correlated with many other features of social setting (both cross-sectionally and over time) that are potentially functionally equivalent. It may be especially challenging to address these complexities because people cannot be randomly assigned to environmental conditions and then their tissue-specific epigenetic and transcriptional profiles examined (as is the case with non-human animals).

Second, beyond relatively discrete windows of sensitivity, what social experiences need to happen throughout the life course to maintain or disrupt continuity? As noted, it is not entirely clear that the individual-based sensitive period model actually accounts for many observed associations between early experience and later health because studies have thus far not examined the intervening years. Empirical research suggests several possibilities, however. Perhaps a sensitive period can create a behavioral tendency (e.g. involving stress reactivity, as suggested by Meany, Tsankova, Miller, and Cole) that combines with subsequent stressors over long periods of time (the context-based accumulation model) to increase the likelihood of disease processes, although diverse forms of capital throughout life are capable of disrupting this invidious chain of events (the context-based pathway model). A variant of this pattern is that the behavioral tendency resulting from the sensitive period actually contributes to the accumulation of subsequent deleterious experiences (e.g. high stress reactivity creates chains of stressors and decreases the likelihood of social supports). Or perhaps individual-based sensitive periods are not actually necessary; rather, functionally equivalent experiences accumulate and, when coupled with genetic mechanisms and absent significant compensatory factors, increase the likelihood of disease in later life.

Space precludes a full consideration of the possible variations suggested by Table 10.1. But, in summary, there is presently a strong tendency in the literature that favors the individual-based sensitivity model. However, the evidence does not necessarily lead to this interpretation and indeed the context-based models of sensitivity, accumulation, and pathways are likely highly relevant in connecting early (perhaps intra-uterine or infant) programming with health through adulthood. Only longitudinal data characterizing the person and context and extending from birth into old age can begin to address these complexities.

Nevertheless, despite the growing relevance of molecular genetics to studies of life course sociology and aging, several cautionary points are appropriate. First, behavioral science conducted with little reference to molecular genetics is perfectly legitimate science. The division of labor comprises scientists engaged in "pure" genetics or life course sociology, with distinctly fewer scientists drawing on both of these bodies of research in attempts at cross-fertilization. Genetically informed life course studies of aging depend on well-developed knowledge bases and paradigmatic models in both fields. Our concern in this chapter is with attempts to build bridges, but such bridges depend on imaginative and careful research in both fields. In short, not every social scientist must "re-tool" to become proficient in molecular biology.

Second, research that explores the intricacies of molecular genetic mechanisms is on-going and, indeed, basic foundational discoveries (e.g. micro RNA) have been made relatively recently and will undoubtedly continue to be made. Virtually all of the links between molecular processes and behaviors are thus provisional, exploratory, and suggestive of future research. Indeed, many social scientists believe that mature integrations of molecular genetics and social models of aging will only be realized after many years, perhaps decades, of further research. This may well be true, although such integrations will profit greatly from exchanges with the social sciences in these early formative years. In this sense, behavioral studies of aging that are informed by molecular genetics present exciting challenges to the technical and creative skills of a new generation of scientists.

ACKNOWLEDGMENTS

The authors gratefully acknowledge support from NICHD through a subproject to the Add Health Wave IV Program Project (Grant 3P01 HD031921) (Shanahan) and from NIA R01AG026453 (Hofer). The authors thank the editors and Angela O'Rand for very constructive comments.

REFERENCES

Alamian, A., & Paradis, G. (2009). Clustering of chronic disease behavioral risk factors in Canadian children and adolescents. *Preventive Medicine*, 48(5), 493–499.

Barker, D. J. P., Bull, A. R., Osmond, C., & Simmonds, S. J. (1990). Fetal and placental size and risk of hypertension in adult life. *British Medical Journal*, 301, 259–262.

Bet, P. M., Penninx, B. W., Bochdanovits, Z., Uitterlinden, A. G., Beekman, A. T., van Schoor, N. M., et al. (2009). Glucocorticoid receptor gene polymorphisms and childhood adversity are associated with depression: New evidence for a gene-environment interaction. *American Journal of Medical Genetics. Part B, Neuropsychiatric Genetics: The Official Publication of the International Society of Psychiatric Genetics*, 150B(5), 660–669.

Bjornsson, H. T., Sigurdsson, M. I., Fallin, M. D., Irizarry, R. A., Aspelund, T., Cui, H., et al. (2008). Intra-individual change over time in DNA methylation with familial clustering. *JAMA*, 299(24), 2877–2883.

Butcher, L. M., & Plomin, R. (2008). The nature of nurture: A genomewide association scan for family chaos. *Behavior Genetics*, 38(4), 361–371.

Calvanese, V., Lara, E., Kahn, A., & Fraga, M. F. (2009). The role of epigenetics in aging and age-related diseases. *Ageing Research Reviews*, 8(4), 268–276.

Casey, B. J., Glatt, C. E., Tottenham, N., Soliman, F., Bath, K., Amso, D., et al. (2009). Brain-derived neurotrophic factor as a model system for examining gene by environment interactions across development. *Neuroscience*, 164(1), 108–120.

Caspi, A., McClay, J., Moffitt, T. E., Mill, J., Martin, J., Craig, I. W., et al. (2002). Role of genotype in the cycle of violence in maltreated children. *Science (New York, NY)*, 297(5582), 851–854.

Charles, S. T., & Almeida, D. M. (2007). Genetic and environmental effects on daily life stressors: More evidence for greater variation in later life. *Psychology and Aging*, 22(2), 331–340.

Cole, S. W. (2008). Social regulation of leukocyte homeostasis: The role of glucocorticoid sensitivity. *Brain, Behavior, and Immunity*, 22(7), 1049–1055.

Cole, S. W., Hawkley, L. C., Arevalo, J. M., Sung, C. Y., Rose, R. M., & Cacioppo, J. T. (2007). Social regulation of gene expression in human leukocytes. *Genome Biology*, 8(9), R189.

Copeland, W., Shanahan, L., Costello, E. J., & Angold, A. (2009). Configurations of common childhood psychosocial risk factors. *Journal of Child Psychology and Psychiatry*, 50(4), 451–459.

Davey Smith, G., & Ebrahim, S. (2003). 'Mendelian randomization': Can genetic epidemiology contribute to understanding environmental determinants of disease? *International Journal of Epidemiology*, 32(1), 1–22.

Davey Smith, G., & Ebrahim, S. (2004). Mendelian randomization: Prospects, potentials, and limitations. *International Journal of Epidemiology*, 33, 30–42.

deFur, P. L., Evans, G. W., Cohen Hubai, E. A., Kyle, A. D., Morello-Frosch, R. A., & Williams, D. R. (2007). Vulnerability as a function of individual and group resources in cumulative risk assessment. *Environmental Health Perspectives*, 115(5), 817–824.

Diorio, J., & Meaney, M. J. (2007). Maternal programming of defensive responses through sustained effects on gene expression. *Journal of Psychiatry and Neuroscience: JPN*, 32(4), 275–284.

Dolinoy, D. C., & Jirtle, R. L. (2008). Environmental epigenomics in human health and disease. *Environmental and Molecular Mutagenesis*, 49(1), 4–8.

Elder, G. H., Jr., & Shanahan, M. J. (2006). The life course and human development. In R. Lerner (Ed.), *Handbook of Child Psychology* (Volume 1, Theory, pp. 615–775). Hoboken, NJ: John Wiley & Sons.

Evans, G. W. (2006). Child development and the physical environment. *Annual Review of Psychology*, 57, 423–451.

Filippini, N., MacIntosh, B. J., Hough, M. G., Goodwin, G. M., Frisoni, G. B., Smith, S. M., et al. (2009). Distinct patterns of brain activity in young carriers of the APOE-epsilon4 allele. *Proceedings of the National Academy of Sciences of the United States of America*, 106(17), 7209–7214.

Fischer, A., Sananbenesi, F., Wang, X., Dobbin, M., & Tsai, L. H. (2007). Recovery of learning and memory is associated with chromatin remodelling. *Nature*, 447(7141), 178–182.

Foley, D. L., Craig, J. M., Morley, R., Olsson, C. A., Dwyer, T., Smith, K., et al. (2009). Prospects for epigenetic epidemiology. *American Journal of Epidemiology*, 169(4), 389–400.

Fowler, J. H., Dawes, C. T., & Christakis, N. A. (2009). Model of genetic variation in human social networks. *Proceedings of the National Academy of Sciences of the United States of America*, 106(6), 1720–1724.

Fraga, M. F., Ballestar, E., Paz, M. F., Ropero, S., Setien, F., Ballestar, M. L., et al. (2005). Epigenetic differences arise during the lifetime of monozygotic twins. *Proceedings of the National Academy of Sciences of the United States of America*, 102(30), 10604–10609.

Frank, M. J., Moustafa, A. A., Haughey, H. M., Curran, T., & Hutchison, K. E. (2007). Genetic triple dissociation reveals multiple roles for dopamine in reinforcement learning. *Proceedings of the National Academy of Sciences of the United States of America*, 104(41), 16311–16316.

Gatt, J. M., Nemeroff, C. B., Dobson-Stone, C., Paul, R. H., Bryant, R. A., Schofield, P. R., et al. (2009). Interactions between BDNF Val66Met polymorphism and early life stress predict brain and arousal pathways to syndromal depression and anxiety. *Molecular Psychiatry, 14*(7), 681–695.

Harden, K. P., Hill, J. E., Turkheimer, E., & Emery, R. E. (2008). Gene-environment correlation and interaction in peer effects on adolescent alcohol and tobacco use. *Behavior Genetics, 38*(4), 339–347.

Hayward, M. D., & Gorman, B. K. (2004). The long arm of childhood: The influence of early-life conditions on men's mortality. *Demography, 41*(4), 87–107.

Heijmans, B. T., Tobi, E. W., Stein, A. D., Putter, H., Blauw, G. J., Susser, E. S., et al. (2008). Persistent epigenetic differences associated with prenatal exposure to famine in humans. *Proceedings of the National Academy of Sciences, 105*(44), 17046–17049.

Hertzman, C., & Power, C. (2003). Health and human development: Understandings from life-course research. *Developmental Neuropsychology, 24*(2–3), 719–744.

Houlihan, L. M., Harris, S. E., Luciano, M., Gow, A. J., Starr, J. M., Visscher, P. M., et al. (2009). Replication study of candidate genes for cognitive abilities: The Lothian Birth Cohort 1936. *Genes, Brains and Behavior, 8*, 238–247.

Jaffee, S. R., & Price, T. S. (2007). Gene-environment correlations: A review of the evidence and implications for prevention of mental illness. *Molecular Psychiatry, 12*(5), 432–442.

Jiang, Y., Langley, B., Lubin, F. D., Renthal, W., Wood, M. A., Yasui, D. H., et al. (2008). Epigenetics in the nervous system. *The Journal of Neuroscience: The Official Journal of the Society for Neuroscience, 28*(46), 11753–11759.

Jirtle, R. L., & Skinner, M. K. (2007). Environmental epigenomics and disease susceptibility. *Nature Reviews Genetics, 8*(4), 253–262.

Johnson, W. (2007). Genetic and environmental influences on behavior: Capturing all the interplay. *Psychological Review, 114*, 423–440.

Kendler, K. S., Gardner, C. O., Fiske, A., & Gatz, M. (2009). Major depression and coronary artery disease in the Swedish Twin Registry: Phenotypic, genotypic, and environmental sources of comorbidity. *Archives of General Psychiatry, 66*, 857–863.

Kendler, K., Jaffee, S., & Romer, D. (Eds.). (in press). The dynamic genome and mental health: The role of genes and environments in development. New York: Oxford University Press.

Kuh, D., The New Dynamics of Ageing Preparatory Network (2007). A life course approach to healthy aging, frailty, and capability. *Journal of Gerontology: Medical Sciences, 62A*(7), 717–721.

Kuh, D., Ben-Shlomo, Y., Lynch, J., Hallqvist, J., & Power, C. (2003). Life course epidemiology. *Journal of Epidemiology and Community Health, 57*, 778–783.

Kuzawa, C. W., & Sweet, E. (2009). Epigenetics and the embodiment of race: Developmental origins of US racial disparities in cardiovascular health. *American Journal of Human Biology: The Official Journal of the Human Biology Council, 21*(1), 2–15.

Laub, J. H. (2003). Shared beginnings divergent lives: Delinquent boys to age 70. Cambridge: Harvard University Press.

Levenson, J. M., O'Riordan, K. J., Brown, K. D., Trinh, M. A., Molfese, D. L., & Sweatt, J. D. (2004). Regulation of histone-acetylation during memory formation in the hippocampus. *The Journal of Biological Chemistry, 279*(39), 40545–40559.

Lynch, J., & Smith, G. D. (2005). A life course approach to chronic disease epidemiology. *Annual Review of Public Health, 26*, 1–35.

McGowan, P. O., Sasaki, A., D'Alessio, A. C., Dymov, S., Labonte, B., Szyf, M., et al. (2009). Epigenetic regulation of the glucocorticoid receptor in human brain associates with childhood abuse. *Nature Neuroscience, 12*(3), 342–348.

Meaney, M. J., & Szyf, M. (2005). Environmental programming of stress responses through DNA methylation: Life at the interface between a dynamic environment and a fixed genome. *Dialogues in Clinical Neuroscience, 7*(2), 103–123.

McClearn, G. E., Vogler, G. M., & Hofer, S. M. (2001). Gene-gene and gene-environment interactions. In E. J. Masoro & S. N. Austad (Eds.), *Handbook of the Biology of Aging* (pp. 423–444) (5th Edn). San Diego: Academic Press.

McLeod, J. D., & Almazan, E. P. (2003). Connections between childhood and adulthood. In J. T. Mortimer & M. J. Shanahan (Eds.), *Handbook of the Life Course* (pp. 391–411). New York: Kluwer-Plenum.

Miller, G. E., Chen, E., Sze, J., Marin, T., Arevalo, J. M., Doll, R., et al. (2008). A functional genomic fingerprint of chronic stress in humans: Blunted glucocorticoid and increased NF-kappa-B signaling. *Biological Psychiatry, 64*(4), 266–272.

Miller, G. E., Chen, E., Fok, A. K., Walker, H., Lim, A., Nicholls, E. F., et al. (2009). Low early-life social class leaves a biological residue manifested by decreased glucocorticoid and increased proinflammatory signaling. *Proceedings of the National Academy of Sciences of the United States of America, 106*(34), 14716–14721.

O'Rand, A. M. (2006). Stratification and the life course: Life course capital, life course risks, and social inequality. In R. H. Binstock & L. K. George (Eds.), *Handbook of Aging and the Social Sciences* (pp. 145–162) (6th Edn). San Diego: Academic Press.

Power, C., & Hertzman, C. (1997). Social and biological pathways linking early life and adult disease. *British Medical Bulletin, 53*(1), 210–221.

Price, T. S., & Jaffee, S. R. (2008). Effects of the family environment: Gene-environment interaction and passive gene-environment correlation. *Developmental Psychology, 44*(2), 305–315.

Robins, L. N., & Rutter, M. (Eds.), (1992). *Straight and devious pathways from childhood to adulthood*. New York: Cambridge University Press.

Rutter, M. (2007). Gene-environment interdependence. *Developmental Science, 10*, 12–18.

Rutter, M. (2008). Biological implications of gene-environment interaction. *Journal of Abnormal Child Psychology, 36*(7), 969–975.

Sampson, R. J., & Laub, J. H. (1993). *Crime in the Making: Pathways and turning points through life.*

Cambridge: Harvard University Press.

Schuit, A. J., van Loon, A. J., Tijhuis, M., & Ocke, M. (2002). Clustering of lifestyle risk factors in a general adult population. *Preventive Medicine, 35*(3), 219–224.

Shanahan, M. J., & Boardman, J. (2009). Genetics and behavior in the life course: A promising frontier. In G. H. Elder, Jr. & J. Z. Giele (Eds.), *The Craft of Life Course Research* (pp. 215–235). New York: Guilford.

Shanahan, M. J., & Hofer, S. M. (2005). Social context in gene–environment interactions: Retrospect and prospect. *Journal of Gerontology B Psychological Science and Social Science, 60*, 65–76.

Shostak, S., & Freese, J. (2009). Genetics and social inquiry. *Annual Review of Sociology, 35*, 107–128.

Tollefsbol, T. O. (Ed.), (2009). *Epigenetics of Aging*. New York: Springer.

Tsankova, N. M., Berton, O., Renthal, W., Kumar, A., Neve, R. L., & Nestler, E. J. (2006). Sustained hippocampal chromatin regulation in a mouse model of depression and antidepressant action. *Nature Neuroscience, 9*(4), 519–525.

Waterland, R. A. (2009). Is epigenetics an important link between early life events and adult disease? *Hormone Research, 71*(Suppl 1), 13–16.

Waterland, R. A., & Michels, K. B. (2007). Epigenetic epidemiology of the developmental origins hypothesis. *Annual Review of Nutrition, 27*(Suppl 1), 363–388.

Weaver, I. C., Cervoni, N., Champagne, F. A., D'Alessio, A. C., Sharma, S., Seckl, J. R., et al. (2004). Epigenetic programming by maternal behavior. *Nature Neuroscience, 7*(8), 847–854.

Weaver, I. C., Meaney, M. J., & Szyf, M. (2006). Maternal care effects on the hippocampal transcriptome and anxiety-mediated behaviors in the offspring that are reversible in adulthood. *Proceedings of the National Academy of Sciences of the United States of America, 103*(9), 3480–3485.

World Health Organization. (1948). Preamble to the Constitution of the World Health Organization. *Official Records of the World Health Organization, 2*, 100.

Yaffe, K., Haan, M., Byers, A., Tangen, C., & Kuller, L. (2000). Estrogen use, APOE, and cognitive decline. *Neurology, 54*, 1949–1954.

Chapter | 11 |

Social Factors, Depression, and Aging

Linda K. George

Department of Sociology and Center for the Study of Aging, Duke University, Durham, North Carolina

INTRODUCTION

Depression is the most prevalent psychiatric disorder in the older population (e.g. Blazer, 2002). An even larger proportion of older adults suffer from significant numbers of depressive symptoms that do not meet the criteria for a psychiatric diagnosis but impair functioning and quality of life. There is scientific consensus that depression results from social, psychological, biological, and genetic causes. This chapter examines the role of social factors in the distribution, antecedents, and consequences of depression in later life. The next two sections examine issues and controversies in defining depression and methods of measuring depression. The following section examines the epidemiology of depression in later life. This is followed by a review of the wide range of social factors that both increase the risk of depression in later life and protect against it. The final sections address the consequences of depression in late life and priority issues for future research.

DEPRESSION IN LATER LIFE: DEFINITIONS REMAIN CONTENTIOUS

There is long-standing controversy about whether depression is best conceptualized as a disease or as psychological distress. The controversy reflects, in part, disciplinary allegiances. Psychiatry conceptualizes depression as a disease with the formal diagnostic label of major depressive disorder (MDD) (American Psychiatric Association, 2000). As such it is defined dichotomously – one either has or does not have the disorder, although "subclinical" or "mild" depression also is recognized. Psychiatrists pay close attention to transitions in and out of illness episodes and use the language of recovery and remission. Most social scientists conceptualize depression in terms of symptoms, typically using continuous symptom counts (e.g. Mirowsky & Ross, 2002). In contrast to psychiatrists, social scientists do not use a diagnostic label, preferring the terms "depressive symptoms" or "psychological distress." In terms of dynamics, they study increases and decreases in symptoms. Although these disciplinary patterns are clear, they are not universal. Psychiatrists often use symptom counts to assess disease severity and some social scientists study MDD.

Advocates of both conceptualizations of depression offer strong justifications for their choice. Psychiatrists generally adopt the medical model in which psychiatric disorders are assumed to be analogous to physical illnesses. Contrary to the accusations of some social scientists, however, psychiatric nomenclature does recognize that (1) *severity* of illness is best measured by continuous symptom counts, (2) persons with high levels of symptoms but who do not meet the criteria for diagnosis are at greatest risk for onset of mental illness, and (3) symptoms of depression that do not meet the diagnostic criteria may nonetheless generate suffering and functional impairment (APA, 2000).

Mental health professionals and social scientists usually have different goals. Psychiatrists diagnose and treat illnesses; their primary interest is not the whole population, only that part of it that is their responsibility to treat. Social scientists, on the other hand, are often interested in the total burden that mental health problems generate in a population and convincingly argue that much of that burden is experienced by persons who are symptomatic, but do not meet the criteria for a psychiatric diagnosis. Reflecting the legacy of labeling theory, social scientists also are aware of the stigma associated with mental illness. Despite substantial public education, most Americans prefer to distance themselves from the mentally ill and being a former or a current mental patient remains a basis for discrimination and social isolation (Link et al., 1999). Symptom counts avoid stigmatizing labels.

In practical terms, the preference for diagnostic measures is compelling. Third-party payers want mental health benefits to be used for mental illnesses rather than "lots of symptoms." Policymakers want evidence that publicly funded programs prevent mental illness or treat it effectively. They understand research results stating that 40% of the patients treated with a given therapy recovered from mental illness; they don't understand what it means if treatment decreased symptoms half of a standard deviation.

Both symptom counts and psychiatric diagnoses are legitimate and important measures of mental health problems. Therefore, this chapter reviews studies of both continuous and dichotomous measures of depression.

MEASURING DEPRESSIVE SYMPTOMS AND MAJOR DEPRESSIVE DISORDER

In contrast to dissension concerning the appropriate conceptualization of depression, measurement of depressive symptoms and MDD is relatively straightforward.

Depressive Symptoms

The CES-D

Introduced to the field more than 30 years ago, the Center for Epidemiologic Studies – Depression Scale (CES-D) has become the near universal measure of depressive symptoms (Radloff, 1977). The CES-D includes 20 items measuring depressive symptoms; respondents report the frequency (from "rarely or none of the time" to "most or all the time") of experiencing the symptoms in the past week. Items are summed (item range = 0–3) and the scale range is from 0 to 60. Careful psychometric assessment of the CES-D was performed during its development (Radloff, 1977) and more recent studies confirm its reliability (e.g. Li, 2005). Although most investigators score the CES-D in continuous form, Radloff established a cut-point of 16 and above as evidence of "clinically significant depression." The cut-point was established by comparing CES-D scores of non-depressed and depressed adults as determined by psychiatric interviews. Note, however, that the CES-D cut-point does not identify "cases" of MDD.

Modifications of the CES-D

Although the CES-D is a relatively concise instrument, many surveys use abbreviated forms of the scale. For example, an 11-item version of the CES-D was included in the ACL study (e.g. Yang & Lee, 2009) and a 12-item version was used in the National Survey of Families and

Households (e.g. Simon & Marcussen, 1999). Although the internal consistency reliability of the original CES-D is very high, ranging from 0.85–0.90 in most studies (e.g. Li, 2005; Radloff, 1977), Krause et al. (1992) report that the CES-D includes four factors: depressed affect, somatic affect, positive affect (reverse coded), and interpersonal strains. It appears that most abbreviations of the CES-D were motivated solely to reduce the time of administration. In some cases, however, the choice of discarded items was based on conceptual grounds (e.g. to eliminate symptoms that are most likely to reflect physical illness) or on Krause's factor analysis results. Little psychometric work appears to have accompanied development of the abbreviated CES-D measures, although some investigators report high correlations between the abbreviated and total scale scores (e.g. r = 0.92; Walsemann et al., 2009).

Another modification involves collapsing the response categories for the symptoms. In its original form, four response categories are used to measure symptom frequency. Some respondents, especially older adults, find it difficult to distinguish between the categories (e.g. "some or a little of the time" vs "occasionally or a moderate amount of the time") (Blazer et al., 1987). Consequently, some investigators simplify the response categories to a yes–no format in which respondents report the presence or absence of the symptom during the past week.

Other Measures

The primary alternative to the CES-D is the 12-item depressive subscale of the Hopkins Symptom Checklist (Derogatis et al., 1974). See Aneshensel et al., 2004 and Lorenz et al., 2006 for studies of late-life depression using the Hopkins Symptom Checklist.

Major Depressive Disorder

Beginning with DSM-III (APA, 1980), the criteria for psychiatric disorders were specified in a way that permits lay interviewers to administer standardized diagnostic interviews that can ascertain the presence of psychiatric disorders. The first instrument to measure specific psychiatric disorders, including MDD, was the Diagnostic Interview Schedule (DIS) (Robins et al., 1981). The DIS was used in the landmark Epidemiologic Catchment Area Studies, which provided the first prevalence estimates of specific psychiatric disorders in the US (e.g. Robins & Regier, 1991).

During the 1990s, after the publication of DSM-IV, a modified version of the DIS was developed. The revised instrument was named the Composite International Diagnostic Interview (CIDI) (Kessler et al., 1998). The CIDI has become the gold standard for measuring specific DSM-IV psychiatric disorders using a standardized interview. For detailed information about the CIDI, including the full interview schedule, see WHO (2004).

The criteria for MDD are nearly identical in DSM-III and DSM-IV.

The DIS and CIDI are more complex than symptom scales such as the CES-D. Complex sets of probes are used to exclude symptoms that do not meet DSM criteria. Probes are used to ensure that the symptom is of psychogenic origin and not due to physical illness or use of medications, and that it interferes with daily functioning. If the minimum number of depressive symptoms is reported, additional probes are used to determine that the symptoms occurred at the same time and persisted for two weeks or more – both of the latter are DSM criteria for MDD. "Recency probes" are used so that the prevalence of MDD can be calculated for several timeframes: current, past month, past six months, past year, and ever in lifetime.

THE EPIDEMIOLOGY OF DEPRESSION AND PSYCHOLOGICAL DISTRESS IN LATER LIFE

Overall, older adults have lower rates of psychiatric disorder in general and MDD in particular than young and middle-aged adults (Gum et al., 2009; Kessler et al., 2005). Although the precise effects of age, cohort, and selective mortality remain unclear, all of them are implicated. With regard to age, there is consistent evidence over the past 50 years that the incidence of depression peaks in adolescence and young adulthood. In addition, each successive cohort appears to have higher rates of depression than its predecessors (Kessler et al., 2005). Depression also is an established risk factor for mortality (Schulz et al., 2002), which also contributes to the lower prevalence among older adults.

The pattern for symptom counts, however, is neither clear-cut nor consistent. Comparing three broad age groups – young, middle-aged, and older adults – some investigators report that older adults have the highest number of depressive symptoms (e.g. Mirowsky & Ross, 1992) and others report that they have the lowest (e.g. Schieman et al., 2002). There is no easy or obvious way to reconcile these discrepancies. These studies are cross-sectional, however; as a consequence, age and cohort differences are confounded.

MDD is characterized by two primary kinds of symptoms: disordered mood (e.g. feelings of sadness, hopelessness) and vegetative symptoms (loss of interest, exhaustion) (APA, 2000). Compared to their younger counterparts, older adults are more likely to experience vegetative symptoms and less likely to experience disordered mood. This poses a significant diagnostic challenge because the vegetative symptoms of MDD also can result from physical illnesses that are prevalent in later life (e.g. Blazer, 2002). The course of MDD takes multiple paths. Some individuals have a single episode from which they permanently recover. More common, however, are recurrent and chronic MDD (APA, 2000). Although estimates vary, most report that 2–4% of Americans aged 65 and older have MDD (e.g. Blazer, 2002; Gum et al., 2009). Prevalence estimates from other countries are generally larger; e.g. 7.9% in Sweden (Forsell et al., 1995) and 6% in China (Chen et al., 2005). The reasons for cross-national differences in the prevalence of MDD are not known. Structural arrangements may account for some of the variation. It also is likely that there are national differences in diagnostic decision-making, although most countries now state that the American DSM system is their official psychiatric nomenclature. Incidence studies are rare, especially those that report age-specific incidence rates. The most frequently reported incidence rate in the US for older adults is 0.15% (or about 3/1000) per year (e.g. Blazer, 2002). Neither prevalence nor incidence studies distinguish among single-episode, recurrent, and chronic MDD, but chronic cases contribute disproportionately to prevalence estimates and are excluded from incidence rates. Henceforth, the term "psychological distress" or "distress" will be used as synonyms for depressive symptoms; MDD will be used to refer to the psychiatric diagnosis. The more general term "depression" will be used when the issues or research findings apply to both dichotomous and continuous measures.

SOCIAL FACTORS AND DEPRESSION IN LATER LIFE: THEORETICAL FOUNDATIONS

Many studies of the relationships between social factors and depression are not based on a specific theoretical paradigm. Rather, most implicitly or explicitly rest on one or more of three primary theoretical perspectives. Each will be briefly described.

Stress Process Theory

The primary theoretical framework used to derive hypotheses about social factors and depression is stress process theory. In a classic article, Pearlin et al. (1981) developed a model that focuses on stressors, factors that mediate or moderate the effects of stress, and health outcomes. Stressors are events (i.e. acute stressors) and conditions (i.e. chronic stressors) that challenge individuals' coping skills, threaten to overwhelm them physically and/or mentally, and increase the risk of illness onset. Stressors are viewed as causally linked to social structural location, including both demographic characteristics (e.g. gender, race/ethnicity, and socioeconomic status (SES)) and social roles (e.g. work, marital, and

parenting roles). Individuals of lower social status are exposed to higher levels of stress and, thus, are at greater risk of health problems. Social resources also are important – adequate resources (e.g. high-quality social support) can prevent or mitigate the effects of stressors on health. Social-psychological resources, such as self-esteem and a sense of control or mastery, also can mediate the harmful effects of stress. Lower status individuals typically have fewer resources with which to confront stressors. As a result they are both exposed to higher levels of stress and more vulnerable to it. The stress process model is viewed as especially important in understanding depression in later life both because of age- or cohort-related declines in resources and because older adults are physiologically more vulnerable. The stress process model has been empirically supported in literally hundreds of studies (Folkman, 2010).

SES as a Fundamental Cause of Illness

A strong relationship between SES and health was first observed in the nineteenth century. Despite fundamental changes in public health measures, leading causes of death, and medical knowledge and technology, this relationship remains. It is true in developed and developing countries. The size of the "gap" between rich and poor varies substantially across nations. Among developed nations, the US is among those with the largest SES and racial/ethnic health disparities – and the gap has grown substantially since the 1980s (see Chapter 9).

The consistency of the relationship between SES and health across time, place, and health outcomes has led to widespread endorsement of the fundamental cause of disease theory (Link & Phelan, 1995). A fundamental cause of illness is a cause that persists despite advances in the prevention and management of specific diseases and for a wide variety of health outcomes. SES is widely viewed as a fundamental cause of illness, disability, and death in all societies. It is an "upstream" causal agent. More proximal or "downstream" causes may mediate the effects of SES on specific health outcomes, but SES is the engine driving the process and, even if the mediators (i.e. risk factors) are eliminated (e.g. by the development of a vaccine for a specific illness), SES remains a robust predictor of overall mortality and morbidity.

There is no conflict between fundamental cause theory and stress process theory. Stress theorists have always posited that stress exposure is, in large part, a result of social stratification. Fundamental cause scholars are neither surprised nor discouraged when empirical results indicate that stress mediates much of the relationship between SES and mental health. The same models support both theories. What differs is interpretive emphasis. Stress process scholars typically urge health policy to target resources that can ameliorate the harmful effects of stress (e.g. health behaviors, social support). From the fundamental cause perspective, the most effective ways to improve population health are those that narrow the gap between the poorest and the richest strata in society through education policy and income redistribution.

The Life Course Perspective

Over the past two decades, the life course perspective has become increasingly influential in the social sciences in general and research on social factors and depression in particular. As detailed elsewhere (e.g. George, 2007), the life course perspective is not an integrated theory, but consists of several principles that can be used to enrich many theories. Four principles are central to the life course perspective. First, and most obviously, is an emphasis on the long view of human lives – the assumption that events and conditions experienced early in the life course often have persisting effects on outcomes later in life, either directly or indirectly (i.e. by influencing mediating processes) (see Chapter 24). Second, the life course perspective focuses on the intersection of personal biography and historical context. Cohorts experience very different historical events and conditions that, in turn, differentially affect life course opportunities and constraints. Individuals within cohorts also are differentially affected by historical context. Third, the life course perspective emphasizes the importance of linked lives and their importance for personal biography (e.g. the effects of family roles on occupational careers). Fourth is the attention paid to human agency.

The life course perspective augments stress process theory in valuable ways. The recognition that childhood traumas are antecedents of depression not only in childhood but throughout life illustrates the successful integration of the life course perspective with stress process theory (e.g. Kessler & Magee, 1994; Shaw & Krause, 2002). Another example is the increased attention to the ways that historical events such as the Great Depression and combat experience during war put specific cohorts and specific groups of individuals within cohorts at increased risk for mental health problems (e.g. Elder, 1974; Elder et al., 1994). Strong relationships between social support and the risk of depression highlight the role of linked lives. And coping strategies reflect at least in part the role of human agency in overcoming adversity or succumbing to it. For a recent examination of the links between stress process theory and the life course perspective, see Pearlin (2010).

SOCIAL FACTORS AND DEPRESSION IN LATER LIFE: EMPIRICAL FINDINGS

Numerous social factors are established risk and protective factors for depression in later life. They are described in categories that are widely assumed to represent increasingly proximate antecedents of depression. Attention also is paid to the extent to which more proximate factors mediate the effects of more distal antecedents. Unless stated otherwise, studies cited are based on samples of older adults.

Demographic Variables

Age differences in depressive symptoms and diagnoses were reviewed above. Here, the associations of gender and race/ethnicity are examined.

Gender

The most consistent correlate of depressive symptoms and MDD is gender, with women at substantially greater risk than men of both. This sex differential holds true for whites, blacks, and Latinos (e.g. Kessler et al., 2005) and for the native-born and immigrants (Wilmoth & Chen, 2003). Cross-sectional comparisons of age differences suggest that the gender differential narrows in later life (e.g. Miech et al., 2005). Although longitudinal data covering all of adulthood are lacking, this pattern has been observed in studies spanning 40 years, suggesting that it is not a cohort effect. A full explanation for the gender gap in depression remains elusive, with sociologists, psychologists, and biologists all offering potential partial explanations. The primary hypotheses offered for the narrowing gender gap in depression across the life course are biological (i.e. that hormonal changes in women make them less susceptible to depression; e.g. Avis et al., 2001) and social (i.e. that gender roles are less pervasive and rigid in later life; e.g. Jorm, 1987).

Race/Ethnicity

In contrast to gender, relationships between race/ethnicity and depression remain ambiguous. US studies comparing blacks and whites variously report that blacks have more depressive symptoms than whites (e.g. Skarupski et al., 2005), have fewer symptoms than whites (e.g. Kubzansky et al., 2000), and that blacks and whites do not differ (e.g. George, 1992). Latinos, on average, have higher levels of depressive symptoms than whites (Chiriboga et al., 2002). With regard to MDD, substantial evidence indicates that blacks and whites do not differ in the prevalence of MDD (e.g. Kessler et al., 2005; Kubzansky et al., 2000). Stable estimates of rates of MDD among Latinos are lacking.

SES

Researchers usually operationalize SES in terms of one or more of three indicators: education, income, and occupational prestige. Education and income – one or both – are the standard indicators of SES in studies of depression in later life. From a life course perspective, education and income, although significantly correlated, differ substantially in interpretation. Education is typically completed in young adulthood; as such, the temporal order between education and depression is generally non-problematic (i.e. education was completed long before depression is assessed). The relationship between income and late-life depression is less temporally clear. A plausible case can be made for the "social causation" hypothesis that low income increases risk of psychiatric problems, but a credible case also can be made for the "social selection" hypothesis that income is determined, in part, by psychiatric status (i.e. chronic mental illness leads to lower-income jobs, to disorderly work histories, or to early retirement in which Social Security and pension benefits are reduced). Longitudinal data can help sort out the temporal associations between income and depression, but it is not a panacea because income and psychiatric status tend to be highly correlated at baseline.

Substantial evidence supports the conclusion that low levels of education and low income – whether or not they are included in the same predictive models – are significantly related to depressive symptoms and MDD in late life (e.g. Kubzansky et al., 2000; Miech et al., 2005; see especially the meta-analysis by Lorant et al., 2003). These associations hold across gender and race/ethnicity.

Women and racial/ethnic minorities have, on average, lower levels of education and income than men and whites. Thus, researchers often determine the extent to which SES mediates the relationships between gender and race/ethnicity and depressive symptoms. In general, findings suggest that SES *partially* mediates the effects of race/ethnicity on depressive symptoms (e.g. Skarupski et al., 2005), although race/ethnicity usually continues to have a direct effect on depression. We are aware of no evidence that education and income explain gender differences in depressive symptoms or MDD.

Stressors

Social stress is the social risk factor that has been studied most frequently and has the strongest empirical support. Two types of stressors are strong and consistent predictors of depressive symptoms and MDD: negative life events and chronic stressors.

Life events are discrete changes in life circumstances that have the potential to challenge one's adaptive capacities and trigger psychological distress – sometimes to the point of full-blown psychiatric disorder. Negative life events are measured in one of two ways: based either on investigators' assumptions that certain events are, by definition, negative (e.g. death of significant others, divorce) or on respondents' self-reports that the event negatively affected them. *No single event* is rated as negative by everyone who experiences it (e.g. Hughes et al., 1988); thus, the self-reports from respondents are more valid. Chronic stressors are long-term conditions that pose persistent challenges to individuals (e.g. chronic financial strain). Unfortunately, chronic stressors tend to be measured quite poorly, with unreliable assessments of the chronicity of the stressful situation (e.g. if a respondent reports current financial strain, this is typically viewed as evidence of a chronic stressor).

Negative Life Events (NLEs)

Two strategies are employed in investigations of NLEs. Some investigators create summary scales of the number of NLEs experienced during a defined interval (e.g. one year, three years); others examine the effects of single, specific NLEs. Both strategies generate evidence that NLEs are significant predictors of both depressive symptoms and MDD (e.g. Adams et al., 2004; Fiske et al., 2003; Moos et al., 2005). In a meta-analysis, Kraaij et al. (2002) concluded that the effects of individual NLEs on depression are typically significant, but modest in size, whereas the effects of aggregate counts of NLEs have much stronger effects.

Growth curve models and related techniques that permit investigators to examine within-person trajectories of stability and change are only beginning to appear in research on depression in later life. Lynch and George (2002) examined trajectories of loss events (deaths and disruptions in social relationships) and trajectories of depressive symptoms over six years. Their results showed that loss events increase over time in this age group (age 65 and older) and that "growth" in loss events predicts "growth" in depressive symptoms. Although the findings parallel those reported for between-person statistical analyses, such as those cited in the previous paragraph, the two analytic strategies answer distinct questions. Traditional between-person analyses determine whether people who experience higher numbers of NLEs are more depressed than people who experience no or low numbers of NLEs. Growth curve techniques ascertain whether an individual who experiences NLEs subsequently becomes more depressed. Li (2005) used growth curve modeling to examine trajectories of bereavement among caregivers over four years. All of the participants were active caregivers at baseline; over the course of the study, many of their care recipients died. The average trajectory for these caregivers indicated that depressive symptoms increased over time until the care recipient's death and then declined over time. Li found that several variables moderated the shape of the trajectory. Among caregivers whose care recipients had more behavior problems before death, who reported higher levels of overload before the care recipient's death, and/or had lower incomes, depression symptoms exhibited a steeper and more rapid decline after bereavement, suggesting that bereavement is counterbalanced to some degree by relief.

The social causation vs social selection debate is relevant to the relationship between NLEs and depression. The social causation perspective posits that stressors have a causal effect on depressive symptoms and MDD. The social selection hypothesis contends that being depressed leads to the experience of NLEs. Two studies examined the reciprocal effects of NLEs and depression (Fiske et al., 2003; Moos et al., 2005). Both studies found evidence of both social causation and social selection – but the effects of NLEs on depression were stronger than those of depression on NLEs.

Chronic Stressors

The relationships between several chronic stressors and depression in late life have been studied. Because of space limitations, we will focus only on the stress of caring for an impaired older adult. Caregiving is the best chronic stressor to discuss because of (1) the large volume of research, (2) the fact that both depressive symptoms and MDD have been studied extensively, and (3) the fact that there are sufficient longitudinal studies to insure that it is typically a chronic stressor lasting months or years. Many investigators also conceptualize physical illness and disability as chronic stressors; these factors are addressed below as a separate category.

Longitudinal studies document that caregiving is a long-term stressor that is strongly related to both depressive symptoms and MDD. Two meta-analyses report that 22–33% of caregivers meet the criteria for a diagnosis of MDD (Cuijpers, 2005; Pinquart & Sorensen, 2006). Another significant proportion of care-givers report high levels of depressive symptoms, but either do not meet the criteria for MDD or participated in studies that only examined symptoms. It should be noted that a large proportion of caregiving studies focus on caregivers for older adults with dementia, which has the potential to bias the results of the meta-analyses. Nonetheless, non-dementia caregivers also report high levels of depressive symptoms.

Expanding the Stress Universe

During the past 10–15 years, expanding the "stress universe" – i.e. developing more comprehensive stress inventories that better capture the full burden of stressors that individuals experience – has been a prominent theme. NLEs and chronic stressors are components of the stress universe. Major additions to the universe of stressors include childhood traumas (e.g. sexual or physical abuse, parental divorce) and other severe traumas regardless of the age at which they occurred (e.g. sexual assault, combat experience). Studies using this expanded view of stress report stronger relationships between stress and depression than more restricted definitions (e.g. Turner & Avison, 2003). In addition, although traditional stress measures mediate little of the associations of demographic variables and SES with depression, expanded measures exhibit strong mediating effects for race/ethnicity and SES, although not for gender (Turner & Avison, 2003). That is, large proportions of the associations of race/ethnicity and SES with depression operate through the higher levels of stress experienced by minorities and low-SES individuals. Unfortunately, virtually all research examining the effects of more comprehensive measures of stress has been conducted in age-heterogeneous samples. We are aware of no studies based exclusively on older adults or that test age interactions.

Another factor in the stress universe is discrimination. The focus to date has been on demonstrating that discrimination partially mediates the relationship between race and depression (e.g. Williams et al., 1997), although this research is based solely on age-heterogeneous samples. Multiple forms of discrimination (e.g. gender, religious) are also potentially important. The life course perspective can be usefully applied to this issue. Presumably, racial and ethnic discrimination are initially experienced early in life. In some cases, discrimination is chronic; in others, it is episodic or time-limited. An important topic for future research is determining whether time-limited and chronic discrimination have persistent effects on depression, even in later life. Age discrimination is of potential importance as well. We do not yet know whether age discrimination affects mental health or whether the combination of age discrimination with other forms of unfair treatment has synergistic effects on depression.

Social Integration

Social integration exists at two levels. At the individual level, social integration refers to attachments to the social structure, generally via roles. Individuals typically lose more attachments to social structure than they gain during later life, as a result of retirement and widowhood. At the aggregate level, residential neighborhoods can be characterized by level of social integration. Socially integrated neighborhoods are characterized by frequent, pleasant interaction among residents, investments in personal property and community resources, and, if needed, collective action to address problems.

Individual-Level Social Integration

At the individual level, two primary forms of social integration have been studied in relation to depression in later life: religious participation and volunteering. Frequent attendance at religious services prospectively predicts both lower levels of depressive symptoms and lower risk of MDD in the US (e.g. Chatters et al., 2008; Norton et al., 2008) and Europe (e.g. Braam et al., 2004). Based on a meta-analysis of 147 studies examining the relationships between religious involvement and depression, Smith et al. (2003) concluded that religiousness, in aggregate, is significantly, but modestly, associated with lower levels of depression. Religious participation takes a variety of forms. Service attendance is consistently the dimension of religious participation most strongly related to depression and other health outcomes.

Two additional issues merit attention. First, the effects of religious attendance on depression have been examined with a wide array of potential confounding factors statistically controlled (e.g. social support, race/ethnicity). Second, the causal order between service attendance and depression is theoretically ambiguous. The social selection hypothesis is of special concern because physically or mentally ill individuals may be unable to attend religious services. There now is sufficient evidence to conclude that the dominant direction of influence is from attendance to disability, rather than the reverse (e.g. Idler & Kasl, 1997). Evidence is lacking, however, for the relationship between attendance and depression.

Volunteering also is associated with fewer depressive symptoms (e.g. Adams et al., 2004) and with declines in depressive symptoms over time (e.g. Morrow-Howell et al., 2003). There also is evidence that volunteering reduces depression in vulnerable groups. Li (2007) found that widowed older adults who began or increased volunteering exhibited more rapid declines in depressive symptoms than their non-volunteer counterparts. Hao (2008) examined the effects of employment and volunteering over eight years, using growth curve models. The overall trajectory in the sample was of gradually increasing depressive symptoms over time. Both employment and volunteering, however, predicted lower depressive symptoms at baseline and slower growth in depressive symptoms over time.

Aggregate-Level Social Integration

Although multi-level models of the effects of neighborhood characteristics on depression during late life hold much promise, there has been almost no research to date. In a review of neighborhood effects studies, Kim (2008) reports that social disorder (e.g. high crime, high proportions of empty dwellings) is the neighborhood characteristic most strongly associated with residents' depression. This conclusion is compatible with social integration theory. Unfortunately, none of the studies reviewed examined depression specifically in late life. Although older adults are included in age-heterogeneous studies, age interactions were not tested to determine whether the effects of neighborhood disorder differed in magnitude for older adults. The one multi-level study of the effects of aggregate characteristics on late-life depression of which we are aware examined the effects of income inequality, measured at the county level, on depressive symptoms of adults aged 70 and older. Muramatsu (2003) reports that higher levels of income inequality significantly predicted depressive symptoms with the individual-level predictors of income, demographic characteristics, and physical health statistically controlled. Clearly this topic is ripe for further inquiry.

Social Relationships and Social Support

It is virtually a truism that married individuals enjoy better health and longer lives than the unmarried. As is often the case, however, the "devil is in the details." Although many studies report that married older adults are less depressed, on average, than the unmarried (e.g. Adams et al., 2004), comparisons of specific marital states paint a less simplistic picture. First, the largest differences in depressive symptoms are between the married, on the one hand, and the divorced or separated, on the other hand (Cairney & Krause, 2005). Never-married men also are significantly more depressed than married men, but married and never-married women do not differ in depressive symptoms. Comparisons of married and widowed older men and women are especially interesting (Lee et al., 2001). Married men report significantly fewer depressive symptoms than widowed men, widowed women, and married women. In contrast, married women report no fewer depressive symptoms than widowed women.

Marital status is often confounded with living arrangements. Spouses overwhelmingly live together; older adults in other marital states usually live alone or, less frequently, with other relatives. This raises the question of whether it is living alone or being married that accounts for marital status differences in depression. Few studies address this issue with regard to depression. A study by Brown et al. (2005), however, partially addresses this issue. Brown et al. compared depressive symptoms among married and cohabiting older men and women. Results indicated that married men were significantly less depressed than cohabiting men, married women, and cohabiting women. The latter three groups did not differ in levels of depressive symptoms. These results suggest that for men it is being married rather than living with a romantic partner that protects against depression.

Another dimension of social relationships is the social network. Two aspects of older adults' social networks have been linked to risk of depression. First, very small social networks are associated with increased risk of depression (e.g. Adams et al., 2004). Second, social network composition matters as well. Fiori et al. (2006) created a typology of older adults' social networks. Networks that included multiple family members and friends were labeled "diverse networks." Networks composed of all or almost all family members were labeled "family networks" and those composed of all or almost all friends were labeled "friend networks." Depressive symptoms differed significantly across the three types of networks. Individuals with diverse networks reported the lowest levels of symptoms, those with family networks reported the highest levels of symptoms, and those with friend networks were intermediate.

The aspect of social relationships most frequently studied in relation to depression is social support, especially subjective social support. Subjective social support refers to the extent to which individuals are satisfied with the quality and availability of support available to them from family and friends. In some studies, subjective social support is referred to as anticipated support and is contrasted with received support (i.e. the amount of social support received within a specified time interval). For some research questions, subjective and received support are further disaggregated into emotional support (e.g. sympathizing, confiding) and instrumental support (tangible forms of assistance).

Numerous studies report that high levels of subjective social support protect older adults from depressive symptoms and MDD (e.g. Adams et al., 2004; George, 1992). This is the direct effect of subjective social support. Subjective social support also buffers the effects of stress on depression (e.g. George, 1992; Hashimoto et al., 1999). That is, the protective effects of subjective social support are stronger under conditions of high than low stress.

Although subjective (or anticipated) social support consistently protects older adults from depression, the effects of received support are more ambiguous. In a study of Chinese older adults, Krause et al. (1998) found that anticipated financial support (i.e. support was available if needed) reduced the effect of financial strain on depression. In contrast, receipt of financial assistance from family was associated with higher levels of depressive symptoms. It appears that the belief that assistance is available if needed provides older adults with a sense of security. In contrast, relying on family for assistance threatens independence and autonomy.

The temporal ordering of subjective social support and depression has received considerable attention. Does social support help older adults avoid depression? Or are depressed individuals predisposed to view the support available to them as deficient? Both processes occur, but the dominant influence is from social support to depression (e.g. Cronkite & Moos, 1984).

Health and Disability

Physical health and disability are strongly related to depressive symptoms and MDD (e.g. Turvey et al., 2009; Yang, 2006). As expected, older adults with health problems and especially those who are impaired in ADLs report higher levels of depression than their more robust peers. The major issue of concern is social causation vs social selection. Are physical illness and disability risk factors for depressive symptoms and MDD? Or is depression a risk factor for the onset of physical illnesses and/or disability? With regard to disability, evidence indicates that, although there are clear reciprocal effects, the dominant direction of influence is from disability to depression (e.g. Yang & George, 2005). Whether this is true for physical illness and depression is unknown.

Psychosocial Resources

Several psychosocial resources are robustly related to depression in later life and partially mediate the effects of other risk and protective factors. In general, two types of psychosocial resources have received the most attention: self-worth and self-efficacy. Self-worth is virtually always operationalized as global self-esteem – the extent to which individuals believe that they are basically good and valued. Self-efficacy, sense of control, and mastery are conceptually similar. Their common denominator is the sense that one is competent and able to control important domains of life experience.

Self-esteem and self-efficacy are negatively related to depression both cross-sectionally and longitudinally (e.g. Holahan & Moos, 1991; Orth et al., 2009). They also mediate several other risk and protective factors. Self-esteem and self-efficacy partially mediate the effects of stress on depression (e.g. Holahan & Moos, 1991; Yang, 2006). That is, stress generally erodes feelings of self-worth and competence, although the relationships of self-esteem and self-efficacy with depression remain significant. In contrast, high levels of subjective social support have positive effects on self-esteem and self-efficacy. Thus, one of the mechanisms by which social support protects against depression is enhanced self-attributions. Self-esteem and self-efficacy also partially mediate the effects of gender and SES on depression (e.g. Holahan & Moos, 1991).

Some researchers argue that low self-esteem is a symptom of depression rather than a distinct concept. This concern appears to be unfounded. Using two longitudinal data sets, Orth et al. (2009) demonstrated that self-esteem predicts subsequent depression, but depression does not predict later self-esteem.

SOCIAL FACTORS AND RECOVERY FROM DEPRESSIVE DISORDER

Social factors also play a role in recovery from MDD. Although the research base is small, evidence is consistent for several social factors and inconsistent for others.

Factors Consistently Related to Recovery from MDD

Disability

Disabled adults are less likely to recover from MDD than their non-disabled peers, even when both groups receive psychiatric treatment (e.g. Bosworth et al., 2002; Oxman & Hull, 2001). Explanations for this pattern remain ambiguous. Hypothesized mechanisms include less efficacious treatment response and compromised coping skills among disabled older adults.

Chronic Stressors

Number of chronic stressors also is inversely related to the odds of recovery from MDD in later life (e.g. Dew et al., 1997). In these studies, chronic stressors are measured during the index episode of depression. Consequently, it is unclear whether the stressors predated the onset of MDD.

Religious Involvement

Religious involvement consistently predicts higher odds of recovery and shorter time until recovery among clinically depressed older adults (Bosworth et al., 2002; Koenig et al., 1998). Recall that religious service attendance is the dimension of religious participation most strongly protective against the *onset* of MDD. With regard to *recovery* from MDD, however, religious coping, which is defined as using religious beliefs and practices to cope with stress, has the strongest protective effect.

Subjective Social Support

The social factor most strongly related to recovery from MDD in later life is subjective social support (e.g. Bosworth et al., 2002; George et al., 1989; Harris et al., 2003; Oxman & Hull, 2001). In these studies, baseline social support is measured early in the illness episode. Thus, levels of social support that predate the MDD are not known, and this pattern can best be interpreted as representing perceptions of social support during the depressive episode.

Social Factors for Which Evidence is Uncertain

The roles, if any, of several social factors in recovery from late-life MDD remain unclear. Evidence is mixed for *gender*, with some studies reporting no gender difference (e.g. Dew et al., 1997) and others reporting higher rates of recovery among men (e.g. George et al., 1989). Evidence also is inconsistent for negative *life events*, with about half the studies reporting no relationship between number of life events and odds of recovery (e.g. George et al., 1989) and the other half indicating that recovery is slower or less likely among those who experience stressful life events (e.g. Dew et al., 1997). The relationship between marital status and recovery from MDD in late life is particularly interesting. Several studies report no relationship between marital status and recovery (e.g. Andrew et al., 1993). Others report that the married are *less* likely to recover than the unmarried (e.g. Bosworth et al., 2002). The possibility that being married reduces the odds of recovery, when it is related to many other positive health outcomes, suggests that the marriages of depressed older adults are of poor quality. That is, low-quality marriage is probably a risk factor for both the onset of MDD and a stressor that reduces the odds of recovery.

To date, education and income appear to be unrelated to recovery from MDD in later life (e.g. Andrew et al., 1993; George et al., 1989). Given the importance of SES for recovery from depressive disorder at earlier ages, however, additional research is needed.

LOOKING TO THE FUTURE

The fields of medical sociology and social epidemiology rest on the premise that morbidity and mortality are, to a significant degree, a function of individuals' social structural locations, related social advantage or disadvantage, the stressors that they experience, and the social resources with which they confront disadvantage and stressors. Much of the strongest evidence supporting this premise is based on social factors and mental health, especially MDD and psychological distress. The fact that many of the articles demonstrating the effects of social factors on depression are published in medical rather than social science journals testifies to the acceptance of a biopsychosocial model of mental illness in psychiatry. This accomplishment alone is a victory for social science.

Despite the substantial progress to date, important issues remain for future research. First, social scientists need to focus more of their energies on MDD, where there is the potential to study transitions into and out of illness episodes – and the effects of social factors on those transitions. We know a great deal about how social factors affect depressive symptoms that do not meet diagnostic thresholds. We know much less about how they affect MDD. Expanding research on MDD will make demands beyond the conceptualization and measurement of depression. Because of low incidence and prevalence, community samples are of limited utility for studying MDD. Social scientists need to focus more effort on clinical and high-risk samples to secure the sample sizes needed for meaningful inquiry. They also will need to build treatment variables into their models to estimate the effects of social factors with access to and amount of treatment statistically controlled. Increasing the attention paid to MDD will be required before social scientists will be asked to participate in health and public policy planning for persons suffering from depression and other mental disorders.

Second, although the life course perspective is receiving increasing attention in the study of late-life depression, additional research is needed. We need to better understand the pathways of resilience and vulnerability that affect depression in later life. As important as identifying early life experiences that constitute risk factors for MDD or depressive symptoms are efforts to understand how it is that most individuals who experience substantial social disadvantage and stress, with limited resources to compensate for those risk factors, nonetheless avoid depression. What does it take, in terms of social assets, to "beat the odds" and sustain mental health in the face of adversity? One promising line of inquiry is to search for "critical periods" – i.e. stages of the life course in which events and experiences have unusually strong effects and become persisting risk factors for illness onset. For example, several studies suggest that childhood traumas not only have direct effects on mental health decades later but also interact with later stressors, increasing vulnerability to MDD (e.g. Landerman et al., 1991).

Latent growth curve analysis and latent class analysis (also called mixture models) have great potential to model trajectories of depression and risk/protective factors across the life course. Admittedly, few data sets allow the study of such long-term dynamics. Nonetheless, these are important avenues for future research. At this point, we lack even rudimentary information about life course patterns of depression and the ways in which those trajectories are shaped by social adversity and advantage. Of special importance are studies that examine the role of social factors in single-episode vs recurrent or chronic trajectories of MDD.

Blazer (2005) describes this as "the age of melancholy," citing the rapid increase in depressive symptoms and disorder in the US and throughout the world. Similarly, according to the WHO (2008), "Unipolar depression makes a large contribution to the burden of disease, being at third place worldwide and eighth place in low-income countries, but at first place in middle- and high income countries" (p. 43). There is much to learn if social scientists are willing to study depressive disorder as well as depressive symptoms and the long-term pathways of vulnerability and resilience that characterize them. These are tasks worthy of our efforts.

REFERENCES

Adams, K. B., Sanders, S., & Auth, E. A. (2004). Loneliness and depression in independent living retirement communities: Risk and resilience factors. *Aging & Mental Health, 8*, 475–485.

American Psychiatric Association (1980). *Diagnostic and statistical manual of mental disorders* (3rd Ed.). Washington, DC: American Psychiatric Association.

American Psychiatric Association (2000). *Diagnostic and statistical manual of mental disorders* (4th Ed, text revision.). Washington, DC: American Psychiatric Association.

Andrew, B., Hawton, K., Fagg, J., & Westbrook, D. (1993). Do psychological factors influence outcome in severely depressed female psychiatric inpatients? *British Journal of Psychiatry, 163*, 747–754.

Aneshensel, C. S., Botticello, A. L., & Yamamoto-Mitani, N. (2004). When caregiving ends: The course of depressive symptoms after bereavement. *Journal of Health and Social Behavior, 45*, 422–440.

Avis, N. E., Crawford, S., Stellato, R., & Longcope, C. (2001). Longitudinal study of hormone levels and depression among women transitioning through menopause. *Climacteric, 4*, 243–249.

Blazer, D. G. (2002). *Depression in late life.* New York: Springer.

Blazer, D. G. (2005). *The age of melancholy: Major depression and its social origins.* New York: Routledge.

Blazer, D. G., Hughes, D. C., & George, L. K. (1987). The epidemiology of depression in an elderly community population. *The Gerontologist, 27*, 281–287.

Bosworth, H. B., McQuoid, D. R., George, L. K., & Steffens, D. C. (2002). Time-to-remission from geriatric depression. *American Journal of Geriatric Psychiatry, 10*, 551–559.

Braam, A. W., Hein, E., Deeg, D. J. H., Twisk, J. W. R., Beekman, A. T. F., & Van Tilburg, W. (2004). Religious involvement and 6-year course of depressive symptoms in older Dutch citizens. *Journal of Aging and Health, 16*, 467–489.

Brown, S. L., Bulanda, J. R., & Lee, G. R. (2005). The significance of nonmarital cohabitation: Marital status and mental health benefits among middle-aged and older adults. *Journal of Gerontology: Social Sciences, 60*, S21–S29.

Cairney, J., & Krause, N. (2005). The social distribution of psychological distress and depression in older adults. *Journal of Aging and Health, 17,* 807–835.

Chatters, L. M., Bullard, K. M., Taylor, R. J., Woodward, A. T., Neighbors, H. W., & Jackson, J. S. (2008). Religious participation and DSM-IV disorders among older African Americans. *American Journal of Geriatric Psychiatry, 16,* 957–965.

Chen, R., Wei, L., Hu, X., Qin, X., Copeland, J. R. M., & Hemingway, H. (2005). Depression in older people in rural China. *Archives of Internal Medicine, 165,* 2019–2025.

Chiriboga, D. A., Black, S. A., Aranda, M., & Markides, K. (2002). Stress and depressive symptoms among Mexican American elders. *Journal of Gerontology: Psychological Sciences, 57,* P559–P568.

Cronkite, R. C., & Moos, R. H. (1984). The role of predisposing and moderating factors in the stress-illness relationship. *Journal of Health and Social Behavior, 25,* 372–393.

Cuijpers, P. (2005). Depressive disorders in caregivers of dementia patients: A systematic review. *Aging & Mental Health, 9,* 325–330.

Derogatis, L. R., Lipman, R. S., Rickels, K., Uhlenhuth, E. H., & Covi, L. (1974). The Hopkins Symptom Checklist: A self-report symptom inventory. *Behavioral Science, 19,* 1–15.

Dew, M. A., Reynolds, C. F., III, Houck, P. R., Hall, M., Buysse, D. J., Frank, E., et al. (1997). Temporal profiles of the course of depression during treatment – Predictors of pathways toward recovery in the elderly. *Archives of General Psychiatry, 54,* 1016–1024.

Elder, G. H., Jr. (1974). *Children of the great depression.* Chicago: University of Chicago Press.

Elder, G. H., Jr., Shanahan, M. J., & Clipp, E. C. (1994). When war comes to men's lives: Life-course patterns in family, work, and health. *Psychology and Aging, 9,* 5–16.

Fiori, K. L., Antonucci, T. C., & Cortina, K. S. (2006). Social network typologies and mental health among older adults. *Journal of Gerontology: Psychological Sciences, 61,* P25–P32.

Fiske, A., Gatz, M., & Pederson, N. L. (2003). Depressive symptoms and aging: The effects of illness and non-health-related events. *Journal of Gerontology: Psychological Sciences, 58,* P320–P328.

Folkman, S. (Ed.), (2010). *The Oxford handbook of stress, health, and coping.* New York: Oxford University Press.

Forsell, Y., Jorm, A. F., Von Strauss, E., & Winblad, B. (1995). Prevalence and correlates of depression in a population of nonagenarians. *British Journal of Psychiatry, 167,* 61–64.

George, L. K. (1992). Social factors and the onset and outcome of depression. In K. W. Schaie, J. S. House & D. G. Blazer (Eds.), *Aging, health behaviors and health outcomes* (pp. 137–159). Hillsdale, NJ: Lawrence Erlbaum.

George, L. K. (2007). Life course perspectives on social factors and mental illness. In W. R. Avison, J. D. McLeod & B. A. Pescosolido (Eds.), *Mental health, social mirror* (pp. 191–218). New York: Springer Publishing Company.

George, L. K., Blazer, D. G., Hughes, D. C., & Fowler, N. (1989). Social support and the outcome of major depression. *British Journal of Psychiatry, 154,* 478–485.

Gum, A. M., King-Kallimanis, B., & Kohn, R. (2009). Prevalence of mood, anxiety, and substance-abuse disorders for older Americans in the national comorbidity survey – Replication. *American Journal of Geriatric Psychiatry, 17,* 769–781.

Hao, Y. (2008). Productive activities and psychological well-being among older adults. *Journal of Gerontology: Social Sciences, 63,* S64–S72.

Harris, T., Cook, D. G., Victor, C., Rink, E., Mann, A. H., Shah, S., et al. (2003). Predictors of depressive symptoms in older people. *Age and Ageing, 32,* 510–518.

Hashimoto, K., Kurita, H., Haratani, T., Fujii, K., & Ishibashi, T. (1999). Direct and buffering effects of social support on depressive symptoms of the elderly with home help. *Psychiatry and Clinical Neuroscience, 53,* 95–100.

Holahan, C. J., & Moos, R. H. (1991). Life stressors, personal and social resources, and depression: A 4-year structural model. *Journal of Abnormal Psychology, 100,* 31–38.

Hughes, D. C., George, L. K., & Blazer, D. G. (1988). Age differences in life events qualities: Multivariate controlled analyses. *Journal of Community Psychology, 16,* 161–174.

Idler, E. L., & Kasl, S. V. (1997). Religion among disabled and nondisabled persons, II: Attendance at religious services as a predictor of the course of disability. *Journal of Gerontology: Social Sciences, 52,* S306–S315.

Jorm, A. F. (1987). Sex and age differences in depression. *Australian and New Zealand Journal of Psychiatry, 21,* 46–53.

Kessler, R. C., & Magee, W. J. (1994). Childhood family violence and adult recurrent depression. *Journal of Health and Social Behavior, 35,* 13–27.

Kessler, R. C., Wittchen, H. U., Abelson, J. M., McGonagle, K. A., Schwartz, N., Kendler, K. S., et al. (1998). Methodological studies of the Composite International Diagnostic Interview (CIDI) in the U.S. National Comorbidity Study. *International Journal of Methods in Psychiatric Research, 7,* 171–185.

Kessler, R. C., Chiu, W. T., Demler, O., & Walters, E. E. (2005). Prevalence, severity, and comorbidity of twelve-month DSM-IV disorders in the National Comorbidity Survey Replication. *Archives of General Psychiatry, 62,* 617–627.

Kim, D. (2008). Blues from the neighborhood? Neighborhood characteristics and depression. *Epidemiologic Reviews, 30,* 101–117.

Koenig, H. G., George, L. K., & Peterson, B. L. (1998). Religiosity and remission of depression in medically ill older patients. *American Journal of Psychiatry, 155,* 536–542.

Kraaij, V., Arensman, E., & Spinhoven, P. (2002). Negative life events and depression in elderly persons: A meta-analysis. *Journal of Gerontology: Psychological Sciences, 57,* P87–P94.

Krause, N., Herzog, A. R., & Baker, E. (1992). Providing support to others and well-being in later life. *Journal of Gerontology: Psychological Sciences, 47,* P300–P311.

Krause, N., Liang, J., & Gu, S. (1998). Financial strain, received support, anticipated support, and depressive symptoms in the People's Republic of China. *Psychology and Aging, 13,* 58–68.

Kubzansky, L. D., Berkman, L. F., & Seeman, T. E. (2000). Social conditions and distress in elderly persons. *Journal of Gerontology: Social Sciences, 55,* S238–S246.

Landerman, R., George, L. K., & Blazer, D. G. (1991). Adult vulnerability for psychiatric disorders: Interactive effects of negative childhood experiences and recent stress. *Journal of Nervous and Mental Disease, 179,* 656–663.

Lee, G. R., DeMaris, A., Bavin, S., & Sullivan, R. (2001). Gender differences in the depressive effect of widowhood in later life. *Journal of Gerontology: Social Sciences, 56,* S56–S61.

Li, L. W. (2005). From caregiving to bereavement: Trajectories of depressive symptoms among wife and daughter caregivers. *Journal of Gerontology: Psychological Sciences, 60,* P190–P198.

Li, Y. (2007). Recovering from spousal bereavement in late life: Does volunteer participation play a role? *Journal of Gerontology: Social Sciences, 62,* S257–S266.

Link, B. G., & Phelan, J. C. (1995). Social conditions as fundamental causes of distress. *Journal of Health and Social Behavior, extra issue,* 80–94.

Link, B. G., Phelan, J. C., Bresnahan, M., Stueve, A., & Pescosolido, B. (1999). Public conceptions of mental illness: Labels, causes, dangerousness, and social distance. *American Journal of Public Health, 89,* 1328–1333.

Lorant, V., Deliege, D., Eaton, W., Robert, A., Philippot, P., & Ansseau, M. (2003). Socioeconomic inequalities in depression: A meta-analysis. *American Journal of Epidemiology, 157,* 98–112.

Lorenz, F. O., Wickrama, K. A. S., Conger, R. D., & Elder, G. H., Jr. (2006). The short-term and decade-long effects of divorce of women's midlife health. *Journal of Health and Social Behavior, 47,* 111–125.

Lynch, S. M., & George, L. K. (2002). Interlocking trajectories of loss-related events and depressive symptoms among elders. *Journal of Gerontology: Social Sciences, 57,* S117–S123.

Miech, R. A., Eaton, W. W., & Brennan, K. (2005). Mental health disparities across education and sex. *Journal of Gerontology: Social Sciences, 60,* S93–S98.

Mirowsky, J., & Ross, C. E. (1992). Age and depression. *Journal of Health and Social Behavior, 33,* 187–205.

Mirowsky, J., & Ross, C. E. (2002). Measurement for a human science. *Journal of Health and Social Behavior, 43,* 152–170.

Moos, R. H., Schutte, K. K., Brenan, P. L., & Moos, B. S. (2005). The interplay between life stressors and depressive symptoms among older adults. *Journal of Gerontology: Psychological Sciences, 60,* P199–P206.

Morrow-Howell, N., Hinterlong, J., Rozario, P. A., & Tang, F. (2003). Effects of volunteering on the well-being of older adults. *Journal of Gerontology: Social Sciences, 58,* S137–S145.

Muramatsu, N. (2003). County-level income inequality and depression among older Americans. *Health Services Research, 38,* 1863–1883.

Norton, M. C., Singh, A., Skoog, I., Corcoran, C., Tschanze, J. T., Zandi, P. P., et al. (2008). Church attendance and new episodes of major depression in a community study of older adults: The Cache County study. *Journal of Gerontology: Psychological Sciences, 63,* P129–P137.

Orth, U., Robins, R. W., Trzesniewski, K. H., Maes, J., & Schmitt, M. (2009). Low self-esteem is a risk factor for depression from young adulthood to old age. *Journal of Abnormal Psychology, 118,* 472–478.

Oxman, T. E., & Hull, J. G. (2001). Social support and treatment response in older depressed primary care patients. *Journal of Gerontology: Psychological Sciences, 56B,* P35–P45.

Pearlin, L. I. (2010). The life course and the stress process: Some conceptual comparisons. *Journal of Gerontology: Social Sciences, 65,* 207–215.

Pearlin, L. I., Menaghan, E. G., Lieberman, M. A., & Mullan, J. T. (1981). The stress process. *Journal of Health and Social Behavior, 22,* 337–356.

Pinquart, M., & Sorensen, S. (2006). Gender differences in caregiver stressors, social resources, and health: An updated meta-analysis. *Journal of Gerontology: Psychological Sciences, 61,* P33–P44.

Radloff, L. S. (1977). The CES-D Scale: A self-report depression scale for research in the general population. *Applied Psychological Measurement, 1,* 385–401.

Robins, L. N., & Regier, R. A. (1991). *Psychiatric disorders in America: The epidemiologic catchment area study.* New York: The Free Press.

Robins, L. N., Helzer, J. E., Croughan, J., & Ratcliff, K. S. (1981). The National Institute of Mental Health Diagnostic Interview Schedule: Its history, characteristics, and validity. *Archives of General Psychiatry, 38,* 381–389.

Schieman, S., Van Gundy, K., & Taylor, J. (2002). The relationship between age and depressive symptoms: A test of competing explanatory and suppression influences. *Journal of Aging and Health, 14,* 260–285.

Schulz, R., Drayer, R., & Rothman, B. (2002). Depression as a risk factor for non-suicide mortality in the elderly. *Biological Psychology, 52,* 205–225.

Shaw, B. A., & Krause, N. (2002). Exposure to physical violence during childhood, aging, and health. *Journal of Aging and Health, 14,* 467–494.

Simon, R. W., & Marcussen, K. (1999). Marital transitions, marital beliefs, and mental health. *Journal of Health and Social Behavior, 40,* 111–125.

Skarupski, K. A., Mendes de Leon, C. F., Bienias, J. L., Barnes, L. L., Everson-Rose, S. A., Wilson, R. S., et al. (2005). Black-white differences in depressive symptoms among older adults over time. *Journal of Gerontology:*

Psychological Sciences, 60, P136–P142.

Smith, T. B., McCullough, M. E., & Poll, J. (2003). Religiousness and depression: Evidence for a main effect and the moderating influence of stressful life events. *Psychological Bulletin, 129,* 614–636.

Turner, R. J., & Avison, W. R. (2003). Status variations in stress exposure: Implications for the interpretation of research on race, socioeconomic status, and gender. *Journal of Health and Social Behavior, 44,* 488–505.

Turvey, C. L., Schultz, S. K., Beglinger, L., & Klein, D. M. (2009). A longitudinal community-based study of chronic illness, cognitive and physical function, and depression. *American Journal of Geriatric Psychiatry, 17,* 632–641.

Walsemann, K. M., Gee, G. G., & Geronimus, A. T. (2009). Ethnic differences in trajectories of depressive symptoms: Disadvantage in family background, high school experiences, and adult characteristics. *Journal of Health and Social Behavior, 50,* 82–98.

Williams, D. R., Yu, Y., Jackson, J. S., & Anderson, N. B. (1997). Racial differences in physical and mental health. *Journal of Health Psychology, 2,* 335–351.

Wilmoth, J. M., & Chen, P. (2003). Immigrant status, living arrangements, and depressive symptoms among middle-aged and older adults. *Journal of Gerontology: Social Sciences, 58,* S305–S313.

World Health Organization. (2004). The World Mental Health Composite International Diagnostic Interview available at www.hcp.med.harvard.edu/wmhcidi/resources.php. Accessed April 10, 2009.

World Health Organization. (2008). *The global burden of disease – 2004 update.* Geneva: WHO Press.

Yang, Y. (2006). How does functional disability affect depressive symptoms in late life? The role of perceived social support and psychological resources. *Journal of Health and Social Behavior, 47,* 355–372.

Yang, Y., & George, L. K. (2005). Functional disability, disability transitions, and depressive symptoms in late life. *Journal of Aging and Health, 17,* 263–292.

Yang, Y., & Lee, L. C. (2009). Sex and race disparities in health: Cohort variations in life course patterns. *Social Forces, 87,* 2093–2124.

Chapter | 12 |

Aging, Inheritance, and Gift-Giving

Jacqueline L. Angel[1], Stipica Mudrazija[2]

[1]Department of Sociology, Lyndon B. Johnson School of Public Affairs, Population Research Center, University of Texas, Austin, Texas, [2]Lyndon B. Johnson School of Public Affairs, Population Research Center, University of Texas, Austin, Texas

CHAPTER CONTENTS

INTRODUCTION

The transfer of material wealth through inheritance is a practice with deep cultural roots. In early agrarian societies, the rules surrounding gifts, inheritance, and bequests defined kinship and status and in large part determined the boundaries of family and community (Laslett, 1991). Over time, such intergenerational wealth transfers have remained important for many reasons. It has long been recognized that inter-vivos transfers (transfers of assets, usually to a child or a spouse, while one is living) and bequests (gifts made through a person's will or living trust and distributed after one's death) play a highly significant role in sustaining the social system. The parent–child bond is a primordial one, and the giving and receiving of material gifts between these two generations is a fundamental characteristic of the relationship.

In recent years the topic of inheritance has taken on new meaning in social discourses on aging within numerous disciplines in the social and behavioral sciences (Munnell, 2003). Gerontologists, taking cues from anthropologists, are giving the issue particular attention because a confluence of social, psychological, economic, and health care factors related to inheritance has serious consequences for the aging population (Hashimoto, 1996). Inheritance and inter-vivo giving influence what the younger generation expects to receive from the older generation in building their own future. The older generation has traditionally shared this expectation, but new economic realities have introduced uncertainty. Understanding the social dimensions of giving across generations is key to understanding how changes in traditional expectations and practices will affect family life in general, and how adult children and their elderly parents will receive support as they grow older (Angel, 2008).

From a policy perspective, family inheritance determines aspects of our social welfare and those institutions linked to the means of transmission of property and other rights in late life (Lee & Mason, 2007). The level of intergenerational transfers affects the distribution of financial assets in a society and can perpetuate wealth inequality across generations (Hurd et al., 2007). Inheritance and bequests can have a significant impact on retirement security and quality of life as people grow older (Hogan et al., 1993). This situation is not limited to the US. A recent UK study shows that a large inheritance plays an important role in the timing of retirement. Approximately one in three British adults is planning to substantially support their retirement years with a family inheritance (Friends Provident, 2009).

On a societal level, this impact is potentially huge (Kotlikoff & Burns, 2005). The largest transfer of wealth in history is expected to occur over the next several decades, and is very likely to change the social fabric of the US. Various sources have predicted that between $10 trillion and $40 trillion will be bequeathed, with up to $25 trillion going to heirs

DOI: 10.1016/B978-0-12-380880-6.00012-5

and the rest to charitable organizations (see Havens & Schervish, 2009).

The last few decades of the lifespan bring an entirely new set of issues for the elderly person to confront. The long, protracted period of aging combined with the increased percentage of adult children in the baby boomer generation with a living parent will no doubt alter the meaning of gifts passed on to grown children, many of whom themselves are on the cusp of deep old age (Dannefer & Shura, 2009; Hurd & Smith, 2002). The ability to give to a child is a reflection of an elderly parent's own success (Cox, 2003). Gifts of equity (either housing or money) from parents can significantly improve their children's lives and provide opportunities for generations into the future (Shapiro, 2003).

On the other side of the coin, the cost of providing financial support for grown children may be high, threatening the standard of living of an elderly parent after retirement from active work (Putnam Investments, 2006). The onset of cognitive and physical frailty and disabilities give rise to higher medical and long-term care costs (Altman et al., 1998), and a steady flow of money is needed to cover these services, constraining the preference to give (Stone, 2000). Further, it is not uncommon for a major catastrophic life event such as a disabling medical illness to undermine one's inheritance intentions (Mitchell & Moore, 1998; Munnell et al., 2003). The financial consequences of such events may be substantial, especially when the assets are spent on long-term care (French et al., 2006). One of the major conundrums of the new era, then, is balancing older persons' desire to pass on as much wealth as possible to their grown children against the need to ensure their personal retirement security (Fetterman, 2007).

For the past 60 years or so, most people could depend on augmenting their personal retirement income with government benefits. Today, however, social security systems in developed countries are facing mounting challenges to their sustainability as a consequence of profound demographic, socioeconomic, and political changes (see Chapters 3 and 18). Coupled with the rising trend in divorce since the 1970s, evaporating private retirement accounts have unexpectedly influenced the retirement plans of many adult children, especially for women and minorities (Angel & Angel, 2009; Angel et al., 2007). More than half of the American population once thought they could rely mostly on their private pensions to supplement their Social Security benefits during retirement. For those lucky enough to have good private pensions, there is now the very real prospect that adequate funds might not be there when they reach retirement age and other sources of money must be found to fill this gap. As noted earlier, even the traditional safety net promised by the Social Security system is being threatened by demographic trends, so planning for the future is difficult. In addition to pressures on Social Security, another issue complicating the ability to pass on wealth is the 2008 global economic recession.

Population aging, then, will have a serious impact on gift-giving practices between parents and their children, and between adult children. This demographic phenomenon will transform the character of American social policies, including pension reform and the future of intergenerational transfer programs such as Social Security (Binstock, 2005). In this chapter, we expand upon these themes, summarizing what is known about the role of gifts and bequests in an aging society. We begin with a brief overview of theoretical explanations of how societies pass on wealth in the US and with some international comparisons, and then move to a discussion of intergenerational financial exchanges in the context of sources of retirement security. To do this, we look at aspects of inheritance as well as inter-vivos gift-giving, This latter type of wealth transfer consists of taking one's property and gifting it away; for example, to pay for a child's or grandchild's college.

We then focus on aspects of private wealth transfers and the changing nature of family gift-giving measured in terms of inter-vivos transfers and bequests in the US, and identify why inheritance will be an even more important part of family life in years to come. Toward that end, we look at the changing nature of property and moral ties between the generations and how the links between them are defined by material exchanges. The chapter concludes with a discussion of the implications for aging policy and identifies some future research priorities.

COMPETING EXPLANATIONS OF INTERGENERATIONAL WEALTH TRANSFERS

Before discussing various hypotheses regarding motivations for intergenerational transfers, it is important to understand the difference in character between inter-vivos transfers and bequests, with particular emphasis on the latter. Inter-vivos transfers happen earlier in the lives of recipients, are often part of a continuing relationship between generations, and are positively related to recipients' needs (Kohli, 2003). Bequests are more significant in size, representing about three quarters of all transfers, are unidirectional, usually happen later in recipients' lives, and are usually divided equally among all children (if they are bequest recipients) regardless of possible differences in needs (Kohli, 2003), although about a fifth of parents treat their children unequally even when making bequests (Light & McGarry, 2004).

Another key difference between inter-vivos transfers and bequests is that the former are intended, while the latter might be intended or accidental. Accidental bequests are very different in character. They are part of the life-cycle model of consumption, in which people save during their working lives and spend their savings during retirement, but, due to uncertainties associated with the length of life, they tend to "over-save" and therefore "accidentally" leave bequests. The following overview of motives for intergenerational transfers broadly applies only to inter-vivos and intended bequests.

Historically, the most commonly held view of the character of private intergenerational wealth transfers in a world with either no, or at most only rudimentary, retirement programs was that parents invest in children so that they can provide them with some sort of old-age security. Although developed countries have since introduced various comprehensive retirement schemes, for a number of developing countries these conditions have not substantially altered. However, the "old-age security" hypothesis has received fairly little scholarly attention. The basic argument that increased fertility is an effective strategy for securing the livelihood of the elderly is straightforward. If wealth is (predominantly) transferred from children to parents, having multiple offspring is a rational strategy to pursue, as hypothesized by Caldwell (1976), although a similar line of reasoning can be found even earlier in the work of Leibenstein (1957). From this basic insight Nugent (1985) developed a list of conditions under which the old-age security hypothesis is considered to be valid. They include either no or insufficient government-provided social security schemes, rudimentary or nonexistent financial institutions and capital markets, and a number of factors related to culture and (family) tradition characterizing different societies.

Closely related to the old-age security hypothesis is the "parental repayment hypothesis," where parents finance human capital investment in their children, who implicitly repay their parents by providing old-age support (Becker & Tomes, 1976). Under this hypothesis, parents would invest more in the human capital of better-endowed children, as this would maximize their future earnings and consequently their family's earnings and consumption. Simultaneously, parents compensate less-endowed children by providing more non-human capital investments.

Perhaps most important for our discussion is the seminal work by Becker (1974) and Barro (1974), who introduced the theory of altruism as the dominant explanation of motivation for intergenerational transfers. The "altruism" hypothesis posits that family is a highly interrelated institution where consumption is equalized among its members regardless of their individual income. Therefore, whoever in the family is in a better financial position will compensate those who have less. While altruism is the dominant and most widely discussed hypothesis on the motives for intergenerational wealth transfers, there is ample evidence that altruism alone may be a necessary but not sufficient condition to explain such a complex process. Low-income households tend to exhibit a behavior consistent with the altruism hypothesis, but this pattern has the tendency to be limited at higher levels of income (Cox et al., 2004).

A major competing hypothesis to altruism emphasizes the "exchange motive" for giving, originally advanced by Bernheim et al. (1985) and Cox (1987). In this model, transfers between parents and children are a form of exchange and represent payments to the recipient for the provision of services or some other form of help. An example is that the likelihood that children will provide financial assistance to their parents rises with the expectation of receiving an inheritance in return (Caputo, 2002). A detailed discussion of altruism and exchange motives can be found in Silverstein (2006).

Among other motives for intergenerational transfers is insurance against (potential) financial adversities. The most important distinction between family and public systems as insurance mechanisms is that the latter are designed to spread the risk across all taxpayers. Among different types of transfers, financial transfers seem to correspond better to the insurance motivation than do non-financial transfers (Silverstein et al., 2002). Another motive for intergenerational transfers is family tradition, which refers to intrafamilial giving, guided by an implicit social contract ensuring long-term reciprocity between family generations (Hashimoto, 1996; Silverstein et al., 2002). In practice this could mean that, all else being equal, the larger an inheritance that a family member receives, the larger inheritance that he or she will pass down to the next generation. However, for inter-vivos transfers it seems that intergenerational reciprocity is not as clearly exhibited as for bequests. In this context, needs (Ikkink et al., 1999) and social norms (Caputo, 2002) are at least as important, if not more important, than straightforward intergenerational reciprocity. Actually, the provision of help according to needs can be viewed as being part of the implicit social contract in the sense that reciprocation might be provided from one generation to the next, not in the form of equal giving but rather in the form of assurance that help would be available when and if it is needed.

One interesting explanation of how the implicit social contract might be upheld and traditional values perpetuated across generations is the so-called demonstration effect (Cox & Stark, 2005). The concept originally referred to parents providing their adult children with the financial help (down payment) to buy a house or an apartment, a so-called "tied transfer" because this provides a model of behavior and encourages the adult children to transition into young adulthood. In turn, grown children would have an incentive to help their parents and to show their young children the desired way to care for elderly parents. The "demonstration effect" can be expanded to include bequest motives. The exchange of care and money between adult children and elderly parents at the end of life in later years is not only motivated by altruism or exchange motives for gift-giving, but because it demonstrates to future generations filial expectations and obligations regarding long-term care.

PUBLIC–PRIVATE NEXUS OF WEALTH TRANSFERS

The two dominant explanations of motivations for intergenerational transfers (altruism and exchange) have interesting implications for the expected relationship between public and private transfers before and after death. If altruism was the only, or at least the main, explanation of intergenerational transfers, the implication for public transfers would be that they ineffectively target particular individuals. Regardless of how much family members earn, personal consumption could be evenly spread across family members and, as a result, public transfers completely substitute or "crowd-out" private transfers. Of course, due to the multifaceted character of intrafamilial relationships and transfers as an integral part of them, it would be hard to expect a full displacement. Therefore, the validity of the altruism hypothesis and its relative importance vis-à-vis other related hypotheses effectively depends on the magnitude of the crowding-out effect. For example, in the "warm-glow" hypothesis, both donors and recipients derive personal benefits from the act of giving, resulting in a partial crowding-out effect (Andreoni, 1990; Chan et al., 2002).

Researchers estimate the magnitude of the crowding out of private by public transfers ranges from 8% to 40% depending on the type of public transfer and the country of interest (Jensen, 2003; Schoeni, 2002; Villanueva, 2005). Overall, however, it is apparent that the complete offset of public transfers by private intrafamilial flows can happen only under very specific circumstances (Kotlikoff et al., 1990), and therefore government programs can be an effective redistribution tool.

On the other hand, the major implication of the exchange hypothesis is a lack of consumption smoothing (i.e. balancing of spending and saving) across family members and consequently no crowding out of private transfers by public ones. This factor has been used by researchers to test the validity of the exchange hypothesis. Studies such as that of Künemund & Rein (1999) fail to find any evidence of crowding out of private transfers, and in fact find some evidence of crowding in, where public transfers might actually increase intrafamilial intergenerational solidarity, an

implication in accordance with the exchange hypothesis. Overall, familial help (formal and informal) is substantially higher in countries with strong welfare regimes, which implicitly supports the crowding in hypothesis.

Another important aspect of the public–private nexus of wealth transfers is the role of transfer taxes, as illustrated by the situation in the US. Transfer taxes are highly progressive, affecting only the richest individuals because sizeable portions of estates are worth substantially below the 2009 exemption level of $3.5 million established by the Economic Growth and Tax Relief Reconciliation Act of 2001 (EGTRRA). Even the much lower pre-EGTRRA level of $675 000 (to which the personal exemption will return in 2011 unless Congress extends EGTRRA) was rather high. According to Gale and Slemrod (2001), only 2% of decedents in 1998 had taxable estates and, even among them, only 6% of the richest (or 0.012% of the total) decedents accounted for 53% of all transfer taxes paid. Therefore, transfer taxes seem to satisfy the vertical equity principle of taxation that those who are better off should pay more in taxes. The horizontal equity principle – that people of similar ability to pay should pay similar taxes – is not that clearly satisfied due to the fact that the current consumption, charitable giving, inter-vivos transfers, and other alternatives to leaving bequests enjoy favorable tax treatment relative to bequests. Also, the estate tax provides a "marriage bonus" due to unlimited deductions for transfers to the surviving spouse, therefore treating them more favorably than single individuals with the same ability to pay the tax.

The main distinction with respect to the response of individuals on the imposition of a transfer tax is between unintended and intended bequests. If individuals tend to "over-save" during their lifetime due to uncertainties associated with the timing of death, possible high out-of-pocket health-related expenditures, and other considerations, there is no reason to expect that establishing a tax on transfers of wealth after they die would in any way change their behavior with respect to accumulation and wealth transfers.

If, however, individuals amass wealth over the life course with the intention of passing it on to their heirs, then the imposition of transfer taxes can alter their behavior in different ways, depending on the prevailing motive for making such transfers. Generally, in the case of both the altruism and the warm-glow giving hypotheses there would be less than socially optimal provision of transfers. On the other hand, if the exchange hypothesis is true and transfers between generations are just a payment parents make for provision of different services by children, then the critical consideration becomes whether parents care more about the price of services they need or about the person providing help, regardless of the price. This consideration ultimately determines what the socially most desirable level of taxation would be (Gale & Slemrod, 2001). For example, if parents do not care whether they get help with different chores from their children or someone else, then the desirable transfer tax level is likely to be relatively low. If, however, parents particularly value the fact that the help and attention is provided by their children, then the demand for children's services will be fairly strong and consequently socially desirable tax level will be relatively high.

McGarry (2001) and Poterba (2001) estimated the extent to which parents respond to preferential tax treatment of inter-vivos gifts compared to bequests, as well as the fact that unequal transfers to children might be preferred to equal giving in terms of minimizing the loss of utility due to the payment of taxes. Although parents somewhat alter their behavior due to estate taxes, they largely continue with the practice of equal giving and do not use to a large extent the tax advantages of inter-vivos transfers, as a substitute for bequests. Poterba (2001) estimated that almost two thirds of households that would increase the net amount passed to their heirs by making inter-vivos transfers chose not to do so. Together, these findings suggest either that bequests have a very substantial unintended component or that the norm of equal giving, and arguably the stronger influence parents have over children if they keep the possession of their wealth until they die, are considered by parents more valuable than the loss their heirs incur due to unfavorable tax treatment of bequests. On the other hand, Bernheim et al. (2004) find substantial decrease in inter-vivos transfers associated with the policy changes that decreased the tax disadvantage of bequests relative to inter-vivos transfers. Other research shows that in the absence of estate taxes around two-thirds of inter-vivos gifts would not take place (Joulfaian, 2005).

DEMOGRAPHY OF FAMILY GIFTING AND WILLS

In the US, only a minority of adult children actually receive bequests. For example, fewer than one-fifth of American baby boomers have ever inherited money and only 15% of others still expect to receive any (Hurd & Smith, 2002). Most of the wealth transfers go to the wealthiest people. Estimates vary, but data from the Survey of Consumer Finances (SCF) indicate that, for most baby boomers who receive an inheritance, the median value is about $47 000 in 2002 dollars (Ng-Baumhackl et al., 2003).

We now examine in great detail the extent and amount of gift-giving, measured in terms of bequests and estate distribution. Data from the University of Michigan Health and Retirement Study (HRS) provide a unique opportunity to examine demographic characteristics with regard to bequest intentions of older adults who plan to transfer wealth (McGarry & Schoeni, 1997). Launched in 1992, the HRS surveyed Americans who were aged 51 to 61 along with their spouses (University of Michigan, 2009). Respondents were interviewed with regard to their physical and mental health, insurance coverage, financial situations, family support systems, work status, and retirement situations. The study selected 7939 respondents in the 2006 HRS who were AHEAD-eligible (individuals aged 70 years or older) during that year and harmonized these data with calculations of annual income and household assets (RAND Center for the Study of Aging, 2007).

Table 12.1 provides a detailed portrait of the sample's demographic characteristics. What the data reveal is that older-household respondents were more likely to have a will than younger-household respondents. Predictably, those with greater annual income and greater amounts of household assets were also more likely to have a will. The gap between men and women with wills was not large, with 73.9% of men and 68.7% of women holding a will. Racial gaps were larger, with 79% of non-Hispanic whites holding a will, but only 29.5% of non-Hispanic blacks and 46.1% of Hispanics holding a will. Having a will was most likely among those who were married or widowed (77.1% and 71.1%, respectively), compared to those who were separated or divorced (53%) or who had never been married (51.1%). Similar findings have emerged in previous HRS/AHEAD cohort studies (e.g. O'Connor, 1996).

Numerous studies over the years have shown that the most common beneficiaries of wills are children and spouses. For example, Rossi and Rossi (1990) found that men and women respondents both named children and spouses as their primary beneficiaries, but that women were more likely to provide for non-family members. Contemporary data in Table 12.2 show that most fathers (97.6%) and most mothers (97.5%) who had a will reported providing for a child or stepchild in 2006. Most men with wills (86.3%) and most women with wills (87.6%) reported providing for all of their children equally. Fewer men and women with wills (14.1% and 15.8%, respectively) reported providing for a grandchild, and only about 1% of men and 4.1% of women reported providing for all grandchildren.

Several studies have reached similar conclusions (e.g. Hurd & Smith, 2002; Simon et al., 1982). What they show is that most respondents would provide for spouses and children regardless of survivorship scenario. Most respondents report they would provide for all children equally, regardless of whether the child was from a former marriage or a non-marital relationship. Hurd and Smith (2002) found that 80% of parents with more than one family expect to leave the same amount of inheritance to each of their children.

Table 12.1 Characteristics of US household respondents over age 70 with wills.

DEMOGRAPHIC CHARACTERISTIC	PERCENT WITH A WILL
Age	
70 to 75	65.5
76 to 80	70.1
81 to 85	74.8
Over 86	78.7
Household Annual Income	
Less than 11 521	44.9
11 521 to 18 420	64.2
18 421 to 29 012	74.9
29 013 to 48 300	81.9
48 301 to 5 039 892	85.0
Household Assets*	
Less than 10 001	34.8
10 001 to 98 850	62.3
98 851 to 253 200	76.1
253 201 to 563 500	83.4
563 501 to 81 847 260	90.6
Gender	
Male	73.9
Female	68.7
Race	
Non-Hispanic white	78.5
Non-Hispanic black	29.5
Hispanic	46.1
Other races	26.7
Marital/Family Status	
Married	77.1
Separated or divorced	53.0
Widowed	71.1
Never married	51.1
Living together, not married	81.2

Source: University of Michigan, 2006.
Note. Based on 7939 respondents and 5977 households. One age-eligible person was selected at random from each household; however, if that person was married, information on the entire household was obtained only once. Percentages have been weighted with household-level weights.
*Assets include home value, real estate, transportation, business, IRA, stocks, bonds, CDs, checking and savings, and other assets, minus debt.

Table 12.2 Distributive preferences among respondents over age 70 with wills.

CHARACTERISTICS OF RESPONDENTS AND BENEFICIARIES	PERCENT IN CATEGORY (WEIGHTED)
Overall ($n = 3781$)	
Will provides for child or stepchild	97.6
Will provides for all children equally	87.0
Will provides for a grandchild	15.4
Will provides for all grandchildren	2.8
Will provides for charity	8.8
Men ($n = 1572$)	
Will provides for child or stepchild	97.6
Will provides for all children equally	86.3
Will provides for a grandchild	14.1
Will provides for all grandchildren	0.9
Will provides for charity	9.6
Women ($n = 2209$)	
Will provides for child or stepchild	97.5
Will provides for all children equally	87.6
Will provides for a grandchild	15.8
Will provides for all grandchildren	4.1
Will provides for charity	8.2

Source: University of Michigan, 2006.

In addition to family bequests, Table 12.2 reveals that a seemingly small fraction of elderly Americans intend to leave an estate to philanthropic organizations when they die. About 10% of men and 8% of women with wills provided for a charity, as shown in the last row of Table 12.2. Supplemental analyses revealed that 25% of respondents who gave to charity reported having no children. However, this was true of only about 6% of those who did *not* give to charity. These results highlight the need to examine the effect of changing family structure on bequests. Frumkin (2006) argues that donors, in general, need to think carefully about their personal legacy in terms of, first, the time horizon of the public problem they want to address and, second, the significance and permanence they attach to their own charitable motive. These two issues related to inheritance decisions are particularly salient for the current generation of retirees, and especially the large number of women and childless couples of the baby boom generation. According to the US CB the percentage of childless women aged 40–44 almost doubled between 1976 and 2002, reaching about two million or 18% of women in that birth cohort (Downs, 2003).

THE MORAL DIMENSIONS OF INTERGENERATIONAL TRANSFERS IN LATE LIFE

We now address the social implications of wealth transfers in families. Unlike in traditional societies where inheritance was based on tradition and common law, in the US and other Western nations, one is free to divide one's estate as one wishes (Finch, 2004). However, in the event one dies without a will, US intestate law is set up by the state to determine the distribution of the estate to heirs.

What keeps lawyers busy and can separate families for years are the economic possessions, because these are the assets that in Western society are considered to be of greatest value, and needed for personal success and social reputation. In the absence of clearly established social norms for intergenerational exchanges, especially prior to death, what accounts for differences among various parents and their adult children? Gift-giving behaviors are a result of ideas and examples passed from one generation to the next (Finch, 2004). Based on family history and behavior, each generation develops expectations of what gifts should be passed on or received. On the other hand, a person's own experiences with earning, saving, and spending, as well as one's own personality, also affect attitudes about money. Differences in gift-giving within the family also reflect the intensity and emotional content of family members' interactions. They are very often colored by the past and by life events (e.g. divorce) that happened long ago or by problems that persist into the present.

Gift-giving within families is influenced by a complex set of interactions and emotional exchanges, or what some refer to as "family ideologies" (Angel, 2008). If all emotional ties have been severed, gift-giving may also cease. In very close families, gift-giving may be more common and the size and value of gifts may be larger. But gift-giving is also related to other aspects of a family's emotional interaction. As research shows, for instance, the relationship between a parent's intentions of gift-giving to their adult children and plans for their health care and retirement needs is not completely predictable (Angel, 2008).

In order for parents to give their children gifts of money or valuable goods, they must have adequate material resources. Yet even poor parents often give substantial gifts to their children, and those gifts can represent far more than what may be immediately apparent. One study of family inheritance practices based on in-depth interviews of late-life families examined differences based on social characteristics in exchange patterns, the feelings of commitment toward performing roles and to meeting filial obligations, and the extent to which economic factors constrain the decision to give gifts in later life (Angel, 2008). The interviewees discussed some of the unwritten rules they followed in their money habits. They also described the lessons they were imparting to their children. Myriad childhood experiences help to shape the core values that parents teach their children about gifting, not so much in terms of specific memories about who gave what to whom, but in the positive experiences and conflicts that erupted in the family and (extended) household. How families think about managing money (e.g. using or not using credit cards) and the ways in which to deal with daily hassles and crises, influence the families' money dynamic.

For those who inherit money or property from parents, relatives, or non-kin, the bequest can also profoundly alter their financial situation. Even relatively modest amounts of money that are above and beyond what one earns can have a measurable impact on one's financial situation. For this reason the occasion of distributing a parent's estate can prove conflict-ridden and traumatic for many families, even to the point that it is often fodder for popular drama. One person's good fortune in receiving a tidy bequest is another's loss, and resentments and jealousies even among close family members are not unusual. Occasionally the division of a parent's estate tears a family apart, and family members can harbor resentments against deceased parents and siblings for years.

Further, estate issues can also create financial hardships. It is a dire state of financial affairs when a husband leaves his wife without income or assets in the event of widowhood. A study by Angel et al. (2007) found a substantial financial widowhood penalty. Black women who became widowed suffered a loss in assets that was five times greater and Hispanic women a loss that was four times greater than non-Hispanic white women. Women who have not had careers or who worked in jobs in which they were unable to vest a pension are almost totally dependent on their husbands' income and limited community assets. Even if their absolute drop in income is less than that of more affluent non-Hispanic white women, minority widows can end up far worse off financially if they have few assets to liquidate or borrow against. In the traditional bread-winner model, where husbands are the primary source of family income, it is traumatic both emotionally and financially when a husband leaves his estate in disarray after his death (Stum, 2008).

The vast majority of Americans express a deep desire to pass on wealth to their children with the caveat of not sacrificing their own retirement security. These attitudes and opinions toward financial exchanges in adulthood inform empirical research that suggests that parents allocate transfers to children on the basis of several criteria (Bernheim & Severinov, 2000). On balance, parents who have money give equally to their children upon their death. The notion that parents expect services in return for their financial gifts is not revealed by the respondents in a study of family inheritance in Austin, Texas (Angel, 2008). On the other hand, elderly parents indicate that their personal concerns about a child in dire need of assistance lead to greater financial support for poorer children.

Arguably, inter-vivos transfers are often dictated by a child's economic needs and are not distributed equally across children. Most middle-class parents today provide for all or most of their children's college education, and many feel that such a gift is sufficient (McGarry & Schoeni, 1997). Economists point to the fact that inter-vivos transfers and permanent loans are channeled to those children who are "liquidity constrained" (Cox, 2003). Some even help with the purchase of a home, but they often view such money as a loan, perhaps repayable at favorable interest rates. Some parents plainly see money as one promising means of cementing the bonds with their children. Others, however, separate the meaning of money from emotional ties and do not give gifts to their adult children.

home equity (Havens & Schervish, 2009). For most individuals, the vast majority of what they earn over the life course is consumed. Large, and even moderate, estates are usually the result of property that is passed down from one generation to the next. Of course, the opportunities parents provide their children for educational and occupational advancement during their childhood and early adulthood represent bequests in the form of additions to young people's human capital that are as real as money. A lack of education and material resources of the sort that keep people from accumulating even a modest estate during their lifetime not only places them at risk of poverty in old age, but keeps them from passing material wealth or opportunities for economic and social advancement on to their children.

In the long run, this lack of intergenerational asset accumulation prevents families from caring for their most vulnerable members and also threatens to undermine the traditional bonds between the older and younger generations. We should remain continually aware of the very real possibility that the loss of that tie between the old and the young could lead to resentment and a decreasing willingness among working-age adults to provide for the elderly (Hudson, 1999). Although some may object to the materialistic basis on which we ground the pact between the generations, it would be naive to think that human motivations are solely altruistic or that we possess an unlimited capacity for self-sacrifice. A more materialistic view leads us to the realization that a system in which the accumulation of assets ties one generation to the next is one in which bonds of generational reciprocity and affection are maximized. Conversely, a system in which the material ties between children and parents are weak faces the risk of turning the young and the old into strangers.

INHERITANCE AND INTERGENERATIONAL FINANCIAL EXCHANGES IN AN AGING SOCIETY

As the population ages, financial linkages across generations may become increasingly strained (Angel, 2008). Uncertainty about retirement security will raise many questions about what is possible. The research we have reviewed makes it clear that income from assets and accumulated wealth are major factors separating those who are well-off in retirement from those who are not. Because of the importance of accumulated wealth in determining the overall welfare of any group, we must emphasize the role of inheritances and bequests in structuring the relations between the generations.

In the US, inheritances and bequests account for the largest fraction of aggregate personal wealth and

CONCLUSION AND AREAS FOR FUTURE RESEARCH

This chapter provides a basic understanding of what is known about the concept of inheritance and gift-giving in terms of how older people balance the competing claims of helping family members during their lifetimes, saving for old age, and leaving a meaningful inheritance. What is abundantly clear is that the size and nature of gifts varies by socioeconomic status. The rich can transfer a great deal of their wealth to their children during their own lifetimes and still have enough resources to enjoy a full life during retirement and bequeath the remainder to their heirs. Those in the middle class have less to share, but intergenerational inter-vivos transfers and bequests can still make a difference in their families' well-being. At the same time, serious disparities in wealth accumulation create considerable inequality in the estimates of expected bequests in low-income families, and as a result hinder the child in living a better life than the parents did (Hurd & Smith, 2002; Shapiro, 2003).

Further, gender inequities in retirement security will also affect the possibility of helping grown children. For women, retirement security has traditionally been provided through marriage. Traditional gender role expectations and the domestic division of labor associated with the male breadwinner model meant that many women never worked or did so only part time. Entrance of women into the paid labor force and the high degree of marital instability over the latter part of the twentieth century, however, mean that women are increasingly responsible for their own retirement security. Women are at a disadvantage relative to men in terms of private pension coverage during retirement, and minority-group women are far less likely than any other group to have retirement coverage from any source. These differences have important implications for the economic security among the large cohorts of women currently approaching or in retirement and on their capacity to pass on wealth to their children.

In addition to social class differences in wealth transfers across generations, the literature and data indicate that present trends in late-life giving before death can be explained in large part by altruistic behavior. On the other hand, decisions about inheritance are predominantly governed by family traditions and ideology. Researchers also find some limited support for other potential explanations. Whether or not these transfers continue to occur will depend on a host of factors, including family ideology concerning money, gifts, altruism, and reciprocity. Increasingly, however, the state of the economy as well as public policy and legal factors, such as inheritance laws related to estate taxes, will be shaping the nature and character of family inheritance.

Upon entering the twenty-first century, we left behind a time that was ruled by tradition and inherited norms concerning both the material and affective aspects of life. Such norms are undergoing ever-faster change and may play an increasingly smaller role in inheritance and financial exchanges between generations in the future. For minority Americans, as for many majority Americans, family life is far different today from how it was either in their countries of origin or in this country only a few decades ago. The pact between the generations that was based on tradition has inevitably been weakened, and a new pact will have to be negotiated on the basis of the new material, as well as social realities that characterize developed nations today.

There may be substantial cuts in US elderly entitlement programs or even reductions in their rates of increase in the years ahead (see Chapter 25), and the consequences could be significant. For instance, the middle class will feel the pinch if Social Security benefits are fully taxed and higher deductibles and co-payments are required for Medicare. Moreover, aging Americans with wealth will almost certainly need to liquidate at least a large fraction of those assets to pay for long-term care.

Middle-class families have traditionally attempted to preserve their estates for their children. But this tradition is in jeopardy. Examining the role of gifts, bequests, and inheritance in old-age support systems and in public policy design in particular is critical. Ongoing investigation into how these changes in inheritance are affecting our society is warranted. Further study of the social implications of inheritance for baby boomers and generations to come is also needed, including analyses of the impact of wealth transfers among family members during their lifetimes as well as at death. These are fertile areas for research, and they deserve serious scholarly attention.

ACKNOWLEDGMENTS

We would like to thank Lisa Yarnell for her help with the data analysis. This research was supported by an LBJ Policy Research Institute grant awarded to the first author.

REFERENCES

Altman, S. H., Reinhardt, U. E., & Shields, A. E. (1998). *The future U.S. healthcare system: Who will care for the poor and uninsured?* Chicago, IL: Health Administration Press.

Andreoni, J. (1990). Impure altruism and donations to public goods: A theory of warm glow giving. *Economic Journal, 100,* 464–477.

Angel, J. L. (2008). *Inheritance in contemporary America: The social dimensions of giving across generations.* Baltimore, MD: Johns Hopkins University Press.

Angel, R. J., & Angel, J. L. (2009). *Hispanic families at risk: The new economy, work, and the welfare state.* New York, NY: Springer.

Angel, J. L., Jiménez, M., & Angel, R. J. (2007). The economic consequences of widowhood for older minority women. *The Gerontologist, 47*(3), 222–234.

Barro, R. J. (1974). Are government bonds net wealth? *Journal of Political Economy, 82*(6), 1095–1117.

Becker, G. S. (1974). A theory of social interactions. *Journal of Political Economy, 82*(6), 1063–1093.

Becker, G. S., & Tomes, N. (1976). Child endowments and the

quantity and quality of children. *Journal of Political Economy*, 84(suppl), 142–163.

Bernheim, B. D., & Severinov, S. (2000). Bequests as signals: An explanation for the equal division. NBER Working Papers (No. 7791). Cambridge, MA: National Bureau of Economic Research, Inc.

Bernheim, B. D., Shleifer, A., & Summers, L. H. (1985). The strategic bequest motive. *Journal of Political Economy*, 93(6), 1045–1076.

Bernheim, B. D., Lemke, R. J., & Scholz, J. K. (2004). Do estate and gift taxes affect the timing of private transfers? *Journal of Public Economics*, 88, 2617–2634.

Binstock, R. H. (2005). The contemporary politics of old age policies. In R. B. Hudson (Ed.), *The New Politics of Old Age Policy* (pp. 265–293). Baltimore, MD: Johns Hopkins University Press.

Caldwell, J. C. (1976). Toward a restatement of demographic transition theory. *Population and Development Review*, 2(3–4), 321–366.

Caputo, R. K. (2002). Adult daughters as parental caregivers: Rational actors versus rational agents. *Journal of Family and Economic Issues*, 23(1), 27–50.

Chan, K. S., Godby, R., Mestelman, S., & Muller, R. A. (2002). Crowding-out voluntary contributions to public goods. *Journal of Economic Behavior & Organization*, 48, 305–317.

Cox, D. (1987). Motives for private income transfers. *Journal of Political Economy*, 95(3), 509–546.

Cox, D. (2003). Private transfers within the family: Mothers, fathers, sons and daughters. In A. Munnell & A. Sundén (Eds.), *Death and Dollars* (pp. 168–197). Washington, DC: The Brookings Institution Press.

Cox, D., & Stark, O. (2005). On the demand for grandchildren: Tied transfers and the demonstration effect. *Journal of Public Economics*, 89, 1665–1697.

Cox, D., Hansen, B. E., & Jimenez, E. (2004). How responsive are private transfers to income? Evidence from a laissez-faire economy. *Journal of Public Economics*, 88(9–10), 2193–2219.

Dannefer, D., & Shura, R. (2009). Experience, social structure and later life: Meaning and old age in an aging society. In P. Uhlenberg (Ed.), *International Handbook of Population Aging* (pp. 747–755). Dordrecht, Netherlands: Springer.

Downs, B. (2003). Fertility of American Women: 2002. *Current Population Reports*, Table 1, P20–P548, 1–11.

Fetterman, M. (2007). *Survey of Inheritance and Giving While Living*. USA TODAY/Gallup survey. Retrieved August 3, 2009 http://www.usatoday.com/money/2007-08-23-inheritance_N.htm

Finch, J. (2004). Inheritance and intergenerational relationships in English families. In S. Harper (Ed.), *Families in ageing societies: A multi-disciplinary approach* (pp. 164–175). New York: Oxford University Press.

French, E., De Nardi, M., Jones, J. B., Baker, O., & Doctor, P. (2006). Right before the end: Asset decumulation at the end of life. *Economic Perspectives*, QIII, 2–13.

Friends Provident. (2009). *As recession erodes family inheritances, Brits face uncertain future*. Milford, England http://www.friendsprovident.com/news/fp/newslink.jhtml?newsItemId=fpcouk%2Fpressreleases%3Afppr050509recessionerodesinheritances.

Frumkin, P. (2006). *Strategic giving: The art and science of philanthropy*. Chicago, IL: University of Chicago.

Gale, W. G., & Slemrod, J. B. (2001). *Rethinking the estate and gift tax: Overview*. (Working paper no. 8205). Cambridge, MA: National Bureau of Economic Research. Retrieved October 17, 2009 from http://www.nber.org.ezproxy.lib.utexas.edu/papers/w8205.

Havens, J. J., & Schervish, P. G. (2009). *New estimates of the forthcoming wealth transfer and the prospects for a golden age of philanthropy*. Chestnut Hill, MA: Social Welfare Research Institute at Boston College. Table 1. Lower level estimates.

Hashimoto, A. (1996). *The gift of generations: Japanese and American perspectives on aging and the social contract*. New York: Cambridge University Press.

Hogan, D., Eggebeen, D., & Clogg, C. (1993). The structure of intergenerational exchange in American families. *American Journal of Sociology*, 98, 1429–1458.

Hudson, R. B. (1999). Conflict in aging politics: New population encounters old ideology. *Social Service Review*, 73, 358–379.

Hurd, M. D., & Smith, J. P. (2002). *Expected bequests and their distributions* (Working Paper No. 9142). Cambridge, MA: National Bureau of Economic Research. Retrieved July 7, 2004 from www.nber.org/papers/W9142.

Hurd, M., Smith, J. P, & Zissimopoulos, J. (2007). *Inter-vivo giving over the lifecycle* (Working Paper #WR-524). Santa Monica, CA: Rand Population Research Center.

Ikkink, K. K., van Tilburg, T., & Knipscheer, K. C. P. M. (1999). Perceived instrumental support exchanges in relationships between elderly parents and their adult children: Normative and structural explanations. *Journal of Marriage and the Family*, 61,(4), 831–844.

Jensen, R. T. (2003). Do private transfers 'displace' the benefits of public transfers? Evidence from South Africa. *Journal of Public Economics*, 88, 89–112.

Joulfaian, D. (2005). Choosing between gifts and bequests: How taxes affect the timing of wealth transfers. *Journal of Public Economics*, 89, 2069–2091.

Kohli, M. (2003). *Intergenerational family transfers in aging societies*. Section on Aging & the Life Course Distinguished Scholar Lecture, 98th Annual Meeting of the American Sociological Association, Atlanta, Georgia, August 19.

Kotlikoff, L. J., & Burns, S. (2005). *The coming generational storm. What you need to know*. Cambridge, MA: MIT Press.

Kotlikoff, L. J., Razin, A., & Rosenthal, R. W. (1990). A strategic altruism model in which Ricardian equivalence does not hold. *The Economic Journal*, 100(403), 1261–1268.

Künemund, H., & Rein, M. (1999). There is more to receiving than needing: Theoretical arguments and empirical explorations of crowding in and crowding out. *Ageing and Society*, 19, 93–121.

Laslett, P. (1991). *Fresh map of life: The emergence of the third age*. Cambridge, MA: Harvard University Press.

Lee, R., & Mason, A. (2007). *Population aging, wealth, and economic growth: Demographic dividends and public policy* (Background paper for the World Economic and Social Survey). New York, NY: Department of Economic and Social Affairs, United Nations.

Leibenstein, H. (1957). *Economic Backwardness and Economic Growth*. New York: John Wiley.

Light, A., & McGarry, K. (2004). Why parents play favorites: Explanations for unequal bequests. *The American Economic Review*, 94(5), 1669–1681.

McGarry, K. (2001). The cost of equality: Unequal bequests and tax avoidance. *Journal of Public Economics*, 79, 179–204.

McGarry, K., & Schoeni, R. F. (1997). Transfer behavior within the family: Results from the Asset and Health Dynamics Study. *The Journals of Gerontology*, 52B, 82–92.

Mitchell, O. S., & Moore, J. F. (1998). Can Americans afford to retire? New evidence on retirement saving adequacy. *The Journal of Risk and Insurance*, 65, 371–400.

Munnell, A. H. (2003). Introduction. In A. H. Munnell & A. Sundén (Eds.), *Death and Dollars* (pp. 1–29). Washington, DC: The Brookings Institution.

Munnell, A., Sundén, A., Soto, M., & Taylor, C. (2003). The impact of defined contribution plans on bequests. In A. H. Munnell & A. Sundén (Eds.), *Death and Dollars* (pp. 265–306). Washington, DC: Brookings Institution.

Ng-Baumhackl, M., Gist, J., & Figueiredo, C. (2003). *Pennies from heaven: Will inheritance bail out the baby boomers?* Washington, DC: AARP Public Policy Institute.

Nugent, J. B. (1985). The old-age security motive for fertility. *Population and Development Review*, 11(1), 75–97.

O'Connor, C. (1996). Empirical research on how the elderly handle their estates. *Generations*, 20, 13–19.

Poterba, J. (2001). Estate and gift taxes and incentives for inter vivos giving in the US. *Journal of Public Economics*, 79, 237–264.

Putnam Investments. (2006). The "we generation": Supporting elderly parents and grown children brings retirement surprises for many. Retrieved August 28, 2009 http://www.thefreelibrary.com/The+%22We+Generation%22%3a+Supporting+Elderly+Parents+and+Grown+Children...-a0154510722

RAND Center for the Study of Aging (2007). *RAND HRS 2006 income and wealth imputations*. Santa Monica, CA: Labor & Population Program.

Rossi, A. S., & Rossi, P. H. (1990). *Of human bonding: Parent–child relations across the life course*. New York, NY: Aldine de Gruyter.

Schoeni, R. F. (2002). Does unemployment insurance displace familial assistance? *Public Choice*, 110(1–2), 99–119.

Shapiro, T. M. (2003). *The hidden cost of being African American: How wealth perpetuates inequality*. New York: Oxford University Press.

Silverstein, M. (2006). Intergenerational family transfers in social context. In R. H. Binstock & L. K. George (Eds.), *Handbook of Aging and the Social Sciences* (pp. 165–180) (6th Edn). San Diego: Academic Press.

Silverstein, M., Conroy, S. J., Wang, H., Giarrusso, R., & Bengtson, V. L. (2002). Reciprocity in parent-child relations over the adult life course. *Journal of Gerontology: Social Sciences*, 57B(1), S3–S13.

Simon, R. J., Fellows, M. L., & Rau, W. (1982). Public opinion about property distribution at death. *Marriage and Family Review*, 5, 25–38.

Stone, R. (2000). *Long-term care for the elderly with disabilities: Current policy, emerging trends, and implications for the twenty-first century*. New York: Milbank Memorial Fund.

Stum, M. (2008). Families and inheritance decisions: Examining non-titled property transfers. *Journal of Family and Economic Issues*, 21, 177–202.

University of Michigan (2006). *Health and Retirement Survey*. Ann Arbor, MI: The University of Michigan.

University of Michigan (2009). *Health and Retirement Study sample evolution: 1992–1998*. Ann Arbor, MI: The University of Michigan.

Villanueva, E. (2005). Inter-vivos transfers and bequests in three OECD countries. *Economic Policy*, 20(43), 505–565.

Chapter | 13 |

Economic Status of the Aged in the United States

Virginia P. Reno, Ben Veghte

National Academy of Social Insurance, Washington, DC

INTRODUCTION

This chapter provides an overview of the economic status of the elderly in the US. We first compare older and younger Americans in terms of median household incomes and poverty over time, and then consider how updated measures of poverty affect conclusions about the economic well-being of older Americans. We then examine the roles of particular sources of income – Social Security, pensions, earnings, and asset income – in supporting older Americans today. Retirement income replacement rates – tools to assess how well retirees are able to maintain their preretirement standard of living – are covered next. Wealth holdings of American households, such as retirement accounts, home equity, and total net worth, are analyzed using the 2007 Survey of Consumer Finances and subsequent ballpark estimates of how the market collapse and housing debacle in 2008/09 eroded these resources. We then view prospects for the economic well-being of retirees in the future, drawing on a retirement risk index developed by the Retirement Research

DOI: 10.1016/B978-0-12-380880-6.00013-7

Center at Boston College and official projections of Social Security's long-term future. The chapter concludes by comparing the US with other industrialized nations in terms of the economic well-being of our older citizens and our prospects for meeting the fiscal challenge of an aging society.

ELDERS AND YOUNGER FAMILIES OVER TIME

How has the economic security of seniors changed relative to that of younger families over the past several decades? This section briefly reviews trends in household median income and poverty by age.

Change in Median Income of Households

We consider median incomes of households over nearly four decades – from 1969 through 2007 – by

age, taking account of household composition. We first compare married couples without children by age to see how elders compare with their younger counterparts. We then compare men and women living alone, again by age, to see how elders in one-person households compare with their younger counterparts. Finally, families with children under age 18 are included, for comparison with childless households, to see how families with children fared over the nearly four decades since 1969. All median incomes are expressed in 2007 dollars and hence are adjusted for inflation (Table 13.1).

Amongst married couples without children, the elderly had the largest percentage gain in median income (73% since 1969). Yet, their income remains far below that of younger couples. Elderly couples' median income of $42390 in 2007 was barely more than half that of their younger counterparts ($73000 for those under age 40 and $82600 for those aged 40–64).

Amongst one-person households, seniors also showed large gains in median income since 1969. Yet, their incomes remain well below those of their younger counterparts. Among men living alone in

Table 13.1 Median income of US households, 1969, 1989, 2007 (in 2007 dollars) by presence of children under age 18, marital status, and age of householder.

HOUSEHOLD TYPE	MEDIAN INCOME ($)			PERCENT CHANGE		
	1969	1989	2007	1969–1989	1989–2007	1969–2007
All households	43700	48360	50000	11	3	14
Couples: no children under 18						
Under age 40	50160	67060	73000	34	9	46
Age 40–64	57680	77160	82600	34	7	43
Age 65 and older	24120	38630	42390	57	10	73
One-person households						
Men under age 65	31570	36810	34400	17	−6	9
Men age 65 and older	11810	18880	22310	60	18	89
Women under age 65	21050	30100	30000	43	(a)	42
Women age 65 and older	9280	15050	15790	62	5	70
Families with children under 18						
Married couples	54780	66880	76630	22	15	40
Unmarried men	44600	45780	45200	3	−1	1
Unmarried women	21580	23320	28380	8	22	32

Tabulations of the March supplement to the U.S. Census Bureau 2008 Current Population Survey by staff of the National Academy of Social Insurance.
(a) Less than ½ of 1%.

2007, seniors had median income of $22 300 compared to $34 400 for younger men. Senior women living alone had median income of $16 000, barely more than half that of younger women living alone: $30 000.

Families with children fared differently depending on the marital status and sex of the householders. Married couples with children saw real incomes rise at roughly the same rate (and level) as did nonelderly couples without children. Median income for two-parent families with children rose by about 40% between 1969 and 2007. At $76 630, their median income was in the same ballpark as that of couples under age 65 without children. Amongst unmarried women with children, median income rose by about one third since 1969. Yet their median amount of $28 340 in 2007 remained far below that of couples with children ($76 630) and of unmarried men with children ($45 200).

Most of the income gains for the elderly occurred during the 1970s. The gains were due in large part to legislated increases in Social Security benefits. Congress enacted ad hoc benefit increases that took effect in 1970, 1971, 1972, and 1974, and then indexed benefits to keep pace with inflation (Clark & Quinn, 1999). Driven by real increases in Social Security benefits in the 1970s and by a greater percentage of the elderly being eligible for benefits, total incomes of seniors rose by roughly 60% between 1969 and 1989. Increases since then have been more modest.

Changes in Poverty Over Time

Poverty among the elderly was widespread during the Great Depression; it is estimated to have exceeded 50% in 1934 (Altman, 2005). The Social Security Act of 1935 brought immediate grants to states to support needy seniors and families with children. The same law created the social insurance program (Old-Age and Survivors Insurance, or Social Security) to prevent seniors from falling into poverty in the future. By 1959, the first year in which the Bureau of the Census officially counted the poor, 35% of elders were poor.

Poverty among older Americans declined in the 1960s and 1970s for the same reasons that their median incomes rose: more of them had worked long enough in covered jobs to qualify for Social Security benefits, and the level of these benefits was increased by Congress. The elderly poverty rate dropped to 25% in 1970 and to 15% in 1975, then gradually declined to about 10% in 2000, where it has hovered since. Engelhardt and Gruber (2006) found that the increase in Social Security benefits between 1967 and 2000 can explain all of the decline in elderly poverty during this period. They conclude that higher benefits have led some elderly people

to live independently rather than with family members, and that the effect of Social Security in reducing poverty would have been even more dramatic in the absence of these changes in living arrangements.

While just one in ten elders is officially counted as poor, many elders have incomes just above the poverty threshold. Those with incomes below 125% of the poverty threshold are characterized as "near-poor." Certain demographic groups are more likely to be poor or near-poor than others. Among seniors, 28% of unmarried women, 33% of African Americans, and 28% of Latinos were poor or near-poor in 2007 (Table 13.2). Moreover, poverty in old age is, in large part, a "women's issue" (Schulz, 2001), as roughly seven out of ten elderly poor and near-poor are female (US Social Security Administration, 2010). Unmarried women of color have particularly high poverty rates.

Poverty among children under 18 also dropped sharply during the 1960s from 27% in 1959 to an all-time low of 14% in 1973. After that, childhood poverty gradually rose and hovered around 20% during much of the 1980s and the first half of the 1990s. Childhood poverty gradually declined to 15–16% at the turn of the century, but was back up to 18% in 2008.

The Welfare Reform Law of 1996 ended Aid to Families with Dependent Children and replaced it with Temporary Assistance for Needy Families. The new program set a five-year lifetime limit on receipt of federally funded cash assistance, imposed strong work requirements, and allowed states to impose sanctions reducing or denying benefits to families who fail to comply with these requirements (Gabe,

Table 13.2 Percent of elders who are poor or near-poor (2007) by marital status, sex, and ethnicity.

CHARACTERISTICS	PERCENT	
	POOR	POOR OR NEAR-POOR
All persons 65 and older	6	16
Married	4	8
Unmarried men	12	21
Unmarried women	18	28
White	8	14
Black	23	33
Hispanic	17	28

Source: US Social Security Administration (2009).

2009). Many other policies that sought to improve economic security for families with children did not translate directly into reductions in poverty as officially measured. This occurred in large part because many of those provisions – the Earned Income Tax Credit (EITC), Food Stamps, housing assistance, and expanded eligibility for health coverage through Medicaid and the Children's State Health Insurance Program – are not counted in the official poverty measures (Blank & Greenberg, 2008). We turn next to issues in defining and measuring poverty.

MEASURING POVERTY OR ADEQUACY

US Social Security Administration researcher Mollie Orshansky (1963, 1965) developed the original methodology for counting poor people in the US. She set the poverty threshold at three times a subsistence food budget for a family of four because the average family of three or more spent one-third of their after-tax income on food, according to the 1955 Household Food Consumption Survey. Her groundbreaking efforts were based on the best data available in the early 1960s. Since then, the thresholds have been updated only for inflation. They do not reflect changes in expenditure patterns or food costs. Ruggles (1990) and Schwarz (2005) replicated Orshansky's methods with more recent data and concluded that the poverty line would be about 70% higher if more recent data were used. When the poverty line for a family of four is compared to the median income of such families, we find that the poverty line has fallen from just under 50% of median income in the early 1960s to 28% in 2007 (Blank & Greenberg, 2008).

National Academy of Sciences Recommendations

In response to a request from Congress, the National Academy of Sciences convened a group of experts to update and improve the measurement of poverty. Its 1995 report (Citro & Michaels, 1995) recommended a broader definition of necessary expenditures (that includes food, housing, out-of-pocket health care expenses, child support expenses, and work-related expenses such as transportation and childcare) and a more refined measure of income (that takes into account taxes, tax credits, and in-kind benefits such as food stamps and housing subsidies).

The CB is using the new measure on an experimental basis, and New York City is using it to assess progress toward reducing poverty. For 2008, the new measure resulted in a slight increase in the count of Americans who are poor – 16% instead of 13% (Table 13.3). Childhood poverty declined slightly (from 19% to 18%), reflecting the net effect of counting in-kind benefits as income and counting necessary expenses associated with children. Poverty among seniors increased sharply (from 10% to 19%), due in large part to recognition of out-of-pocket health spending as a basic necessity.

When New York City used the new methods to count its poor, 23% of the city's residents were found to be poor in 2006. They included 27% of the city's children and 32% of its elders (Center for Economic Opportunity, 2008). Finding that seniors were as economically vulnerable as children (or even more so), Mayor Bloomberg, who had previously pushed for cuts in programs for the elderly, initiated pilot programs for older residents that would reduce taxi costs, provide free bus services to get to grocery stores, and offer legal aid to those at risk of eviction from their homes (Yen, 2009).

Relative Poverty

The OECD defines poverty relative to a society's current living standards, using a threshold that is 50% of median income (after taxes and benefits) for households of similar size. This relative standard reflects a concern for social integration and cohesion by defining poverty as the inability to afford the basic elements of a lifestyle that is typical in one's society.

Table 13.3 Poverty rates: Official and NAS measures: United States, 2008; New York City, 2006.		
AREA AND AGE	**OFFICIAL MEASURE**	**NAS MEASURE**
United States, 2008		
All Ages	13	16
Under age 18	19	18
Age 18–64	12	14
Age 65 and older	10	19
New York City, 2006		
All Ages	18	23
Under age 18	27	27
Age 18–64	14	20
Age 65 and older	18	32
Sources: Center for Economic Opportunity (2008) and US Census Bureau (2009).		

Hence, this measure tracks growth in wages, not just prices. By this measure, the 17% of Americans who were poor in 2005 included 21% of children, 24% of elders, and 15% of other adults (OECD, 2008). In brief, both the updated US poverty measures and the OECD measures of relative poverty find that older Americans are as likely as (or even more likely than) children to experience economic deprivation.

Making Ends Meet: An Economic Security Threshold

Wider Opportunities for Women (WOW) is developing a new Elder Economic Security Standard Index to measure the minimum income older adults need to remain secure, given prevailing costs where they live. Different budgets apply to elders based on their living arrangements, health status, and geographic location. The national average index provides a benchmark for economic security to compare with official poverty thresholds. While the poverty threshold for a person living alone was $10 400 in 2008, the WOW measure finds that an older American in good health living alone would need about $16 300 to make ends meet if she or he owned a home mortgage-free. A renter in good health would need more, about $20 250, while a homeowner still paying off a mortgage would need about $24 000 to make ends meet (Wider Opportunities for Women, 2009). These standards are tools for policymakers and advocates to use in assessing priorities in support of economic security for seniors. They suggest that incomes well above the poverty threshold are needed to make ends meet and age in place. At the same time, updated measures of poverty show that many American elders have incomes below subsistence levels.

COMPONENTS OF INCOME OF THE ELDERLY TODAY

This section examines the composition of the income of the elderly and the role of various sources in the economic status of the elderly today. What are the respective roles of Social Security, pensions, earnings from work, and asset income in undergirding the finances of today's seniors? Do these sources fill different roles for upper- and lower- income elders? To what extent do recipients of Social Security rely on these benefits for most of their income? How does reliance on Social Security differ between married couples and unmarried beneficiaries? How does it differ among racial and ethnic groups? This section addresses these questions, drawing on data from the annual income supplement to the CPS.

How Many Elders Receive Key Sources of Income?

Social Security is the foundation of income for almost all older Americans: about nine in ten elders receive it (Table 13.4). Employer-sponsored pensions – including private pensions and payments from public plans for government employees – are less common. Roughly half of married couples have pension income, as do about one-third of unmarried elders. Income from assets includes interest, dividends, rental income, and income from estates or trusts. About two-thirds of married couples have some income from assets, as do nearly half of unmarried men and women. For many, asset income is small. Earnings and self-employment income are important sources of income for those

Table 13.4   Percentage receiving sources of income, 2008; couples and unmarried persons age 65 and older.

TYPE OF INCOME	TOTAL	MARRIED COUPLES	UNMARRIED PERSONS
Social Security	87	88	86
Pensions – total	41	49	35
Public employee pensions	15	18	13
Private pensions	28	35	23
Income from assets	54	66	47
Earnings from work	26	41	13
Supplemental security income	4	2	5
Source: US Social Security Administration (2010).			

who are still working. About four in ten married elderly couples and 16% of unmarried elders had earned income in 2008. SSI, which provides means-tested payments to those with very low income and limited asset holdings, is received by about 5% of unmarried elders and 2% of married elderly cou-ples. The maximum federal SSI payment for an older person living alone in 2009–2010 is $674 a month, which amounts to about 75% of the official poverty guidelines.

How Do Shares of Income Differ by Income Level?

Income "shares" represent the fraction of the aggregate dollars of income for a group that comes from a par-ticular source. For example, Social Security represented 37% of the aggregate dollars of income received by all aged couples and unmarried individuals in the 2008 CPS (US Social Security Administration, 2010).

The shares of various sources differ markedly by the size of household income. In Figure 13.1, elders are divided into five equal groups (quintiles) based on their total incomes. Each pie chart shows the share of the group's total income that comes from each source.

Social Security is an important share of income for middle- and upper-middle-income elders as well as for low-income retirees. Those in the bottom two fifths of the income distribution (with incomes below $19 880) received more than 80% of their total income from Social Security in 2008. Those

in the middle income group (between $19 880 and $31 300) received nearly two thirds of their income from Social Security; pensions were their next larg-est source at 16% of the total. Those in the next-to-highest income group (with between $31 300 and $55 890) relied on Social Security for nearly half their income (44%) while pensions were their second larg-est source and earnings from work were third. Only in the top income group (with incomes over $55 890) was Social Security not the largest source of income. Because most high-income elders were not yet fully retired, earnings from worker were their largest source of income. When and if they do retire, their incomes might come in relatively equal shares from Social Security, pensions, and income from assets – the pro-verbial "three-legged stool" of retirement income. For all other income groups, Social Security is far more important than pensions or asset income in support-ing older Americans.

Who Relies on Social Security for Most of their Income?

In contrast with "shares" of income, "reliance on Social Security" counts the fraction of recipients who rely on their benefit for half or more of their total income. Grad and Foster (1979) reported the first estimates of this measure more than 30 years ago. In 1976, just over half of elderly couples (56%) and nearly three quarters of elderly unmarried recipients (73%) received half or more of their total income

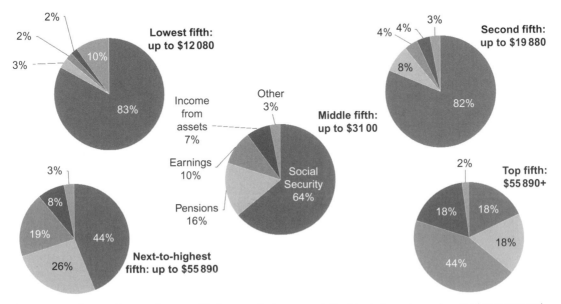

Figure 13.1 Shares of income from specified sources by income quintile. Married couples and married persons aged 65 and order.
Source: US Social Security Administration, 2010; Income of the Population 55 and Over, 2008.

Table 13.5 Percent relying on Social Security for half or more of total income, 2008; married couple and unmarried beneficiaries by race and ethnicity.

GROUP TYPE	TOTAL	MARRIED COUPLES	UNMARRIED PERSONS
All beneficiaries	64	52	73
African Americans	71	54	77
Hispanics	74	61	82
Asian Americans	68	53	82
White (non-Hispanic)	63	51	72

Source: US Social Security Administration (2010).

from Social Security. Similar proportions of beneficiaries rely on Social Security today (see Table 13.5). Reliance on Social Security is greater among communities of color and among the unmarried – widowed, divorced, separated, or never married. Beneficiaries without spouses who relied on Social Security for at least half of their incomes made up 82% of Hispanic and of Asian elders, 77% of African American elders, and 72% of white elders.

RETIREMENT INCOME REPLACEMENT RATES

To assess how well income in retirement will allow a worker to maintain his or her prior standard of living, financial advisors often use replacement rates; i.e. the ratio of retirement benefits to preretirement earnings. Because some expenses are reduced or eliminated in retirement (such as taxes on wages, work-related expenses, and saving for retirement), experts generally advise that replacement of 70% to 80% of prior earnings could produce a comparable standard of living (Fidelity Research Institute, 2007; Palmer et al., 2008).

Social Security Replacement Rates Today

Social Security is designed to provide a foundation of retirement income that will be supplemented by pensions and savings. It has a progressive benefit formula that replaces a larger share of past earnings for low earners than for high earners. This feature recognizes two realities: first, low earners need higher levels of wage replacement in order to meet basic needs, and, second, low earners are less likely to have been covered by an employer-sponsored retirement plan or to have discretionary income to save over their working

lives. Figure 13.2 shows replacement rates for four hypothetical 65-year-olds retiring in 2009 with different lifetime earnings histories (Board of Trustees, 2009). For the illustrative average earner, benefits replace 40% of average lifetime earnings.

Actual retirees often do not fare as well as these illustrative replacement rates suggest, for two reasons (Thompson, 1994). First, many retirees incur reductions in their benefits because they claim them early. Benefits claimed at 62 (the earliest eligibility age) are reduced by 25% below the level payable at the full-benefit age, which is 66 for people born between 1943 and 1954. The full-benefit age will gradually rise to 67 for those born in 1960 and later. Then, benefits claimed at age 62 will be reduced by 30%. Second, many retirees do not have steady work histories like those assumed for the illustrative workers. Women, in particular, are likely to experience gaps or spells of reduced hours of work while caring for young children, aging parents, or other relatives. Those breaks in employment would generally cause retirees to receive lower benefits than would similar earners with steady work. Another measure of the typical Social Security benefit in relation to earnings is the average retired worker benefit ($13 860) as a percentage of the average earnings of all workers ($42 040), which was 33% in 2009. Clearly, if workers need 70% to 80% of their prior earnings to maintain their standard of living, Social Security provides only a foundation.

Counting Pensions in Replacement Rates

Munnell and Soto (2005) have estimated replacement rates for retiree households using the HRS. They take account of income from pensions and financial assets as well as Social Security. Replacement rates are generally higher for retiree households with pensions in addition to Social Security. Replacement rates differ

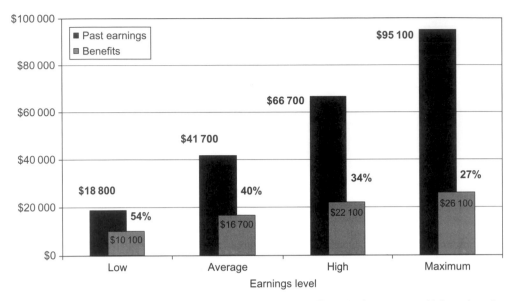

Figure 13.2   Social Security benefits compared to past earnings, 2009; illustrative low, average, high, and maximum earners retiring at age 65.
Source: Board of Trustees, 2009. Low earnings are 45% of the average wage; high earnings are 160% of the average wage.

INCOME IN NUMERATOR	MARRIED COUPLES		UNMARRIED PERSONS	
	WITHOUT PENSIONS	WITH PENSIONS[a]	WITHOUT PENSIONS	WITH PENSIONS
Denominator = Career average wage-indexed earnings + return on financial assets[b]				
Retirement benefits (SS+pensions)	43	63	46	70
Retirement benefits+financial assets[c]	55	74	58	86
Denominator = CPI-indexed high 5 of last 10 years earnings + return on financial assets				
Retirement benefits (SS+pensions)	34	52	33	56
Retirement benefits+financial assets	45	60	44	67

Table 13.6   Median replacement rates for households by marital status, pension status, and measure of pre-retirement income.

[a]Pensions include defined benefit plans and defined contribution plans.
[b]Return on financial assets in the denominator includes income from stocks, bonds, savings and checking accounts, and certificates of deposit before retirement.
[c]Assumes that all financial assets (listed in (b) above) are turned into life annuities to provide income in retirement.
Source: Munnell & Soto (2005).

depending on how the retirees' preretirement income is counted (Table 13.6).

The first measure of preretirement income uses average earnings over the entire career (indexed to wage levels near retirement), plus preretirement income from financial assets, such as interest and dividends. With this measure, married couples without pensions had a median replacement rate of 43% from Social Security alone, while couples with pensions

had a median replacement rate from Social Security and pensions of 63%. Comparable figures for unmarried retirees were a 46% replacement rate for those with only Social Security and 70% for those with pensions in addition to Social Security. A broader measure of retirement income shown in Table 13.6 converts all financial assets – checking and savings accounts, stocks, bonds, certificates of deposit, and so forth – into annuitized income in retirement. This

Table 13.7 Social Security replacement rate for illustrative average earner at age 65 in 1986, 2005, 2030.

YEAR	REPLACEMENT RATE (PERCENT)	
	GROSS	AFTER PART B
1986	42	41
2005	42	39
2030	36	32

Source: Munnell & Sass (2006).

assumption raises median replacement rates by about 10 percentage points. This estimate assumes that retirees devote all their liquid assets to retirement annuities, leaving no cushion to cover emergencies or other unexpected costs.

The alternative measure of preretirement earnings uses the high five of the last ten years of earnings before retirement (instead of career average earnings) to more closely reflect living standards in the decade before retirement. With this measure of higher preretirement earnings, replacement rates are lower – about 10 to 15 percentage points lower than those cited above. Munnell and Soto (2005) concluded that about two-thirds of recent retirees were entering retirement in pretty good financial condition, with replacement rates in the 65%–75% threshold range of adequacy. But they also saw several reasons for caution. First, the one-third of households without pensions is not faring well. Second, over time, the replacement rates of those with private pensions will decline, for these are rarely if ever indexed for inflation. Third, the replacement rate estimates assume that people buy life annuities with their DC retirement accounts, yet few do. And finally, the retirement income landscape is changing for future retirees in ways that reduce the adequacy of both Social Security and private retirement plans.

Social Security Replacement Rates in the Future

Without a change in current Social Security law, 65-year-old retirees will get less adequate net wage replacement from Social Security in coming decades than has been the case for retirees over the past 25 years (Table 13.7). The replacement rates for a medium earner retiring at age 65 in 1986 and 2005 were about 41% and 39%, respectively, after deducting from Social Security benefits premiums for Medicare Part B, which pay for doctors' bills. By 2030, the net replacement rate for a similar 65-year-old retiree will drop to about 32%. Reasons for this

decline include the legislated increase in the 'full-benefit age' for receiving Social Security benefits and rising Medicare premiums that are deducted directly from Social Security benefits. Social Security benefit reductions already in law and rising Medicare premiums mean that benefit increases would be needed just to maintain the net Social Security replacement rates retirees have experienced over the past 25 years (Munnell & Sass, 2006; Reno, 2007).

The Shift to Defined Contribution Plans

About half (49%) of all workers under age 65 in the US participate in some kind of employer-sponsored retirement plan (Purcell, 2009). That portion has remained relatively stable over the past 30 years. Yet the nature of these plans has shifted markedly. In the early 1980s, employers started moving away from traditional pensions – or DB plans – to DC plans, such as those authorized under section 401(k) of the Internal Revenue Code. By law, tax-favored DB pension plans are required to offer benefits to retirees in the form of monthly benefits for life or annuities. In contrast, 401(k)-type plans give the worker a lump sum payout when he/she leaves a job, which he/she can either take in hand or roll over into a tax-favored individual retirement account (IRA) or a tax-favored account with another employer. Upon retirement, 401(k) plans give the worker the option of receiving a lump-sum payout as well.

While coverage under 401(k) plans is growing, recent studies find that workers fail to take full advantage of them to achieve retirement security. In particular, workers may postpone joining the plan; contribute less than the optimal amount; fail to adequately diversify their investments; invest too much in the employer's company stock; borrow from their plan and thus forego asset appreciation; and cash out accumulations when they change jobs (Munnell, 2007). Assess of the role of employer-sponsored retirement plans in the future well-being of retirees requires a look at the size of retirement savings accounts of American households.

WEALTH HOLDINGS IN 2007 AND LOSSES IN 2008–09

Asset holdings are an increasingly important component of economic security for seniors as more retirement plans take the form of individual savings accounts rather than contractual benefit promises from employers. This section examines the retirement savings account accumulations of working households, the role of homeownership, and the net worth

Table 13.8 Household retirement savings account balances by age, 2007: Defined contribution accounts, IRAs, and Keogh plans.

AGE OF HOUSEHOLDER	NUMBER OF HOUSEHOLDS (IN THOUSANDS)	PERCENTAGE WITH ACCOUNTS	MEAN VALUE OF ACCOUNTS ($)	MEDIAN VALUE OF ACCOUNTS ($)
All households	116 122	54	148 580	45 000
Under age 35	25 148	45	25 280	9 600
35 to 44	22 745	58	81 310	37 000
45 to 54	24 120	66	156 120	63 000
55 to 64	19 564	62	271 920	100 000
65 and older	24 545	41	207 320	60 800

Source: Purcell (2009)

of US households based on the most recent findings of the 2007 SCF. We then cite estimates of how the stock market meltdown and collapse of the housing market in 2008/09 affected the wealth of American households.

Retirement Savings Accounts

Altogether just over half (53%) of all households have some funds set aside for the householder or spouse in tax-favored retirement savings accounts, which include employer-sponsored DC accounts, IRAs, and Keogh plans for the self-employed. For households that had such accounts, the median value was $45 000 in 2007. Households approaching retirement had larger accumulations. The median value for account holders aged 55 to 64 was $100 000 (Table 13.8).

The mean value of accounts was much higher than the median ($272 000 compared to $100 000 for 55- to 64-year-olds) indicating that retirement account wealth is highly concentrated at the top. The median is the amount where half of account holders have more and half have less. If households with a zero account balance are included (38% of 55–64-year-olds), then fully 69% of all households aged 55 to 64 had less than $100 000 in retirement account savings in 2007 (Pilon, 2009; Purcell, 2009). Purcell estimates that with an accumulation of $100 000 a 65-year-old man could buy a life annuity (with no inflation protection and no provision for dependents or survivors) of about $700 a month, based on interest rates current in April 2009. Because women live longer than men, the same sum would buy a 65-year-old woman a smaller annuity (about $650).

The concentration of retirement savings accounts at the top of the distribution becomes a concern as

employers, workers, and the federal government rely increasingly on them – together with Social Security – to serve as the twin pillars of retirement income security over the long term, replacing the traditional three-legged stool of Social Security, occupational DB pensions, and individual savings. In 2007 the long-term costs of the subsidy provided by the federal government for such retirement plans was $135 billion (US Office of Management and Budget, 2009). According to the Urban-Brookings Tax Policy Center, roughly 70% of these subsidies go to those in the top 20% of the income distribution, and almost half go to the top 10% (Eisenbrey, 2008).

Household Net Worth

Household net worth represents the value of all of a household's assets minus its liabilities. The SCF is the leading source of data on household wealth. It defines net worth as financial assets plus non-financial assets (e.g. the value of vehicles, residences, and businesses), minus debt (Bucks et al., 2009). Household net worth rises with age as workers accumulate retirement savings, home equity, and other assets over their lifetimes (Table 13.9). For many elder households, the home is the most important asset.

Homeownership

Homeownership increases with age; just over eight in ten households headed by a person between the ages of 55 and 74 are homeowners. After age 75 the homeownership rate declines slightly to 77% as some elders may move to other living arrangements at advanced ages. Many seniors are still paying off debt on their homes. About half of homeowners

Table 13.9 Household net worth and homeownership, 2007; families by age of householder.

AGE	MEDIAN NET WORTH ($)	PERCENT			MEDIAN	
		OWNING HOME	WITH DEBT ON HOME	DEBT-FREE HOME	HOME VALUE ($)	HOME DEBT ($)
Total	120 300	69	49	20	200 000	107 000
Under 35	11 800	41	37	3	175 000	135 000
35 to 44	86 600	66	60	7	205 000	128 000
45 to 54	182 500	77	65	12	230 000	110 000
55 to 64	253 700	81	55	26	210 000	85 000
65 to 74	329 400	85	43	43	200 000	69 000
75 and older	213 500	77	14	63	150 000	40 000

Source: Bucks et al. (2009)

aged 65–74 still had home debt in 2007. The median home value for homeowners aged 65–74 was $200 000, while the median debt for the half of those homeowners who were still paying for their homes was $69 000. In 2007, as in prior years, the home remained the main asset of most households approaching retirement.

The critical role of the home in the asset holdings of typical households approaching retirement is shown in Table 13.10. Munnell et al. (2009) estimate the wealth for households aged 55 to 64 using the mean value for the middle 10% of such households.

Total wealth excluding the value of defined benefits amounted to $255 500 for this typical household. Home equity (the value of the home minus debt on the home) accounted for just over half that wealth, while retirement savings accounts and other financial assets made up about one third. If expected lifetime payments from Social Security and DB pensions are expressed as asset values for this typical household, then total wealth rises to $675 500 and Social Security is the largest component of that wealth (44%), while the home is the second largest component (20%) and DB pensions rank third (18%).

The Financial Crisis and the Housing Bubble

The latest data from the SCF are for 2007, before the market fell and the housing bubble burst in 2008/09. The next round of SCF data will be collected for 2010 and likely become available early in 2012. In the meantime, what are scholars estimating to be the impact of the economic downturn on the status of retirees now and in the future?

Using SCF data from 2007 and national price indices, Bosworth and Smart (2009) simulated the size and distribution of wealth losses from the 2008/09 financial crisis. They found that the collapse of the housing market triggered a broad decline in asset prices that greatly reduced the wealth of all categories of households. Older households mitigated their real estate and stock market losses with Social Security and DB pensions. Yet, no demographic group was left unscathed. As Bosworth & Smart (2009, p. 1) note,

Prior to the financial crisis, our study and others had concluded that the current baby boom cohort of near retirees were surprisingly well-prepared for retirement compared with similarly aged households over the past quarter century. Unless there is a strong recovery of asset values in the next few years, that favorable assessment is no longer true.

They continue (p. 17):

Since younger families have a larger share of their net wealth in housing and hold larger mortgages as a share of home value, they typically suffered a larger percentage loss in net worth. In contrast, older households were hit harder by the decline in stock prices. Overall … [o]lder households lost much of their presumed gains relative to earlier cohorts, and they will have less time to recover.

By projecting housing and stock values, Rosnick and Baker (2009) estimated three possible scenarios about how baby boom wealth changed between 2004 and 2009. They concluded that the "loss of wealth due to the collapse of the housing bubble and the plunge in the stock market will make baby boom

Table 13.10   Wealth of a typical household approaching retirement[a], 2007.

SOURCE OF WEALTH	AMOUNT ($)	PERCENT DISTRIBUTION	
		TOTAL WEALTH	WEALTH OTHER THAN DEFINED BENEFITS
Total wealth	676 500	100	–
Wealth other than defined benefits:	255 500	38	100
Primary house	138 600	20	54
Business assets	15 900	2	6
Financial assets	29 600	4	12
401(k), IRA, and other retirement savings	50 500	7	20
Other non-financial assets	21 000	3	8
Defined benefits:	421 000	62	–
Social Security	298 900	44	–
Other pension plans	122 100	18	–

[a]"Typical household approaching retirement" refers to the mean value for the middle 10% of households headed by a person aged 55–64.
Source: Munnell et al. (2009).

far more dependent on Social Security and Medicare than prior generations" (p. 2).

Munnell et al. (2009) assessed the role of 401(k) plans after the 2007 SCF in light of the collapse of financial markets in 2008, which spread to the real economy in 2009. They estimated that 401(k) balances lost about 30% of their value in the 12 months following the market peak in October 2007. Moreover, employers, faced with declining revenues and the prospect of laying-off workers, cut back on their 401(k) matching or suspended matching altogether (Munnell & Soto, 2010).

OUTLOOK FOR THE FUTURE

This section examines how the financial crisis and housing market collapse have put more Americans at risk of falling far short of maintaining their pre-retirement standards of living in retirement. These projections assume no changes in Social Security beyond the scheduled increase in the full benefit age that is phasing in. Stories in the popular media raise questions about the capacity of the system to pay scheduled benefits. What do official Social Security projections show for the future? What sorts of policy changes would be needed to ensure that it remains in long-term financial balance? What options could

be adopted to improve the adequacy of benefits and what would they cost?

Households at Risk After the Crises

The Center for Retirement Research at Boston College has developed a National Retirement Risk Index to estimate how many retirees in the future are at risk of falling short of maintaining their preretirement living standards. The index was constructed using the 2004 SCFs to estimate how many households are on track to maintain their living standards in retirement. Similar tabulations from prior versions of the triennial SCFs reveal that the fraction of households at risk had risen – from 30% in 1989 to 43% in 2004. Updating the index with the 2007 SCFs showed little change in the overall index. But updating the index to reflect the housing market collapse and financial market meltdown after 2007 brought a sharp and unprecedented increase in the portion of households at risk. By the end of the second quarter of 2009, the combined effect of declining retirement accounts and home equity, declining interest rates, and the continuing increase in the Social Security full benefit age meant that 51% of households were estimated to be at risk of falling more than 10% short of maintaining their living standards in retirement (Munnell, et al., 2009). Because middle and upper income

Table 13.11 Percent of households at risk by income group and by cohort, 2004, 2007, and 2009.

	2004	2007	2009
All	43	44	51
By income			
Low income	53	57	60
Middle income	40	40	47
High income	36	35	42
By age cohort			
Early boom	35	37	41
Late boom	44	43	48
Gen Xers	49	49	56

Source: Munnell et al. (2009).

households hold more assets, they experienced greater losses (Table 13.11). When viewed by age cohort, younger groups (late boom and Generation Xers) are at greater risk than are early boom.

These estimates assume that Social Security will continue to pay benefits as called for in the law – including phasing in the increase in the full benefit age to 67 for persons born in 1960 and later – a change that gradually lowers benefits. Yet, some policymakers are calling for further cuts in future benefits to balance program finances. What is the financial outlook for Social Security and what can be done to address it?

Social Security in the Future

Social Security trustees assess its future finances every year using updated assumptions about birth and death rates, wage and price growth, employment, interest rates, and so forth. Recognizing the great uncertainty of 75-year forecasts, they project three scenarios: low-cost; high-cost; and intermediate. The intermediate scenario is considered the best estimate and is most often used. In 2009, it showed that Social Security has been running surpluses for 25 years and will have surpluses in each of the next 14 years (2010–2023). Reserves, held in federal government bonds, are projected to grow to $4.3 trillion by the end of 2023. After 2023, reserves will have to be gradually drawn down to pay benefits. By 2037, without changes, reserves will be depleted. Income coming into the fund after 2037 will cover about three fourths of benefit payments due then.

The long-range actuarial deficit is 2.0% of taxable payroll. This means that to close the 75-year financing gap solely with a contribution rate increase would require raising the rate paid by workers and employers from 6.2% to 7.2%, which would yield a combined increase from 12.4% to 14.4%, or 2.0% of payroll.

In a recent report, *Fixing Social Security: Adequate Benefits, Adequate Finances,* the National Academy of Social Insurance examined a variety of policy options to improve the adequacy of benefits for vulnerable groups, such as the oldest old (those over age 85); widowed spouses of low-income couples; retirees (usually women) with low benefits because of gaps in paid work while they cared for children; and low-paid, long-service workers whose benefits fall short of meeting the poverty line (Reno & Lavery, 2009). The report also examined 18 different options to increase program revenues in the future to levels that would securely finance current benefits and pay for benefit improvements, if desired.

By exposing the vulnerability of average Americans to the risks of a market economy, the financial crisis shines a new light on the critical role of Social Security in maintaining economic security for elders. The next and final section of this chapter examines how the US compares with other industrialized countries in the economic well-being of our elders and our capacity to meet the financial challenges of an aging society.

INTERNATIONAL COMPARISONS

In the sixth edition of this handbook, Schulz and Borowski (2006) discussed pension reforms in other countries and how the push for "privatization" of retirement benefits has worked out. In this section we compare the economic status of the aged in the US with that of elders in other industrialized countries and assess the challenge of financing pensions for aging societies both here and abroad.

Comparing Well-Being of the Aged

Indicators of the relative well-being of elders include prevalence of poverty, the level at which Social Security benefits replace prior earnings, the role of employer-sponsored pensions, and out-of-pocket health care spending.

For cross-national comparisons we use the OECD definition of relative poverty; that is, spendable income of less than 50% of the median for households of similar size. By this measure, 24% of US seniors are poor. That is nearly twice the average poverty rate across 30 OECD countries (13%). This US poverty rate looms particularly high relative to Canada and key Western European countries (Table 13.12).

Social Security replacement rates in the US are modest when compared with those in other OECD countries. Replacement rates for the 30 countries studied are calculated for low-, average-, and high-wage workers, using each country's benefit formula. Of the 30 countries studied, US replacement rates ranked fourth from the bottom for low earners (at 50%), fifth from the bottom for average earners (at 39%), and ninth from the bottom for high earners (at 28%) (OECD, 2005a, 2005b). In contrast, average replacement rates for the 30 nations were 72% for low earners, 57% for average earners, and 49% for high earners.

Income from employer-sponsored retirement plans, personal savings, and earnings from work supplement Social Security and other public benefits in other countries as well as in the US. Table 13.12 shows shares of aggregate income of elders from public benefits (Social Security and public assistance), earnings from work, and income from capital, which includes employer-sponsored pensions and returns on individual savings. In the aggregate, US elders rely less on public benefits and more on earned income and income from capital than is the case in Canada and key Western European countries. But when we consider the distribution of employer-sponsored pension income, we find that it is highly skewed toward the top in the US.

The average annual pension income in the top quintile ($16 000) was about 150 times the average for the bottom quintile ($100) for the years 2004–06 (Employee Benefit Research Institute, 2010). Those in the bottom three-fifths of the income spectrum received less than about $1700 a year. Based on these findings, Baily and Kirkegaard (2009) concluded that

the seeming inability of the voluntary US employment-based pension system to expand much beyond the top income echelons is a powerful

reminder that there are few if any effective voluntary replacements for the Social Security system to provide retirement income to the majority of Americans. (p. 436)

In brief, employer-based pensions in the US do not alleviate the problem of low replacement rates from Social Security for low- and moderate earners. The highly skewed distribution of employer-based pensions together with low-replacement rates from Social Security suggest that in the coming decades the top quintile of the aged in the US stands to fare much better than its counterparts in most other OECD countries, while the lower quintiles are likely to fare worse (Baily and Kierkegaard, 2009).

Health care is largely free for retirees in many OECD countries. Despite the existence of Medicare and Medicaid, older Americans pay far more out-of-pocket than do their counterparts in other OECD countries (OECD, 2009b). A recent study by the Employee Benefits Research Institute (Fronstin et al., 2009) found that

men retiring at age 65 in 2009 will need anywhere from $68 000 to $173 000 in savings to cover health insurance premiums and out-of-pocket expenses in retirement if they want a 50–50 chance of being able to have enough money, and $134 000 to $378 000 if they prefer a 90 percent chance. With their greater longevity, women will need more: a woman retiring at age 65 in 2009 will need anywhere from $98 000 to $242 000 in savings to cover health insurance premiums and out-of-pocket expenses in retirement for a 50–50 chance of having enough money, and $164 000 to $450 000 for a 90 percent chance. (p. 9)

These estimates do not include the cost of long-term care, which in several OECD countries is covered by social insurance or other (non-means-tested) government programs (Lundsgaard, 2005).

Table 13.12 Elderly poverty rate and shares of income from key sources: Six countries, Mid-2000s.

COUNTRY	PERCENT POOR	SHARES OF INCOME			
		PUBLIC BENEFITS	WORK	CAPITAL	TOTAL
Canada	4	41	18	42	100
Sweden	6	69	10	22	100
France	9	85	7	8	100
Germany	10	73	12	19	100
United Kingdom	10	49	12	39	100
US	24	36	34	30	100

Source: OECD (2009b).

Challenge of Aging Societies

How does the US demographic outlook compare to that of other OECD countries? Whilst the number of older Americans is growing, the share of our future population over age 65 will not be as large as in many other OECD countries because the number of younger Americans is also growing due to higher fertility rates and more net immigration. Americans aged 65 and older are projected to increase from about 13% of the population today to about 21% by 2050. In contrast, Germany and Japan are already coping with aging populations of 20% and 23%, respectively. By 2050 seniors are projected to make up 26% of the population in Canada, 32% in Germany, and 40% in Japan (OECD, 2009a). Still, the growing number of older Americans poses a challenge to funding the US Social Security system. Mitigating this demographic shift are two other US developments. First, even though the US standard retirement age over the next 50 years is scheduled to remain about average in the OECD and to reach 67 by 2027, the effective retirement ages in the US for men and women are higher than elsewhere – fourth and fifth highest, respectively, among OECD countries (Baily & Kirkegaard, 2009). Since the mid-1980s, labor force participation among older Americans has been increasing (Quinn, 2002). Second, as already noted, Social Security benefits are modest by international standards and, as discussed earlier in this chapter, US replacement rates will decline in the future as the age for full-benefit receipt rises to 67.

The best summary measure of the affordability of a society's Social Security system is expenditures as a share of the country's GDP. The US Social Security program in 2009 amounted to about 4.8% of GDP, a share that is projected to rise to 6.2% in 2035 after all the baby boom have retired, and then stabilize at about 5.8% of GDP for the rest of the next 75 years (Board of Trustees, 2009). Many of our trading partners spend considerably more on their Social Security programs today than is projected for the US in the future (Table 13.13). Peterson Institute economists Baily and Kirkegaard (2009) concur:

The US – with only a moderately poor fiscal starting point, moderate current costs of pension

Table 13.13 Social Security spending as a share of GDP in 2005; selected OECD countries.

COUNTRY	PERCENTAGE OF GDP
Austria	12.6
Canada	4.5
Finland	8.4
France	12.4
Germany	11.4
Japan	8.7
Sweden	7.7
United Kingdom	5.7

Source: OECD (2009c).

provision, low levels of future pension promises, […] and only moderate demographic pressure […] is in the category of OECD countries that can expect to be only moderately affected. This is an important point when trying to filter the occasionally overly gloomy commentary regarding the outlook for the US economy and its future ability to provide for its retiring baby boom. Most OECD countries face more immediate and severe future challenges to the sustainability of their [public] pension systems than does the US. (p. 90)

In summary, the US faces a modest financial challenge to ensure that scheduled Social Security benefits will be maintained (or even improved) in the long-term future. By international standards, the US has higher rates of poverty among elders and provides lower levels of wage-replacement from Social Security. The recent financial crisis exposes the vulnerability of American workers and retirees to losses in private sector savings, pensions, home equity, and employment earnings. Those losses shed a bright light on the critical importance of ensuring an adequate foundation of economic security through social insurance.

REFERENCES

Altman, N. J. (2005). *The battle for social security: From FDR's vision to Bush's gamble.* Hoboken: John Wiley & Sons, Inc.

Baily, M. N., & Kirkegaard, J. F. (2009). *US pension reform: Lessons from other countries.* Washington, DC: Peterson Institute for International Economics.

Blank, R. M., & Greenberg, M. H. (2008). *Improving the measure of poverty.* Washington, DC: The Brookings Institution.

Board of Trustees. (2009). *Annual report of the Board of Trustees of the Federal Old-Age and Survivors Insurance and Federal Disability Insurance Trust Funds.*

Washington, DC: US Social Security Administration.

Bosworth, B., & Smart, R. (2009). *The wealth of older Americans and the sub-prime debacle.* Chestnut Hill, MA: Center for Retirement Research at Boston College.

Bucks, B. K., Kennickell, A. B., Mach, T. L., & Moore, K. B.

(2009). Changes in U.S. family finances from 2004 to 2007: Evidence from the survey of consumer finances. *Federal Reserve Bulletin, February*, A1–A56.

Center for Economic Opportunity (2008). *The CEO poverty measure: A working paper by the New York City center for economic opportunity.* New York: The New York City Center for Economic Opportunity.

Citro, C. F., & Michaels, R. T. (Eds.), (1995). *Measuring poverty: A new approach.* Washington, DC: National Academy Press.

Clark, R. L., & Quinn, J. F. (1999). *The economic status of the elderly.* Medicare Brief, Number 4. Washington, DC: National Academy of Social Insurance.

Eisenbrey, R. (2008). Testimony before the Subcommittee on Select Revenue Measures of the House Committee on Ways and Means. June 26. Retrieved January 15, 2010 from http://www.epi.org/publications/entry/webfeatures_testimony_waymeans_20080626/.

Employee Benefit Research Institute. (2010). Databook on employee benefits. Retrieved January 28, 2010 from http://www.ebri.org/publications/books/index.cfm?fa=databook

Engelhardt, G. V., & Gruber, J. (2006). Social Security and the evolution of elderly poverty. In A. Auerbach, D. Card & J. Quigley (Eds.), *Public policy and the income distribution* (pp. 259–287). New York: Russell Sage Foundation.

Fidelity Research Institute. (2007). The Fidelity Research Institute Retirement Index. *Research Insights Brief*, March.

Fronstin, P., Salisbury, D. L., & VanDerhei, J. (2009). Savings needed for health expenses in retirement: An examination of persons ages 55 and 65 in 2009. *EBRI Notes*, 30(6), 2–11.

Gabe, T. (2009). *Poverty in the United States: 2008.* Washington, DC: Congressional Research Service.

Grad, S., & Foster, K. (1979). *Income of the population 55 or older, 1976.* Washington, DC: U.S. Government Printing Office.

Lundsgaard, J. (2005). Consumer direction and choice in long-term care for older persons, including payments for informal care. How can it improve care outcomes, employment, and fiscal sustainability? *OECD Health Working Papers No. 20.*

Munnell, A. H. (2007). The declining players in the retirement income game: Lecture 1 – The withdrawal of employers, Storrs Lecture, Yale Law School March 5–6.

Munnell, A. H., & Sass, S. A. (2006). *Social security and the stock market: How the pursuit of market magic shapes the system.* Kalamazoo, MI: W.E. Upjohn Institute for Employment Research.

Munnell, A. H., & Soto, M. (2005). *What replacement rates do households actually experience in retirement?* Chestnut Hill, MA: Center for Retirement Research at Boston College.

Munnell, A. H., & Soto, M. (2010). *Why did some employers suspend their 401(k) match?* Chestnut Hill, MA: Center for Retirement Research at Boston College. 10(2).

Munnell, A. H., Golub-Sass, F., & Muldoon, D. (2009). *An update on 401(k) plans: Insights from the 2007 survey of consumer finance.* Chestnut Hill, MA: Center for Retirement Research at Boston College. 9(5).

Organisation for Economic Co-operation and Development (OECD). (2005a). *Pensions at a glance: Public policies across OECD countries.* Paris: OECD.

Organisation for Economic Co-operation and Development (OECD). (2005b). *Society at a glance 2005: OECD social indicators.* Paris: OECD.

Organisation for Economic Co-operation and Development (OECD). (2008). *Growing unequal? income distribution and poverty in OECD countries.* Paris: OECD.

Organisation for Economic Co-operation and Development (OECD). (2009a). *OECD country statistical profiles 2009.* Retrieved February 14, 2010 from http://stats.oecd.org/Index.aspx?QueryName=254&QueryType=View.

Organisation for Economic Co-operation and Development (OECD). (2009b). *OECD health*

data 2009: Statistics and indicators for 30 countries. Paris: OECD.

Organisation for Economic Co-operation and Development (OECD). (2009c). *Pensions at a glance: Public policies across OECD countries.* Paris: OECD.

Orshansky, M. (1963). Children of the poor. *Social Security Bulletin, 26(7)*, 3–13.

Orshansky, M. (1965). Counting the poor: Another look at the poverty profile. *Social Security Bulletin, 28(1)*, 3–29.

Palmer, B., DeStefano, R., Schachet, M., & Paciero, J. (2008). *Replacement ratio study: A measurement tool for retirement planning: Aon Consulting.* Retrieved February 13, 2010 from http://www.aon.com/about-aon/intellectual-capital/attachments/human-capital-consulting/RRStudy070308.pdf.

Pilon, M. (2009). Crunching some new numbers on retirement savings. *Wall Street Journal* (April 23). Retrieved January 24, 2010 from www.wsj.com

Purcell, P. (2009). *Retirement savings and household wealth in 2007.* Washington, DC: Congressional Research Service.

Quinn, J. (2002). Retirement trends and patterns among older American Workers. In S. Altman & D. Shactmen (Eds.), *Policies for an aging society* (pp. 293–315). Baltimore: Johns Hopkins University Press.

Reno, V. P. (2007). *Building on Social Security's success.* EPI Briefing Paper #208. Washington, DC: Economic Policy Institute.

Reno, V. P., & Lavery, J. I. (2009). *Fixing social security: Adequate benefits, adequate financing.* Washington, DC: National Academy of Social Insurance.

Rosnick, D., & Baker, D. (2009). *The wealth of the baby boom cohorts after the collapse of the housing bubble.* Washington, DC: Center for Economic and Policy Research.

Ruggles, P. (1990). *Drawing the line: Alternative poverty measures and their implications for public policy.* Washington, DC: The Urban Institute Press.

Schulz, J. H. (2001). *The economics of Aging.* Westport, CT: Auburn House.

Schulz, J. H., & Borowski, A. (2006). Economic security in retirement: Reshaping the public-private pension mix. In R. H. Binstock & L. K. George (Eds.), *Handook of aging and the social sciences* (pp. 360–379) (6th ed.). San Diego: Academic Press.

Schwarz, J. E. (2005). *Freedom reclaimed: Rediscovering the American vision*. Baltimore: Johns Hopkins University Press.

Thompson, L. H. (1994). Social Security reform and benefit adequacy. *The Retirement Project Brief Series, No. 17* (The Urban Institute).

US Census Bureau. (2009). Current population survey, 2009 annual social and economic supplement.

US Office of Management and Budget. (2009). Analytical Perspectives, FY 2009 Budget Table 19–4. Retrieved December 15, 2009 from http://www.whitehouse.gov/omb/rewrite/budget/fy2009/apers.html.

US Social Security Administration. (2009). *Fast facts and figures about social security 2009*. Washington, DC: U.S. Government Printing Office.

US Social Security Administration. (2010). *Income of the population 55 or older, 2008*. Washington, DC: U.S. Government Printing Office.

Wider Opportunities for Women. (2009). Single women's retirement income falls short of the Elder Economic Security Standard Index. Washington, DC. Retrieved February 20, 2010 from http://www.wowonline.org/ourprograms/eesi/documents/NationalEESIfactsheet_single_March2009FINAL.pdf.

Yen, H. (2009). Hidden pockets of elderly said to be in poverty. *AARP Bulletin Today*. Retrieved January 12, 2010 from http://bulletin.aarp.org/yourmoney/personalfinance/articles/hidden_pockets_of_elderly_said_to_be_in_poverty.html.

Chapter | 14 |

Employment and Aging

Sara E. Rix[1]
AARP, Washington, DC

CHAPTER CONTENTS

INTRODUCTION

This chapter on employment and aging largely focuses on historical, present, and possible future labor force experiences of older persons in the US. It also provides a broader perspective with a brief discussion of older worker trends and policies in Europe.

FROM MORE TO LESS TO MORE AGAIN: US LABOR FORCE TRENDS SINCE WORLD WAR II

Older Workers in the Early Post-War Decades

Paid employment is probably not the first thing that leaps to mind when the subject of older Americans comes up. Yet many people remain in the labor force well into old age (Figure 14.1), and their numbers are increasing. In numerous surveys over more than a decade, preretirees have been insisting that they expect to work during their so-called "retirement years," both because they want to remain active and because they need the income or health insurance that employment provides (Helman et al., 2008; Yakoboski & Dickemper, 1997). Although there is considerable evidence that workers tend to retire earlier than they expected to (Helman et al., 2008), many signs point to prolonged worklives for a sizable portion of the labor force.

Longer work lives would represent a reversal of the trend toward seemingly ever-earlier retirement that characterized the labor force behavior of men for about four decades following World War II. In 1948,

---

[1]The views in this chapter are those of the author and do not necessarily represent the official policy of AARP.

DOI: 10.1016/B978-0-12-380880-6.00014-9

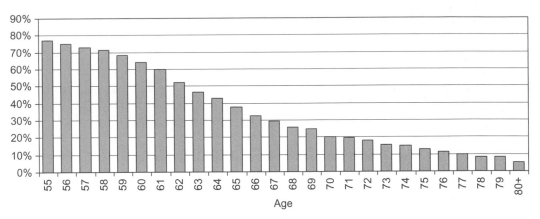

Figure 14.1 Labor force participation rates for persons aged 55 and over by single years of age, 2008 (annual average in percentages).
Source: US Department of Labor, Bureau of Labor Statistics, unpublished data from the Current Population Survey.

nearly half of men aged 65 and over were in the labor force; that is, they were either working or looking for work. By 1985, that was the case for about one in six – a decline of more than 30 percentage points. Over the same period, the participation rate for men aged 55 to 64 plummeted as well. Nine out of ten men in this age group were in the labor force in 1948, a number that fell by almost 22 percentage points to just two out of three by 1985.

It was during this period that Social Security coverage increased, the benefit eligibility age was lowered to 62 (in 1956 for women and 1961 for men), Medicare was enacted (1965), automatic cost-of-living increases to Social Security benefits were introduced (as of 1975), and employer-provided pension coverage expanded. Retirement became more affordable for more workers at younger ages. Employers, many of whom harbored cost concerns as well as negative attitudes about the technological competence and learning ability of older workers (AARP, 1995), had little need to stand in the way of the retirement of their older employees. They could turn instead to the huge cohort of baby boomers and growing numbers of married women entering the workforce. The early retirement incentives in many private pension plans enabled employers to divest themselves of their older workers in a relatively humane way and made the transition to retirement less painful.

The picture for women – notably those aged 55 to 64, who are now perhaps more appropriately described as "middle-aged" – was considerably different. The labor force participation rate for these women rose (Table 14.1) as succeeding cohorts of younger women entered and remained longer in the workforce and as older women returned to work after caregiving. The rate increased by nearly 18 percentage points from 1948 to 1985, or from 24.3% to 42%.

Women aged 65 and over, on the other hand, had rather limited labor force attachment to begin with, a fact that changed little from the late-1940s to the mid-1980s – only 9.1% of women in this age group were in the labor force in 1948, a figure that reached 10.8% in 1960 before falling to 7.3% in 1985.

Labor force trend data also highlight the narrowing discrepancy by sex in labor force participation rates at older ages during this same period. Among the middle-aged, convergence occurred as a result of the declining participation of men and the rising participation of women. Among those aged 65 and over, convergence up to 1985 was due largely to men's labor force withdrawal.

Why Work?

Widespread, voluntary late life leisure in reasonable financial comfort is a fairly recent phenomenon made possible by the expansion and enhancement of public and private pensions, the availability of retiree health benefits (notably Medicare), and growing economic wealth. Even so, many older workers left the labor force before such security was widely available. In 1900, about one-third of men aged 65 and over were no longer in the labor force. This figure increased over the next several decades and reversed only briefly during World War II (US Department of Commerce, 1975). Historian David Hackett Fischer (1978) attributes the acceleration of retirement to, at least in part, the growth of manufacturing and the assumption that older workers could not keep pace with the work in the factories. In the early twentieth century, aging was associated with productivity loss (Costa, 1998). Young men were presumed to be better suited to the work demands of the industrial age. Such sentiments have been held by both employers

Table 14.1 Labor force participation rates for women and men aged 25–64, by age group, 1948–2008 (annual averages).

SEX AND YEAR	AGE			
	25–34	35–44	45–54	55–64
Women				
1948	33.2	36.9	35.0	24.3
1958	35.6	43.4	47.8	35.2
1968	42.6	48.9	52.3	42.4
1978	62.2	61.6	57.1	41.3
1988	72.7	75.2	69.0	43.5
1998	76.3	77.1	76.2	51.2
2008	75.2	76.1	76.1	59.1
Men				
1948	95.9	97.9	95.8	89.5
1958	97.1	97.9	96.3	87.8
1968	96.9	97.1	94.9	84.3
1978	95.3	95.7	91.3	73.3
1988	94.3	94.5	90.9	67.0
1998	93.2	92.6	89.2	68.1
2008	91.5	92.2	88.0	70.4

Source: US Department of Labor, Bureau of Labor Statistics (2010b).

and workers and reflect still-common ageist opinions and attitudes (AARP, 1995; Brown, 2005) that have not augured well for older Americans who need to work.

Without an assured source of retirement income, older workers had little choice but to continue working as long they could hold onto their jobs unless they had saved enough to live on without working, controlled the family wealth, and/or had family members who could and would care for them financially. Life was hard on the farm and in the arduous manual jobs held by so many older Americans. Workers wore out, and health problems propelled many of them out of the labor force.

Over time, the reported reasons for retirement changed, and health issues became a less dominant factor. For example, only 29% of new male Social Security beneficiaries aged 62 to 64 gave health problems as the primary reason for leaving their last job in 1982, in contrast to more than half (54%) in 1968 (Sherman, 1985). Eventually, workers began to look forward to retirement, and the proportion indicating that they had left their last job because of a *desire*

to retire increased substantially. One reason for that may have been the proliferation of affordable leisure activities (Costa, 1998) that proved that retirement could be fun.

Signs of Change in the 1980s

Whatever the appeal of retirement, the situation began to change around the mid-1980s to the mid-1990s as the long, steady decline in older men's participation came to an end. Rates of participation started rising, particularly among men aged 65 and over.

There is no single explanation for this turnabout among men. The fact that mandatory retirement was federally outlawed for most occupations in 1986 might have kept some workers in the labor force longer. Liberalization of the Social Security earnings test in the 1980s and 1990s and its elimination for workers over the age of eligibility for full Social Security benefits in 2000 reduced the "penalty" workers paid for continuing to earn while collecting retirement benefits. These developments might have provided an incentive to continue working, although one would expect a greater impact on hours worked than on participation itself.

The educational attainment of the older population had risen, and better-educated workers tend to remain longer in the labor force (Haider & Loughran, 2001). Disability rates were falling, health status seemed to be improving, and a smaller proportion of older persons was reporting poor health (Manton & Gu, 2001; Martin et al., 2007). At the same time, jobs themselves were less demanding than they had been a generation earlier (Steuerle et al., 1999). Thus, some of the physical impediments to prolonging work live were mitigated or eliminated.

In addition, the private pension system was undergoing significant change. On-the-job pension coverage began to stagnate, and DC pension plans started to replace DB plans. It would not be long before DC plans would eclipse DB plans in terms of worker coverage. Workers fortunate enough to be employed in firms offering a retirement income plan would see the burden of ensuring adequate income in retirement shift from employers to employees. Between 1985 and 1990 alone, the number of DB pension plans fell by 34% while the number of DC plans rose by 30% (*Abstract of 5500 Annual Reports* cited in AARP, 2009, Table 2.1). For those whose investments prove inadequate and who have not saved enough to supplement Social Security, who lack other investments or a handsome inheritance, or who are unwilling to retire to a lower standard of living, working longer may be the only feasible option. Workers with DC plans retire, on average, from one to two years later than those with DB plans (Friedberg & Webb, 2005; Munnell et al., 2003).

Johnson (2002) and Schirle (2008) question the validity of common explanations for older men's growing attachment to the labor force. They argue, for example, that some presumed causal factors such as declining mortality, improved health status, and the spread of DC plans could not have caused the shift. This is because mortality rates were falling and educational attainment was rising as participation rates were declining. Johnson (2002) also contends that the drop in DB plan participation began too early to view it as a main cause of the marked change in older men's labor force participation in the mid-1980s. He does not, apparently, consider the possibility of a lag effect due to workers' growing awareness of the consequences of pension plan developments.

Spousal employment may also have had an impact on men's work and retirement decisions. Schirle (2008) attributes "a substantial portion" of the increase in the labor force participation of married men aged 55 to 64 to their wives, estimating that a wife in the labor force increases the likelihood of her husband's participation by 19 percentage points. Solitary leisure, it seems, lacks the appeal of shared leisure for these men, presumably prompting them to work until their wives are ready to retire.

Given the heterogeneity of the population aged 55 and older, it is likely that different workers have been affected by different factors and in different ways. Although there might not be a single trigger for the reversal in participation – which not all experts are convinced is permanent (e.g. Laitner & Silverman, 2007) – financial factors have played an important role. Access to health insurance (largely employer-provided in the US) has been another reason older Americans remain at work, at least prior to becoming eligible for Medicare at age 65. As employers seek to control their health care costs, retiree health benefits, which help workers bridge an insurance gap between early retirement and Medicare eligibility, are less available than they once were.

Workers do not have complete control over whether they remain on the job or retire. Ill health, an accident, job loss, and/or caregiving responsibilities can throw a wrench into the most carefully planned decisions. But they do have more say over the timing of retirement than, for example, the performance of the stock market or whether their employers will continue to offer retiree health benefits.

When Times Get Tough

Unemployment rates tend to be lower among older workers than among younger ones, even in recessions. Employers may let their less experienced – generally younger – workers go first, although the higher wages and benefits of older employees can work against them when costs must be cut. Seniority clauses in union contracts have protected some older workers, but many are losing that protection as a result of the sharp decline in union membership. Another reason for their lower unemployment is that older workers are more likely than their younger counterparts to drop out of the labor force – that is, to stop looking for employment – after becoming displaced (US Department of Labor, 2008b) and are then no longer classified by the Bureau of Labor Statistics (BLS) as unemployed. Once unemployed, older workers typically remain out of work longer than those who are younger; they are also more likely to be found among the long-term unemployed.

The recession that began in December 2007 was deep and painful for workers of all ages. Throughout the recession, the unemployment rate remained lower for persons aged 55 and over than it was for workers under that age, but it rose sharply – from 3.2% to 7.2% between December 2007 and December 2009 (US Department of Labor, 2010b). Half of the older unemployed population had been out of work for six months or more in December 2009, up from one in five at the start of the recession (US Department of Labor, 2008a, 2010a). Involuntary part-time work and job-seeking discouragement also increased. Perhaps as a result of the economic impact of the recession on older workers, more older Americans opted for Social Security benefits at the earliest eligibility age of 62 in fiscal year 2009 than had been expected (Goss, 2009).

At the same time, however, the number employed and the labor force participation rate rose for older persons but not for those under age 55. Some of this increase was due to the increase in the number of "older" workers as more baby boomers moved into and through their fifties, but some of it appears to be a postponement of retirement, perhaps in response to the economic downturn. For older individuals who want to work in retirement, deciding not to retire may be a wise decision in a recession.

Although working longer in the face of a downturn in the stock market and an uncertain economy seems to make a great deal of sense, today's near-retirees do not appear to be so heavily invested in equities that stock losses, including those of the recent recession, would alter their retirement plans substantially (e.g. Aaronson et al., 2006). And, even if such losses do encourage people to work longer (Brown, 2009), plans and expectations may be thwarted by rising unemployment, which can make keeping or finding a job difficult or impossible. Analyses of 30 years of data from the CPS led Coile and Levine (2009) to predict an increase in retirement due to rising unemployment almost 50% greater than any decrease in retirement attributable to the stock market decline.

OLDER AMERICAN WORKERS IN THE GLOBAL ECONOMY

Labor Shortages

How older workers fare in coming decades in the US workforce will depend in part on what happens in the global economy. On the one hand, with technology creating fluid worksites, opportunities for older workers could expand by, for example, enabling people to work at home, in satellite offices, or under a variety of flexible work arrangements. On the other hand, because people in so many jobs can work almost anywhere, older US workers could face growing competition from cheaper, and perhaps better-trained, workers abroad. Nonetheless, the retirement of the baby boomers, coupled with slowing labor force growth, is expected to create labor and skills shortages and open up employment opportunities for older workers (Aspen Institute, 2002; US General Accounting Office, 2003). Although the BLS refrains from projecting labor shortages or surpluses, it does forecast sizable job growth in some fields such as health and social assistance (Figueroa & Woods, 2007) that have been experiencing labor shortages in recent years.

Not all labor experts anticipate wide-spread labor shortages (e.g. Blinder, 2006; Freeman, 2006). Globalization makes forecasting more difficult as the potential supply of accessible labor has become so much larger. Blinder (2006), for one, warns that in the future considerably more jobs will move offshore, with adverse consequences for American workers.

Employers who are confronted with a shortage of workers have many options; in addition to offshoring jobs, these include increasing the hours of current workers, lobbying to ease immigration restrictions, investing in labor-saving technologies, *and* retaining and hiring more older workers. Examples of efforts to hire and retain older workers by making work more appealing to, and feasible for, aging employees can be found in the health industry, which has experienced difficulties in finding and retaining workers. Should employers in other industries face shortages, they will likely respond similarly.

Cappelli (2005) suggests that boomers themselves may play a key role in mitigating any labor shortages by remaining longer at work. If ample numbers of boomers do push back the date of full retirement, the very workers expected to create labor shortages through their retirement would help prevent them.

Older Workers Abroad

Labor force participation rates for the older segments of the population in the US are high compared to those in many other developed countries. However, trends in labor force participation over time have tended to be similar. After World War II, participation rates for older men fell in most developed nations, while those for older women rose.

Generous pensions and policies designed to expand employment opportunities for younger workers via the retirement of older workers encouraged many people to leave the labor force at relatively young ages in countries such as Germany and France. In recent years, however, the EU has directed attention to older worker retention in light of the precariously financed public pension programs in many countries in Europe (Rix, 2005). Toward that end, the European Council – an assembly of the heads of the EU member states, which initiates policies and sets common objectives – established two targets for EU nations to reach by 2010. These were an increase to 50% in the employment rate of persons aged 55 to 64 (the Stockholm target in 2001) and a five-year increase in the effective retirement age, or age at which workers leave the labor force (the Barcelona target in 2002).

Although the two goals were extremely ambitious and the time frame for their realization encompassed a severe recession, considerable progress was made up through 2008 by many countries in raising the employment rate among the targeted group (Figure 14.2). As of 2008, the current 27 countries of the EU

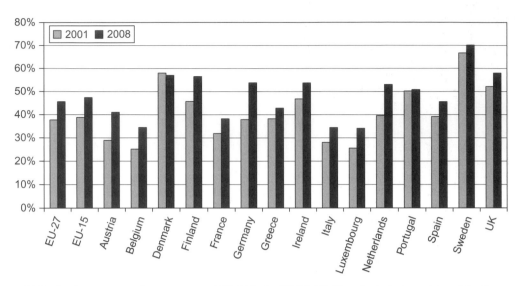

Figure 14.2 Employment rates for persons aged 55–64 in the EU-27, EU-15, and selected countries of the European Union, 2001 and 2008.
Source: European Commission, Eurostat (2010).

had a combined employment rate of nearly 46% for persons aged 55 to 64, an increase of almost 8 percentage points since 2001. There was, however, wide variation across countries. Sweden's 2008 employment rate for the 55-to-64-year-old population, for example, was 70.1%, while those for France and Luxembourg were, respectively, only 38.2% and 34.1% (European Commission, 2010).

EU countries have also seen a rise in the effective retirement age. Six years after the Barcelona target was announced, the age at which workers leave the labor force had risen by 1.3 years for the EU-27 (European Union, 2010, preliminary estimates).

Countries in the EU have responded to the Stockholm and Barcelona challenges in different ways, and some governments have gotten closer to the targets than others. Policymakers have resorted to both retirement-discouraging "sticks" (such as increases in the age of pension eligibility to make retirement less attractive) and work-enhancing "carrots" (such as more phased or partial retirement opportunities and reduced Social Security contributions for workers above a certain age to make work more appealing). By 2008, the member states of the EU were still some distance from the targets, especially the five-year increase in the effective retirement age. Nonetheless, the high-level government focus directed to older workers has been in striking contrast to the US.

Older workers have not been featured anywhere near as prominently in public policy debate or discussion in the US. In America, employment targets, which might be seen as leading to quotas, would likely prove unpopular among policymakers, employers, and the public. Moreover, the need for such targets is less evident in the US. The employment rate of persons aged 55 to 64 currently exceeds the 50% target set by the Stockholm initiative. In addition, employment rates in the population aged 55 and older have been rising. The increase has been quite sharp among some segments of that older population, such as those aged 65 to 69 – conventionally thought of as retirement age. The employment-to-population ratio for this age group rose from 17.8% in 1985 to 29% in 2009, a 63% increase (US Department of Labor, 2010b). Also, the US Social Security system provides less generous benefits than do the public pension systems in many European countries, so it provides comparatively less incentive to retire. Finally, serious financial problems for the US Social Security system remain some years away. Consequently, there is less immediate pressure than in Europe to get workers to delay retirement.

Nonetheless, some attention *has* been paid to encouraging longer worklives in the US. Like their European counterparts, American policymakers have employed carrot and stick approaches to fostering the employment of older workers. These include an increase in the age of eligibility for full Social Security benefits, more actuarially fair delayed retirement credits under Social Security, and elimination of the Social Security earnings penalty for workers above the full benefit eligibility age. Moreover, age discrimination in employment became illegal in the US more than forty years ago, and mandatory retirement was abolished for most occupations about twenty-five years ago, presumably making it easier for US older workers who want to work to do so.

WHERE OLDER AMERICANS WORK

Industry and Occupation

Older persons may be less likely than workers in most younger age groups to be in the labor force; however, age differences in where older people work and what they do are less pronounced. Older workers can be found in virtually every industry and occupation broadly classified, although they are more likely to be in the services sector than any other. The same is true of younger workers. America's oldest workers (65 and over) are better represented in agriculture and related industries than are their younger peers, but this sector is hardly a major source of employment. Differences in industry distribution by sex are more evident those than by age.

Age differences in occupational distribution are also modest. Representation in management and business rises with age, which is logical given the experience and maturity that such jobs tend to require. As with industry, differences in occupational distribution by sex are more apparent than age differences. As might be expected, older women tend to be concentrated in traditionally female-dominated occupations.

Self-Employment

The large majority of US workers are wage and salary workers, but older workers are more likely than younger ones to be self-employed – 6% of workers under age 55, compared with 10% of workers aged 55 to 64, and 17% of those aged 65 and over in 2008 (US Department of Labor, 2009). These figures exclude the incorporated self-employed because the BLS treats such workers as employees of their businesses and hence classifies them as wage and salary workers.

Most self-employed older workers have been self-employed in earlier years. However, a significant number move into self-employment for the first time in later life. About one-third of self-employed workers aged 50 and older become self-employed at or after that age (Karoly & Zissimopoulos, 2004). These newly self-employed workers might be phasing into retirement in a bridge job, embarking on a new career, or opting to become consultants following job loss and a fruitless search for re-employment.

Self-employment may appeal to older wage and salary workers who have always wanted to be their own boss, parlay a hobby or talent into income, or get away from the grind of a 40-hour work week. Surveys indicate that about one in six or seven baby boomers expects to start a business or go into business for themselves when they retire (e.g. AARP, 2004).

Despite the fact that self-employment can make it easier for older workers to scale back their work hours as health conditions or interests dictate, workers eyeing self-employment may paint too rosy a picture of the time commitment and financial investment that working for oneself often entails. This may be one reason why older workers are more likely to move from self-employment to wage and salary work than vice versa (Karoly & Zissimopoulos, 2004).

TRANSITIONS FROM WORK TO RETIREMENT – AND BACK

The retirement transition stereotype has workers going directly from long-term jobs or careers into full-time retirement in a single step, accepting good wishes and a gold watch or other token of long tenure after which they move on to other activities that exclude paid employment. Many workers do leave the labor force this way, but the retirement transition appears to be more nuanced for as many or more workers and often involves more employment than the word "retirement" typically conjures up.

Estimates vary, depending on definition, worker age, and timeframe, but it seems that the majority of older workers do not fully retire directly from career jobs. Rather, they get to full retirement via some form of transitional employment or bridge job, which may be self-employment (Cahill et al., 2007; Johnson et al., 2009). These "post-career" transitions may involve a voluntary career change, follow a job loss, or represent an attempt to phase or ease into retirement that requires a job change. Although such employment has been studied in some detail only in recent years (Giandrea et al., 2007; Quinn, 1999), it was also common among workers retiring more than thirty years ago (Ruhm, 1990).

Leaving a job at older ages weakens labor force attachment, and the longer workers remain out of the workforce, the less likely they are to return. Age discrimination, atrophied skills, inertia, and increasing comfort with the retirement lifestyle all conspire against retirees who think of getting back into the labor force. Thus, retention, rather than efforts to entice workers back into the labor force, may be the best way to keep people working longer. Nevertheless, a substantial percentage of workers do re-enter the workforce for any number of reasons – the money, the social contacts, the work itself, or to get out of the house. Several studies suggest that as many as one-quarter of older labor force exiters "unretire" (Maestas, 2007; Ruhm, 1990). In fact, some of them appear to have planned to re-enter before retiring in the first place (Maestas, 2007).

THE MEANING OF WORK FOR OLDER WORKERS

Older persons work for the money and, in the case of pre-Medicare-eligible workers, for the health insurance that employment may provide (AARP, 2003). However, as mentioned above, they work for other reasons as well – enjoyment, sociability, and/or an interest in making a contribution (AARP, 2003). In short, they remain in the labor force because they need to and because of employment's social and psychological returns. Although financial reasons top the list when older workers are pressed to identify the *main* reason that they are now working or plan to work in retirement (AARP, 2003), non-pecuniary reasons are also important to the majority of older workers.

HEALTH STATUS AND WORK ABILITY

Age is a poor predictor of performance and work ability (Sterns & Huyck, 2001). Yet, many older persons leave the labor force because of health problems (Uccello, 1998). This suggests that, on the whole, the workforce left behind may be healthier and perhaps more productive than it would be if more retirees had chosen to keep working. If rising retirement ages, escalating medical costs, and inadequate retirement savings compel less-healthy preretirees to work longer, the average health status and productivity of the older workforce could deteriorate.

Are health impediments a barrier to prolonging the worklives of large numbers of Americans? The answer to this question may become clear if further increases in the retirement age are implemented in order to restore solvency to the Social Security system. Life expectancy has risen sharply over the past century, but years at work has not shown a comparable increase. Indeed, people worked considerably later in life when life expectancy was far shorter.

To what extent has rising life expectancy been accompanied by improved health status? Declining disability rates at upper ages (Manton & Gu, 2001) indicate that health status and greater work ability in old age have improved. Nonetheless, some potentially work-limiting conditions such as hypertension, heart disease, and diabetes rise with age and affect a sizable portion of the older population, as do hearing and vision impairments. The percentage of older persons reporting only fair or poor health has fallen, but more than one-fifth of persons aged 55 and over nonetheless maintain that their health is less than good (Schoenborn & Heyman, 2009).

Thus, the extent to which added years of life are healthy years becomes an important and relevant question as far as prolonging work is concerned. Munnell et al. (2008) estimate that, although life expectancy for 50-year-old men increased by 4.3 years from 1970 to 2000, *healthy* life expectancy – a measure of disability-free remaining years they developed using data in the NHIS – increased by somewhat less than three years. Moreover, this improvement was primarily associated with increased educational attainment. Large differences in healthy life expectancy by educational attainment exist. In 2000, college-educated white males at age 50 had a healthy life expectancy of 22.8 years; those with less than a high school education could expect only 13.3 more years of healthy life. What troubles Munnell and her colleagues is that improvement in educational attainment has plateaued. The proportion of 50-to-54-year-old men with high school diplomas and college degrees is expected to remain fairly stable for the next 20 years. If so, further improvements in healthy life expectancy are problematic.

Regardless of whether today's older persons are less healthy than those of a generation or more ago, at least as healthy, or perhaps healthier, health conditions today are being managed more effectively than in the past (Weir, 2007). Consequently, most older people probably could work longer than they now do. However, as Munnell et al. (2008) point out, "many of those who need to work longer – low-wage workers dependent on Social Security – are precisely the individuals who have onerous jobs that stress their health and lack the education to manage their care."

An aging workforce also raises questions about mental functioning. Aging is associated with some decline in cognitive ability, namely that involving what is known as "fluid knowledge" or flexibility in solving novel problems (Wegman & McGee, 2004). However, "crystallized knowledge," which is based on experience and thus accumulated over time, fails to show the same deterioration. It is also generally more evident among older workers than among younger workers.

One quarter of the workforce is projected to be aged 55 or older in 2018 (Toossi, 2009), and a growing number will be in their seventies or older. Some changes (e.g. enhanced crystallized knowledge) should make older workers increasingly valuable to their employers; other changes may impede their ability to perform certain jobs. For the most part, however, aging should not unduly affect ability to perform for, as Sterns and Huyck (2001) point out, most people remain "mentally competent with normal aging" and "most jobs do not require maximal mental or physical performance." Nevertheless, growth in the number and proportion of older workers means that "maintaining the health and safety of older workers will become increasingly challenging" (Wegman & McGee, 2004), a challenge that employers must be prepared to address to sustain the performance and productivity of their aging workforces.

THE CHANGING NATURE OF WORK AND ITS IMPLICATIONS FOR OLDER WORKERS

Physical vs Cognitive Job Demands

The nature of work has changed dramatically over the past century for workers of all ages. The country has moved from a largely agricultural economy to a manufacturing one to the knowledge-based society of today. This has had significant implications, both positive and negative, for older workers. In 1900, more than one-third of workers were employed in agriculture; by 2000 that was so for fewer than 3% (US Department of Commerce, 1975; US Department of Labor, 2001). With the shift to a knowledge-based, information economy, physically demanding jobs have declined. Few workers aged 50 and older today hold jobs that are highly physical, although nearly half of them are in occupations with some such demands, among them bending or twisting, kneeling or crouching, or standing (Johnson et al., 2007). At the same time, work is becoming more cognitively challenging.

Physical demands are not the only aspect of work that may make some jobs unappealing or intolerable. Many jobs are stressful, involve inflexible work schedules, and/or subject workers to difficult co-workers or customers, all of which can lessen the appeal of continued employment if other options are available.

Workers aged 50 and older have experienced sharper declines in physically demanding work than younger workers and steeper increases in stressful cognitively demanding work, according to Johnson et al. (2007), who contend that, if occupational growth trends continue as projected and if job attributes remain constant, job demands themselves should change little over the next 35 years. Should that be the case, the types of demands placed on workers by their jobs would not be that much different from – and certainly no worse than – today.

To the extent that people in physically demanding jobs retire earlier than other workers when they can afford to do so (Hayward et al., 1989), the decline in the proportion of arduous jobs should facilitate continued employment. However, stress and other job-related factors (such as inflexible work schedules) may foster early retirement even if the work is not physically taxing. More than one-third of older workers are in jobs requiring high cognitive ability. Cognitively demanding jobs that place significantly greater training/retraining demands on workers could, on the one hand, make work more stimulating and attractive and, on the other hand, continue to push workers into retirement at relatively early ages.

Keeping Workers Job-Ready

The global economy means that there is an expanding pool of available workers, which therefore increases the potential competition for workers in the US and underscores the need for continuous training and retraining, particularly in the emerging technologies that employers may require for their firms to remain viable. Declining job tenure for some age groups (US Department of Labor, 2008c), frequent job turnover (Johnson et al., 2009), and technological change also highlight a growing need for continuous training and retraining, or lifelong education. This is even more crucial in the case of older workers, whose formal training may have taken place decades ago. These workers may face continuing employer concerns about their trainability or the wisdom of training them near the end of their careers. Charness and Czaja (2006) point out that rapid technological developments and an accelerating pace of change in the workplace require repeated training not only in new systems but in new ways to do things; this may prove a challenge to aging workers, who have to keep up.

Recent research reveals considerable interest on the part of older workers in training (Towers Perrin, 2008), but it also indicates that those workers do not necessarily get as much training as wanted or needed. Not only do older workers seem to engage in less training, but their training is more likely to be informal compared to the training received by younger workers (Frazis et al., 1998).

The available evidence indicates that people can learn well into old age. However, physiological changes that occur with age, including declines in hearing, vision, and memory, could make learning new skills more taxing for older workers than for younger ones (Charness & Czaja, 2006). Moreover, older workers might take longer to master new skills (Charness & Czaja, 2006; Sterns & McDaniel, 1994), which could have implications for the development, implementation, and cost of training programs.

The good news is that productivity appears to be only weakly related to age. The bad news, however, is that there is a paucity of studies on training outcomes in the workplace (as opposed to laboratory or other non-work settings) for workers at upper ages. Additional research is needed on the effectiveness of various training techniques, particularly for the "oldest" segments of the older population, whose numbers are increasing but who have been underrepresented in both the workforce and in training studies to date.

Most job-training in the US is employer-provided. Older workers who require training to get a job, whether they are displaced workers or seeking to return to the labor force, have relatively few options unless they are able to pay for training themselves. Only one federal program, the Senior Community Service Employment Program, is focused exclusively on older worker training, and this is mainly a job placement program for economically disadvantaged persons aged 55 and over. The country's major training program, the Workforce Investment Act, has largely emphasized re-employment rather than the training or skills acquisition that might enable older workers, among others, to adapt better to a changing world of work.

AGE DISCRIMINATION IN EMPLOYMENT

In 1967, Congress enacted the Age Discrimination in Employment Act (ADEA), banning discrimination against workers aged 40 to 65 in all terms of employment. Subsequent amendments outlawed mandatory retirement before the age of 70 and ultimately eliminated it altogether. Legally, older workers are protected from age discrimination in employment, but they do not necessarily feel that they have escaped it. In 2007, for example, 6 out of 10 workers aged 45 to 74 maintained that they had either observed or been a victim of age discrimination in the workplace (AARP, 2008). It is unknown just how valid such observations are. Age discrimination is all but impossible to document, as few employers are going to admit that they engage in illegal behavior. Age discrimination may be especially difficult to detect in hiring, when the qualifications of competitors are likely not known. This may be one reason that age discrimination complaints involving terminations are much more common than those dealing with hirings among the charges filed with the Equal Employment Opportunity Commission (EEOC), the federal agency with jurisdiction to enforce the ADEA (Peeler, 2009).

The number of charges filed with the EEOC provides some indication of discriminatory behavior or perceptions of it; however, not all charges filed with the EEOC are deemed to offer sufficient evidence of discrimination. In addition, much age discrimination may go unrecognized or never lead to the filing of charges. Some sizable financial agreements and judgments against employers in age cases nevertheless underscore the reality of age discrimination for older workers (Neumark, 2008). In early 2010, for example, 165 older television scriptwriters resolved a class-action age discrimination suit against major networks, production studios, and talent agencies for $70 million.

The use of "testers" who apply for jobs supports claims that age discrimination is widespread and serves as a barrier to older workers in their search for employment (Bendick et al., 1999). Older job applicants are far less likely than younger applicants to make it through the screening process to an interview (Lahey, 2006).

In his assessment of the effectiveness of age discrimination laws, Neumark (2008) concludes that the ADEA probably does help older workers retain their jobs. It does not, however, seem to have helped them get hired. The law may even, in fact, have reduced the hiring of older workers because it has increased the costs of terminating them.

ACCOMMODATIONS FOR AN AGING WORKFORCE

Workplace Modifications

There is little evidence, outside of the field of health care, that many employers have done much to accommodate older workers (see Eyster et al., 2008). To be fair, however, if older workers are generally healthy it may not be clear what employers should be doing beyond ensuring a safe, clean, properly lit, and ergonomically correct work environment – which workers of all ages should have access to. Health and wellness information and preventive health programs might forestall or alleviate problems associated with some age-related conditions such as arthritis. Older workers in more physically demanding jobs might benefit from special equipment designed to ease some of the burdens or from work teams that can share them. Serious cognitive decline or early-onset Alzheimer's disease will confront some employers but will likely affect a small number of workers. On the whole, workplace modifications may best be handled on a case-by-case basis. Modifications could be greatly appreciated by older workers or they could be viewed as stigmatizing and consequently place employers at risk of lawsuits.

Workplace Flexibility

More flexible work arrangements, including opportunities to phase into full-time retirement from full-time work, might encourage employees – especially those who are no longer willing or able to work full time – to push back the date of retirement. Many older workers report that they would be interested in shifting to part-time work (AARP, 2004) or phasing into retirement (Mulvey & Nyce, 2005).

Despite the apparent interest in fewer hours and/or more flexibility – and the fact that older individuals are more likely than all but the youngest to work part time – the work hours of older workers have been increasing (Gendell, 2008). Seventy-eight percent of workers aged 55 or over were employed full time in 2008, an increase from 74% ten years earlier (US Department of Labor, 2010b).

Older workers who do manage to achieve more access to workplace flexibility seem to have to "pay" for it. Haider and Loughran (2001) found that workers who remained in the labor force after age 65 were better educated, healthier, and wealthier than their nonworking peers but had relatively low wages – perhaps, as the researchers speculated, because they were willing to (or had to) trade wages for flexibility. Older (aged 50-plus) career changers are apparently more likely to have flexible work schedules in their new jobs than in their old, but their wages are substantially lower and their benefits fewer (Johnson et al., 2009).

On the whole, most workers still lack access to workplace flexibility, and very few can telecommute (Hardy, 2008). Part-time employment is widespread, but much part-time work is low wage, with few benefits and often less-than-appealing duties. Formal phased retirement programs are rare, but informal and ad hoc arrangements that facilitate an easing into retirement are common (Hutchens, 2003). So, too, is the rehiring of retirees, which may also function as a form of gradual retirement. In their study of "re-careering" at later ages, Johnson et al. (2009) observed that older workers appear to have to change careers to get more workplace flexibility. It is unclear whether workers would be better off easing into retirement in the jobs that they have long held, but maintaining institutional knowledge would seem to be a benefit of phased retirement for their employers.

One goal of phased retirement is to keep people in the workforce longer. However, there is some concern that workers might instead scale back their work hours sooner if they are able to combine partial wages with partial retirement benefits. The result could be a later retirement age with no appreciable increase in time spent actually working (Munnell & Sass, 2008).

RECONCILING THE NEEDS OF WORKERS, EMPLOYERS, AND THE ECONOMY: TOWARD AN AGE-NEUTRAL WORKFORCE?

Many older workers contend that they want or need and expect to work in retirement, and a growing number seem to be doing just that. A further push may come from any Congressional action to increase the age of eligibility for full Social Security benefits beyond age 67, index benefit receipt to improvements in life expectancy, or add more work incentives or retirement disincentives to Social Security. More years at work would mean added earnings, additional opportunities to contribute to 401(k) plans, the possible replacement of zero- or very-low earning years under Social Security with higher-earning years, and fewer years to finance with retirement savings. All of

this points to a more financially secure retirement for workers. Prolonged employment would also be good for the economy. Delaying Social Security receipt beyond the presently established age of eligibility for full benefits could help restore the system's solvency. People with earnings pay more in taxes. Longer work lives on the part of experienced, dependable employees could be good for employers as well.

If labor and skills shortages begin to materialize, employers will do what is needed to attract and retain workers. Many of those workers will be older simply because population growth will be greatest for the older age groups. This pool of potential labor will be very diverse. The 55-year-old worker and the 75-year-old worker may both be "old" under the ADEA, but they will likely differ greatly in terms of interests, needs, and abilities. Potential employers will have to deal with these differences, as well as with those of much younger workers.

Reconciling the needs of various parties may not be all that difficult. If it takes more workplace modifications and flexibility, more phased retirement, or more and better-paying part-time jobs to attract and retain older workers, employers will respond with the necessary inducements. Many of these arrangements can also benefit younger workers. It is true that some impediments seem to stand in the way of employers offering certain programs such as formal phased retirement (e.g. Penner et al., 2002), so legislative action may be required in some instances.

With more workers deciding to remain longer in the labor force, employers will face the challenge of dealing with some workers who are no longer up to the job. Consistently applied performance evaluation systems for workers of all ages can help employers resolve this problem in ways that do not discriminate against older workers.

Most workers will eventually retire, and employers must look to the future to identify labor replacement needs and engage in succession planning. Employers thus cannot be truly age blind. Nor are workers themselves age blind – they do and will continue to make work and retirement decisions in response to their financial circumstances, family situations, health status, *and* advancing age.

ISSUES FOR FUTURE RESEARCH

Knowledge and understanding of employment and aging have benefited enormously from a growing body of research on older workers in recent years. However, there remain many issues for further research. For example,

- Under what circumstances are older workers pushing back the date of retirement, and how long are they likely to remain at work?

- Do workers who "re-career" voluntarily in later life remain in the workforce longer than those who do not re-career or who were pushed into changing careers as a result of job loss?
- How do bridge jobs and re-careering affect eventual retirement security?
- Who and how many of the preretirees who say they expect to work during their retirement years actually do so?
- Does phased retirement extend working life or does it encourage workers to reduce their work hours earlier than they otherwise would have?
- Does the type of phased retirement – scaling back with one's current employer, finding part-time work with another employer, or signing on with a temporary agency – make a difference?
- What are the implications of extended working lives for the performance, productivity, and health of the older labor force?
- What policies and programs facilitate the employment of older workers and encourage them to continue their working lives?

Even without employer or legislative efforts to keep more people at work for longer periods or additional research that enhances understanding of who pushes back the date of retirement, for how long, and under what circumstances, the workforce is projected to age substantially. With more older workers proving by example that they are capable, adaptable, and willing and able to learn new technology, doubts about these workers may dissipate, thus opening up even more opportunities for older individuals. Older workers may then simply be viewed as just another important component of an increasingly multigenerational workforce. In any case, "old age" and "employed" seem certain to remain paired for more years than in the recent past. And when one in four labor force participants is at least age 55, as can be expected by 2018, work may be something that does leap to mind when the subject of old age arises.

REFERENCES

Aaronson, S., Fallick, B., Figura, A., Pingle, J., & Wascher, W. (2006). The recent decline in the labor force participation rate and its implications for potential labor supply. *Brookings Papers on Economic Activity, 2006*(1), 69–134.

AARP (1995). *American business and older workers: A road map to the 21st century*. Washington, DC: AARP.

AARP (2003). *Staying ahead of the curve 2003: The AARP working in retirement study*. Washington, DC: AARP.

AARP (2004). *Baby boomers envision retirement: II*. Washington, DC: AARP.

AARP (2008). *Staying ahead of the curve 2007: The AARP work and career study*. Washington, DC: AARP.

AARP (2009). *The social compact in the twenty-first century*. Washington, DC: AARP.

Aspen Institute (2002). *Grow faster together. Or grow slowly apart*. Washington, DC: Aspen Institute Domestic Strategy Group. Retrieved December 3, 2002 from http://www.pwib.org/downloads/GrowFast.pdf.

Bendick, M., Brown, L. E., & Wall, K. (1999). No foot in the door: An experimental study of employment discrimination against older workers. *Journal of Aging & Social Policy, 10*(4), 5–23.

Blinder, A. S. (2006). Offshoring: The next industrial revolution? *Foreign Affairs, 85*, 113–128.

Brown, S. K. (2005). *American business and older employees: A focus on midwest employees*. Washington, DC: AARP.

Brown, S. K. (2009). *A year-end look at the economic slowdown's impact on middle-aged and older Americans*. Washington, DC: AARP.

Cahill, K. E., Giandrea, M. D., & Quinn, J. F. (2007). *Down shifting: The role of bridge jobs after career employment*. Issue Brief 06. Chestnut Hill, MA: The Center on Aging and Work/Workplace Flexibility at Boston College.

Cappelli, P. (2005). Will there really be a labor shortage? In M. Losey, S. Meisinger & D. Ulrich (Eds.), *The future of human resource management* (pp. 5–14). New York: John Wiley & Sons, Inc.

Charness, N., & Czaja, S. J. (2006). *Older worker training: What we know and don't know*. Washington, DC: AARP.

Coile, C., & Levine, P. B. (2009). *The market crash and mass layoffs: How the current economic crisis may affect retirement*. NBER Working Paper 15395. Cambridge, MA: National Bureau of Economic Research.

Costa, D. L. (1998). *The evolution of retirement*. Chicago: University of Chicago Press.

European Commission, Eurostat. (2010). Employment data: Employment rate of older workers by gender. Retrieved February 21, 2010 from http://epp.eurostat.ec.europa.eu/portal/page/portal/employment_unemployment_lfs/data/main_tables

Eyster, L., Johnson, R. W., & Toder, E. (2008). *Current strategies to employ and retain older workers*. Washington, DC: Urban Institute.

Figueroa, E. B., & Woods, R. A. (2007). Industry output and employment projections to 2016. *Monthly Labor Review, 130*(11), 53–85.

Fischer, D. H. (1978). *Growing old in America*. Oxford: Oxford University Press.

Frazis, H., Gittleman, M., Horrigan, M., & Joyce, M. (1998). Results from the 1995 survey of employer-provided training. *Monthly Labor Review, 121*(6), 3–13.

Freeman, R. B. (2006). *Is a great labor shortage coming? Replacement demand in the global economy.* NBER Working Paper 12541. Cambridge, MA: National Bureau of Economic Research.

Friedberg, L., & Webb, A. (2005). Retirement and the evolution of pension structure. *The Journal of Human Resources, 40*(2), 281–308.

Gendell, M. (2008). Older workers: Increasing their labor force participation and hours of work. *Monthly Labor Review, 131*(1), 41–54.

Giandrea, M. D., Cahill, K. E., & Quinn, J. F. (2007). *An update on bridge jobs: The HRS war babies.* BLS Working Paper 407. Washington, DC: U.S. Department of Labor, Bureau of Labor Statistics, Office of Productivity and Technology.

Goss, S. C. (2009). Applications for social security retired worker benefits in fiscal year 2009. Memo from the Chief Actuary of the Social Security Administration, May 28.

Haider, S., & Loughran, D. (2001). *Elderly labor supply: Work or play?* RAND Working Paper DRU-2582. Santa Monica, CA: RAND.

Hardy, M. (2008). *Making work more flexible: Opportunities and evidence. Insight on the Issues 11.* Washington, DC: AARP Public Policy Institute.

Hayward, M. D., Grady, W. R., Hardy, M. A., & Sommers, D. (1989). Occupational influences on retirement, disability, and death. *Demography, 26*(3), 393–409.

Helman, R., Mathew Greenwald & Associates, VanDerhei, J., & Copeland, C. (2008). *The 2008 Retirement Confidence Survey: Americans much more worried about retirement, health costs a big concern.* EBRI Issue Brief #316. Washington, DC: Employee Benefit Research Institute.

Hutchens, R. M. (2003). *The Cornell study of employer phased retirement policies: A report on key findings.* Ithaca, NY: Cornell University School of Industrial and Labor Relations.

Johnson, R. (2002). The puzzle of later male retirement. *Economic Review, Third Quarter*, 5–26.

Johnson, R. W., Mermin, G. B. T. & Resseger, M. (2007). *Employment at older ages and the changing nature of work.* Washington, DC: AARP.

Johnson, R. W., Kawachi, J., & Lewis, E. K. (2009). *Older workers on the move: Recareering in later life.* Washington, DC: AARP.

Karoly, L. A., & Zissimopoulos, J. (2004). *Self-employment and the 50+ population.* Washington, DC: AARP.

Lahey, J. (2006). *Age, women, and hiring: An experimental study.* CRR WP 2006-23. Chestnut Hill, MA: Center for Retirement Research at Boston College.

Laitner, J., & Silverman, D. (2007). *Life-cycle models: Lifetime earnings and the timing of retirement.* Working Paper 2007-165. Ann Arbor: University of Michigan Retirement Research Center.

Maestas, N. (2007). *Back to work: Expectations and realizations of work after retirement.* WR-196-2. Santa Monica, CA: RAND.

Manton, K. G., & Gu, X. (2001). Changes in the prevalence of chronic disability in the United States black and non-black population above age 65 from 1982 to 1999. *Proceedings of the National Academy of Sciences of the United States of America, 98*(11), 6354–6359.

Martin, L. G., Schoeni, R. F., Freedman, V. A., & Andreski, P. (2007). Feeling better? Trends in general health status. *The Journals of Gerontology: Social Sciences, 62B,* S11–S21.

Mulvey, J., & Nyce, S. (2005). Strategies to retain older workers. In R. L. Clark & O. S. Mitchell (Eds.), *Reinventing the retirement paradigm* (pp. 111–132). Oxford: Oxford University Press.

Munnell, A. H., & Sass, S. A. (2008). *Working longer: The solution to the retirement income challenge.* Washington, DC: Brookings Institution Press.

Munnell, A. H., Cahill, K. E., & Jivan, N. A. (2003). *How has the shift to 401(k)s affected the retirement age? An Issue in Brief 13.* Chestnut Hill, MA: Center for Retirement Research at Boston College.

Munnell, A. H., Soto, M., & Golub-Sass, A. (2008). *Will people be healthy enough to work longer?* CRR WP 2008-11. Chestnut Hill, MA: Center for Retirement Research at Boston College.

Neumark, D. (2008). *Reassessing the age discrimination in employment act.* Washington, DC: AARP.

Peeler, R. L. (2009). Comments presented at the National Council on Aging webinar, age discrimination and the economic downturn. Washington, DC: NCOA, July 21.

Penner, R. G., Peron, P., & Steuerle, E. (2002). *Legal and institutional impediments to partial retirement and part-time work by older workers.* Washington, DC: Urban Institute.

Quinn, J. F. (1999). *Retirement patterns and bridge jobs in the 1990s.* EBRI Issue Brief #206. Washington, DC: Employee Benefit Research Institute.

Rix, S. E. (2005). *Rethinking the role of older workers: Promoting older worker employment in Europe and Japan.* Issue Brief #77. Washington, DC: AARP Public Policy Institute.

Ruhm, C. J. (1990). Bridge jobs and partial retirement. *Journal of Labor Economics, 8*(4), 482–501.

Schirle, T. (2008). Why have the labor force participation rates of older men increased since the mid-1990s? *Journal of Labor Economics, 26*(4), 549–594.

Schoenborn, C. A., & Heyman, K. M. (2009). Health characteristics of adults aged 55 years and over: United States, 2004–2007. *National Health Statistics Reports 16.* Hyattsville, MD: National Center for Health Statistics.

Sherman, S. R. (1985). Reported reasons retired workers left their last job: Findings from the New Beneficiary Survey. *Social Security Bulletin, 48*(3), 22–30.

Steuerle, E., Sprio, C., & Johnson, R.W. (1999). *Can Americans work longer? Straight talk on Social Security and Retirement Policy, 5.* Washington, DC: Urban Institute.

Sterns, H. L., & Huyck, M. H. (2001). The role of work in midlife. In M. E. Lachman (Ed.), *Handbook of midlife development* (pp. 447–486). New York: John Wiley & Sons, Inc.

Sterns, H. L. & McDaniel, M. A. (1994). Job performance and the older worker. In S. E. Rix (Ed.), *Older workers: How do they measure* up? An overview of age differences in employee costs and performance. Washington, DC: AARP.

Toossi, M. (2009). Labor force projections to 2018: Older workers staying more active. *Monthly Labor Review, 132*(11), 30–51.

Towers Perrin (2008). *Investing in training 50+ workers: A talent management strategy.* Washington, DC: AARP.

Uccello, C. E. (1998). *Factors influencing retirement: Their implications for raising retirement age.* Washington, DC: AARP.

US Department of Commerce, Bureau of the Census (1975). *Historical statistics of the United States, colonial times to 1970, part 1.* Washington, DC: U.S. Government Printing Office.

US Department of Labor (2001). *Employment and earnings, 48*(1). Retrieved July 12, 2010 from http://www.bls.gov/opub/ee/empeam200901.pdf.

US Department of Labor (2008a). *Employment and earnings, 55*(1).

Retrieved July 12, 2010 from http://www.bls.gov/opub/ee/empearn200801.pdf

US Department of Labor, Bureau of Labor Statistics (2008b). Worker displacement, 2005–2007. *News* USDL 08-1183.

US Department of Labor, Bureau of Labor Statistics (2008c). Employee tenure in 2008. *News* USDL 08-1344.

US Department of Labor, Bureau of Labor Statistics (2009). *Employment and earnings, 56*(1). Retrieved February 5, 2010 from http://www.bls.gov/opub/ee/empearn200901.pdf.

US Department of Labor, Bureau of Labor Statistics (2010a). The employment situation – December 2009. *News* USDL-09-1583.

US Department of Labor, Bureau of Labor Statistics (2010b). Labor force statistics from the Current Population Survey. Retrieved February 7, 2010 from http://data.bls.gov/PDQ/outside.jsp?survey=ln.

US General Accounting Office (2003). *Older workers: Employment assistance focuses on subsidized jobs and job search, but revised performance measures could improve access to other services.* GAO-03-350. Washington, DC: US General Accounting Office.

Wegman, D. H., & McGee, J. P. (Eds.), (2004). *Health and safety needs of older workers.* Washington, DC: The National Academies Press.

Weir, D. R. (2007). Are baby boomers living well longer? In B. Madrian, O. S. Mitchell & B. J. Soldo (Eds.), *Redefining retirement: How will boomers fare?* (pp. 95–111). Oxford: Oxford University Press.

Yakoboski, P., & Dickemper, J. (1997). *Increased saving but little planning: Results of the 1997 Retirement Confidence Survey.* EBRI Issue Brief #191. Washington, DC: Employee Benefit Research Institute.

Chapter | 15 |

The Changing Residential Environments of Older People

Stephen M. Golant

Department of Geography, University of Florida, Gainesville, Florida

CHAPTER CONTENTS

THE INCREASING DEMANDS MADE OF THE RESIDENTIAL ENVIRONMENT

Older Americans are now asking more of their residential environments than at any time in history. They always hoped to live in affordable, safe, and comfortable places in good repair, where they could easily reach their workplaces, neighbors, friends, shopping, recreational pursuits, doctors, and places of prayer. Now many seek to be continually entertained and stimulated in residential settings such as planned active adult communities, intellectually inspired in university communities, and civically engaged in communities rich in social capital. Their most pressing and unquestionably ambitious demand, however, is to maintain as much *normalcy* as possible in their residential arrangements, even as they are afflicted with worsening chronic health conditions and debilitating declines in their physical and cognitive capabilities. This implies living in places where they experience overall pleasurable, hassle-free, memorable feelings and activities that have relevance to them; and where they feel both competent and in control – that is, they do not have to behave in personally objectionable ways or to unduly surrender mastery of their lives or environments to others.

Thus, it is hardly surprising that most older Americans have turned away from residential care settings that look, feel, or operate like nursing homes with their sterile and controlling medical-like environs. Rather, achieving residential normalcy usually means staying put in dwellings and neighborhoods that that they have occupied for a good part of their adult lives. But this means they are asking their residential environments to guarantee much more than

DOI: 10.1016/B978-0-12-380880-6.00015-0

an enjoyable lifestyle. Aging in place successfully has now become a far more complicated and ambitious quest. It requires that older persons cope with their chronic health problems and impairments by proactively introducing into their dwellings some combination of physical or structural modifications, assistive devices, medical monitoring, diagnostic and home security technologies, and personal assistance and care solutions, either from family members or paid workers (Golant, 2009). It requires that they live in neighborhoods and communities with independence-supporting and health-related services that enable them to cope with their vulnerabilities and maintain their autonomy. Conventional places of residence must offer more than the shelter and amenities that are appropriate for active, healthy, and functionally intact older occupants. They must also help their older occupants compensate for the effects of their chronic health problems, physical and cognitive limitations, and absent social supports.

What a vast literature on the appropriateness of residential environments tells us, however, is that, except for their disdain for institutional settings, older people are open to aging in place in many different residential settings. There is no one-size-fits-all set of optimum residential activities, experiences, and situations. Normalcy is very much an individual affair. A growing number of elders are discovering that they feel comfortable, secure, and independent in less familiar residential variants, known as NORC (naturally occurring retirement community) supportive service programs, elder villages, cohousing communities, and in places that have been made especially "livable" or "healthy" for seniors. A small but growing number of older persons have turned to the more supportive and residential-like environments of planned senior housing options, such as independent living communities (aka congregate housing), assisted living, and continuing care retirement communities (Golant, 2008c).

The private sector has capitalized on these demands for residential normalcy by older people. Service providers have greatly increased their home modification and care offerings (Golant, 2008c). Home-based technologies are now pitched as "a tool that helps a person with disabilities to accomplish activities or get the support they need and want" (Kutzik et al., 2008, p. 224). The insurance industry has created more comprehensive and flexible long-term-care insurance products with coverage in both conventional homes and assisted living (Doty, 2008). Financial institutions have created reverse mortgages so that older homeowners can receive a reliable cash income stream from the equity in their dwellings (Foote, 2007). And senior housing developers now offer many varieties of residential care settings for less independent elders.

Many public sector stakeholders also now believe that they can reduce their long-term care expenditures when they satisfy these normalcy needs. The Medicaid program now gives state governments more opportunities and incentives to offer community-based long-term care programs affordable for lower-income seniors wanting to stay put (Doty, 2008). The Older Americans Act has created State Aging and Disability Resource Centers (single point of entry information and referral centers) and the National Family Caregiver Support Program offers caregiver counseling, training, and respite care. Owners or sponsors of publicly subsidized and affordable multi-unit rental housing projects are relying on multiple service strategies to bring health and supportive services to their low-income seniors (Golant, 2008a).

Presented with these aging-in-place possibilities, older persons are now questioning once-taken-for-granted assumptions about where they live. As a poignant example, residents of continuing care retirement communities who recognize the feasibility of their aging in place in their independent quarters are rebelling against managements who are demanding that they move to their assisted living sections. They fear that, by moving to the next "level," they would be identified as "needy" or "dying," thus threatening their self-worth (Shippee, 2009) – even as enabling this residential transition has been the raison d'être for this type of senior housing.

As conventional residential environments have become fulcrums of care delivery, a smaller share of older persons have occupied nursing homes (Doty, 2008). However, even these venerable establishments are evolving. Nursing homes known by such labels as the Eden Alternative and Green Houses are now attempting to shed their institutional image by modifying their physical settings and operations to more resemble our contemporary assisted-living residences (Calkins & Keane, 2008; Rabig et al., 2006).

These new aging-in-place realities are not occurring without downsides. Studies now reveal that older persons sometimes live in inhospitable dwellings with physical features and designs that are incongruent with their functional limitations or in neighborhoods that lack needed services and are inaccessible to key destinations. There is more evidence of older adults receiving poor-quality care, and sometimes being abused by their family caregivers (Golant, 2008b).

A large and multidisciplinary literature is now focusing on the aging-in-place capabilities and downsides of older people's residential environments, the potential of different residential transformations, the feasibility of environmental interventions, and the difficulties of achieving residential normalcy in places that are responsible for the care of more vulnerable older people. All these studies agree that judgments concerning older persons aging successfully are increasingly less credible if they do not consider the role played by their place of residence. They also share the belief that their findings can contribute to positive changes. They assume that the residential settings of older people can be changed or modified to achieve better outcomes. To examine these issues, this chapter focuses on three broad categories of residential environments: dwelling or home environments; neighborhood and community environments; and the planned residential care environments of assisted-living facilities.

DWELLING OR HOME ENVIRONMENTS

The Physical Environment as a Risk Factor

The longer durations of dwelling occupancy of older persons – especially by the eight out of ten who are homeowners – increase the likelihood that they occupy older buildings (Golant, 2008d). In 2007, about 73% of owners and 68% of renters lived in dwellings built before 1980 and about 22% of both groups lived in dwellings built before 1950 (US Census Bureau, 2008). Thus, older persons must sometimes cope with threats to their residential normalcy resulting from the aging of their dwellings. Older buildings are more likely to have equipment or structural components that are technologically or stylistically obsolete or to have simply worn out. They may have, for example, outdated and inefficient lighting, poor insulation, deteriorated wood siding, hard-to-open windows, water leaks, impractical room designs, and inefficient heating and cooling systems (Golant, 2008d). These are not inevitable consequences of aging dwellings, but older persons are less likely than younger occupants to perform routine home maintenance or make structural improvements (Davidoff, 2004). Lower-income older persons in particular have difficulties because large expenditures are often necessary to eliminate these deficiencies. Finding reliable, affordable, and honest professional labor is also challenging. Older persons may also be less motivated to make costly changes because they have shorter remaining lifespans to enjoy any returns on their investment and because of expectations that the values of their dwellings will not appreciate greatly in the future.

Failure to remedy such physical inadequacies may simply result in less energy-efficient, comfortable, usable, or physically attractive living situations. But these defects also increase their risk of negative health outcomes, such as hypothermia or hyperthermia, environmental and mold allergies, and breathing problems because of poor air quality.

Even if dwellings do not suffer from these problems, however, they will often be incompatible with older occupants because architects designed them for a younger and more able population of consumers.

Although the Rehabilitation Act of 1973 (Section 504) required housing constructed with public funds to have accessible dwelling units and the Fair Housing Amendments Act of 1988 required that all new multi-family housing must be accessible to mobility-limited persons, the single-family structures occupied by most older households are exempt from these requirements. Consequently, older persons may confront various environmental barriers: difficult-to-use stairs to access a dwelling's front door or its second floor, narrow door poorly located electrical and plumbing controls, and shelves and cupboards out of easy reach. Their dwellings also may contain potential walking and tripping hazards: poor or inadequate lighting, slippery and high-gloss floor surfaces, uneven paths and surfaces, clutter, wires and cables, poorly place furniture or throw rugs; and inadequate physical supports, such as grab bars and hand rails (Iwarsson et al., 2006; Pynoos et al., 2006).

Environmental Gerontology: Linking Theory with Practice

Several studies by environmental gerontologists in the US and Europe over the past decade have focused on these environmental problems and have assessed the effectiveness of different types of dwelling- or home-based solutions (Gitlin, 2003; Iwarsson, 2003; Oswald et al., 2007a). Research conducted in five European countries between 2002 and 2004 by a Lund University occupational science team (the ENABLE-AGE Project) focused on how to make the home environments of older residents with vision difficulties or lower and upper body limitations more "accessible" and "usable," as measured by their activity performance (Carlsson et al., 2009). In the US, Gitlin (2003) has conducted research on home environments to evaluate strategies designed to reduce environmental barriers and dwelling-based accidents, and to increase the capacity of older people to live independently for longer.

The overarching aim of these studies has been to optimize the fit or congruence between aging persons and their physical-social environments (Iwarsson et al., 2007; Scheidt & Windley, 2006; Wahl & Oswald, 2009) and they are typically guided by Lawton's (1998) ecological (or competence-press) theory of aging. He argued that older people's behavioral outcomes and psychological well-being depend not just on the demands or stresses of their external worlds, but also on their level of competence (that is, biological health, sensory and motor skills, and cognitive functioning). As Diehl and Willis (2003, p. 130) generalize, "competent behavior in everyday life always reflects the confluence, or interaction, of personal and environmental factors and focuses on individuals' abilities to adapt to the challenges of different environmental conditions." The ENABLE-AGE researchers, for example, introduced the concept of "accessibility" to denote person–environment (P–E) fit: "that is the relationship between a person's functional capacity and the prevalence of physical environmental barriers in the home" (Nygren et al., 2007, p. 86). Thus, for older people with arthritic hands, turning a faucet is an *inaccessible* behavior only when it is poorly designed.

Practical Applications: Reducing Home Accidents and Mobility Limitations

Annually, about one-third of adults aged 65 and older fall, with the incidence of episodes being higher among the very old (Centers for Disease Control and Prevention, 2008). Injuries mostly occur in or around the outside of their dwellings and nearly one-third of those who fall subsequently need help with their everyday self-care or IADLs (Pynoos et al., 2006; Schiller et al., 2007). Even minor injuries can be psychologically devastating because they increase fears of falling, thereby leading to reduced activities, depression, and social isolation.

Researchers and practitioners have argued that these falling accidents are more probable when older persons occupy dwellings with the environmental hazards described earlier. Establishing causality, however, is far more difficult because there are so many individual risk factors, including disorders of the sensory–nervous or musculoskeletal systems (e.g. gait and balance disorders), the effects of various acute and chronic diseases, and medication side-effects (Pynoos et al., 2006; Wahl et al., 2009). The activities and personalities of older persons also matter. Paradoxically, it is not always the more vulnerable who fall more frequently, but rather those engaged in more vigorous dwelling-related tasks such as housework, gardening, and home repairs, or who have more risk-taking or impulsive personalities (Chan et al., 2007).

This multifaceted etiology helps explain why home assessment intervention strategies designed to reduce fall-related outcomes often have inconsistent results. However, environmental interventions designed more generally to help older people compensate for their mobility limitations have produced more compelling results. These are most successful when they target older people with a history of falls, mobility limitations, and depressive symptoms, and when they are environment-targeted; for example, focused only on bathroom hazards (Salminen et al., 2009; Wahl et al., 2009). Outcomes are also better for older persons with internal locus of control personalities, who perceive they have more control over their behaviors and environments (Oswald et al., 2007b).

The quality and scope of home intervention strategies are also key. Better outcomes result from using trained professionals and multiple types of interventions (e.g. comprehensive assessments, dwelling modifications, participant instruction and guidance, balance and muscle strengthening exercises, and fall recovery strategies). The multifaceted ABLE (Advancing Better Living for Elders) occupational and physical therapy intervention conducted by Gitlin et al. (2009) reduced the functional difficulties of the occupants and their fear of falling, increased their self-efficacy, and, most notably, reduced their 3.5-year mortality rates.

NEIGHBORHOOD AND COMMUNITY ENVIRONMENTS

Multiple Influences of Older People's Neighborhoods

A growing number of studies, especially by epidemiologists and sociologists, have focused on how the neighborhood environments of older people can account for reported variations in their mobility levels and activities and their physical, mental, or functional health (Krause, 2003; Northridge et al., 2003). They argue that the functional limitations and more restricted transportation options of older people result in their spending more time (with more exposure) in their neighborhoods and put them at greater risk of being adversely affected by their poor physical, social, or economic conditions or inadequate supportive services. These investigations are often framed by the sociomedical model of disability – the Disablement Process (Freedman et al., 2008). Disablement encompasses how the chronic and acute health conditions of individuals affect their "abilities to act in necessary, usual, expected and personally desired ways in their society" (Verbrugge & Jette, 1994, p. 3). These limitations make it more difficult for individuals to perform their physical and/or mental actions. Disabilities only result, however, when their physical settings, assistive devices and social supports do not mediate or compensate for their limitations.

These studies have consistently found that poor neighborhood conditions of older people are significantly correlated with their restricted activities and poorer health. After controlling for individual-level risk factors, however, they offer mixed findings regarding neighborhood effects and their statistical associations become weaker, insignificant, and/or are only applicable to individuals with certain individual attributes.

Various methodological challenges complicate the interpretations of these findings:

- the possibilities of omitting, misinterpreting, or confounding individual-level (e.g. demographic) and contextual (i.e. neighborhood or community) effects (Oakes, 2004);

- the dangers of overemphasizing objective environmental indicators (e.g. police-reported crime rates) as opposed to respondents' subjective interpretations (e.g. fear of crime) (Clark et al., 2009);
- the difficulties of disentangling dwelling and neighborhood effects;
- the questionable validity of relying on small-area data units, such as census tracts and their aggregated data, as proxies of neighborhood;
- the possibility that cross-sectional (as opposed to longitudinal) research designs fail to capture a neighborhood's effects over time (Basta et al., 2008; Glass & Balfour, 2003; Golant, 2003).

Neighborhood Influences on Activities and Mobility Levels

When older people cannot drive, their ability to use walking pathways and transit routes becomes more important – even as these modes of transportation represent very small shares of their total travel. Older people who occupy less population-dense neighborhoods dominated by residential as opposed to mixed (with commercial) land uses, and that have less reliable public transit, poorer quality walking environments, and poorer street connectivity (e.g. cul-de-sac streets) have more difficulty accessing needed goods and services (Beard et al., 2009a; Clarke et al., 2008; Yeom et al., 2008). They also walk less in unsafe and physically neglected neighborhoods such as those with trash, litter, and crumbling sidewalks (Mendes de Leon et al., 2009).

Certain groups of older persons are more disadvantaged: those living alone without spouses or other family who can provide transportation; those without driver licenses, such as older ethnic and racial minorities and lower-income women over age 75; those in their eighties and above of both genders with age-related visual, cognitive, or psychomotor function declines; and those living in states with more stringent driver licensing standards for older persons. A significant share of our future older baby boom will be at risk of being transportation-challenged because they will live in auto-dependent suburban locations (Golant, 2008b).

Neighborhood Influences on Health

Studies have linked the cognitive declines and depressive symptoms of older occupants with their occupancy of socioeconomically disadvantaged places and their chronically stressful and fearful conditions. These places have more social disorders, such as crime and drug use, and physical problems, such as vandalized, abandoned, and rundown buildings

(Krause, 2003). They are more likely to be occupied by less-educated and lower-income populations and higher concentrations of minorities (Basta et al., 2008; Beard et al., 2009b; Sheffield & Peek, 2009). Their older occupants have poorer access to supportive or stimulating physical resources (e.g. parks, gyms, bookstores, libraries, well-lit walkways) and social resources (e.g. social clubs, neighborhood organizations) (Beard et al., 2009b; Krause, 2003). They have a "high toleration for illness which stems from untreated chronic conditions […] elevated exposure to hazards, and limited coping strategies, generating widespread cognitive deficits" (Wight et al., 2006, p. 1076), and weaker collective efficacy – a type of social capital implying trusting and helpful social, professional, and institutional networks (Bowling & Stafford, 2007; Cagney et al., 2005). Older people cope less effectively with these deficient environments when they are more socially isolated or have more unpleasant social interactions, which results in less adequate or protective "stress-buffering support systems" (Beard et al., 2009b, p. 1). On the other hand, the stable support of a marital partner can mitigate their psychological distress (Bierman, 2009), and neighborhoods with ethnically homogeneous older populations (e.g. Mexican Americans) can confer a protective effect and contribute to their occupants' reduced depressive symptoms (Ostir et al., 2003).

Living in socioeconomically disadvantaged neighborhoods also contributes to the poor self-rated physical health and greater self-rated health declines of older adults, particularly black and Mexican American minorities (Cagney et al., 2005; Patel et al., 2003; Yao & Robert, 2008). In contrast, more economically advantaged or affluent neighborhoods have "the capacity to mobilize on behalf of a health-enhancing and health protective environment" (Cagney et al., 2005, p. 187). Older people living in disadvantaged areas also have higher chances of experiencing limitations in their lower body functioning (Freedman et al., 2008). In particular, they are more likely to be obese when they occupy neighborhoods with higher densities of fast food outlets, lower mixed land uses, lower street connectivity, and a greater prevalence of social problems (Grafova et al., 2008; Li et al., 2008).

Optimizing the Neighborhoods or Communities Occupied by Seniors

What is Different?

We can identify four neighborhood or community exemplars that are designed to make it more feasible for older persons to age in place, although studies have yet to rigorously assess the extent to which these are successful solutions. These include:

(1) elder-friendly, livable, healthy, or life-long communities;
(2) NORCs linked with supportive services (NORC-SSPs);
(3) elder villages; and
(4) cohousing communities.

The first three make it easier for their older occupants to access independence-supporting and health-related services; the fourth additionally offers them an especially supportive social situation. They all share three characteristics. First, these residential environments do not substantially differ from those occupied by older persons throughout their adult lives; second, the older occupants make their own choices regarding the extent of their participation; and third, the catalyst for these reinvented neighborhoods are the needs of a *place's* older population for a more supportive physical or social environment. The focus is on the risk factors of a *residential enclave* rather than that of an *individual*. This is a fine distinction, but an important one. Most federal- or state-sponsored service programs attempt to identify the assistance needs of older individuals rather than of geographically defined population aggregations.

Elder-Friendly, Livable, Healthy, or Life-Long Communities

A growing number of local governments and philanthropic groups in the US are making their communities more compatible with the needs of their financially and physically vulnerable older persons. They are known by such labels as "friendly," "livable," "healthy," or "life-long" communities. Their broad mission is to help their older residents to age in place more affordably, safely, and independently in their current dwellings or in close-by locations. Implementation typically involves a governmental jurisdiction (a city, town, municipality, county, planning/service area, or health authority) or community nonprofit organization assessing the readiness of a place's programs and services to support the health and assistance needs of their elderly residents and then formulating an action plan (Alley et al., 2007).

One exemplar, the Advantage Initiative, developed by the Visiting Nurse Service of New York (Feldman et al., 2003), had the following goals:

- address basic population needs (e.g. affordable housing, safety, service information);
- optimize physical and mental health and well-being (e.g. access to preventive health services and medical, social, and palliative services);
- maximize independence (e.g. accessible transportation, support from family and other caregivers);
- promote social and civic engagement (e.g. involvement in community life, opportunities for meaningful paid and voluntary work);
- make aging issues a community-wide priority.

These community responses are also taking place globally. The WHO's (2007, p. 5) idea of an "age-friendly city" builds on its "active ageing framework," which it emphasizes is not just about "healthy aging," but depends also on the material conditions (the physical environment) and social circumstances that "surround individuals, families, and nations." As many as 40 cities internationally have used it as a program framework. The "policies, services, settings and structures" of the WHO's (2007, p. 5) age-friendly city are very similar to those of the Advantage Initiative.

Deciding on what localities are the best candidates for these programs has been somewhat haphazard, however, and currently no consensus even exists as to what constitutes a "community." Somewhat paradoxically, given the emphasis of academic research, neighborhoods are infrequently the geographic focus. One explanation is that most rural and suburban neighborhoods rarely offer the totality of goods, services, or activities likely to benefit less-independent older persons. Nor do neighborhoods usually have the jurisdictional or political power to introduce needed resources. Thus, in larger and politically organized geographic jurisdictions – such as counties, cities, towns, or planning districts – "social capital may be better able to undertake collective action to combat population health threats, and to provide health-promoting public goods for its residents, such as health care" (Kim et al., 2006, p. 1046).

Advocates also rarely offer evidence that the most vulnerable older persons with the most demanding dwelling or neighborhood problems occupy the communities adopting "livable" goals. Rather, the catalysts for these programs seem to have more to do with the efforts of innovative, knowledgeable, and aggressive grass-roots organizers. Leadership qualities – social capital – rather than environmental problem assessments are driving these programmatic efforts.

Naturally Occurring Retirement Community–Supportive Service Programs (NORC–SSPs)

A NORC consists of a building, or cluster of buildings, mostly high-rise rental complexes multi-unit buildings owned as cooperatives or condominiums, but also neighborhood clusters of single-family and low-rise multi-family dwellings. They are occupied by relatively large concentrations of older adults who moved in at a younger age and then simply stayed, or by older persons who moved in recently (Hunt & Gunter-Hunt, 1985). Typically, they are not publicly subsidized, but tend to be affordable to working and middle-class seniors. A product of unplanned demographic influences rather than imposed age restrictions, NORC buildings are usually indistinguishable from other residences and are rarely designed or retrofitted to accommodate the limitations of their older occupants (Ormond et al., 2004).

NORC–SSPs are NORCs that also benefit from an organized program of community-based supportive services and health care to help their residents age in place. The first ones appeared in New York City in the late 1980s and United Jewish Communities launched them as a national initiative in 2001. They are now found throughout the US (Vladeck, 2008). The program participation of their residents is voluntary and they have more say in their operation than seniors in other care settings. Moody (2008, p. 8) observes that these programs generally respond to "middle-class people who are not sick enough for Medicare, who have too much income for Medicaid services, and who are not rich enough for private individual care." Some places, however, will have larger concentrations of poor residents than others.

Many NORCs do not participate in these supportive service programs because they are not top-heavy with very old residents or have not self-defined themselves as having a population in need. Others believe their participation in an SSP would stigmatize their building as a "nursing home" or as a dwelling for charity cases. Still others are in communities that do not have the leadership or service infrastructure to mount such a program.

In some NORCs, the initiative for program participation comes from the building's residents or their condominium or cooperative board, which see the benefits of an organized delivery of health-related and independence-supporting services. In other instances, the catalyst is an assessment by an outside community-based nonprofit aging services organization (often with religious or ethnic affiliations). Typically, a housing development or a neighborhood group partners with a lead organization – a social service or health care provider (from the aging network) – to offer an array of supportive and health-related services. A network of contracted service providers performs individual needs assessments, offer information and referrals, provide program oversight, and arrange and coordinate the delivery of services, which may include case management, preventive health screening and chronic care management, meals, transportation, personal care, financial/legal counseling, home modifications, and educational/recreational activities. Residents often function in an advisory capacity or volunteer their assistance to others who require escort, monitoring, transportation, and other non-licensed services.

NORC–SSPs allow vendors, merchants, and care agencies to offer a more comprehensive and coordinated package of services more regularly and less expensively (lower per-unit cost). A single management organization (rather than multiple older consumers) arranges for service delivery and providers enjoy economies-of-scale benefits by offering services to a sizable cluster of older residents with comparable needs. For example, the transportation costs of a social worker visiting a single building are the same whether she sees one or multiple residents, but on a per-client basis are obviously less in the latter instance. She can also see more residents, and in more flexible time slots, than if she traveled to geographically dispersed clients.

NORC–SSP programs rely on funding from multiple sources including the general revenues of state and local government, the Older Americans Act, nonprofit charitable organizations, private philanthropic contributions, building owners/management firms, and, less frequently, resident fees (Ormond et al., 2004).

Elder Villages – The Beacon Hill Prototype

Beacon Hill is an upscale neighborhood in a historic downtown district of Boston. A core group of long-time civic-minded residents recognized that they needed various supportive and health-related services to make independent living more feasible and so organized Beacon Hill Village as a nonprofit membership organization in 2002. Whereas outside stakeholders play a central role in the initiation and operation of NORC-SSPs, "intentional communities" like Beacon Hill are more of a grass-roots neighborhood-based effort. Compared with NORC–SSPs, the residents have stronger leadership roles and greater responsibility for organizing and running the program. It now has about 460 members ranging in age from 51 to 99 (average age is the early seventies). Members pay an annual membership charge set by the village's Board of Directors ranging from $500 to $1000 per household. The poorest members may pay lower rates. Resident dues account for about half of the village's budget with the other half covered by foundations and nonprofit groups. This service organization model (with variations) has been widely replicated throughout the country.

The umbrella organization sees itself as a consolidator of existing community services. On the request of its resident members (emphasizing a consumer-driven philosophy), it offers information about a wide range of services relying on a prescreened list of providers and partnerships with outside service and health care organizations. The residents can also rely on a group of staff members (e.g. geriatric social workers, nurses) screened and employed by the organization, who respond to their requests for services and who can talk them through problems (Gross, 2006). Their dues cover a select group of limited services such as information and referral, assistance with grocery shopping, discounts from service providers, rides for medical appointments, and group exercise and walking classes. They receive most services from outside vendors at discounted prices (e.g. taxicabs, food providers, cleaning, cooking, geriatric care management, handyman services, home inspections, and home health care services).

The village model appears to work best when there is not only a critical mass of residents with similar needs – which allows for volume purchasing and service discounts – but when the residents are well-educated and have the ability to function as leaders. This is because, unlike most NORC–SSPs, the initiative for services typically comes from the residents rather than the organizations that provide the social services (Moody, 2008).

Cohousing Communities

Senior cohousing communities are custom-designed neighborhoods that nurture a strong sense of social community and thus share some of the qualities of traditional small towns and villages. They are occupied by a very self-selected group of persons (over the age of 50) who often know each other very well even before occupying their new homes because they were earlier friends or members of the same organization. Moreover, they have typically spent their prior two to three years in multiple planning sessions together, deciding (often in deliberations with a developer) how their community will look, operate, and support their preferred way of life. They have a common goal: "to recreate an old-fashioned neighborhood that supports friendly cooperation, socialization, and mutual support" (Durrett, 2009, p. 5).

Cohousing communities originated in Denmark in the late 1960s, but those dedicated for seniors were built only in the late 1980s. Most of the 250 cohousing developments – existing or in development – in the US are also predominantly intergenerational. The first US senior developments were not built here until 2005; e.g. Glacier Circle in Davis, California (Durrett, 2009).

Senior cohousing communities are compact developments typically consisting of 15 to 30 attached single-family dwellings (although as few as 9 in at least one instance) tightly arranged along a pedestrian street or clustered around a courtyard in a very residential-like setting. The dwellings and their lots are typically smaller than those found in new construction generally. Residents usually own their houses as condominiums, but may also rent. The architectural design of the cohousing development – its buildings and site layout – is intended to ensure the safety of the residents and maximize their visual participation and social interactions, even as it also satisfies their needs for privacy.

An integral component of a cohousing development is its "common house." This detached single-family dwelling functions as the hub of their common activities, such as group meals, workshop and hobby activities, fitness classes, and all types of social gatherings. It specifically contains large guest rooms or apartments to accommodate family or hired caregivers.

The residents of a cohousing community enjoy living in a very close-knit community where they never have to feel isolated or alone, where they participate in group-organized everyday activities (e.g. meals, social gatherings), and share responsibilities for their community's management and maintenance. The division of labor, however, "is based on what each person feels he or she can fairly contribute. No one person, however, dominates the decisions or the community-building process, and no one person should become excessively taxed by the process" (Durrett, 2009, p. 27). They are empowered to make this residential arrangement whatever they want it to be.

Although not usually affordable to the poor, cohousing communities are priced competitively with other comparable housing developments. Moreover, their overall upkeep and maintenance costs tend to be lower because of their smaller size, typically well-designed energy-efficient dwellings, and, "by cooperating on upkeep and by pooling their resources, cohousers reduce some of their cost-of-living expenses, including those involved in hiring and housing outside caregivers" (Durrett, 2009, p. 32).

Cohousing arrangements appear able to accommodate older persons who require a safe and secure place to live, need help during a short-term medical or illness episode, and who will not be alone in a crisis situation such as a falling accident or medical emergency. These developments typically follow the Principles of Universal Design (Center for Universal Design, 2006) to ensure their buildings and sites are accessible to those with functional limitations.

This option may also be well suited to older persons who only require light care, such as meal preparation, transportation assistance, and help with housekeeping, shopping, and laundry. What share of the residents will need this assistance at any given time much depends on the community's initial age composition, which in turn will reflect decisions by its first occupants.

How well these cohousing communities will accommodate older persons with more severe functional limitations or cognitive declines is unclear. Much will depend on how a given community's residents feel about serving as caregivers or accommodating hired workers. They must agree about how they will cope with a very disabled older resident and the issue of "when does someone become too sick to remain?" And this will "all depend on the group and their individual and collective sensibilities" (Durrett, 2009, p. 199).

LONG-TERM CARE ARRANGEMENTS AS RESIDENTIAL SETTINGS

Assisted Living: Integrating Planned Residential and Care Environments

Assisted living facilities in the US showcase the challenges of achieving residential normalcy in a setting that also offers long-term care. On entry, occupants have an average age of just under 85 (Assisted Living Federation of America, 2009). They often suffer from multiple physical or cognitive deficits, chronic illnesses, and sometimes depressive symptoms. Higher percentages of the residents now also have dementia (such as Alzheimer's disease), requiring them to be housed in a separate wing or floor that has extra security because of their wandering or disruptive behaviors (Hyde et al., 2008).

Forty-three states and the District of Columbia now license or statutorily label over 38 000 facilities with a total of almost one million units/beds as assisted living. They include "virtually every type of group residential care on the continuum between home care and nursing homes" (Mollica et al., 2007, p. 1-1) – residential care facilities, adult or personal care homes, board and care, homes for the aged, adult foster care, and retirement homes.

This diversity makes it difficult to generalize either about the residential or care qualities of assisted living. Some operate in freestanding buildings, while others are part of a larger building or campus complex that includes an independent living community or a nursing home. Although some look more like vacation resorts, others resemble boarding houses or dormitories. They have different rules regarding physical infrastructure requirements, the care requirements of the residents they can admit or retain, and their operating and service procedures (Golant, 2004).

As long as they meet their state's minimum requirements, providers also have discretion regarding how their facilities look and operate and the frailty levels of their elder residents. This may reflect when their properties were built – that is, what was once fashionable, marketable, and financially feasible; whether they are owned by families, nonprofit-organizations, or are part of large corporate chains; and whether they are occupied by the very affluent or Medicaid-eligible residents (Doty, 2008).

The Ideal Residential Environment and its Quality of Care Tradeoffs

Many proponents of assisted living argue that these facilities should ideally subscribe to the core values of a social model of care or service philosophy – or person-centered care approach – as opposed to the medical model practiced in nursing homes (Kane, 2001; Polivka & Salmon, 2008). Consequently, they should have the physical design, scale, comfort, and social ambience of the conventional home; eliminate "institution-like paraphernalia" (Calkins & Keane, 2008, p. 115); and guarantee the safety, security, and good-quality care of their residents without infringing on their privacy, autonomy, and individuality (Cutler, 2007; Regnier, 2002).

Advocates argue that private rooms and bathrooms, individual room temperature controls, and locking doors are essential, and care settings should avoid "long corridors, drab and utilitarian materials, furnishings, fixtures, and décor" (Kane & Cutler, 2009, p. 18). Stakeholders in the assisted living industry, however, do not all agree on the feasibility of a social model of care. Critics retort that requiring assisted living providers to offer only private single-occupancy apartments would discriminate against lower- or moderate-income elders (seeking more affordable shared accommodations) and "would have very little impact on quality" (US Senate Special Committee on Aging, 2003, p. 14).

They also argue that implementing a social model can threaten the quality of care. The operators of a small family-owned board and care residence, for example, might offer a more congenial residential environment, but may not have the financial resources to hire the best-trained staff or to install the most technologically sophisticated monitoring devices that would lead to better resident assessments and safety outcomes (Carder et al., 2008; Zimmerman et al., 2008). Even as rules may result in less resident autonomy and satisfaction – such as what or when to eat or drink, or when to sleep or participate in community activities – they also can assure good-quality care. Thus, allowing the diabetic resident to have a less restrictive diet and respecting the privacy of the physically impaired resident who wants to shower alone may result in bad outcomes.

Both the quality of life and care of residents will depend on the qualifications, experience, and training of the staff. They influence whether residents can satisfy their self-care needs, and also whether they are treated as the "faceless old" as opposed to "paying customers" with individual wants, purchasing powers, and consumer rights (Wylde, 2008, p. 191).

A stable group of employees is also important, but assisted living facilities have average annual staff turnover rates of 42% (Sikorska-Simmons,

2005). Both good-quality care and residential satisfaction are more likely with a less changeable staffing environment. High staff turnover saps a setting of experienced and trained workers and disrupts the continuity of supportive staff–resident relationships. Along with the effects of high-quality service, resident satisfaction is also higher when staff persons have "good interpersonal skills and a warm and friendly personality" (Mitchell & Kemp, 2000, p. 125). Less obviously, favorable reports by residents have been attributed to their deference to the staff and the fear of retribution (Beel-Bates et al., 2007).

In addition, family members will be influential in at least three ways. First, they can "supplement or supplant" (Gaugler & Kane, 2007, p. 83) various types of instrumental care provided by assisted living staff (e.g. laundry, cleaning, grooming, and participating in doctor's visits); second, they can function as resident advocates by expressing care concerns and monitoring and drawing attention to their family member's medical and emotional problems; and third, they are an important source of socioemotional support.

The influence of family members, however, may not always be positive. Older residents may become stressed when family members disagree on care responses. Also, assisted living providers may be more responsive to the needs of family members, who they view as the customers to please because they pay the bills and make the occupancy decisions. Yet, most research shows that family members are more satisfied than residents (Gaugler & Kane, 2007).

How long older persons live in assisted living facilities may also influence their views. On average, they stay just over two years and it is unclear whether they can become emotionally attached to their environments in this short time. Further, assisted living facilities can have relatively unstable social contexts, with average annual resident turnover rates of 43% (Assisted Living Federation of America, 2009). Others argue, however, that residents' "involvement in activities" better predicts feelings of hominess (Cutchin et al., 2003, p. 242).

CONCLUSION

As aging-in-place opportunities become ubiquitous, the level of competence of older persons is no longer a reliable indicator of where they can or will live. The variety of accommodating residential environments is a confirmation of the ecological theory of aging and the sociomedical model of disability. They both interpret the older person's competence as an adaptational response to the interactions or confluence of individual and environmental factors.

Because the mission statements of older people's residential environments have become more ambitious and multifaceted, it has also become more difficult to judge their appropriateness. Older persons who achieve normalcy in their residential way of life find that their housing arrangement has deficiencies as a care setting or that, even as it offers good care and assistance, it falls short as a home environment. When residential and care environments are out of sync, older persons are forced to make difficult trade-off decisions regarding whether their QOL or quality of care is more important.

Methodologically, it is difficult to disentangle the individual-level and environmental (or contextual) risk factors that influence QOL or care outcomes. This will demand more comprehensive and collaborative evaluations that measure the residential qualities of a place, the quality of its independence-supporting and health-related services, and how they reinforce, complement, or conflict with each other. These assessments will profitably distinguish a place's dwelling, neighborhood, and community environments, and their separate and interdependent influences. These evaluations will also require more comprehensive portrayals of both the residential lifestyles and competence of older persons – measured by both objective and subjective indicators – and that encompass their past life histories, current status, and future expectations and trajectories (Golant, 2003). The following will be key research inquiries:

- Who are the older persons adopting the less mainstream or more innovative housing-care strategies? Can they be distinguished by their demographic characteristics, personality traits, past lifestyles, family support networks, or the extent of their functional limitations and health problems?
- Why do the less mainstream or more innovative housing-care alternatives emerge in some communities and neighborhoods, but not in others? To what extent is their appearance more closely linked with the resourcefulness of private- and public-sector stakeholders as opposed to the location of older persons who need help to maintain their independence?
- Will older persons with incomes too high to qualify for most public programs, but too low to afford the costs of most private sector housing or care options, be able to afford these less mainstream or more innovative housing-care alternatives?
- As we increasingly offer independence-supporting and health-related services in conventional residential-like settings, should we require the same regulatory oversight of these private households as we do of assisted living facilities or even nursing homes?
- How do the results of home intervention programs to reduce falls and increase the

dwelling's usability and accessibility inform our efforts to introduce independence-supporting and health-related services to the elder public at large?

- What outcomes should we measure when judging the QOL or care found in residential settings? Should we focus on the outcomes experienced by residents or family members (relieved of their caregiving roles), or by communities or governments (experiencing lower public health or long-term care costs)? Should we rely more on objective indicators – lower accident rates, fewer hospitalizations and emergency room visits, longer periods of independence – or on the subjective assessments of key stakeholders such as residents, workers, managements, and government agencies?
- What is the most appropriate geographic scale – dwellings, neighborhoods, communities, service areas, planning districts, states – on which to assess these outcomes or introduce solutions?
- How incomplete, distorted, and inaccurate are our current residence-care assessments because we do not examine older people's idiosyncratic environmental histories including their previous residential lifestyles, care experiences, and family relationships?
- What are the unintended downsides of delivering long-term care into conventional residential settings? If hospital beds, highly structured medical and therapeutic regimens, 24-7 staffing, electronic monitoring systems, eligibility and reimbursement procedures, and family members with paternalistic attitudes are introduced into conventional homes, is there a danger that that they will turn into institutional-like living environments?

REFERENCES

Alley, D ., Liebig, P., Pynoos, J., Banerjee, T., & Choi, I. H. (2007). Creating elder-friendly communities: Preparations for an aging society. *Journal of Gerontological Social Work, 49*, 1–18.

Assisted Living Federation of America (2009). *2009 overview of assisted living*. Washington, DC: Assisted Living Federation of America.

Basta, N. E., Matthews, F. E., Chatfield, M. D., Brayne, C., & Mrc, C. (2008). Community-level socio economic status and cognitive and functional impairment in the older population. *European Journal of Public Health, 18*(1), 48–54.

Beard, J. R., Blaney, S., Cerda, M., Frye, V., Lovasi, G. S., Ompad, D., et al. (2009a). Neighborhood characteristics and disability in older adults. *Journal of Gerontology: Social Sciences, 64B*(2), 252–257.

Beard, J. R., Cerda, M., Blaney, S., Ahern, J., Vlahov, D., & Galea, S. (2009b). Neighborhood characteristics and change in depressive symptoms among older residents of New York city. *American Journal of Public Health, 99*(1), 1–7.

Beel-Bates, C. A., Ingersoll-Dayton, B., & Nelson, E. (2007). Deference as a form of reciprocity among residents in assisted living. *Research on Aging, 29*(6), 626–643.

Bierman, A. (2009). Marital status as contingency for the effects of neighborhood disorder on older adults' mental health. *Journal of Gerontology: Social Sciences, 64*(3), 425–434.

Bowling, A., & Stafford, M. (2007). How do objective and subjective assessments of neighbourhood influence social and physical functioning in older age? Findings from a British survey of ageing. *Social Science & Medicine, 64*(12), 2533–2549.

Cagney, K. A., Browning, C. R., & Wen, M. (2005). Racial disparities in self-rated health at older ages: What difference does the neighborhood make? *Journal of Gerontology: Social Sciences, 60*(4), S181–190.

Calkins, M., & Keane, W. (2008). Tomorrow's assisted living and nursing homes: The converging worlds of residential long-term care. In S. M. Golant & J. Hyde (Eds.), *The assisted living residence: A vision for the future* (pp. 86–118). Baltimore, MD: The John Hopkins University Press.

Carder, P. C., Morgan, L. A., & Eckert, J. K. (2008). Small board-and-care homes: A fragile future. In S. M. Golant & J. Hyde (Eds.), *The assisted living residence: A vision for the future* (pp. 143–168). Baltimore, MD: The John Hopkins University Press.

Carlsson, G., Schilling, O., Slaug, B., Fange, A., Stahl, A., Nygren, C., et al. (2009). Toward a screening tool for housing accessibility problems: A reduced version of the housing enabler. *Journal of Applied Gerontology, 28*(1), 59–80.

Center for Universal Design. (2006). *Universal design in housing*. Raleigh, NC: The Center for Universal Design, North Carolina State University, College of Design.

Centers for Disease Control and Prevention. (2008). Self-reported falls and fall-related injuries among persons aged ≥ 65 years – United States, 2006. *Morbidity and Mortality Weekly Report, 57*(9), 225–229.

Chan, B. K., Marshall, L. M., Winters, K. M., Faulkner, K. A., Schwartz, A. V., & Orwoll, E. S. (2007). Incident fall risk and physical activity and physical performance among older men: The osteoporotic fractures in men study. *American Journal of Epidemiology, 165*(6), 696–703.

Clark, C. R., Kawachi, I., Ryan, L., Ertel, K., Fay, M. E., & Berkman, L. F. (2009). Perceived neighborhood safety and incident mobility disability among elders: The hazards of poverty. *BMC Public Health, 9*, 162.

Clarke, P., Ailshire, J. A., Bader, M., Morenoff, J. D., & House, J. S. (2008). Mobility disability and the urban built environment. *American Journal of Epidemiology, 168*(5), 506–513.

Cutchin, M. P., Owen, S. V., & Chang, P. F. (2003). Becoming 'at home' in assisted living residences: Exploring place integration processes. *Journal of Gerontology: Social Sciences, 58*(4), S234–S243.

Cutler, L. J. (2007). Physical environments of assisted living: Research needs and challenges. *The Gerontologist, 43*, 68–82.

Davidoff, T. (2004). *Maintenance and the home equity of the elderly.* Berkeley, CA: University of California, Berkeley, Haas School of Business, Fisher Center for Real Estate and Urban Economics, Paper No. 03-288.

Diehl, M., & Willis, S. L. (2003). Everyday competence and everyday problem solving in aging adults: The role of physical and social context. In H.-W. Wahl, R. J. Scheidt & P. G. Windley (Eds.), *Annual review of gerontology and geriatrics: Aging in context: Socio-physical environments* (pp. 130–166). New York: Springer.

Doty, P. (2008). The influence of public and private financing on assisted living and nursing home care: The past, present, and possible futures. In S. M. Golant & J. Hyde (Eds.), *The assisted living residence: A vision for the future* (pp. 299–328). Baltimore, MD: The John Hopkins University Press.

Durrett, C. (2009). *The senior cohousing handbook: A community approach to independent living.* Gabriola Island, BC: New Society Publishers.

Feldman, P. H., Oberlink, M., Rudin, D., Clay, J., Edwards, B., & Stafford, P. B. (2003). *Best practices: Lessons for communities in supporting the health, well-being, and independence of older people.* New York: Visiting Nurse Service of New York, Center for Home Care Policy and Research.

Foote, B. E. (2007). *Reverse mortgages, background and issues: CRS report for congress.* Washington, DC: Congressional Research Service.

Freedman, V. A., Grafova, I. B., Schoeni, R. F., & Rogowski, J. (2008). Neighborhoods and disability in later life. *Social Science & Medicine, 66*(11), 2253–2267.

Gaugler, J. E., & Kane, R. L. (2007). Families and assisted living. *The Gerontologist, 47*, 83–99.

Gitlin, L. N. (2003). Conducting research on home environments: Lessons learned and new directions. *The Gerontologist, 43*(5), 628–637.

Gitlin, L. N., Hauck, W. W., Dennis, M. P., Winter, L., Hodgson, N., & Schinfeld, S. (2009). Long-term effect on mortality of a home intervention that reduces functional difficulties in older adults: Results from a randomized trial. *Journal of American Geriatrics Society, 57*(3), 476–481.

Glass, T. A., & Balfour, J. L. (2003). Neighborhoods, aging, and functional health. In I. Kawachi & L. F. Berkman (Eds.), *Neighborhoods and Health* (pp. 303–334). Oxford, UK: Oxford University Press.

Golant, S. M. (2003). Conceptualizing time and space in environmental gerontology: A pair of old issues deserving new thought. *The Gerontologist, 43*(5), 638–648.

Golant, S. M. (2004). Do impaired older persons with health care needs occupy U.S. assisted living facilities? *Journal of Gerontology: Social Sciences, 59*(2), S68–79.

Golant, S. M. (2008a). Affordable clustered housing-care: A category of long-term care options for the elderly poor. *Journal of Housing for the Elderly, 22*(1–2), 3–44.

Golant, S. M. (2008b). Commentary: Irrational exuberance for the aging in place of vulnerable low-income older homeowners. *Journal of Aging and Social Policy, 20*(4), 379–397.

Golant, S. M. (2008c). The future of assisted living residences: A response to uncertainty. In S. M. Golant & J. Hyde (Eds.), *The assisted living residence: A vision for the future* (pp. 3–45). Baltimore, MD: The John Hopkins University Press.

Golant, S. M. (2008d). Low-income elderly homeowners in very old dwellings: The need for public policy debate. *Journal of Aging and Social Policy, 20*(1), 1–28.

Golant, S. M. (2009). Aging in place solutions for older Americans: Groupthink responses not always in their best interests. *Public Policy & Aging Report, 19*(1), 33–39.

Grafova, I. B., Freedman, V. A., Kumar, R., & Rogowski, J. (2008). Neighborhoods and obesity in later life. *American Journal of Public Health, 98*(11), 2065–2071.

Gross, J. (2006). Aging at home: For a lucky few, a wish come true. *The New York Times,* 9 February.

Hunt, M. E., & Gunter-Hunt, G. (1985). Naturally occurring retirement communities. *Journal of Housing for the Elderly, 3*(3–4), 3–21.

Hyde, J., Perez, R., & Reed, P. S. (2008). The old road is rapidly aging: A social model for cognitively or physically impaired elders in assisted living's future. In S. M. Golant & J. Hyde (Eds.), *The assisted living residence: A vision for the future* (pp. 46–85). Baltimore, MD: The John Hopkins University Press.

Iwarsson, S. (2003). Assessing the fit between older people and their physical home environments: An occupational therapy research perspective. In H.-W. Wahl, R. J. Scheidt & P. G. Windley (Eds.), *Annual review of gerontology and geriatrics: Aging in context: Socio-physical environments* (pp. 85–109). New York: Springer.

Iwarsson, S., Nygren, C., Oswald, F., Wahl, H.-W., & Tomsone, S. (2006). Environmental barriers and housing accessibility problems over a one-year period in later life in three European countries. *Journal of Housing for the Elderly, 20*(3), 23–43.

Iwarsson, S., Wahl, H.-W., Nygren, C., Oswald, F., Sixsmith, A., Sixsmith, J., et al. (2007). Importance of the home environment for healthy aging: Conceptual and methodological background of the European ENABLE-AGE project. *The Gerontologist, 47*(1), 78–84.

Kane, R. A. (2001). Long-term care and a good quality of life: Bringing them closer together. *The Gerontologist, 41*(3), 293–304.

Kane, R. A., & Cutler, L. J. (2009). Promoting homelike characteristics and eliminating institutional characteristics in community-based residential care settings: Insights from an 8-state study. *Seniors Housing & Care Journal, 17*(1), 15–37.

Kim, D., Subramanian, S. V., Gortmaker, S. L., & Kawachi, I. (2006). US state- and county-level social capital in relation to obesity and physical inactivity: A multilevel, multivariable analysis. *Social Science & Medicine, 63*(4), 1045–1059.

Krause, N. (2003). Neighborhoods, health, and well-being in late life. In H. W. Wahl, R. J. Scheidt & P. G. Windley (Eds.), *Annual review of gerontology and geriatrics: Focus on aging in context, socio-physical environments* (pp. 223–249). New York: Springer Publishing Co.

Kutzik, D., Glascock, A. P., Lundberg, L., & York, J. (2008). Technological tools of the future: Contributing to appropriate care in assisted living. In S. M. Golant & J. Hyde (Eds.), *The assisted living residence: A vision for the future* (pp. 223–247). Baltimore, MD: The John Hopkins University Press.

Lawton, M. P. (1998). Environment and aging: Theory revisited. In R. J. Scheidt & P. G. Windley (Eds.), *Environment and aging theory: A focus on housing* (pp. 1–31). Westport, CN: Greenwood Press.

Li, F., Harmer, P. A., Cardinal, B. J., Bosworth, M., Acock, A., Johnson-Shelton, D., et al. (2008). Built environment, adiposity, and physical activity in adults aged 50-75. *American Journal of Preventive Medicine, 35*(1), 38–46.

Mendes de Leon, C. F., Cagney, K. A., Bienias, J. L., Barnes, L. L., Skarupski, K. A., Scherr, P. A., et al. (2009). Neighborhood social cohesion and disorder in relation to walking in community-dwelling older adults: A multilevel analysis. *Journal of Aging Health, 21*(1), 155–171.

Mitchell, J. M., & Kemp, B. J. (2000). Quality of life in assisted living homes: A multidimensional analysis. *Journal of Gerontology: Social Sciences, 55*(2), P117–P127.

Mollica, R. L., Sims-Kastelein, K., & O'Keeffe, J. (2007). *Residential care and assisted living compendium.* Washington, DC: US Department

of Health and Human Services, Office of Disability, Aging and Long-Term Care Policy.

Moody, H. R. (2008). *The new aging enterprise.* Washington, DC: AARP, Office of Academic Affairs.

Northridge, M. E., Sclar, E. D., & Biswas, P. (2003). Sorting out the connections between the built environment and health: A conceptual framework for navigating pathways and planning healthy cities. *Journal of Urban Health, 80*(4), 556–568.

Nygren, C., Oswald, F., Iwarsson, S., Fange, A., Sixsmith, J., Schilling, O., et al. (2007). Relationships between objective and perceived housing in very old age. *The Gerontologist, 47*(1), 85–95.

Oakes, J. M. (2004). The (mis) estimation of neighborhood effects: Causal inference for a practicable social epidemiology. *Social Science & Medicine, 58*(10), 1929–1952.

Ormond, B. A., Black, K. J., Tilly, J., & Thomas, S. (2004). *Supportive services programs in naturally occurring retirement communities.* Washington, DC: Office of Disability, Aging and Long-Term Care Policy.

Ostir, G. V., Eschbach, K., Markides, K. S., & Goodwin, J. S. (2003). Neighbourhood composition and depressive symptoms among older Mexican Americans. *Journal of Epidemiology & Community Health, 57*(12), 987–992.

Oswald, F., Wahl, H. -W., Schilling, O., Nygren, C., Fange, A., Sixsmith, A., et al. (2007a). Relationships between housing and healthy aging in very old age. *The Gerontologist, 47*(1), 96–107.

Oswald, F., Wahl, H. W., Schilling, O., & Iwarsson, S. (2007b). Housing-related control beliefs and independence in activities of daily living in very old age. *Scandanavian Journal of Occupational Therapy, 14*(1), 33–43.

Patel, K. V., Eschbach, K., Rudkin, L. L., Peek, M. K., & Markides, K. S. (2003). Neighborhood context and self-rated health in older Mexican Americans. *Annals of Epidemiology, 13*(9), 620–628.

Polivka, L., & Salmon, J. R. (2008). Assisted living: What it should

be and why. In S. M. Golant & J. Hyde (Eds.), *The assisted living residence: A vision for the future* (pp. 397–418). Baltimore, MD: The John Hopkins University Press.

Pynoos, J., Rose, D., Rubenstein, L., Choi, I. H., & Sabata, D. (2006). Evidence-based interventions in fall prevention. *Home Health Care Services Quarterly, 25*(1–2), 55–73.

Rabig, J., Thomas, W., Kane, R. A., Cutler, L. J., & McAlilly, S. (2006). Radical redesign of nursing homes: Applying the green house concept in Tupelo, Mississippi. *The Gerontologist, 46*(4), 533–539.

Regnier, V. (2002). *Design for assisted living: Guidelines for housing the physically and mentally frail.* New York: John Wiley & Sons.

Salminen, M., Vahlberg, T., Salonoja, M. T., Piertti, T. T., Aarnio, P., & Kivela, S. L. (2009). Effects of risk-based multifactorial fall prevention program on the incidence of falls. *Journal of the American Geriatrics Society, 57*, 612–619.

Scheidt, R. J., & Windley, P. (2006). Environmental gerontology: Progress in the post-Lawton era. In J. Birren & K. W. Schaie (Eds.), *Handbook of the psychology of aging* (pp. 105–125) (6th Edn). New York: Academic Press.

Schiller, J. S., Kramarow, E. A., & Dey, A. N. (2007). Fall injury episodes among noninstitutionalized older adults: United States, 2001–2003. *Advance Data from Vital and Health Statistics, 392*, 1–16.

Sheffield, K. M., & Peek, M. K. (2009). Neighborhood context and cognitive decline in older Mexican Americans: Results from the Hispanic established populations for epidemiologic studies of the elderly. *American Journal of Epidemiology, 169*(9), 1092–1101.

Shippee, T. P. (2009). "But I am not moving": Residents' perspectives on transitions within a continuing care retirement community. *The Gerontologist, 49*(3), 418–427.

Sikorska-Simmons, E. (2005). Predictors of organizational commitment among staff in assisted living. *The Gerontologist, 45*(2), 196–205.

US Census Bureau. (2008). American Housing Survey for

the United States: 2007 Current Housing Reports, Series H50/07. Washington, DC: US Government Printing Office.

US Senate Special Committee on Aging (2003). *Assisted living: Examining the assisted living workgroup final report, hearing.* Washington, DC: US Government Printing Office.

Verbrugge, L. M., & Jette, A. M. (1994). The disablement process. *Social Science & Medicine, 38*(11), 1–14.

Vladeck, F. (2008). Naturally occurring retirement communities. *Designer Builder, January/February,* 43–47.

Wahl, H.-W., & Oswald, F. (2009). Environmental perspectives on aging. In D. Dannefer & C. Phillipson (Eds.), *International handbook of social gerontology* (pp. 111–124). Thousand Oaks, CA: Sage.

Wahl, H. -W., Fange, A., Oswald, F., Gitlin, L. N., & Iwarsson, S.

(2009). The home environment and disability-related outcomes in aging individuals: What is the empirical evidence? *The Gerontologist, 49*(3), 355–367.

Wight, R. G., Aneshensel, C. S., Miller-Martinez, D., Botticello, A. L., Cummings, J. R., Karlamangla, A. S., et al. (2006). Urban neighborhood context, educational attainment, and cognitive function among older adults. *American Journal of Epidemiology, 163*(12), 1071–1078.

World Health Organization. (2007). *Global age-friendly cities: A guide.* Geneva: World Health Organization.

Wylde, M. A. (2008). The future of assisted living: Residents' perspectives. In S. M. Golant & J. Hyde (Eds.), *The Assisted living residence: A vision for the future* (pp. 169–197). Baltimore, MD: The John Hopkins University Press.

Yao, L., & Robert, S. A. (2008). The contributions of race, individual socioeconomic status, and neighborhood socioeconomic context on the self-rated health trajectories and mortality of older adults. *Research on Aging, 30*(2), 251–273.

Yeom, H. A., Fleury, J., & Keller, C. (2008). Risk factors for mobility limitation in community-dwelling older adults: A social ecological perspective. *Geriatric Nursing, 29*(2), 133–140.

Zimmerman, S., Sloane, P. D., & Fletcher, S. K. (2008). The measurement and importance of quality: A collaborative effort. In S. M. Golant & J. Hyde (Eds.), *The assisted living residence: A vision for the future* (pp. 119–142). Baltimore, MD: The John Hopkins University Press.

Chapter | 16 |

Civic Engagement and Aging

Stephen J. Cutler[1], Jon Hendricks[2], Greg O'Neill[3]

[1]Emeritus, Department of Sociology, University of Vermont, Burlington, Vermont, [2]Emeritus, Honors College, Oregon State University, Corvallis, Oregon, [3]National Academy on an Aging Society, Gerontological Society of America, Washington, DC

CHAPTER CONTENTS

INTRODUCTION

In recent years, interest in the civic engagement of older Americans has increased considerably among social scientists, policymakers, and governmental and nonprofit leaders for several reasons. First, dramatic gains in health, education, and longevity over the past half century have increased individuals' capacity for civic roles and contributions in later life. Second, Putnam's (2000) provocative commentary in *Bowling Alone* spurred social scientists to explore Americans' actual and potential civic contributions; gerontologists have delved into older adults' economic and social contributions to counter negative aging stereotypes. Third, prompted by research linking civic engagement with healthy, successful aging, policymakers and government officials are interested in promoting service opportunities for older Americans that can benefit society as well as the volunteers themselves. Finally, facing an escalating demand for social services and concerns about the loss of traditional volunteers – especially housewives – nonprofit sector leaders have stepped up efforts to enlist the growing population of older persons to help fill the gap.

Civic engagement is generally said to be good for one and all. Despite such hearty endorsements, a great deal of ambiguity surrounds the concept and its application. Here we examine civic engagement in greater detail from the perspectives of conceptual and theoretical issues and then measurement issues. The next section provides an overview of findings on trends and life course variation in civic engagement; subsequent sections discuss implications of civic engagement for older adults and for society, respectively; and the final section considers directions for further work on civic engagement.

DOI: 10.1016/B978-0-12-380880-6.00016-2

DEFINITIONS AND CONCEPTUAL FOUNDATIONS

The Search for a Common Definition

There is no prevailing definition of "civic engagement" although many have been offered (National Academy on an Aging Society, 2009a). The term has been applied to a range of activities "[f]rom volunteering to voting, from community organizing to political advocacy." Central to most characterizations is the notion that civic engagement is *action* contributing "to the improvement of one's community, neighborhood and nation" (Philanthropy for Active Civic Engagement, 2009, p. 7). The types of activities identified as civic engagement fall into two broad categories: social (including most behaviors classified as volunteering and public service) and political (including participation in all facets of the political process) (McBride, 2006–2007).

The multifaceted character of civic engagement is likely responsible for a lack of consensus regarding its definition. Not only does the concept cover a lot of ground, but it encompasses volunteering done on behalf of formal organizations, including schools, churches, hospitals, and nonprofit organizations, as well as informal engagements such as helping friends, neighbors, and relatives (Putnam, 2000).

Further complicating matters is the propensity for some observers to include both paid and unpaid contributions under the same rubric. The advent of incentive programs, such as educational vouchers, stipends, and other forms of compensation, has blurred the line between paid and unpaid participation. Moreover, some scholars argue that unpaid caregiving constitutes a vital form of civic engagement (Martinson & Minkler, 2006). Others suggest that the portrayal of civic engagement even includes the acquisition of knowledge and skills required to perform various civic actions (Fisher et al., 2005).

To date, research on older adults' civic engagement has focused primarily on formal volunteering – specifically, membership in voluntary associations and volunteer activities done through or for an organization. Because this chapter deals largely with the research literature in this emerging field, we limit our focus to formal volunteering. But, given widespread efforts to promote civic engagement, we explore issues of labeling further because the term's definition carries significant implications for determining which activities receive public and private support.

Conceptual Foundations

To understand the ramifications of civic engagement, it is important to recognize that it yields both social and personal benefits. Taylor and Bengtson (2001) caution that macro-level and micro-level perspectives need to be disentangled lest all aspects of productive aging – including civic engagement – be relegated to individualistic explanations without attending to institutional barriers or macro-level considerations. Attention to macro-level factors will reveal the broader social forces underlying differences between diverse groups of older persons and will shed light on the public policies promoting or inhibiting productive engagement. Taylor and Bengtson conclude by noting that there is a need at the macro-level to consider underlying social inequalities when classifying older people as productive or not. Below we speak to macro- as well as micro-level frames with which to examine civic engagement.

Social Integration

The French sociologist Durkheim directed his attention to issues of collective consciousness and its effect on individual behavior. He was concerned with social integration at the turn of the twentieth century, and it may be that civic engagement offers a means of maintaining moral integration and social solidarity via shared experiences in the twenty-first century. Beyond redressing financial retrenchments by providing voluntary contributions, civic engagement proffers a vehicle for promoting socially integrated belief systems among those participating in civic relations.

In developing an analytic frame, a number of additional questions arise: How are shared meanings and social ties created and sustained? What factors determine why some groups or individuals are more involved than others in creating shared meanings? Shared meanings may result from both incentives to engage and the experience of common events. For example, incentives (such as stipends) that are increasingly included in public policies fostering civic engagement could encourage individuals to engage. In addition, significant events can create social ties that inspire engagement. An AARP (2003) survey reported that, following the attacks of 9/11, 30% of volunteers reported a stronger desire than before to volunteer in their communities. Once engaged, individuals experience greater attachment and loyalty towards their communities, and therefore are more likely to sustain their participation.

In response to the second question, Zedlewski (2007) identifies factors that determine why some groups or individuals are more likely than others to create shared meanings. She concludes that the majority of older adults who miss opportunities to volunteer have lifestyles that make it unlikely they will become aware of such opportunities in the first place. Her data reveal that higher education, managerial experience, marriage to a volunteer, and religiosity all lead to greater awareness of and access to meaningful volunteer opportunities.

Self and Identity

The literature on volunteering and civic engagement is replete with references to improved physical or psychological health and subjective well-being (see below). In nearly every instance, civic engagement is identified as a source of intrinsic rewards, buttressing a sense of self and personal identity (Hendricks & Cutler, 2004). Seemingly, identification with a publicly recognized good has a consistent and positive effect on an individual's sense of self-worth or fulfillment. These findings contribute to a new definition of retirement and strengthen the notion of an emergent third age subsequent to work life, rather than reinforcing retirement as a cultural marker of marginalization.

Selectivity

Participation rates in various forms of civic engagement are not stable, either in terms of time spent or number of activities in which individuals are involved. To make sense of these trends, it helps to apply what Carstensen (1995) terms "socioemotional selectivity." The principle of socioemotional selectivity posits that, as people realize they have relatively little time or energy to give, they make considered connections based on relationships providing the greatest returns. They invest in some areas and distance themselves from others. In terms of civic engagement, not all forms are equal or yield comparable results. Hendricks and Cutler (2004), among others, assert that socioemotional selectivity helps explain why some volunteer involvements are retained as others are discarded, depending on their meaning, relevance for personal identity, and priorities. Accordingly, forms and rates of engagement likely reflect the satisfaction older participants derive from helping others and giving back through meaningful participation. Activities most meaningful to individuals' self-concepts and emotional needs likely are retained, while those more peripheral are jettisoned. With meaningful opportunities, older participants will continue to contribute as long as they are able (Hendricks & Cutler, 2004; Windsor et al., 2008).

MEASURING CIVIC ENGAGEMENT

Measurement Variability

The conceptual ambiguities discussed above are echoed in a lack of consensus regarding measuring civic engagement. A comprehensive and detailed catalog of existing measures is beyond the scope of this chapter, but several examples will point to the array of variations in measurement and will document the absence of a gold standard for measuring civic engagement.

One of the most comprehensive measures of individual-level civic engagement is the National Conference on Citizenship's (2008) "civic health index." Based on 40 indicators, it tracks engagement along nine dimensions: connecting with civic and religious groups; trusting others; connecting to others through family and friends; giving and volunteering; staying informed; understanding politics and government; participating in politics; trusting and feeling connected to major institutions; and expressing political views. Similarly, but tapping a more macro level of engagement (e.g. state- and regional-level variation) is the comprehensive Corporation for National and Community Service's (CNCS) "civic life index" (Grimm et al., 2007a), based on 12 indicators representing four domains. The domains are: (1) volunteering for an organization, (2) neighborhood engagement, (3) voting, and (4) civic and nonprofit infrastructure (i.e. number of nonprofit organizations and religious institutions per capita). Also multidimensional but lacking a composite measure are indicators in the AARP Survey of Civic Involvement (AARP, 1997), which tap civic engagement (e.g. formal and informal volunteering), civic orientations (e.g. trust in government, political efficacy), political involvement, connectedness (e.g. community attachment, neighborhood interaction), and cultural and social orientations (e.g. religious involvement, media use).

Federal data on individual-level civic engagement have been based on two sources. The focus of the American Time Use Survey (ATUS) is on volunteer activities done for, or through, an organization; the reference period is the prior day; and specific voluntary activities are identified via a detailed time diary (US Bureau of Labor Statistics, 2009a). The Current Population Survey's (CPS) September Supplement on Volunteering annually asks whether respondents have done any volunteer activities through or for an organization during the past year, the types and number of organizations for which they volunteered, how much time they spent volunteering, and how they became involved (US Bureau of Labor Statistics, 2009b). Recent refinements enquire about specific activities in the main organization for which individuals volunteered; whether they attended public meetings, made charitable contributions, or fixed or improved something; and whether they volunteered more than 120 miles away from home or abroad. Although evolving and expanding, the thrust of the CPS data has been on formal volunteering. The November 2008 CPS included a new Supplement on Voting and Civic Engagement with questions on voting behavior and, for the first time, broader questions about civic activities, including participation in organized groups, non-electoral political behavior, and extent of connections with other community members. As these data become available, records from households participating in both the September and November 2008 Supplements can be merged, yielding information on a wider variety of civic engagement activities (R. Grimm, Jr., personal communication, August 27, 2009).

Three other data sources often employed in aging research also include measures related to civic engagement, but vary widely in scope. The narrowest is the National Opinion Research Center's GSS (Davis et al., 2009), 16 of those conducted between 1974 and 2008 asked nationally representative samples of adults about membership in 16 specific types of voluntary associations. The four-wave ACL survey (Inter-University Consortium for Political and Social Research, 2009) asks whether respondents have done volunteer work in the last 12 months for a religious organization, a school or educational organization, or for a political group or labor union, as well as the number of hours spent on volunteer work during the past year. The multi-wave HRS (2009) has asked biannually whether respondents have done any volunteer work in the past year for religious, educational, health-related, or other charitable organizations and how many hours they contributed. On a one-time basis in 2000, an expanded HRS included attitudinal items on economic altruism, social altruism, benevolence, and obligation.

Measurement complexities multiply when the focus shifts to comparative international data. For example, the 2007 Canada Survey of Giving, Volunteering, and Participating obtained detailed data on formal volunteering, informal volunteering on behalf of friends, neighbors, and non-household relatives, and charitable donations (Statistics Canada, 2007). The multi-wave, multi-nation Survey of Health, Ageing, and Retirement in Europe (SHARE) (2009) asks in-depth questions about voluntary activities in the past month, how frequently the respondent engaged in these, motivations for doing so, and perceived satisfaction and appreciation. Substantive overlap is present in other major studies (e.g. the English Longitudinal Study of Ageing and the Australian Longitudinal Study of Ageing), but variation in content coverage, question wording, and time referents leave researchers with no agreed-upon set of items to pursue comparative research on civic engagement (Bailie, 2006).

Methodological Pitfalls and New Paradigms

The growing scientific and policy importance of civic engagement, coupled with wide variation in measurement, has led to greater interest in identifying and resolving vexing methodological issues. We note three of them here, beginning with two sources of bias.

First, participating in a survey is itself a form of volunteering, so surveys on civic engagement and volunteering over-represent respondents already inclined to contribute their time, thus inflating survey-based estimates of volunteer rates (Abraham et al., 2009). Second, asking about volunteer activity via "perceptual" surveys (e.g. "have you done any volunteer activities through or for an organization in the past year?") is less space- and time-consuming, but is fraught with ambiguities and elicits substantially lower volunteer rates than surveys utilizing "behavioral" prompted checklists (e.g. "in the past 12 months, did you teach or coach for an organization as an unpaid volunteer?") (Toppe, 2005). Perhaps most challenging is the need to match measurement of civic engagement with its emerging, broader conceptualization. Toppe and Galaskiewicz (2006) propose that civic engagement be conceptualized and measured along four dimensions: (1) helping, including volunteering and neighboring; (2) giving to people, organizations, and causes; (3) influencing, including political and cause-related activities; and (4) participating, as in group memberships or bowling leagues. Their typology includes even more detailed levels of measurement, and it suggests the direction and distance we need to go to reach consensus on conceptualizing and measuring civic engagement.

TRENDS

From de Tocqueville to Putnam and Beyond

The publication of *Bowling Alone: The Collapse and Revival of American Community* (Putnam, 2000) heralded a concern that the distinctively American level of civic engagement, first noted by de Tocqueville in the 1830s, had eroded. The last third of the twentieth century, Putnam argued, brought a decline in social capital and a weakening of ties binding people to one another and to their communities. Space limitations preclude a detailed review of Putnam's conclusions, but three points are worth noting.

First, the decline appears to be a phenomenon occurring primarily in the US. Andersen et al. (2006) examined time-use data on association activities from four countries from the mid-1960s through the late 1990s and found a clear decline only in the US; associational participation was stable in Canada, the Netherlands, and the United Kingdom. Further, the US decline was evident only among women, a result attributed by the authors to the increasing labor force participation of women over this period.

Second, long-term trends in civic engagement over the past three decades appear to conform to a U-shaped curvilinear pattern. Data from the National Conference on Citizenship (2008), the NORC GSS (Rotolo, 1999), and the CPS (Grimm et al., 2006) all show declines in civic engagement in the 1970s and 1980s followed by increases in the 1990s and thereafter. Some evidence suggests that the recent downturn in the US economy precipitated a decline in civic engagement (National Conference on Citizenship, 2009), but other data suggest a significant increase in civic involvement between 2008 and 2009 (Gallup Poll, 2009).

Third, the data demonstrate that elders have contributed significantly to these recent increases. Goss (1999) found that people aged 60 and older were nearly twice as likely to volunteer in the late 1990s as their counterparts in the mid 1970s – an increase that accounted for much of the overall rise in the frequency of volunteering over the 24-year period examined in the analysis. CPS trend data reveal that the volunteer rate of older adults (aged 65 and older) rose by 64% between 1974 and 2005, and the proportion of older volunteers contributing more than 100 hours per year rose by 46% – both increases representing the largest of any of the several age groups examined in the analysis (Grimm et al., 2006). Einolf (2009), using 1995 and 2005 waves of the Midlife in the US panel study and comparing cohorts at the same age, finds a steady increase in volunteering from the "long civic" generation (born 1926 to 1935), to the "silent" generation (born 1936 to 1945), to the "early baby boom" generation (born 1946 to 1955).

Life Course Patterns

Research has identified reasonably consistent patterns of age differences in aspects of volunteerism. CPS data show a consistent curvilinear pattern of volunteer rates by age (US Bureau of Labor Statistics, 2009c), ranging from a low of 18.6% for the 20 to 24 year-old age group to a high of 31.3% among persons aged 35 to 44, and down again to 23.5% among persons aged 65 and older. Investigators have long noted that this curvilinear pattern of age differences is likely due to compositional effects (e.g. education, employment status, marital status, gender, presence of dependent children, self-perceived health). Cutler and Hendricks (2000), for example, utilized NORC GSSs from 1974 to 1994 to illustrate how a curvilinear pattern of age differences in number of association memberships was replaced, when controlling for compositional factors, with a pattern of increasing memberships through ages 55 to 59, a slight decrease in the 60-to-64-year old age group, then generally stable membership levels through the 85-and-older age group. A recent analysis of persons 57 to 85 years of age in the National Social Life, Health, and Aging Project confirms a positive relationship between age and volunteerism and a positive (but nonsignificant) relationship between age and organized group involvement (Cornwell et al., 2008).

Although unadjusted cross-sectional CPS data for 2008 show lower volunteer rates among older persons, the same data indicate the median annual number of hours spent volunteering by older volunteers exceeds that of any other age group (96 hours for persons aged 65 and older compared to 52 hours for the total sample) (US Bureau of Labor Statistics, 2009c, Table 2). Hypothesizing a tendency among older persons to shed peripheral volunteer activities and retain core involvements, Hendricks and Cutler (2004) found the average number of hours of volunteer activities per organization and the total number of hours spent in volunteer activities in the main organization to increase with age, followed by high and stable participation levels at older ages. Thus, the unadjusted rate at which older persons volunteer may be lower than younger age groups, but those who do so appear to make the heaviest investment of time.

It is problematic to reach a conclusion about how civic engagement changes with aging. Civic engagement and volunteer activities have been used in longitudinal studies as predictors of outcomes such as health and well-being, but rarely as time-dependent foci in and of themselves. An early study based on two longitudinal surveys of older persons spanning four years and two and a half years, respectively, found that persons with stable or increasing participation levels outnumbered those with declining levels; persons not participating at the time of the initial interview were unlikely to be participating later; and those participating initially were likely to have continued their participation (Cutler, 1977). A recent study based on five waves of the HRS also found relatively stable patterns: nearly 60% of respondents volunteering at T_1 were still volunteering at most or all of the subsequent waves, while 67% of those not volunteering at T_1 did not volunteer in any of the subsequent waves (Butrica et al., 2009).

IMPLICATIONS OF CIVIC ENGAGEMENT FOR OLDER ADULTS

Predictors of Civic Engagement

Although there is variation, studies generally find that women have higher rates of volunteer participation than men (Rozario, 2006–2007; US Bureau of Labor Statistics, 2009c, Table 1) and married persons have higher rates than non-married (Zedlewski & Schaner, 2005). Research on racial differences has yielded mixed results. Some studies find higher levels of volunteerism among African American elders (Cornwell et al., 2008), but most have found whites to have higher levels (US Bureau of Labor Statistics, 2009c, Table 1). This race effect disappears in many, but not all, studies when socioeconomic factors are controlled (Musick & Wilson, 2008). It is also important to note that forms of civic engagement and volunteering may differ among minorities and other groups, with minorities having a preference "to provide aid on a personal basis, rather than through formal organizations" (Musick & Wilson, 2008, p. 214).

Across a variety of civic engagement indicators, human capital variables are consistent predictors of older-adult participation. Those with higher levels of education and income and those in better health are more likely to be involved in volunteer and civic activities (Choi, 2003; Cornwell et al., 2008; Kaskie et al., 2008; Tang, 2006). These findings have been replicated in many countries (e.g. Erlinghagen & Hank, 2006 for Europe and Kim et al., 2007 for Korea). Higher rates of volunteer participation are found among adults in the labor force than among those who have left the labor force, seemingly because working adults are exposed to volunteer opportunities through their work contacts (Zedlewski, 2007). Studies also indicate that, within occupations, persons in higher status jobs and in self-directed careers have higher levels of volunteer participation (Wilson & Musick, 1997a), as do part-time workers (Choi, 2003).

Further, despite evidence that the trend toward more women working full-time depresses their volunteer rate, the net effect of major structural changes has been stable or even slightly rising rates of volunteering (Musick & Wilson, 2008). These changes include women's increasing education, the decline of the extended family, and the increasing labor force participation of women.

There seems to be general agreement that social activities and religiosity promote formal volunteering (AARP, 1997; Wilson & Musick, 1997b). Whether care-giving results in role overload or role extension into formal volunteering has been the subject of considerable research, with scant consensus. Some studies have found the caregiving role to be associated with higher levels of volunteering (Burr et al., 2005); others maintain that caregiving is unrelated to volunteer activity (Farkas & Himes, 1997); still others note that spousal caregiving reduces volunteering, especially for women (Choi et al., 2007).

In addition, research has identified a wide range of social-psychological and attitudinal variables associated with civic engagement activities (Grano et al., 2008; Kaskie et al., 2008; Okun & Michel, 2006; Okun & Schultz, 2003). These include sense of community and generativity, altruism, values regarding humanitarianism, the adequacy of volunteer opportunities, and self-efficacy. Grano et al. summarize this literature by noting:

> older volunteers are motivated by altruistic and esteem values, such as the desire to feel useful, feel productive, and fulfill moral obligations [...] and motivated, to a lesser extent, by understanding and protective values, such as the opportunity of learning new skills or the opportunity for social interaction. (p. 307)

Finally, data suggest that people volunteer because an organization or someone in their social network has asked them to do so (Rozario, 2006–2007). Surveys conducted by the Independent Sector (2000, 2001) reveal that less than one-third of adults aged 65 and older said they had been asked to volunteer in the past year, compared to about half of all adults over age 21. Compared to adults of all ages, older adults are less likely to volunteer if they are not asked, yet more likely to volunteer if asked. Moreover, recent surveys suggest older adults want to spend more time volunteering (Bridgeland et al., 2008). Previous research found that nearly 40% of adults aged 55 to 74 who did not volunteer said that they would have liked to, and nearly half of those who did report volunteering said that they would have liked to do more (Mutchler et al., 2003).

Micro-Level Benefits of Civic Engagement

A number of researchers have asserted that volunteerism is linked with positive physical and mental health outcomes and successful aging (Grimm et al., 2007b; Hinterlong & Williamson, 2006–2007). Earlier studies on well-being outcomes typically relied on cross-sectional samples, making it impossible to separate selection effects from causation effects. The increasing availability of longitudinal data, together with the results of cross-sectional studies (e.g. Morrow-Howell et al., 2009a), have created a consistent picture of the salutary effects of engaging in civic activities.

Relationships between civic engagement and physical and psychological well-being have been examined using multiple waves of the ACL study (Morrow-Howell et al., 2003; Musick et al., 1999; Musick & Wilson, 2003; Tang, 2009; van Willigen, 2000), the Assets and Health Dynamics among the Oldest Old Study (Lum & Lightfoot, 2005), the National Survey of Families and Households (Greenfield & Marks, 2007), the Wisconsin Longitudinal Study (Piliavin & Siegl, 2007), and the Longitudinal Study of Aging II (Hong et al., 2009). Collectively, these studies suggest that civic engagement, measured by volunteering and net of confounding variables, enhances a variety of measures of well-being: happiness, life satisfaction, self-esteem, sense of control, physical health (including both self-rated health and functional dependency), depression, and longevity. Further, research indicates that the relationship between volunteering and well-being is perhaps best viewed as curvilinear with the greatest benefits accruing to persons with moderate levels of participation (Lum & Lightfoot, 2005; Musick et al., 1999). Similar overall relationships between volunteer activity and well-being are found in studies of elders in Japan (Sugihara et al., 2008), Australia (Windsor et al., 2008), and Israel (Shmotkin et al., 2003).

Greenfield and Marks (2004) and van Willigen (2000) assert that older persons may receive relatively greater returns from volunteering compared to their younger and middle-aged counterparts due to a desire to compensate for role losses accompanying aging and later-life transitions. Further, among older volunteers, those who have experienced the greatest role losses – due to unstable job histories or other adversities – may receive relatively greater benefits. Morrow-Howell and colleagues (2003, 2009a) go so far as to recommend that, because of the benefits reaped, it might make sense to select volunteers based on the likelihood of maximizing returns to the individuals involved. In their study of older African American women volunteering in public schools over a three-year period, Tan et al. (2009) report that volunteers not only burned more calories than a matched group of non-volunteers, but also realized other health benefits. The authors selected their volunteers from a social category believed to be less engaged in civic engagement or physical activities and, therefore, at higher risk of maladies associated with sedentary lifestyles.

Civic Engagement as a Formal Retirement Role for Older People?

It is appropriate to ask whether the civic engagement movement has gained enough momentum to confer a newly recognized retirement role for older people. Increasingly frequent discussions within the scholarly and popular literature identify the third age as a period of active participation in activities that fall under the umbrella of civic engagement, following separation from the labor force and prior to physical decline. Boggs et al. (1995) assert that, among retirees, civic engagement constitutes an important role, provided it is more than busywork, and has the potential to counter some of the negative imagery of retirement as a time of implacable passivity. Given that rates of engagement and volunteering are increasing among successively younger cohorts of older adults (Einolf, 2009), civic engagement likely will expand through the retirement years of the baby boom. In light of the Serve America legislation (see below), growing public attention, and incentives ranging from transportation and hotel vouchers to property tax credits, educational scholarships, and "purpose prizes" (O'Neill, 2006–2007), levels of engagement are not declining, and are providing meaningful participation for those who are so engaged. The sheer size of the baby boom cohort supports the prospect that far greater social capital is waiting in the wings and volunteering is not in steep decline, as some have predicted (Gallup Poll, 2009). These phenomena are at odds with Putnam's (2000) pessimistic predictions of a decline in participation rates, and are supported by Cutler and Hendricks' (2000) findings that compositional characteristics of successive age cohorts

are factors in their volunteerism and that once such factors are controlled, rates hold fairly stable into the eighth decade (see also Sander & Putnam, 2006). With the prolongation of active life expectancy and the length of time following labor force separation, civic participation could become increasingly pertinent and prominent later in life.

IMPLICATIONS OF CIVIC ENGAGEMENT FOR SOCIETY

Providing Infrastructure, Resources, and Incentives

Older adults continue to make vital economic and social contributions to communities and families through unpaid roles, namely volunteering and caregiving (Bass & Caro, 2001). Those receiving services provided by older volunteers also benefit from older adults' engagement with them. Children in educational activities especially benefit (Morrow-Howell et al., 2009b; Rebok et al., 2004). Further, older adults' volunteer activities help governments and nonprofit organizations to meet the growing demand for social services. As we emphasize below, increased volunteerism has a palpable effect on the economy and potentially reduces government costs for health care given the salutary effect of volunteerism on physical and mental health (Zedlewski & Butrica, 2007).

This "win–win" scenario has captured the attention of gerontologists; it advocates promoting civic engagement and has spawned a host of related activities. The major national professional associations in aging – the American Society on Aging, The Gerontological Society of America, and the National Council on Aging – have made civic engagement a programmatic priority. Charitable foundations – especially The Atlantic Philanthropies – and others who fund projects, research, and programs in aging (e.g. AARP) are supporting numerous and varied civic engagement initiatives (see National Academy on an Aging Society, 2009b). And, in recent years, scholarship on older adult civic engagement has increased significantly.

Political interest in the civic engagement of older Americans also has increased perceptibly since the 2005 White House Conference on Aging (WHCoA), where the topic was highlighted (O'Neill, 2006–2007). In the 2006 reauthorization of the Older Americans Act, new authority was granted to the Administration on Aging to develop and implement civic engagement programs (defined by statute as "an individual or collective action designed to address a public concern or an unmet human, educational, health care, environmental, or public safety need") for older Americans ("Unofficial compilation of the Older Americans Act," n.d., § 102,

¶ a12). More recently, the Edward M. Kennedy Serve America Act of 2009 (Serve America Act) – the largest expansion of national civilian service programs since the Depression-era Civilian Conservation Corps – includes several provisions targeting midlife and older adults.

Although the federal government supports a variety of volunteer and employment programs for older adults, the most prominent of these – Foster Grandparent Program, Senior Companion Program, and Senior Community Service Employment Program – are "stipended" programs targeting low-income older adults for mentoring, caregiving, and nonprofit support positions. In contrast, the Serve America Act promotes service by seniors of all socioeconomic backgrounds to address "unmet local, State, and national needs in the areas of education, public safety, emergency and disaster preparedness, relief, and recovery, health and human needs, and the environment" (Edward M. Kennedy Serve America Act, 2009, § 2142, ¶ 1).

The 2009 Serve America Act establishes an Encore Fellowship for individuals aged 55 or older to serve in leadership or management positions in public or private nonprofit organizations for one year; it directs 10% of AmeriCorps' total FY 2010 budget of $372.5 million to organizations enrolling adults aged 55 and older; and it creates Silver Scholarships, which provide a $1000 higher education award – transferable to children and grandchildren – to older volunteers who contribute 350 hours of service annually. The new law stipulates that the nation's 50 State Commissions on National and Community Service provide detailed plans to recruit and leverage the resources of the baby boom generation. It also expands service options for older Americans by lowering the age requirement for the Foster Grandparent and Senior Companion programs from 60 to 55, and increases hourly stipend eligibility for these programs from 125% to 200% of the federal poverty level.

Macro-Level Benefits of Civic Engagement

Freedman (1999) launched the suggestion that a social movement is afoot in which older people are the new trustees of civic life. Weiss and Bass (2002, p. 191) suggest that something akin to a "drive to engage" persists among older people. Further, Adler and Goggin (2005) assert that a civic engagement movement among older adults is proceeding. Morrow-Howell and Freedman (2006–2007) justify the publication of a special issue of *Generations* on the topic for its potential to help shape the civic engagement movement. Recognizing the extensive engagement of older Americans, Binstock et al. (2009–2010) build on Freedman's (2006–2007) concept of "social-purpose encore careers" to prophesize that older persons could become a new force on behalf of society as environmental activists.

Indeed, older adults constitute a significant portion of civic organization membership (Sander & Putnam, 2006; VolunteerMatch, 2007). Moreover, the economic value of older adults' unpaid civic contribution is considerable, partially compensating for declining public and private expenditures. For example, 2008 data provided by the CNCS (2009) indicate that approximately 62 million adult volunteers gave eight billion hours of service to America's communities worth nearly $162 billion. By the same reckoning, the 8.75 million older Americans who in 2008 volunteered an average of 96 hours each (US Bureau of Labor Statistics, 2009c, Table 2) contributed an economic value of $17 billion.

CHALLENGES AND DIRECTIONS FOR FUTURE RESEARCH

Critical Perspectives and Downsides

Evidence to date indicates that civic engagement benefits both participants and the broader community. That fact notwithstanding, concerns remain about current proposals to increase volunteer rates among older adults. Martinson and Minkler (2006) offer a caveat to the burgeoning civic engagement movement by cautioning against possible depreciation of older people who do not participate. During a time of fiscal retrenchment there is pressure on the volunteer community to absorb responsibilities for which funding has disappeared, in effect "letting government off the hook in the provision of basic goods and services for the community and, in particular, for its most vulnerable members" (Martinson & Minkler, 2006, p. 321). They point out that promoting volunteering and other forms of civic engagement among older adults is not politically neutral, regardless of how it is depicted. There are many groups for whom volunteering is not feasible and the diversity of the older population may compound the stigma that might attach to those who do not contribute through civic engagement. Ekerdt (1986) and Holstein (2006) also express concern that coercive social expectations, comparable to the notion of a work ethic or a "busy ethic" around older adult civic engagement, may denigrate those who are too ill, too poor, or otherwise unable to join the movement.

Conceptual Clarification

As we have emphasized throughout this chapter, the lack of a clear-cut definition of civic engagement impedes both conceptual and methodological advances. Perhaps the prime illustration is whether caregiving should be considered a civic activity

(Holstein, 2006). According to some characterizations, caring for a child at a daycare center would be considered civic engagement, but caring for one's own grandchildren at home would not. Although the distinction revolves around work in the private vs public realms, researchers note that contributions of older American caregivers reduce state and federal expenditures on child care and long-term care services, freeing these funds for other public activities. Scholars also have raised provocative questions regarding the tension between self and public interests that arises in any exercise of civic engagement. Consider, for example, the implications of age-segregated and isolated retirement communities for civic life in America. Such "gated" communities may engender higher levels of commitment to volunteer work but also may direct those energies toward private needs such as neighborhood watch, Not in My Backyard (NIMBY) campaigns, or political opposition to school bonds that typically benefit those within their walls (Hinterlong & Williamson, 2006–2007). Although some descriptions of civic engagement exclude forms of collective action that many would consider abhorrent, such as the Ku Klux Klan, other definitions are ambiguous on how to deal with instances in which the voluntary, collective actions of a group of citizens may not serve what other groups consider to be the common good (McBride, 2006–2007).

Recent research has sought to identify civic engagement as a formal retirement role, distinguished in terms of level of commitment that goes beyond the act of volunteering itself. Kaskie et al. (2008) suggest that "by retirement, civic engagement could easily constitute a [normative] role rather than discrete attitudes or behaviors" (p. 369), but further research is needed to address the validity of this construct. How many hours of volunteering a week does it take to differentiate between participating in a civic activity and occupying a civic engagement role? Does it matter what type of civic engagement is pursued? Would doing pro bono legal work for an environmental organization be the same as volunteering to help the same organization pick up trash along a highway? Clearly, additional efforts to establish a precise definition and related behavioral indicators are needed for systematic research (Hinterlong & Williamson, 2006–2007).

Research Needs

The aging of the baby boom generation creates tremendous potential for civic engagement, yet raises questions that researchers and policymakers must address. Will civic engagement by older people decline as the baby boom generation ages, as Putnam (2000) has argued? Or, might civic engagement increase as baby boom move into retirement and other life demands – such as hours spent at work – decrease? How will new work options, such as flexible schedules, retraining, and "bridge jobs," affect civic roles? How will future participation rates of women in the paid labor force affect civic engagement? What kinds of social institutions will improve the ability of older adults to participate in civic life? How will increased economic, racial, and ethnic heterogeneity of baby boom, compared with previous cohorts, affect civic engagement?

Although a corpus of research exists that can help answer these questions, scholars and policymakers are just beginning to consider the implications of these findings. Baby boom could boost the volunteer sector, not just because of the generation's size, but also because of its relatively high levels of education, wealth, and skills. Recent studies find that baby boom are volunteering at higher rates than were previous generations (Einolf, 2009; Rotolo & Wilson, 2004). According to US CB surveys of volunteer activity, an estimated 31% of baby boom volunteered when they were aged 46 to 57, compared with an estimated 25% of the "greatest generation" (born between 1910 and 1930) at the same ages (Foster-Bey et al., 2007).

Researchers are finding the newly retired committed to formal volunteer work. Using data from the HRS, Zedlewski (2007) examined transitions from work to volunteering for adults aged 55 to 64 who retired between 1996 and 2000. About 45% engaged in formal volunteer activities within a four-year post-retirement period, even though only 34% had volunteered while working. Noting that the population aged 55 to 64 will be about 75% larger by 2020 than in 2000, Zedlewski remarks that "nonprofit organizations seem destined to benefit from a significant growth in the services of retirees" (p. 6).

Demographics are changing faster than societal structures can adapt, creating a situation of structural lag. Surveys find that most nonprofit and voluntary organizations are not prepared to engage large numbers of baby boom in meaningful service (Casner-Lotto, 2007). For the last two decades, the voluntary sector has benefited from the substantial contributions of older volunteers whose strong community values were shaped in the World War II era. Despite being placed mostly in routine administrative or fundraising roles, this small cohort of older volunteers has provided a disproportionate share of volunteer hours (Reed & Selbee, 2001). Now the "long civic" generation members are rapidly aging out of the volunteer ranks, leaving gaps to be filled. But a growing body of evidence suggests that baby boom are not willing to perform the traditional "envelope-stuffing" tasks relegated to past and current volunteers. Consistent with their higher levels of education and professionalism, boom seek "interesting, growth-producing, mission-critical, productive, high-level, high-impact work that allows them the freedom to apply their high skills and influence" (Graff, 2007, p. 2). Studies show that baby boom who engage in professional or managerial volunteer roles are the most likely to continue volunteering from one year to the next, while those involved in general labor and routine activities are least likely to continue (Grimm et al., 2007a).

More research is required on older adult civic engagement to inform program and policy development. Evidence asserts that volunteering is good for older adults, but we lack research to determine which programs and policies will maximize older adults' engagement in volunteer roles. We need research to identify: (1) volunteer behaviors and motivations of the baby boom generation, (2) effective strategies to mobilize younger baby boom and older adults, (3) best practices for volunteer program structure and design to attract and retain older volunteers, and (4) how to attract a diverse population of older adults, not only in terms of ethnicity, but also in terms of education, income, and functional abilities. In particular, initiatives targeting lower-socioeconomic-status adults and minorities might have the greatest payoff because these individuals report the lowest levels of volunteer activity; and Musick et al.'s (1999) data show the strongest protective effect of volunteering for those who previously engaged in the least amount of social activity.

Additionally, advocates have argued that outcomes of research identifying the exact economic impact of seniors' civic engagement activities will be critical for building a constituency among legislators and other policymakers to expand civic engagement opportunities for older adults (O'Neill, 2006–2007). Advocates have also emphasized the need to develop strategies to support capacity building by nonprofit groups to attract and retain older adult volunteers. A specific concern is that nonprofit organizations are not ready to take advantage of growing numbers of older volunteers (Freedman, 1999), and recommendations have been made to invest more resources in volunteer management and recognition and to increase the number of professional or leadership volunteer roles within their organizations (Eisner et al., 2009).

Recent interest in civic engagement coincides with a period of strong economic growth, growing numbers of healthy (and often wealthy) people who can expect to live 20 or 30 years past retirement, and a surge in programs and policy innovations advancing civic engagement opportunities for older Americans. Pavalko and Wolfe (2009, p. 27) caution, however, that a potential "caregiving squeeze" among working women could affect the ability of future older adults to participate in civic engagement activities. Further, current and future economic conditions might require older adults to spend more time in the labor force, possibly crowding out civic activities (National Conference on Citizenship, 2009). Thus, we need to follow civic engagement trends closely and continue to develop programs and policies that promote and expand socially focused work and service options for those older adults who aspire to be deeply engaged in the lives of our communities and our country.

REFERENCES

AARP (1997). *Maintaining America's Social Fabric: The AARP survey of civic involvement*. Washington, DC: AARP.

AARP (2003). *Time and money: An in-depth look at 45+ volunteers and donors*. Washington, DC: AARP.

Abraham, K. G., Helms, S., & Presser, S. (2009). How social processes distort measurement: The impact of survey nonresponse on estimates of volunteer work in the United States. *American Journal of Sociology, 114*, 1129–1165.

Adler, R. P., & Goggin, J. (2005). What do we mean by "civic engagement"? *Journal of Transformative Education, 3*, 236–253.

Andersen, R., Curtis, J., & Grabb, E. (2006). Trends in civic association activity in four democracies: The special case of women in the United States. *American Sociological Review, 71*, 376–400.

Bailie, L. (2006). Challenges in social statistics: Standards for defining and measuring volunteer activity. Retrieved July 27, 2009, from the International Association for Official Statistics Web site: http://www.iaos2006conf.ca/pdf/Lorna%20Bailie.pdf

Bass, S., & Caro, F. (2001). Productive aging: A conceptual framework. In N. Morrow-Howell, J. Hinterlong & M. W. Sherraden (Eds.), *Productive aging: Concepts and challenges* (pp. 37–78). Baltimore, MD: The Johns Hopkins University Press.

Binstock, R. H., Sykes, K., & Reilly, S. (2009–2010). Imagining ACES: A reverie for environmentalists and elders. *Generations, 33*(4), 75–81.

Boggs, D., Rocco, T., & Spangler, S. (1995). A framework for understanding older adults' civic behavior. *Educational Gerontology, 91*, 449–465.

Bridgeland, J. M., Putnam, R. D., & Wofford, H. L. (2008). *More to Give: Tapping the talents of the baby boomer, silent and greatest generations*. Washington, DC: AARP.

Burr, J. A., Choi, N. G., Mutchler, J. E., & Caro, F. G. (2005). Caregiving and volunteering: Are private and public helping behaviors linked? *Journal of Gerontology: Social Sciences, 60B*, S247–S256.

Butrica, B. A., Johnson, R. W., & Zedlewski, S. R. (2009). Volunteer dynamics of older Americans. *Journal of Gerontology: Social Sciences, 64B*, 644–655.

Carstensen, L. L. (1995). Evidence for a life-span theory of socioemotional selectivity. *Current Directions in Psychological Science*, 4, 151–156.

Casner-Lotto, J. (2007). Boomers are ready for nonprofits, but are nonprofits ready for them? Washington, DC: The Conference Board. Retrieved July 29, 2009, from http://www.conference-board.org/publications/describe.cfm?id=1319

Choi, L. H. (2003). Factors affecting volunteerism among older adults. *The Journal of Applied Gerontology*, 22, 179–196.

Choi, N. G., Burr, J. A., Mutchler, J. E., & Caro, F. G. (2007). Formal and informal volunteer activity and spousal caregiving among older adults. *Research on Aging*, 29, 99–124.

Cornwell, B., Laumann, E. O., & Schumm, L. P. (2008). The social connectedness of older adults: A national profile. *American Sociological Review*, 73, 185–203.

Corporation for National and Community Service. (2009). Volunteering in America: Research highlights. Retrieved July 29, 2009, from http://www.volunteeringinamerica.gov/assets/resources/VolunteeringInAmericaResearchHighlights.pdf

Cutler, S. J. (1977). Aging and voluntary association participation. *Journal of Gerontology*, 32, 470–479.

Cutler, S. J., & Hendricks, J. (2000). Age differences in voluntary association memberships: Fact or artifact. *Journal of Gerontology: Social Sciences*, 55B, S98–S107.

Davis, J. A., Smith, T. W., & Marsden, P. V. (2009). *General Social Surveys, 1972–2008: Cumulative codebook*. Chicago: National Opinion Research Center.

Edward M. Kennedy Serve America Act, Pub. L. No. 111-13, § 2142. (2009).

Einolf, C. J. (2009). Will the boomers volunteer during retirement? Comparing the baby boom, silent, and long civic cohorts. *Nonprofit and Voluntary Sector Quarterly*, 38, 181–199.

Eisner, D., Grimm, R. T., Maynard, S., & Washburn, S. (2009). The new volunteer workforce. *Stanford Social Innovation Review, Winter*, 32–37.

Ekerdt, D. (1986). The busy ethic: Moral continuity between work and retirement. *The Gerontologist*, 26, 239–244.

Erlinghagen, M., & Hank, K. (2006). The participation of older Europeans in volunteer work. *Ageing & Society*, 26, 567–584.

Farkas, J. I., & Himes, C. L. (1997). The influence of caregiving and employment on the voluntary activities of midlife and older women. *Journal of Gerontology: Social Sciences*, 52B, S180–S189.

Fisher, D., McInerney, P-R., & Petersen, K. (2005). Reconceptualizing the notion of civic engagement. Paper presented at the annual meeting of the American Sociological Association, Philadelphia, PA, August. Retrieved December 22, 2009, from http://www.allacademic.com/meta/p22852_index.html

Foster-Bey, J., Grimm, R., Jr., & Dietz, N. (2007). Keeping baby boomers volunteering: A research brief on volunteer retention and turnover. Retrieved July 28, 2009, from the Corporation for National and Community Service, Office of Research and Policy Development Web site: http://www.nationalservice.gov/pdf/07_0307_boomer_report.pdf

Freedman, M. (1999). *Prime time: How baby boomers will revolutionize retirement and transform America*. New York: Public Affairs.

Freedman, M. (2006–2007). The social-purpose career: Baby boomers, civic engagement and the next stage of work. *Generations*, 30(4), 43–46.

Gallup Poll. (2009). Soul of the community: Knight communities overall. Retrieved October 9, 2009, from http://www.soulofthecommunity.org/files/2009/overall-2009.pdf

Goss, K. A. (1999). Volunteering and the long civic generation. *Nonprofit and Voluntary Sector Quarterly*, 28, 378–415.

Graff, L. (2007). Boom or bust? Will baby boomers save us? Retrieved July 28, 2009, from the Linda Graff And Associates Inc. website: http://www.lindagraff.ca/musings.html#boom

Grano, C., Lucidi, F., Zelli, A., & Violani, C. (2008). Motives and determinants of volunteering in older adults: An integrated model. *The International Journal of Aging and Human Development*, 67, 305–326.

Greenfield, E. A., & Marks, N. F. (2004). Formal volunteering as a protective factor for older adults' psychological well-being. *Journal of Gerontology: Social Science*, 59B, S258–S264.

Greenfield, E. A., & Marks, N. F. (2007). Continuous participation in voluntary groups as a protective factor for the psychological well-being of adults who develop functional limitations: Evidence from the National Survey of Families and Households. *Journal of Gerontology: Social Sciences*, 62B, S60–S68.

Grimm, R., Jr., Dietz, N., Foster-Bey, J., Reingold, D., & Nesbit, R. (2006). Volunteer growth in America: A review of trends since 1974. Retrieved July 27, 2009, from the Corporation for National and Community Service, Office of Research and Policy Development Web site: http://www.nationalservice.gov/pdf/06_1203_volunteer_growth.pdf

Grimm, R., Jr., Cramer, K., Dietz, N., Shelton, L., Dote, L., Manuel, C., et al. (2007a). Volunteering in America: 2007 state trends and rankings in civic life. Retrieved July 27, 2009, from the Corporation for National and Community Service, Office of Research and Policy Development Web site: http://www.nationalservice.gov/pdf/VIA/VIA_fullreport.pdf

Grimm, R., Jr., Spring, K., & Dietz, N. (2007b). The health benefits of volunteering: A review of recent research. Retrieved July 27, 2009, from the Corporation for National and Community Service, Office of Research and Policy Development Web site: http://www.nationalservice.gov/pdf/07_0506_hbr.pdf

Health and Retirement Study. (2009). Documentation: Question concordance. Retrieved July 27, 2009, from http://hrsonline.isr.umich.edu/concord

Hendricks, J., & Cutler, S. J. (2004). Volunteerism and socioemotional selectivity in later life. *Journal of Gerontology: Social Sciences, 59B,* S251–S257.

Hinterlong, J. E., & Williamson, A. (2006–2007). The effects of civic engagement of current and future cohorts of older adults. *Generations, 30*(4), 10–17.

Holstein, M. (2006). A critical reflection on civic engagement. *Public Policy & Aging Report, 16,* 21–26.

Hong, S.-I., Hasche, L., & Bowland, S. (2009). Structural relationships between social activities and longitudinal trajectories of depression among older adults. *The Gerontologist, 49,* 1–11.

Independent Sector (2000). America's senior volunteers. Retrieved August 26, 2009, from http://www.independentsector. org/programs/research/ SeniorVolun.pdf

Independent Sector. (2001). Giving & volunteering in the United Sates: Key findings. Retrieved August 26, 2009, from http://www. independentsector.org/PDFs/ GV01keyfind.pdf

Inter-University Consortium for Political and Social Research. (2009). Americans' Changing Lives: Waves I, II, III, and IV, 1986, 1989, 1994, and 2002. Retrieved July 27, 2009, from http://www. icpsr.umich.edu/cocoon/ICPSR/ STUDY/04690.xml

Kaskie, B., Imhof, S., Cavanaugh, J., & Culp, K. (2008). Civic engagement as a retirement role for aging Americans. *The Gerontologist, 48,* 368–377.

Kim, J., Kang, J.-H., Lee, M.-A., & Lee, Y. (2007). Volunteering among older people in Korea. *Journal of Gerontology: Social Sciences, 62,* S69–S73.

Lum, T. Y., & Lightfoot, E. (2005). The effects of volunteering on the physical and mental health of older people. *Research on Aging, 27,* 31–55.

Martinson, M., & Minkler, M. (2006). Civic engagement and older adults: A critical perspective. *The Gerontologist, 46,* 318–324.

McBride, A. M. (2006–2007). Civic engagement, older adults and inclusion. *Generations, 30*(4), 66–71.

Morrow-Howell, N., Hinterlong, J., Rozario, P. A., & Tang, F. (2003). Effects of volunteering on the well-being of older adults. *Journal of Gerontology: Social Sciences, 58B,* S137–S145.

Morrow-Howell, N., & Freedman, M. (2006–2007). Introduction: Bringing civic engagement into sharper focus. *Generations, 30*(4), 6–9.

Morrow-Howell, N., Hong, S.-I., & Tang, F. (2009a). Who benefits from volunteering? Variations in perceived benefits. *The Gerontologist, 49,* 91–102.

Morrow-Howell, N., Jonson-Reid, M., McCrary, S., Lee, Y., & Spitznagel, E. (2009b). *Evaluation of Experience Corps: Student reading outcomes (Working Paper).* St. Louis: Center for Social Development, Washington University.

Musick, M. A., & Wilson, J. (2003). Volunteering and depression: The role of psychological and social resources in different age groups. *Social Science and Medicine, 56,* 259–269.

Musick, M. A., & Wilson, J. (2008). *Volunteers: A social profile.* Bloomington, IN: Indiana University Press.

Musick, M. A., Herzog, A. R., & House, J. S. (1999). Volunteering and mortality among older adults: Findings from a national sample. *Journal of Gerontology: Social Sciences, 54B,* S173–S180.

Mutchler, J., Burr, J. A., & Caro, F. G. (2003). From paid work to volunteer: Leaving the paid workforce and volunteering in later life. *Social Forces, 81,* 1267–1293.

National Academy on an Aging Society. (2009a). Definitions of civic engagement. Retrieved December 22, 2009, from http://www. civicengagement.org/agingsociety/ links/CEdefinitions.pdf

National Academy on an Aging Society. (2009b). The civic enterprise. Retrieved August 18, 2009, from http://www. agingsociety.org/agingsociety/ civic-engagement-diagram.html.

National Conference on Citizenship. (2008). 2008 civic health index: Beyond the vote. Retrieved July 27, 2009, from http://www.ncoc. net/index.php?tray=series&tid= top5&cid=97

National Conference on Citizenship. (2009). Older Americans may be shifting from volunteering and community work to private helping: The economic downturn is reshaping civic engagement. Retrieved August 31, 2009, from http://www.ncoc.net/index.php? tray=content&tid=top5&cid= 2gp62

Okun, M. A., & Michel, J. (2006). Sense of community and being a volunteer among the young-old. *Journal of Applied Gerontology, 25,* 173–188.

Okun, M. A., & Schultz, A. (2003). Age and motives for volunteering: Testing hypotheses derived from socioemotional selectivity theory. *Psychology and Aging, 18,* 231–239.

O'Neill, G. (2006–2007). Civic engagement on the agenda at the 2005 White House Conference on Aging. *Generations, 30*(4), 101–108.

Pavalko, E. K., & Wolfe, J. D. (2009). Workplace policies, caregiving, and women's long-term income security. *Public Policy & Aging Report, 19*(2), 27–31.

Philanthropy for Active Civic Engagement. (2009). Welcome to PACE - Philanthropy for Active Civic Engagement. Retrieved December 22, 2009, from http:// www.pacefunders.org/index.html

Piliavin, J. A., & Siegl, E. (2007). Health benefits of volunteering in the Wisconsin Longitudinal Study. *Journal of Health and Social Behavior, 48,* 450–464.

Putnam, R. D. (2000). *Bowling alone: The collapse and revival of American community.* New York: Simon & Schuster.

Rebok, G. W., Carlson, M. C., Glass, T. A., McGill, S., Hill, J., Wasik, B. A., et al. (2004). Short-term impact of Experience Corps participation on children and schools: Results from a pilot randomized trial. *Journal of Urban Health, 81,* 79–93.

Reed, P. B., & Selbee, L. K. (2001). The civic core in Canada: Disproportionality in charitable giving, volunteering, and civic participation. *Nonprofit and*

Voluntary Sector Quarterly, 30, 761–780.

Rotolo, T. (1999). Trends in voluntary association participation. *Nonprofit and Voluntary Sector Quarterly, 28,* 199–212.

Rotolo, T., & Wilson, J. (2004). Whatever happened to the long civic generation? Explaining cohort differences in volunteerism. *Social Forces, 82,* 1091–1121.

Rozario, P. A. (2006–2007). Volunteering among current cohorts of older adults and baby boomers. *Generations, 30*(4), 31–36.

Sander, T., & Putnam, R. (2006). Social capital and civic engagement of individuals over age fifty in the United States. In L. Wilson & S. Simson (Eds.), *Civic engagement and the baby boomer generation: Research, policy and proactive perspectives* (pp. 21–41). New York: Haworth Press.

Shmotkin, D., Blumstein, T., & Modan, B. (2003). Beyond keeping active: Concomitants of being a volunteer in old-old age. *Psychology and Aging, 18,* 602–607.

Statistics Canada. (2007). *Caring Canadians, Involved Canadians: Highlights from the 2007 Canada Survey of Giving, Volunteering and Participation.* Retrieved July 27, 2009, from http://www. givingandvolunteering.ca/files/ giving/en/csgvp_highlights_ 2007.pdf

Sugihara, Y., Sugisawa, H., Shibata, H., & Harada, K. (2008). Productive roles, gender, and depressive symptoms: Evidence from a national longitudinal study of late-middle-aged Japanese. *Journal of Gerontology: Psychological Sciences, 63B,* P227–P234.

Survey of Health, Ageing, and Retirement in Europe [SHARE]. (2009). Survey of health, ageing and retirement in Europe. Retrieved July 27, 2009, from http://www.share-project.org/

Tan, E. J., Rebok, G. W., Yu, Q., Frangakis, C. E., Carlson, M. C.,

Wang, T., et al. (2009). The long-term relationship between high-intensity volunteering and physical activity in older African American women. *Journal of Gerontology: Social Sciences, 64B,* 304–311.

Tang, F. (2006). What resources are needed for volunteerism? A life course perspective. *Journal of Applied Gerontology, 25,* 375–390.

Tang, F. (2009). Late-life volunteering and trajectories of physical health. *Journal of Applied Gerontology, 28,* 524–533.

Taylor, B. A., & Bengtson, V. L. (2001). Sociological perspectives on productive aging. In N. Morrow-Howell, J. Hinterlong & M. W. Sherraden (Eds.), *Productive aging: Concepts and challenges* (pp. 120–144). Baltimore, MD: The Johns Hopkins University Press.

Toppe, C. (2005). *Measuring volunteering: A behavioral approach.* Retrieved July 27, 2009, from the Center for Information & Research on Civic Learning & Engagement Web site: http://www.civicyouth. org/PopUps/WorkingPapers/ WP43Toppe.pdf.

Toppe, C., & Galaskiewicz, J. (2006). *Measuring volunteering: Committee report.* Retrieved July 27, 2009, from the Points of Light Foundation web site: http://archive.pointsoflight. org/downloads/pdf/resources/ research/CommitteeReport.pdf

Unofficial compilation of the Older Americans Act of 1965 as amended in 2006 (Public Law 109-365). (n.d). Retrieved July 25, 2009, from the Administration on Aging Web site: http://www. aoa.gov/AoAroot/AoA_Programs/ OAA/oaa_full.asp

US Bureau of Labor Statistics. (2009a). Volunteering in the United States: 2008 technical note. Retrieved July 27, 2009, from http://www.bls.gov/news. release/volun.tn.htm

US Bureau of Labor Statistics (2009b). Charts from the American Time Use Survey. Retrieved July 27, 2009, from

http://www.bls.gov/TUS/CHARTS/ home.htm

US Bureau of Labor Statistics. (2009c). Volunteering in the United States, 2008. Retrieved July 27, 2009, from http://www.bls. gov/news.release/volun.nr0.htm

van Willigen, M. (2000). Differential benefits of volunteering across the life course. *Journal of Gerontology: Social Sciences, 55B,* S308–S318.

VolunteerMatch (2007). *Great Expectations: Boomers and the future of volunteering* (VolunteerMatch User Research Study). San Francisco: MetLife Foundation.

Weiss, R. S., & Bass, S. A. (2002). Epilogue. In R. S. Weiss & S. A. Bass (Eds.), *Challenges of the Third Age: Meaning and purpose in later life* (pp. 189–197). New York: Oxford University Press.

Wilson, J., & Musick, M. (1997a). Work and volunteering: The long arm of the job. *Social Forces, 76,* 251–272.

Wilson, J., & Musick, M. (1997b). Who cares? Toward an integrated theory of volunteer work. *American Sociological Review, 62,* 694–713.

Windsor, T. D., Anstey, K. J., & Rodgers, B. (2008). Volunteering and psychological well-being among young-old adults: How much is too much? *The Gerontologist, 48,* 59–70.

Zedlewski, S. R. (2007). Will retiring boomers form a new army of volunteers? Retrieved July 25, 2009, from the Urban Institute web site: http://www.urban.org/ UploadedPDF/411579_retiring_ boomers.pdf

Zedlewski, S. R., & Butrica, B. A. (2007). *Are we taking full advantage of older adults' potential?* Washington, DC: Urban Institute.

Zedlewski, S. R., & Schaner, S. G. (2005). Older adults' engagement should be recognized and encouraged. Retrieved July 27, 2009, from the Urban Institute Web site: http://www.urban. org/UploadedPDF/311201_ Perspectives1.pdf

Chapter | 17 |

Late-Life Death and Dying in 21st-Century America

Deborah T. Gold

Departments of Psychiatry & Behavioral Sciences and Sociology, Duke University Medical Center, Durham, North Carolina

INTRODUCTION AND BRIEF OVERVIEW

During the twentieth century, life expectancy in the United States nearly doubled. In 1900, death occurred throughout life; in twenty-first century America, death is more likely to occur in late life. Early in the twentieth century, families managed death and dying. Now, America is death-aversive (Becker, 1973; Solomon et al., 2003). Instead of caring for dying family members, we turn this care over to professionals. American norms around death and dying have changed in the last 100 years, perhaps because of improved medical care and technology or the increasing movement from acute to chronic conditions, which can delay death even more. Yet our fear of death has expanded even as death has been delayed (Cicirelli, 2006).

This chapter examines how social factors and institutions affect and contextualize death. All societies must manage death, but cultural responses differ substantially both across and within societies. Age, a critical social factor, influences perceptions about death, as do religiosity and education. In truth, no one can fully model the social experience of death because of its heterogeneity.

DEFINING DEATH AND DYING

Death is the end of life and biological functioning. But medical technology has made it problematic to identify the precise moment at which the transition from life to death takes place (Rosenberg, 2009). In the past, death was the absence of heartbeat and respiration. With the introduction of life-sustaining treatments (LSTs), those endpoints are no longer definitive. In 1968, Harvard Medical School established an ad hoc committee on brain death to establish clinical guidelines for identifying irreversible coma, now usually referred to as "persistent vegetative state" or PVS (Anonymous, 1968). In this classic article, four criteria for brain death were established: unreceptivity and unresponsitivity, no movements or breathing, no reflexes, and flat electroencephalogram. Thirty years later, Wijdicks (2001) gave physicians a clinical definition of brain death, especially important when dying patients were eligible as organ donors. Unfortunately, clinical clarity did not improve our understanding of the dying process, nor did it provide an interpretive model to guide the study of death and dying. Currently, several theories now offer perspectives for understanding and studying death and dying.

Theories of Death and Dying

Stage Theories of Death and Dying

Elisabeth Kubler-Ross (1969) was the first to develop a *stage theory of dying*. This theory proposed five stages of grief: denial, anger, bargaining, depression, and acceptance. Although these stages were viewed as typical for dying patients, Kubler-Ross added the caveats that not all dying patients completed the stages in this exact order and that others may skip stages or "backtrack." She also noted that a constant in all stages was hope, which enabled the dying to find emotional strength to cope with the end of life. Because of the caveats (which imply that the theory cannot be falsified), Kubler-Ross's theory proved ultimately untestable, but it gave physicians and patients permission to talk frankly about mortality and terminal care for the first time.

Buckman (1993) later proposed a *three-stage model of dying* that addressed some of the weaknesses of Kubler-Ross's theory – principally that it focused primarily on psychosocial dynamics and ignored physical and spiritual aspects of dying. Buckman identified three stages of dying: the initial stage (facing the awareness and threat of dying); the chronic stage (the experience of the illness); and the final stage (ultimately accepting death). Buckman also disregarded physical aspects of dying but added spirituality to his model of coping with death.

Awareness of Dying

One of the first sociological perspectives on death and dying was the *theory of awareness contexts* (Glaser & Strauss, 1965). Awareness contexts around dying include what people know about terminal illness and their willingness to discuss this knowledge openly with others (Hellström et al., 2005). Glaser and Strauss reported that most dying hospitalized patients knew little or nothing about their impending deaths; significant others such as friends and family did not know much more. Using a symbolic interactionist perspective, they emphasized that people with identical information about a dying patient processed that information in different ways.

Trajectories of Dying

A third theoretical model of dying emerged from a subsequent collaboration of Glaser and Strauss. In *Time for Dying* (1968), Glaser and Strauss focused on *trajectories of the dying experience*. This perspective emphasizes dying as a process occurring over time and the utility of examining the pathways or trajectories associated with it. The temporal ordering of events in a death trajectory is fluid and varies across individuals. Dying individuals, their significant others, and their medical providers must adjust to the changes that occur during this process. Implicitly, the notion of varying trajectories of dying implies that stage theories of death and dying cannot do justice to the heterogeneity of individual experience. An important illustration of research using trajectories of dying is provided by Lunney and colleagues (2002). They used Medicare claims data to determine whether there are discrete, typical trajectories and whether those trajectories differ in health care utilization and cost during the last year of life. Four trajectories captured most of the variance in the sample. The trajectories also differed substantially in amount and cost of care in the last year of life.

Readiness to Die

Copp (1997) proposed yet another theoretical perspective called *readiness to die*. It too was based on symbolic interactionism and emerged from unstructured interviews with 12 dying cancer patients and their nurses that reflected their symbolic constructions around death. Both nurses and patients segregated the dying body from the person and his or her mind in that body. As a patient's health deteriorated, nurses increasingly emphasized disengagement of the self from the body, although neither nurses nor patients could explain why. Ultimately, nurses constructed a conceptual map on which they could locate each patient. Four patterns emerged from these maps: person ready, body not ready; person ready, body ready; person not ready, body ready; and person not ready, body not ready. These categories allowed nurses to appropriately pace patients' care and encouraged nurses and patients to communicate openly about impending death, thereby reducing potential tensions that might arise in such situations.

Themes of Dying in Late Life

Lloyd-Williams and colleagues (2007) conducted qualitative interviews about death and dying with 20 adults over age 80 from which six key themes associated with end of life in the old-old emerged: *fears surrounding death and dying* (how they would die); *the inevitability of death* (older people knowing death was not far away); *thoughts and wishes surrounding end-of-life care* (especially dying at home); *preparation for death* (causing minimum burden for family); *euthanasia/ assisted dying* (few were advocates for euthanasia); and *after death* (viewing death as an absolute end or belief in an afterlife). These themes differed from themes discussed by younger and middle-aged adults, suggesting that even the oldest-old experience death anxiety.

DEATH AND DYING IN AMERICA: HISTORICAL CHANGES IN SOCIAL NORMS

Prior to, and during, the twentieth century, death occurred in the context of the family, with little intervention from medical practitioners. In the 1800s, 80% of people died at home (Corr et al., 2009). Social norms of the time dictated that all activities surrounding death occur at home, with all family members participating. Deaths were typically not attended by healthcare professionals. Further, adults did not insulate children from the experience of death or protect them from the pain and sadness of the experience. Normalizing death and dying may have diminished children's fear and helped them cope more effectively with loss.

Industrialization and Medical Technology

As the US moved into the twentieth century and industrialization became a powerful driving force, death and dying changed in several ways. The five most frequent causes of death in 1900 were acute conditions: tuberculosis; pneumonia and influenza; diseases of the heart; diarrhea, enteritis, and ulceration of the intestines; and intracranial lesions of vascular origin (Centers for Disease Control (CDC)/National Center for Health Statistics (NCHS), 2003). Cancer was eighth and senility ninth. Most deaths were caused by acute infections that, without antibiotics, could not be cured. Few people had long and lingering deaths, as the pace of decline was rapid. Even if individuals experienced chronic diseases such as cancer or diabetes, acute infections were still likely to be the direct causes of death.

Later in the twentieth century, deaths from infections declined precipitously and deaths from chronic, degenerative diseases rose dramatically. The theory of the epidemiologic transition – which focuses on the relationship between health and disease as well as their sociological, demographic, and economic determinants – explains the dramatic increase in life expectancy observed in the US (Land & Yang, 2006). Because people lived longer before they died, management of death changed as well.

Families and Death

Beginning in the mid-twentieth century, most families no longer took responsibility for the management of death and dying. Instead, funeral homes grew into a multimillion-dollar industry (Laderman, 2003). In addition, there were profits from embalming, burial, and cemetery plots, and millions of dollars went to the florists, casket and vault makers, and other commercial entities. Costs rose dramatically as new expectations emerged: the best coffin, the strongest vault, the prime cemetery plot. And although people were often dismayed by the financial investment that death required, they were also grateful to have no responsibility for caring for the dead (Mitford, 2000). By professionalizing death and dying, Americans distanced themselves from the experience. The social role of the funeral director emerged, and the service provided relieved the family of the more distasteful aspects of death.

Another major change occurred in the usual place of death. Prior to 1900, most people died at home, on the battlefield, or in accidents. By 1949, nearly 50% of deaths occurred in a healthcare institution, primarily a hospital (Corr et al., 2009). Although a large proportion of dying people express the desire to die at home (Hays et al., 1999), others remain in hospitals or other facilities (e.g. nursing home, hospice) (Flory et al., 2004). In 1989, 62% of people with chronic illnesses died in acute care hospitals (Gruneir et al., 2007).

Hospital deaths affect all family members. Hospitalized patients are more likely to die without family members present. Family members, however, may feel relieved at not witnessing terminal suffering. Relief of suffering is perhaps the most important factor for both people who are dying and family members who love them (Shinjo et al., 2010). Being hospitalized ensures better access to pain management and other interventions to maximize comfort and minimize suffering.

Dying older adults would much prefer to be at home than in the hospital. According to Brazil and colleagues (2005), who studied caregivers whose care recipient was over age 50 and died during the study, 63% of terminal patients wanted to die at home, but 30% of them did not. Tang (2003) studied 180 terminal cancer patients; she found that 90% of her sample wanted to die at home, but many fewer actually did so. A few studies have addressed strategies that might improve a patient's odds of dying at a preferred site. For example, Muramatsu and colleagues (2008) found increased state spending on home health services significantly improved the likelihood of home death.

When family members are present during the death of a loved one, they interact with medical personnel in important ways. They are often distressed by the normal physiological indications that death is coming. For example, most family members are distressed at the "death rattle," a gurgling or rattling sound (Wildiers & Menten, 2002). According to several studies, the death rattle does not cause distress to dying patients; as a result, healthcare providers rarely treat it for the patient's sake (Wee & Hillier, 2008). Several studies, however, found that, when family members are present, healthcare personnel use anticholinergic drugs to reduce the death rattle and cause less emotional discomfort to family members (Wee & Hillier, 2008). It is fair to conclude that the presence of family influences the practice of palliative care medicine.

Finally, compared to the first half of the twentieth century, the duration of dying has increased. This is, in part, a result of the primary causes of death changing from acute to chronic conditions. Family members play a role in this as well, especially if they request that physicians "do everything." With sophisticated medical technology and use of LSTs, the duration of dying is frequently extended.

Causes of Death in the 20th and 21st Centuries

The leading causes of death in 2006 were quite different from those in 1900. The largest cause of death in the 21st-century US for both men and women is heart disease; cancer and stroke are second and third. For men, however, unintentional accidents replace stroke in third place. Infections (influenza and pneumonia) are the seventh leading cause of death for men and the eighth for women. Overall, leading causes of death do not vary by race. For whites and blacks, the top three causes of death are heart disease, cancer, and cerebrovascular accidents. For Asians, the leading cause of death is cancer, followed by heart disease and cerebrovascular accidents; and for Hispanics, the three leading causes are heart disease, cerebrovascular accidents, and unintentional injuries (Weaver & Rivollo, 2006–2007).

Increased life expectancy and improved disease prevention and health promotion resulted in another change during the twentieth century. As mentioned earlier, dying has migrated to late life instead of occurring throughout the life course. Overall, age-adjusted death rates dropped substantially between 1900 and 2000. About 17 per 1000 Americans died in 1900; in 2000, the rate was about 9 per 1000. Older Americans also have benefited as the death rate for Americans aged 65 to 74 fell from nearly 7% per year to fewer than 2% per year (Arias, 2007).

Hospitals and the Medical Profession

Changing mortality rates and causes of death were driving forces that increased the use of institutions as places of death. For medical professionals, dying is more manageable and symptoms more controllable in a setting that provides health care on a 24/7 basis. Most dying patients want to avoid severe pain. Physicians can more easily control pain and sedate dying patients in the hospital. Lives can be saved at a moment's notice with Code Blue teams available much more rapidly than in the community. Medications, diagnostic tests, surgical suite accessibility: all are available in hospitals.

Costs of Dying in the 21st-Century US

The costs of the last year of life increased exponentially over the last several decades as medical technology advanced in sophistication and use of LST increased. Scitovsky (2005) asked whether a disproportionate amount of health care dollars is spent on the terminally ill and reached the following conclusions: (1) health care costs at the end of life are substantial; (2) high costs of dying have not necessarily been recent, we may just be more aware of them; and (3) the high medical costs at the end of life do not result from aggressive treatment but rather from the fact that virtually everyone receives high-cost care in the hospital, regardless of their terminal status (Scitovsky, 2005). Zilberberg and Shorr (2008) modeled costs of mechanical ventilation and projected that in 2020 such care would reach an inflation-adjusted cost of more than $64 billion. These findings suggest the US must find ways to limit either cost per service or the number of services provided.

The Study to Understand Prognoses and Preferences for Outcomes and Risks of Treatment (SUPPORT) was a landmark effort to improve end-of-life decisions and to reduce life extension with medical technology (SUPPORT Principal Investigators, 1995). The sample included more than 9000 terminally ill adults. SUPPORT also developed and tested an intervention designed to improve end-of-life care through better doctor–patient communication and greater understanding by physicians of patients' end-of-life wishes. Unfortunately, none of the five sites showed improvements in patient care or outcomes. Did this result from normatively derived behavior that encourages healthcare providers to do all they can, regardless of patient or family wishes? Or are healthcare providers indifferent to any approach that deviates from the way they were originally taught to handle end-of-life care? In addition, there was no reduction in hospital resource use for the intervention group. Perhaps narrowly focused studies that examine components of SUPPORT's hoped-for outcomes could enable researchers to better understand and improve the quality and cost of terminal patient care. Certainly the US economy cannot support the level of resource and human costs that terminal care now requires.

Social Values and Options for the Terminally Ill

Extensive empirical evidence suggests that care for the terminally ill has high human and resource costs. Even with such interventions as hospice and palliative care, terminally ill patients often experience substantial physical and mental pain and suffering. Some propose that physician-assisted suicide (PAS) and euthanasia *are* interventions that can and do terminate end-of-life suffering and should be more widely available.

Euthanasia, the deliberate termination of life carried out by a physician, elicits nearly universal resistance from healthcare professionals, patients, and families in the US. Only two countries – the Netherlands and Belgium – have fully legalized euthanasia, both implemented in 2002. Even in the twenty-first century, euthanasia is unacceptable to the majority of US citizens.

PAS elicits a different and, in some cases, more accepting response. In PAS, a physician provides the prescription for oral barbiturates, but the patient takes responsibility for their use. PAS is legal in many countries, but some nations, including Canada and Australia, explicitly forbid assisted suicide. In other countries such as France and Germany, legislation forbidding PAS does not exist. However, the practice is not tolerated, and practitioners could be brought to trial for failing to assist a person in danger. The Netherlands, Switzerland and Belgium are the only European countries in which PAS is legal. In Switzerland, non-physician-assisted suicide is legal as well (Humphry, 2002).

In the US, euthanasia is illegal in every state, and no federal laws permit PAS. However, in 1997, Oregon passed the first Death with Dignity Act (DWDA) (Lindsay, 2009). This legislation permits terminally ill Oregonians to voluntarily terminate their lives with self-administration of lethal medications prescribed by a physician. The regulations for PAS in Oregon are extensive and stringent. Participants must be residents of Oregon with a terminal diagnosis who request PAS from their physicians twice verbally and once in writing, and only physicians in Oregon can write prescriptions for PAS. Many people, medical and lay alike, believed legalizing PAS would have serious, unanticipated consequences (e.g. influx of non-Oregon residents wanting PAS; requests by non-terminally ill people for PAS) (Lindsay, 2009).

In order to quantify potential consequences, the State of Oregon has kept meticulous records of the Death with Dignity process. Between 1997 and 2008, 401 patients have died using methods described in the DWDA (Hedberg et al., 2009). As documented in all State of Oregon annual reports, many more people requested PAS than used it. In 2008, for example, physicians wrote 88 prescriptions for lethal drugs specifically for PAS. Fifty-four patients took the medications and died; 22 died that year of their underlying disease; and 12 remained alive (http://egov.oregon.gov/DHS/ph/pas/docs/year11.pdf). Examination of the social characteristics of the 401 Oregonians who participated in DWDA between 1997 and 2008 is enlightening. They were between 55 and 84 years of age (87%) and primarily white (98%). African Americans represent 2% of the state's population, but not a single African American has requested PAS. Additionally, these individuals were slightly more likely to be male (53%) and well educated (44% had a college degree or more), and most were dying of cancer (80%). In 75% of the cases, the prescribing physician was not present at the PAS event.

Policy makers and politicians believed that Oregon's electorate was unique in accepting PAS. The State of Washington, however, passed its own Death with Dignity Act-Initiative 1000 in 2009, with more than 60% of the vote. Not long afterward, the Montana Supreme Court ruled 5–2 for the legal right to assisted suicide by upholding a lower court's ruling. The Vermont State Legislature rejected a law permitting PAS in 2007, but it has been refiled and will come up for a vote in 2010. California has a similar bill up for discussion in the legislature. These civil rights debates are occurring more frequently and are more socially diverse than before.

To date we know little about older adults' attitudes toward PAS. Koenig et al. (1996) asked 168 older adults (mean age = 75.8 years) with medical or psychiatric conditions and their family members (n = 146) about their attitudes toward PAS for terminal patients, chronically ill patients, and those with mental incompetence. Support for PAS for the terminally ill differed significantly between older patients and their family members (40% vs 60%, p < 0.001). Differences between older adults and their family members were not significant for chronically ill patients and mentally ill patients (Koenig et al., 1996).

Emanuel and colleagues (2000) examined attitudes toward and desires for PAS and euthanasia among terminally ill patients and their caregivers. Their sample included 988 terminally ill patients (mean age = 66.5, age range: 22–109 years) and 893 caregivers. Sixty percent of the patients had cancer, 78% were white, and 14% were African American. Of the terminally ill patients, 60% supported the idea of PAS or euthanasia in a hypothetical situation. Only 11%, however, said that they had seriously considered either option for themselves. Characteristics associated with being less likely to consider euthanasia or PAS included older age (65+), feeling appreciated, and being African American. Those associated with being more likely to consider these options included depression, substantial caregiving needs, and pain.

Social norms around death and dying in general, and PAS more specifically, continue to change in the twenty-first century. It does appear that options for PAS will be supported in more states. But research has shown that we are far from 100% supportive of hastening death.

INDIVIDUAL-LEVEL ISSUES

Fear of Death: Its Beginnings

In twenty-first century America, fear of death transcends age, place, and race/ethnicity (Lehto & Stein, 2009). How did fear become the overarching attitude toward death in America? Several plausible explanations exist. As death moved into the hands of healthcare professionals, individuals were no longer desensitized from direct contact with death. Ultimately, we have become ignorant about death, and ignorance breeds fear (Hui & Fung, 2009).

Also, as the twentieth century progressed, death happened less frequently. In fact, mortality rates declined at an exceptionally rapid pace, although age differences existed in the mortality reduction. From 1900–1940, 80% of the mortality reductions occurred in people under age 45 (Cutler & Meara, 2004). Between 1960 and 2000, 80% of mortality reduction occurred in people over age 45. Fewer deaths meant that fewer people were exposed to it directly and had less direct knowledge of the processes leading up to it.

Death Anxiety

Research indicates that the relationship between age and death anxiety is curvilinear (Depaola et al., 2003). Specifically, death anxiety is high among younger adults, peaks in middle age, and is lower and more stable in late life (Depaola et al., 2003). That younger and middle-aged adults show greater levels

of fear of death than older adults has been demonstrated in multiple studies (Cicirelli, 2006). One possible explanation for this pattern is that people who have lived longer have also had more time to be aware of their own mortality and to accept it. As individuals lose significant others, death may no longer be terrifying. Some individuals may prefer to die rather than survive when age-peers have predeceased them.

Social Factors and Attitudes Toward Death and Dying

The heterogeneity of the American population – especially in late life – results in wide variability of beliefs and attitudes toward death and dying. Age, race/ethnicity, SES, and gender all influence how people will cope with short-term and long-term consequences of death and dying. These social factors influence people's attitudes about their own deaths as well as the likely duration of their lives. Religious factors also explain substantial variability among Americans (Hui & Fung, 2009).

Race

Demographic research indicates that race is significantly related to mortality rates. From infant mortality to fatal injuries in young children (Pressley et al., 2007) to violent death among youth (Teplin et al., 2005) to racial differences in breast cancer outcomes (Demicheli et al., 2007) to survival of older men after hospitalization (Liu & Sullivan, 2003), African Americans die earlier than their Caucasian counterparts.

In his review, Hummer (1996) noted that racial differences are observed in overall health, overall mortality, life expectancy, and self-reported health. He also described three theoretical explanations for these mortality differences: racial genetic, cultural/behavioral, and socioeconomic. Nonetheless, his analysis indicates that these three factors do not totally account for race differences in mortality. He also takes issue with those who emphasize socioeconomic disadvantage as the primary cause of racial differences in mortality, stating that institutional and individual-level racism must be examined as well (Hummer, 1996).

Over thirty years ago, Bengtson and colleagues (1977) explored age, race, gender, and social class differences in attitudes toward death. They examined similarities and differences in three issues: fear of death, frequency of thinking about death, and awareness of proximity of death. Participants were categorized in three age groups: 45–54 years, 55–64 years, and 65–74 years. Fear of death significantly decreased with age. Although women reported fearing death more than men, the difference was not significant. No differences were found for race or SES. There were virtually no differences for any of the four key characteristics in frequency of thinking about death, although age differences approached significance. Finally, respondents were asked how much time they felt they had before they died. African Americans expressed the greatest longevity expectations at all ages, while elderly whites and Hispanics reported the fewest years left to live. Differences in age and race were highly significant.

How have attitudes about these three facets of death changed over the last 35 years? Although these findings have not been replicated, several related studies have examined racial influences on specific aspects of the end of life. In a study of end-of-life decision making by African American and Caucasian older adults, Allen and colleagues (2008) found that increasing information reduced African Americans' desire for LST and slightly increased Caucasians' desire to initiate LST. Blackhall and colleagues (1999) report African Americans are more likely than whites to want to be kept alive on life support and choose curative rather than palliative care. Their ethnographic interviews suggested that African Americans deeply distrust the white-dominated healthcare system and believe that financial well-being is the key to being kept alive.

Johnson and her colleagues (2008) interviewed black and white adults over age 65 in North Carolina to determine whether attitudes about hospice and use of advance directives significantly differed by race. Whites were more likely to be married, had more education and income, and were four times more likely to have an advance directive than blacks; whites also expressed more positive attitudes toward hospice care. However, when distrust of health care, spirituality, advance care planning beliefs, and end-of-life care preferences were added to the model, the race effect was no longer statistically significant.

In a study using data from the National Longitudinal Mortality Study (NLMS), Howard and colleagues (2000) examined the effects of race, SES, and age on cause-specific mortality. The sample included more than 400 000 blacks and whites and was generally representative of the US population. Strong race by age interactions led them to stratify results by age. Black race accounted for strikingly higher risk of mortality in 38 disease strata. For example, black women had almost twice the excess mortality from ischemic heart disease and diabetes than white women, and black men had twice the excess mortality risk from diabetes, cirrhosis, infections, stomach cancer, and stroke than white men. Controlling for SES, however, explained 40% to 50% of the excess mortality for black women and 20% to 40% for black men. Interestingly, some racial differences in excess mortality decreased with age. Diseases that showed strong associations between race and excess mortality in the younger sample but not for the oldest-old (age 75+) include hypertension, ischemic heart disease, ill-defined heart disease, and stroke.

Gender

Gender also plays an important and complicated role in mortality. Life expectancy in almost every country, including the US, is significantly higher for women than men. In fact, this is true in virtually all mammalian species, although the cause(s) of this gender difference remain unknown. According to Eskes and Haanen (2007), men have earlier onset of cardiovascular disease than women; however, scientists provide no compelling explanation for this difference. No physiological factors appear to cause women to live longer, although higher levels of estrogen might have a cardiovascular protection effect. The Women's Health Initiative studies, however, found no differences in mortality between women on estrogen/estrogen plus progestin and those not on those hormones (Hulley et al., 1998).

It is frequently observed that older men are more susceptible to fatal diseases and accidents while older women are more likely to experience crippling, non-lethal diseases (e.g. osteoporosis, osteoarthritis). Gender differences in longevity have powerful implications for the composition of older cohorts in terms of health care utilization, residential or institutional care, and the experience of dying (Seale, 2003). These differences cause women to have increasing levels of disability as they age. A visit to any long-term care facility reveals the disproportionate proportion of women to men resulting from these longevity gender differences. Gender differences in longevity, especially in developed countries, result in older women substantially outnumbering older men (Seale, 2003). Most older men have wives who serve as caregivers when they require assistance with chronic disease and dying (Navaie-Waliser et al., 2002). The fact that men tend to marry younger women exacerbates this pattern. The experience of death for an older man will likely include care at home, with spouse and other family around him during the dying process. His widow's options for caregiving and dying are dramatically different. Without a spousal caregiver, older women are forced to rely on adult children (primarily daughters), other female relatives, or formal caregivers, none of whom are likely to provide the level of care they gave their husbands (Navaie-Waliser et al., 2002).

Messages that healthcare providers convey to dying patients differ by gender. In a fascinating study of the influence of gender and age on terminal care, Johnson and colleagues (2000) examined whether gender and age influenced patient perceptions of physician recommendations for terminal care. The authors found that women aged 70 and older were more likely to perceive that their physicians recommended palliative rather than life-sustaining care. Although no definitive explanation for this finding exists, physicians' recommendations may arise in part from ageism and sexism.

Age

The Johnson et al. (2000) study suggests one situation in which physicians may recommend less aggressive care to older terminally ill patients. However, age is likely linked to death and dying in other ways. Age is obviously associated with mortality. But does the dying process itself differ by age? As demonstrated by Nuland (1994), death in late life typically does not follow orderly stages such as those proposed by Kubler-Ross (1969). One limitation of Kubler-Ross's and similar models is that they are based on interactions with cognitively intact dying patients and their relatives. In a classic study, Exton-Smith (1961) found that more than 40% of his sample (n = 220) were "mentally confused" at the moment of death, and 88 died in a coma. It is reasonable to conclude that these patients were unaware that death was imminent.

As noted earlier, death typically occurs at older ages than previously, and several diseases causing or contributing to death are linked to cognitive impairment (e.g. Parkinson's disease, Alzheimer's Disease (AD). In 2005, AD was the fifth-leading cause of death in people over age 65 (Heron, 2007). But that number represents a significant under-reporting of dementia-related deaths. Wachterman and colleagues (2008) reviewed death certificates of nursing home patients and found that only 27% of residents diagnosed with dementia had the diagnosis noted on the death certificate. This suggests that more older adults die with diminished cognition or dementia than previously estimated, giving credence to the idea that a methodical and systematic passage from life to death is less probable among the elderly than previously assumed.

Socioeconomic Status

Increasing life expectancy in America over the last century is due in part to increased access to health care, healthier lifestyles (e.g. nutrition, exercise), and increased awareness of health promotion and disease prevention strategies. Low education and income are associated with increased risk of death. Most studies on SES and mortality show significantly worse outcomes for those with low income and low education. Ward and colleagues (2004) examined disparities in all-cancer mortality between those living in poorer counties (≥20% below the poverty line) and those in more affluent counties (<10% below the poverty line). Those living in poorer counties had a higher mortality rate (13% higher for men; 3% higher for women) and a lower five-year survival rate (10%) than residents of more affluent counties.

MEDICAL/TECHNOLOGICAL ISSUES

The increasing fear of death that has emerged in America throughout the last century has resulted in what Kastenbaum (1982) labeled the "death system," which is, "The interpersonal, sociophysical, and symbolic network through which society mediates the individual's relationship with death." Many Americans desire a society without death and keep their distance from people and places routinely associated with death (Solomon et al., 2003). Without the death system in place, the organized handling of death, dying, burial, and mourning might create social uncertainty. This system is an ever-changing complex of places, people, services, and symbols that testifies to the ineluctability of death.

The Formal American Death System: Places

One of the biggest changes in the death system over the last century has been in place of death. As noted earlier, death and dying have moved from the family home to a hospital or other medical institution. Nearly half of all US deaths occur in hospitals, although this rate has decreased steadily since the late 1980s (Teno, 2002). Although usually unspoken, in the medical world, patient death is viewed as failure (Thomas, 1980). The primary social role of physicians and other healthcare providers is to cure illness and sustain life at all costs; the primary purpose of the hospital is to provide a place in which this can occur.

A second prominent place in the death system is the nursing home or extended care facility. In 2004, 22% of deaths in the US occurred in nursing homes (Bern-Klug, 2009). In comparison, approximately 45% died in hospitals (in-patient or emergency department) while 24% died at home (CDC/NCHS, 2004). Weaver and colleagues (2009) found that proximity to death increases the likelihood of nursing home placement by 50%. But providing appropriate end-of-life care in nursing homes is fraught with challenges (Ersek & Wilson, 2003). Trotta (2007) notes that maintaining the personhood and identity of the dying is critical to a good death but difficult to achieve in nursing homes.

Alternatives to Hospitals and Nursing Homes

In the 1950s, Dame Cicely Saunders began her campaign against painful and impersonal institutional death by opening St. Christopher's, the first modern hospice, in 1967. Care at St. Christopher's was palliative, not curative. Managing patients' symptoms and maximizing comfort were its goals. The focus of hospice was on its patients, not on their diseases. Ultimately, the hospice movement flourished in England and has slowly spread elsewhere around the globe.

The first American hospice opened in 1971 and was distinct from those in England. The work of Kubler-Ross may have resulted in an emphasis on psychological preparation for death in US hospice. Entry into hospice in the US is physician-driven and often occurs later in the disease process than in other countries (Connor, 2008; McGorty & Bornstein, 2003).

Social factors influence hospice use as well. Strong geographic differences exist in US hospice use, with south and southwestern hospice use higher than that in the Midwest and northeast. Women are more likely to use hospice than men, and older adults use hospice more than their younger counterparts (Connor et al., 2007). Racial disparities also exist, with African Americans substantially less likely than whites to use hospice services and palliative care (Johnson et al., 2008).

In line with their higher death rates, older adults have always been the most frequent hospice users (Connor, 1998) This trend accelerated, however, when Medicare began to cover hospice services in 1983. Kidder (1992) found that Medicare saved money in the first three years. With increasing healthcare costs overall, however, savings did not continue. In fact, between 2004 and 2005, Medicare expenditures for hospice rose 20% (Neigh, 2008).

Hospice care is widely acknowledged as critical for terminally ill older adults. Palliative care may be best provided in the context of hospice, although some argue for providing palliative care in hospitals. Ultimately, the cost of such care will dictate its availability. For older adults who choose to die at home, hospice and palliative care outside of the hospital is critical.

The Formal American Death System: People

The burden of care for the dying has shifted from informal to paid caregivers. Although those who provide formal care respond emotionally to the dying process, their feelings of loss are surely less intense that those of family members and friends (Redinbaugh et al., 2003). In family care, women bear the burden of caregiving. This is also true in hospice and palliative care where the majority of paid workers and volunteers are women.

Healthcare workers are critical to the success of the death system. Most patients in settings for the terminally ill are older adults. Healthcare professionals may experience less grief at the loss of an older patient than when a child or younger adult dies. Yet little research has examined social factors and their impact on professional caregivers' attitudes and behaviors.

People involved in the death system outside the healthcare arena include morticians, cemetery staff, florists, religious leaders, casket makers, funeral directors, and countless others. It is beyond the scope of this chapter to even mention all of them. The point is that there is a phalanx of professionals ready to step in, with or without a fee, to ensure that death and dying are removed from the daily course of events.

NOT QUITE THE END: LIFE-SUSTAINING TREATMENTS (LSTs)

The belief that patient death is a failure of the physician and medical system is patently false, yet the American public, to some degree, believes that, with enough technology and skill, American physicians can cure all medical ills (Buxton, 2008). Ever-improving medical technologies strengthen this belief, as do popular television shows. The power of this belief clearly affects the use of LSTs, especially with older adults.

LSTs (resuscitation, mechanical ventilation, kidney dialysis, antibiotics, artificial nutrition and hydration) are interventions used to prolong life when a patient is near death. But, when LSTs are initiated for individuals whose underlying conditions are chronic or terminal, they may exacerbate an already emotion-laden situation. Long-term use of LSTs may increase costs simply by keeping a patient in a hospital receiving care longer. Many argue that extending life with poor quality squanders valuable healthcare resources.

Two important questions face healthcare providers, patients, and their families. Who should make the decisions about the initiation and/or continuation of LSTs? Should everyone receive LST indefinitely? In an ideal world, all patients should have access to high-tech treatments and be able to make their own critical decisions about their use. Most, however, are comatose and unable to make these decisions. Exton-Smith (1961) noted that many of his patients were incapable of decision making around the time of their deaths.

Social factors affect decisions about LSTs, as does the individual's physical state and possibility of survival. Religious beliefs may explicitly or implicitly dictate appropriate use of LSTs. Bioethicists and some religions classify medical intervention for the purpose of extending life as either *ordinary* or *extraordinary*. *Ordinary* care is standard or usual medical care. For ethicists, *ordinary* care is morally obligatory and required to preserve life. *Extraordinary* care is non-standard or experimental care. Bioethicists do not view *extraordinary* care as morally required (Watt, 2000). But the differences between *ordinary* and *extraordinary* care are not absolute. For example, for many years, the Roman Catholic Church defined artificial nutrition and hydration as *extraordinary* care, allowing families to withhold or withdraw such care when there was no hope of recovery. In his 2004 allocution, however, Pope John Paul II redefined the provision of food and water as *ordinary* care; therefore, families were required to provide it regardless of potential medical outcomes (Henke, 2007). This Papal dictum had a substantial impact on human behavior and healthcare.

No federal or state laws provide clear guidelines for the use of LSTs. Medicine also fails to provide uniform or straightforward answers. Ideally, these decisions should be made by the person at risk for LSTs, but that is rarely possible. In fact, the only certain way an individual can make decisions about LTSs is through a living will or another advance directive.

An advance directive allows an individual to make decisions about a wide variety of end-of-life choices. Most people believe that medical personnel should follow advance directives. But others believe that patients may change their minds about LSTs at a time that they are unable to say so (Castledine, 2009). They prefer that physicians and other healthcare professionals decide whether or not to implement advance directives. A major practical problem with living wills is that they are often not available when patients most need them. Inpatient hospital stays require people to submit their living will or proxy before being admitted; those admitted from the emergency department ordinarily do not have living wills with them. Gillick (2006) provides an excellent review of advance directive options and their legal foundation.

In 1996, Dr. Joseph Barmakian established The US Living Will Registry on the Internet (http://www.uslivingwillregistry.com/default.asp) as an electronic repository for individuals' living wills, guaranteeing their availability to healthcare providers. Similar registries are in some states and are associated with the national organization (e.g. in Vermont, Washington, and Nevada). Other federal and state sites operate independently. Electronic storage sites for critical documents seem logical in today's world, allowing both patients and their healthcare providers easy access to their advance directives. Participants carry cards from their chosen sites, directing emergency responders how to access the person's end-of-life-care wishes.

The social importance of these sites should not be underestimated. Easy access for providers may make the difference between responding to patients' wishes and being unaware of them. But first, people must post their wishes on such sites and provide access information to relatives, friends, and healthcare personnel. Second, healthcare providers must use these sites to learn patient wishes and let patients make their own decisions.

If disagreement occurs among family, physicians, nurses, and other players, hospital ethics committees have the power to decide to withhold or terminate a patient's treatment (Aulisio & Arnold, 2008; Gavrin, 2007). If the family wants continued care and the ethics committee denies it, the family's only alternative is to transfer the patient to another facility within 10 days of the committee's decision. After that, the hospital has the right to cease such care and is immune from prosecution.

CONCLUSIONS

The social and medical changes of the twentieth century have been remarkable, and expectations for such change in the twenty-first century seem almost without bounds. Medical technology assists physicians to identify ways in which life can be extended. The laws in some states, however, are permitting terminally ill individuals to hasten the end of life. Ethical and moral issues surrounding both life extension and assisted suicide confuse and alienate people. This happens, in part, because of the tremendous heterogeneity of the American people in terms of critical social factors such as gender, age, race, religion, and socioeconomic status. All of these variables play a role in achieving health across the life course; they also play a role in decision making at the end of life. We know little about the causal relationships between social factors and end-of-life decision making, but we do know there are strong correlations between gender and religion and decisions to extend or shorten the life course.

We might conclude that increased access to information about death and dying would result in increased conversations about them as well. We might also expect that talking about death and dying would diminish our fears. This does not appear to be the case. Death and dying have multiple characteristics that cause us to fear them. We do not know when death will come or in what form; we do not know how long dying will last, nor do we know with certainty what happens after death. Neither books nor the Internet answer these conundrums. Both the scholarly literature (Lee, 2008) and many websites portray death as the taboo of the twenty-first century.

Baby boom have the potential to modify American attitudes toward death and dying simply because of the size of this generation. Throughout their lives, many baby boom have been taught to ignore and deny death. But, as the baby boom age, the topic of death and dying has reached center stage in the American policy arena and medical world. Baby boom are watching – or have watched – their parents' decisions about end-of-life care and have faced difficult decisions about do not resuscitate (DNR) orders and living wills and letting go. Yet research has not yet explored the potential outcome of the baby boom experience. If baby boom have observed their parents receiving extraordinary medical interventions at the end of life – despite financial burden or personal suffering – they will likely perpetuate current attitudes about death. On the other hand, if baby boom witness the use of living wills and advance directives that prohibit expensive LSTs and provide palliative care, this may convince them that a battle with death is almost always a losing cause. Ultimately, the personal and policy decisions of this generation can influence decision making for subsequent generations.

Social factors such as race, gender, and education will continue to play critical roles in determining individual decisions about the end of life. Will current racial differences in attitudes toward LSTs and hospice use continue? Future research in this area needs to go beyond the fact of racial differences and help us understand the reasons for such differences. Religious beliefs also shape individual and community attitudes, and future research needs to examine how people integrate individual beliefs based on religion, race, and gender, especially if they do not agree.

Research on death in biological sciences centers around apoptosis, free radicals, and caloric restriction. Research in social sciences must integrate individual and cultural factors and examine relationships among variables difficult to measure. An essential first step toward improved understanding of death and dying is the development of valid and reliable scales to measure the impact of death and dying on individuals and families. Clarification of what we mean by quality of life at the end of life is also essential, and the impact of place of death (hospital, institution, family home) can provide the foundation on which future research rests. Little useful future research will occur, however, if Americans continue their fear of death. Research has confirmed that this fear – or death anxiety or whatever we call it – exists; now research needs to help us conquer it.

REFERENCES

Allen, R. S., Allen, J. Y., Hilgeman, M. M., & DeCoster, J. (2008). End-of-life decision-making, decisional conflict, and enhanced information: Race effects. *Journal of the American Geriatrics Society, 56*(10), 1904–1909.

Anonymous (1968). Definition of irreversible coma: Report of the Ad Hoc Committee of the Harvard Medical School to examine the definition of brain death. *Journal of the American Medical Association, 205*(9), 337–340.

Arias, E. (2007). United States life tables, 2004. *National Vital Statistics Reports.* Hyattsville, MD: National Center for Health Statistics.

Aulisio, M. P., & Arnold, R. M. (2008). Role of the ethics committee. *Chest, 134*(2), 417–424.

Becker, E. (1973). *The denial of death.* New York: Free Press.

Bengtson, V. L., Cuellar, J. B., & Ragan, P. K. (1977). Stratum contrasts and similarities in attitudes toward death. *Journal of Gerontology, 32*(1), 76–88.

Bern-Klug, M. (2009). A framework for categorizing social interactions related to end-of-life care in nursing homes. *The Gerontologist, 49*(4), 495–507.

Blackhall, L. J., Frank, G., Murphy, S. T., Michel, V., Palmer, J. M., & Azen, S. P. (1999). Ethnicity and attitudes towards life sustaining technology. *Social Science and Medicine, 48*(12), 1779–1789.

Brazil, K., Howell, D., Bedard, M., Krueger, P., & Heidebrecht, C. (2005). Preferences for place of care and place of death among informal caregivers of the terminally ill. *Palliative Care, 9*(6), 492–499.

Buckman, R. (1993). Communication in palliative care: A practical guide. In D. Doyle, G. W. C. Hanks & N. MacDonald (Eds.), *Oxford Textbook of Palliative Medicine* (pp. 51–69). Oxford, UK: Oxford Medical Publications.

Buxton, D. (2008). Redefining medical success and failure. *Journal of Palliative Medicine, 11*(10), 1343–1344.

Castledine, S. G. (2009). Contradictions at the end of life. *British Journal of Nursing, 18*(18), 1151.

Centers for Disease Control/National Center for Health Statistics. (2003). Mortality statistics: 1900–1998: United States. Retrieved November 3, 2009 from http://www.cdc.gov/nchs/data/dvs/lead1900_98.pdf.

Centers for Disease Control/National Center for Health Statistics. (2004). Mortality statistics: Work table 309, deaths by place of death, age, race, and sex: United States. Retrieved December 2, 2009 from http://www.cdc.gov/nchs/data/dvs/MortFinal2004_Worktable309.pdf.

Cicirelli, V. G. (2006). Fear of death in mid-old age. *Journal of Gerontology: Psychological Sciences, 61B*(2), P75–P81.

Connor, S. R. (1998). *Hospice: Practice, pitfalls, and promise.* Washington, DC: Taylor & Francis.

Connor, S. R. (2008). Development of hospice and palliative care in the United States. *Omega, 56*(1), 89–99.

Connor, S. R., Elwert, F., Spence, C., & Christakis, N. A. (2007). Geographic variation in hospice use in the United States in 2002. *Journal of Pain and Symptom Management, 34*(3), 277–285.

Copp, G. (1997). Patients' and nurses' constructions of death and dying in a hospice setting. *Journal of Cancer Nursing, 1*(1), 2–13.

Corr, C., Nabe, C. M., & Corr, D. M. (2009). *Death and dying, life and living* (6th ed.). Belmont, CA: Wadsworth.

Cutler, D. M., & Meara, E. (2004). Changes in the age distribution of mortality over the twentieth century. In D. A. Wise (Ed.), *Perspectives on the economics of aging* (pp. 333–366). Chicago: University of Chicago Press.

Demicheli, R., Retsky, M. W., Hrushesky, W. J., Baum, M., Gukas, I. D., & Jatoi, I. (2007). Racial disparities in breast cancer outcome: Insights into host-tumor interactions. *Cancer, 110*(9), 1880–1888.

Depaola, S. J., Griffin, M., Young, J. R., & Neimeyer, R. A. (2003). Death anxiety and attitudes toward the elderly among older adults: The role of gender and ethnicity. *Death Studies, 27*(4), 335–354.

Emanuel, E. J., Fairclough, D. L., & Emanuel, L. L. (2000). Attitudes and desires related to euthanasia and physician-assisted suicide among terminally ill patients and their caregivers. *Journal of the American Medical Association, 284*(19), 2460–2468.

Ersek, M., & Wilson, S. A. (2003). The challenges and opportunities in providing end-of-life care in nursing homes. *Journal of Palliative Medicine, 6*(1), 45–57.

Eskes, T., & Haanen, C. (2007). Why do women live longer than men? *European Journal of Obstetrics & Gynecology and Reproductive Biology, 133*(2), 126–133.

Exton-Smith, A. N. (1961). Terminal illness in the aged. *Lancet, 278*(7192), 305–308.

Flory, J., Yinong, Y. X., Gurol, I., Levinsky, N., Ash, A., & Emanuel, E. (2004). Place of death: U.S. trends since 1980. *Health Affairs, 23*(3), 194–200.

Gavrin, J. R. (2007). Ethical considerations at the end of life in the intensive care unit. *Critical Care Medicine, 35*(2)(Suppl.), S85–S94.

Gillick, M. R. (2006). The use of advance care planning to guide decisions about artificial nutrition and hydration. *Nutrition in Clinical Practice, 21*(2), 126–133.

Glaser, B. G., & Strauss, A. L. (1965). *An awareness of dying.* Chicago: Aldine Publishing.

Glaser, B. G., & Strauss, A. L. (1968). *Time for dying.* Chicago: Aldine Publishing.

Gruneir, A., Mor, V., Weitzen, S., Truchil, R., Teno, J., & Roy, J. (2007). Where people die: A multilevel approach to understanding influences on site of death in America. *Medical Care Research and Review, 64*(4), 351–378.

Hays, J. C., Gold, D. T., Flint, E. P., & Winer, E. P. (1999). Patient preference for place of death: A qualitative approach. In B. de Vries (Ed.), *End of life issues: Interdisciplinary and multidimensional perspectives* (pp. 3–22). New York: Springer.

Hedberg, K., Hopkins, D., Leman, R., & Kohn, M. (2009). The 10-year experience of Oregon's Death with Dignity Act: 1998–2007. *Journal of Clinical Ethics, 20*(2), 124–132.

Hellström, I., Nolan, M., & Lundh, U. (2005). Awareness context theory and the dynamics of dementia. *Dementia, 4*(2), 269–295.

Henke, D. E. (2007). A history of ordinary and extraordinary means. In R. P. Hamel & J. J. Walter (Eds.), *Artificial nutrition and hydration and the permanently unconscious patient: The Catholic debate* (pp. 53–78). Washington, DC: Georgetown University Press.

Heron, M. P. (2007). Deaths: Leading causes for 2004. *National Vital Statistics Reports, 56,* 1–96. Retrieved December 22, 2009 from http://www.cdc.gov/nchs/data/nvsr56/nvsr56_05.pdf.

Howard, G., Anderson, R. T., Russell, G., Howard, V. J., & Burke, G. L. (2000). Race, socioeconomic status, and cause-specific mortality. *Circulation, 102*(10), 42–47.

Hui, V. K., & Fung, H. H. (2009). Mortality anxiety as a function of intrinsic religiosity and perceived purpose in life. *Death Studies, 33*(1), 30–50.

Hulley, S., Grady, D., Bush, T., Furberg, C., Harrington, D., Riggs, B., et al. (1998). For the Heart and Estrogen/progestin Replacement Study Research Group (1998). Randomized trial of estrogen plus progestin for secondary prevention of coronary heart disease in postmenopausal women. *Journal of the American Medical Association, 280*(7), 605–613.

Hummer, R. A. (1996). Black-white differences in health and mortality: A review and conceptual model. *Sociological Quarterly, 37*(1), 105–125.

Humphry, D. (2002). *Final Exit* (3rd ed.). New York: Dell Publishing.

Johnson, K. S., Kuchibhatla, M., & Tulsky, J. A. (2008). What explains racial differences in the use of advance directives and attitudes toward hospice care? *Journal of the American Geriatrics Society, 56*(10), 1953–1958.

Johnson, M. F., Lin, M., Mangalik, S., Murphy, D. J., & Kramer, A. M. (2000). Patients' perceptions of physicians' recommendations for comfort care differ by patient age and gender. *Journal of General Internal Medicine, 15*(4), 248–255.

Kastenbaum, R. (1982). New fantasies in the American death system. *Death Education, 6*(2), 155–166.

Kidder, D. (1992). The effects of hospice coverage on Medicare expenditures. *Health Services Research, 27*(2), 195–217.

Koenig, H. G., Wildman-Hanlon, D., & Schmader, K. (1996). Attitudes of elderly patients and their families toward physician-assisted suicide. *Archives of Internal Medicine, 156*(19), 2240–2248.

Kubler-Ross, E. (1969). *On death and dying.* New York: Macmillan.

Laderman, G. (2003). *Rest in peace: A cultural history of death and the funeral home in twentieth-century America.* New York: Oxford University Press.

Land, K. C., & Yang, Y. (2006). Epidemiologic transition theory and recent trends in adult mortality. In R. H. Binstock & L. K. George (Eds.), *Handbook of aging and the social sciences* (pp. 42–59) (6th ed.). San Diego: Academic Press.

Lee, R. L. M. (2008). Modernity, mortality and re-enchantment: The death taboo revisited. *Sociology, 42*(19), 745–759.

Lehto, R. H., & Stein, K. F. (2009). Death anxiety: An analysis of an evolving concept. *Research & Theory for Nursing Practice, 23*(1), 23–41.

Lindsay, R. A. (2009). Oregon's experience: evaluating the record. *The American Journal of Bioethics, 9*(3), 19–27.

Liu, L., & Sullivan, D. H. (2003). Relationship between social demographic factors and survival within one year of hospital discharge in a cohort of elderly male patients. *Journal of Epidemiology, 13*(4), 203–210.

Lloyd-Williams, M., Kennedy, V., Sixsmith, A., & Sixsmith, J. (2007). The end of life: A qualitative study of the perceptions of people over the age of 80 on issues surrounding death and dying. *Journal of Pain and Symptom Management, 34*(1), 60–66.

Lunney, J. R., Lynn, J., & Hogan, C. (2002). Profiles of older

Medicare decedents. *Journal of the American Geriatrics Society, 50*(6), 1108–1112.

McGorty, E. K., & Bornstein, B. H. (2003). Barriers to physicians' decisions to discuss hospice: Insights gained from the United States hospice model. *Journal of Evaluation in Clinical Practice, 9*(3), 363–372.

Mitford, J. (2000). *The American way of death revisited.* New York: Vintage.

Muramatsu, N., Hoyen, R. L., Yin, H., & Campbell, R. T. (2008). Does state spending on home- and community-based services promote home death? *Medical Care, 46*(8), 829–838.

Navaie-Waliser, M., Feldman, P. H., Gould, D. A., Levine, C. L., Kuerbis, A. N., & Donelan, K. (2002). When the caregiver needs care: The plight of vulnerable caregivers. *American Journal of Public Health, 92*(3), 409–413.

Neigh, J. E. (2008). What does the future hold for hospice in the present environment? *Caring, 27*(11), 6–7.

Nuland, S. B. (1994). *How we die.* London: Chatto and Windus.

Pressley, J. C., Barlow, B., Kendig, T., & Paneth-Pollak, R. (2007). Twenty-year trends in fatal injuries to very young children: The persistence of racial disparities. *Pediatrics, 119*(4), 875–884.

Redinbaugh, E. M., Sullivan, A. M., Block, S. D., Gadmer, N. M., Lakoma, M., Mitchell, A. M., et al. (2003). Doctors' emotional reactions to recent death of a patient: Cross sectional study of hospital doctors. *British Medical Journal, 327*(7408), 185–190.

Rosenberg, R. N. (2009). Consciousness, coma, and brain death. *Journal of the American Medical Association, 301*(11), 1172–1174.

Scitovsky, A. A. (2005). "The high cost of dying": What do the data show? *The Milbank Quarterly, 83*(4), 825–841.

Seale, C. (2003). Global mortality rates: Variations and their consequences for the experience of dying. In C. D. Bryant (Ed.), *Handbook of Death & Dying.* Thousand Oaks, CA: Sage Publications.

Shinjo, T., Morito, T., Hirai, K., Miyashita, M., Sato, K., Tsuneto, S., et al. (2010). Care for imminently dying cancer patients: Family members' experiences and recommendations. *Journal of Clinical Oncology, 28*(1), 142–148.

Solomon, S., Greenberg, J., & Pyszczynski, T. (2003). Fear of death and human destructiveness. *Psychoanalytic Review, 90*(4), 457–474.

SUPPORT Principal Investigators (1995). A controlled trial to improve care for seriously ill hospitalized patients: The Study to Understand Prognoses and Preferences for Outcomes and Risks of Treatments (SUPPORT). *Journal of the American Medical Association, 274*(2), 1591–1598.

Tang, S. T. T. (2003). When death is imminent: Where terminally ill patients with cancer prefer to die and why. *Cancer Nursing, 26*(3), 245–251.

Teno, J.M. (2002). *Facts on dying: Policy relevant data on care at the end of life.* Retrieved November 3, 2009 from http://www.chcr.brown.edu/dying/factsondying.htm.

Teplin, L. A., McClelland, G. M., Abram, K. M., & Milionis, D. (2005). Early violent death among delinquent youth: A prospective longitudinal study. *Pediatrics, 115*(6), 586–593.

Thomas, L. (1980). Dying as failure. *The Annals of the American Academy of Political and Social Science, 447*(1), 1–4.

Trotta, R. L. (2007). Quality of death: A dimensional analysis of palliative care in the nursing home. *Journal of Palliative Medicine, 10*(5), 1116–1127.

Wachterman, M., Kiley, D. K., & Mitchell, S. L. (2008). Reporting dementia on the death certificates of nursing home residents dying with end-stage dementia. *Journal of the American Medical Association, 300*(22), 2608–2610.

Ward, E., Jemal, A., Cokkinides, V., Singh, G. K., Cardinez, C., Ghafoor, A., et al. (2004). Cancer disparities by race/ethnicity and socioeconomic status. *CA Cancer Journal for Clinicians, 54*(2), 78–93.

Watt, H. (2000). *Life and death in healthcare ethics: A short introduction.* New York: Routledge.

Weaver, F., Stearns, S. C., Norton, E. C., & Spector, W. (2009). Proximity to death and participation in the long-term care market. *Health Economics, 18*(8), 867–883.

Weaver, R. R., & Rivello, R. (2006–2007). The distribution of mortality in the United States: The effects of income (inequality), social capital, and race. *Omega, 54*(1), 19–39.

Wee, B., & Hillier, R. (2008). Interventions for noisy breathing in patients near to death. *Cochrane Database of Systematic Reviews,* Issue 1. Art. No.: CD005177. DOI: 10.1002/14651858.CD005177.pub2.

Wijdicks, E. F. M. (2001). The diagnosis of brain death. *New England Journal of Medicine, 344*(16), 1215–1221.

Wildiers, H., & Menten, J. (2002). Death rattle: Prevalence, prevention and treatment. *Journal of Pain Symptoms and Management, 23*(4), 310–317.

Zilberberg, M. D., & Shorr, A. F. (2008). Prolonged acute mechanical ventilation and hospital bed utilization in 2020 in the United States: Implications for budgets, plant and personnel planning. *BMC Health Services Research, 8,* 242.

Part | 4 |

Aging and Society

Chapter | 18 |

The Political Economy of Pension Reform in Europe

Martin Kohli[1], Camila Arza[2]

[1]*Department of Political and Social Sciences, European University Institute, Florence, Italy,* [2]*Latin American School for Social Sciences/CONICET, Buenos Aires, Argentina*

CHAPTER CONTENTS

INTRODUCTION

Since the end of World War II, pension reform has become central to the European social policy agenda – first in terms of construction and expansion, then increasingly in terms of consolidation and retrenchment. The high levels of pension expenditures experienced in the past few years, and the even-higher ones projected for the coming decades, have now become a key issue of concern throughout Europe. At stake are the basic options not only for the welfare state but also for fiscal and labor market policy, and, more generally, for economic growth and social cohesion.

Thus, pension systems (both public and private) need to be viewed in a broader political economy framework (see Arza & Kohli, 2008b). Their major purpose is to provide income security to retirees. In addition to such redistribution (or individual income smoothing) over the life course, they may also aim at redistribution across population groups, such as lifting the low-income elderly out of poverty. But beyond these income goals, pensions are linked up with a range of other issues:

- They are typically the largest public transfer programs, and thus the source of major fiscal pressures (and sometimes opportunities).
- They influence financial markets by favoring or impeding the accumulation of funds and of personal savings.
- They regulate labor markets by facilitating an ordered transition out of employment.

DOI: 10.1016/B978-0-12-380880-6.00018-6

- They enable employers to manage their work force by offering instruments for the shedding or replacement of workers.
- They contribute to the institutionalization of the life course by creating a predictable sequence and timing between work and retirement.
- They provide workers with a legitimate claim to compensation for their "life-long" work, and thus with a stake in the moral economy of work societies.
- They attach citizens to a public community of solidarity, and thus play a part in nation-building.
- They produce new social and political cleavages by creating large groups of actual and potential beneficiaries.
- They structure the agenda of corporatist conflict and negotiation.
- They offer opportunities for administrative offices and jobs.
- They weigh in on election outcomes.

Through all these issues, pension systems form a major part of the political economy of current societies. In this chapter we will not be able to touch on all issues, let alone cover them adequately, but will go into some of them as we discuss the institutional changes that have come to be known under the label of "pension reform."

THE DEVELOPMENT OF PENSIONS IN EUROPE

Origin and Expansion

The origin of public pension systems is conventionally credited to Germany's creation, in 1889, of an old-age insurance program under Bismarck. It was financed by social contributions and managed by public bodies with representatives of owners and workers, and provided modest earnings-related benefits for industrial workers and their surviving families. Many of the issues that have dominated later discussions could already be observed at this historical juncture (Kohli, 1987; Ritter, 1991): the pension system's contribution to the institutionalization of the life course and to workers' integration into the new moral economy of industrial society; its part in nation-building, especially critical in Germany with its late national unification; its impact on administrative and fiscal reform; and its relevance for office-seeking.

Two years later, in 1891, Denmark established the *Alderdomsunderstøttelsen*, a basic benefit for the elderly in need, which was financed by tax revenues and managed by the local government (Abrahamson & Wehner, 2003) – an early forerunner of the type

that later came to be associated with the name of Beveridge. These first two pension schemes thus represented alternative institutional approaches to old-age income protection. They would soon be emulated by other countries, giving form to the pension regimes that have characterized European welfare states ever since.

Over the first decades of the twentieth century, most European countries set up old-age pension systems under different versions of these two broadly defined models. Anglo-Saxon and Scandinavian countries created basic pensions that were originally means-tested but later became universal. This group has been labeled "the Beveridgean family," in recognition of William Beveridge's role in shaping British welfare at the end of World War II (Myles & Quadagno, 1996). Continental and Southern European countries, instead, followed the German model, consisting of work-based earnings-related pensions, and formed the "Bismarckian family" of pension policy. Central and Eastern European countries were also influenced by the Bismarckian design, developing work-related pension schemes somewhat later than Western Europe.

These early schemes tended to provide low benefits at rather high retirement ages (age 70 in Bismarck's design) to limited parts of the population. Pensions were often conceived more as disability allowances than as benefits for retirement in the sense of a new life phase. High retirement ages and low life expectancies meant that the elderly received benefits for only a short period of time, if at all. As a result, pension expenditures remained relatively modest. In 1930, social expenditures (including pensions) were still below 5% of GDP in all European countries (Pierson, 2006).

After World War II, the welfare state, in what has been called its "golden age," fueled by unprecedented economic growth and an active organized labor movement, became the basis of the class compromise of advanced capitalist societies. Pension schemes across Europe were part of a broader welfare system to cover the main social risks, including work injury, sickness, and unemployment. Pension coverage was expanded to most workers and their families. Eligibility became more generous, normal retirement ages were reduced, and early retirement options were introduced in many countries. In Italy, for instance, the retirement age was reduced to 60 for men and 55 for women in 1939 (Brugiavini, 1997), and, in 1968, even earlier retirement was made available for both public and private sector workers. In some cases, easier-to-meet eligibility rules were only applied to particular occupational categories (such as mining), reflecting the hazardous nature of these occupations, but also their political power and influence. By and large, with the expansion of coverage and benefit generosity, pensions became a comprehensive system of income protection in old age. Their role for public policy broadened as they increasingly became a key instrument for industrial restructuring and for managing unemployment (Kohli et al., 1991). Retirement was recognized and institutionalized as a life stage of its own, to be expected by the majority of the population, of considerable length, and structurally set apart from gainful work (Kohli, 1987, 2000). From then on, popular expectations of states' duties for providing and peoples' rights for receiving adequate pensions would guide the political process of pension system transformation and the collective resistance against cutbacks.

Institutional Differentiation

In the political economy of European welfare states, both the Bismarckian and Beveridgean types of pension systems were used for similar purposes, such as for the institutionalization of retirement and the management of the labor market. In many ways, however, their institutional patterns remained distinct, and there was further differentiation as the Scandinavian countries parted ways with the Anglo-Saxon ones. By 1990, pension systems seemed to be an easy fit for the three-fold typology of welfare regimes advanced by Esping-Andersen (1990): the "liberal" (Anglo-Saxon) regime with low public benefits to be topped up by occupational and private schemes; the "social-democratic" (Scandinavian) regime with high universal public benefits; and the "conservative" (Continental European) regime with public benefits aimed at preserving the status differentiation of the labor market.

In the Bismarckian family (most of Continental Europe), public pensions became more generous. Benefits were increased and often indexed to prices and/or wages, so that they offered a level of living more or less in tune with the growth of workers' incomes. This reduced the room for supplementary private schemes, so that the state remained the main provider. In Anglo-Saxon and Scandinavian countries, the expansion of pensions was first done through the transformation of previously means-tested schemes into universal flat-rate programs (Overbye, 1992). In Sweden, means-testing was removed in 1948 and the *folkpension* consolidated as a universal flat-rate benefit covering all the resident population (Olsson, 1987). Norway (1956), Finland (1957), and Denmark (1970) followed the same route. Britain also removed means-testing in 1946 in the wake of the influential Beveridge report (Beveridge, 1942), and the Basic State Pension (BSP) became a universal and flat-rate benefit for all. However, British benefits remained low in comparison to most other European countries. As benefits also depended on contribution records, many workers with incomplete working histories (who could

not get a full BSP entitlement) still needed to resort to supplementary means-tested social assistance.

Another area of transformation in Scandinavian countries was the creation of new earnings-related layers set up to complement basic provision, giving these countries a partial resemblance to the Bismarckian family. For this reason, some authors have labeled them the "second generation" of social insurance systems (Hinrichs, 2001; Natali, 2008). In contrast, Anglo-Saxon countries started to diverge from the Scandinavian group in terms of the public–private mix of old-age protection, with a limited role for the state and a greater role for the market. The UK and Ireland – together with Denmark and the Netherlands – belong to what Myles and Pierson (2001) have called the "latecomer" countries, where public earnings-related pensions were introduced late or not at all. The State Earnings-Related Pension Scheme (SERPS), the first compulsory earnings-related pension in Britain, was only set up in 1975 and implemented in 1978. This late arrival made it politically weak: the SERPS was unable to resist cutbacks in the 1980s and was finally converted into the State Second Pension (S2P) in 2002.

Growing Spending

The long periods involved in the maturation of the new pension rules introduced after World War II meant that in many countries their full financial impact would not be observed immediately, but only some decades later when the generations under these schemes started to retire. More importantly, the age structure was that of a young and growing population, with a broad base of young and a narrow top of older ages. As a result, pension expenditures in the 1950s and 1960s were still rather low (Arza & Kohli, 2008b). By 1980, however, they had grown to over 10% of GDP in Germany and Austria, and over 8% in Belgium, France, Italy, Luxembourg, and Sweden. By 2005, they had passed the 5% threshold in all countries but Ireland and Iceland, and in some cases, such as Italy, France, and Austria (all Bismarckian-type systems), they were already above 12% of GDP (OECD, 2010).

Under the favorable economic and demographic conditions of the 1950s and 1960s, pension expenditures were not yet seen as a problem for public finances. This started to change after the mid-1970s, when economic growth rates fell (sometimes into negative terrain), the demographic outlook clouded, and economic ideas shifted away from Keynesianism. For some time, the expansion of pension schemes still continued, and they were more broadly used for facilitating earlier exit from the labor force as a response to economic downturns and historical transitions such as those of Eastern Europe after 1990 (Kohli et al., 1991). But, over the 1990s, expenditure growth projections came to be generally regarded as a serious risk for the sustainability of public finances and the competitiveness of national economies. Pension reform, often meaning the reduction of benefits and public pension budgets but also the adaptation of existing schemes to changing socioeconomic and labor market contexts, acquired top priority on government agendas.

CURRENT CHALLENGES

There is broad agreement on the list of challenges that pension schemes now face, but disagreement on how these challenges should be interpreted, what impetus for reform they should provide, and, most of all, what the reforms should be (see the next section). First on the list is population aging. The increase in life expectancy (at birth as well as at later ages) has been massive, and has usually been underestimated by official population projections (Oeppen & Vaupel, 2002). This has been one of the great achievements of modern societies, but it comes at a price: of working longer, increasing pension contributions, or decreasing benefits. Barring the advent of a major natural disaster or man-made destruction (which is not something that does, nor should, inform welfare policies), life expectancy growth is likely to continue, and may even accelerate through biomedical advances (see Chapter 4). On the other side, the drop to low and very-low fertility as part of what is usually conceptualized as the Second Demographic Transition has meant that younger cohorts of workers are getting smaller. There are (tentative) arguments about a possible fertility increase in the most advanced societies (Myrskylä et al., 2009), but a return to above-reproduction fertility and thus to natural population growth seems unlikely. Some quantitative easing of population aging can come (and has come) from immigration, but for most European countries the numbers that would be required for keeping the ratio of workers to pensioners constant are clearly above what is politically feasible (United Nations Population Division, 2000).

In terms of pension costs and benefits, it is obviously not crude demography that matters but indeed the ratio of workers (as contributors or tax-payers) to pensioners. Demographic dependency ratios may thus be misleading; what counts is to what extent the "demographic potential" is really at work and how much it produces. Changes in employment rates, productivity per worker, and age of transition from work to retirement will thus modulate the effect of the underlying demographic structure.

The second key challenge is economic transnationalization (and similar macro-economic changes). This has meant, among other things, an increase in the mobility of capital and thus the bargaining power of employers, a shift from banks to financial markets as main providers of credit, and a shift from "stakeholder" to shareholder control with claims for more immediate profits. In such an open economy, the political ability of states to levy the taxes and contributions required for social security is eroding (Scharpf & Schmidt, 2000).

It should be noted that the willingness of citizens to pay taxes still varies widely among nation-states. This may have to do with cultural preferences for redistribution and economic equality. Tax and contribution levels that are accepted, e.g. in Sweden, would be deemed unacceptable in Anglo-Saxon countries and would be subverted in Mediterranean countries. The Anglo-Saxon countries follow the opposite route: They offer generous tax breaks to the finance industry and to employers as an incentive to provide private old-age pensions and health insurance, resulting in a "divided welfare state" that absorbs almost as much public revenue as the welfare arrangements of Germany and France but with less-efficient and less-egalitarian outcomes (see Blackburn, 2008; Hacker, 2002). As a result, welfare state benefit levels also vary. Welfare institutions may be conceived as filters that modify the impact of transnationalization in nation-specific or regime-specific ways (Blossfeld et al., 2006).

At the level of production, the shift has been described as one from a "Fordist" mode, characterized by standardized mass production with high-level wage bargaining and seniority, to a "Post-Fordist" mode, with flexible production and individualized work contracts. The Post-Fordist mode implies a rise of discontinuous careers with more flexibility and insecurity, and, more generally, a destandardization of life course patterns. Karl Ulrich Mayer speaks of the transition from a Fordist to a Post-Fordist life course regime that also extends into the domain of the family (Mayer, 2001). The male breadwinner model gives way to female career employment, and family models shift towards delayed and partial marriage, high divorce rates, low fertility, and, consequently, pluralized family forms. There are obviously other causal factors beyond transnationalization at play here, but the changes seem to coalesce into a consistent pattern.

For the welfare state, this implies a shift from the "old" risks of the Fordist to the "new" risks of the Post-Fordist society. Other observers see a shift from the traditional "passive" welfare state, with its emphasis on social protection from market risks, to a new productivist "workfare" state that activates its citizens by providing them with the skills and motivation for employment; in other words, by increasing their marketability (Jessop, 2002; Vis, 2007). In a broader conceptualization linking social and economic policy, this has been termed the model of the "competition state" (Vukov, 2010), emphasizing "that states are no longer concerned with maximizing citizens' welfare through redistribution, but rather with actively promoting the competitiveness of their territory," through economic policies that attract capital and facilitate enterprise and innovation, and through social policies that foster re-commodification by assuring labor market flexibility and a high supply of a skilled and motivated work force.

Pensions have a peculiar place in this concept as they are the one policy area where a productivist emphasis seems inappropriate and income protection remains paramount. Even here, however, activation is now being promoted, in terms of remaining in the work force as long as possible, of remaining productive in other fields such as volunteering or family care, and of becoming an independent entrepreneur, if not of one's work career, at least of one's investments.

The pension literature has so far not given much attention to these issues. It has until recently stressed continuity, by predicting that pensions would remain stable (or expand further) through the sheer weight of their existence and the political clout of the class of beneficiaries that they created, and that the changes that would occur would remain path-dependent; that is, restricted by the specific principles and policies institutionalized in each welfare regime. As we shall now see, these predictions have been overturned by the dynamics of pension reform.

THE DYNAMICS OF PENSION REFORM

Contrary to most theoretical expectations, reform has been deep and widespread. "Cost-containment" started in the UK in the early 1980s and rapidly expanded across Europe. Most countries changed indexation rules from wages to prices, reduced early retirement options, increased normal retirement ages, and extended the period of reference for the calculation of benefits under earnings-related systems. In virtually all cases, personal pensions were created, either by privatizing parts of the existing system, by setting new mandatory layers, or by establishing incentives (such as tax deductions) for voluntary individual savings. Most countries reformed pensions incrementally, in a step-by-step process that introduced significant innovation but maintained the main architecture of existing systems. Such parametric adjustments allowed governments to contain the projected growth in public pension expenditures for the future. In a number of cases, however, reform was more structural, reshaping the original structure of pension policy, like in Central and Eastern European countries. An illustrative overview of the changes is given in Table 18.1.

Reversing the Early Exit Trend

Early exit from the labor force, long encouraged by consensual strategies of employers and unions with the explicit or implicit collusion of the state (Kohli et al., 1991), has come to be considered one of the central problems facing pension finances. In Germany, it has been calculated to account for almost 25% of the old-age pension budget (Börsch-Supan, 2006). Early exit is also at odds with the emphasis on activation that has become a key feature of European social policy. While raising the retirement age limit beyond the traditional threshold of 65 remains highly contentious, raising the labor force participation below this threshold is now a broadly consensual goal, as stated, for example, in the Lisbon (1999) and Stockholm (2000) agendas of the EU.

The EU has no mandate for pension reform (or any other social policy), but has ventured into this area indirectly through addressing the competitiveness of European economies. Increasing the employment rate of older workers became a centerpiece in the employment strategy agreed upon by the Lisbon summit, to be implemented through the "Open Method of Coordination," a soft policy instrument based on common goal-setting and regular progress reports. The goal set in 2000 for the year 2010, to be achieved by all member states, was an employment rate of at least 50% among the population aged 55–64. To some observers this seemed an overly ambitious goal at the time, given that several countries showed a rate of less than 30% (while Denmark was slightly, and Sweden – in line with countries such as the US, Japan, and Switzerland – already largely above this mark). But, as Table 18.2 shows, by 2008 another six out of the fifteen EU member states of 1997 had reached the goal, some among them (such as the Netherlands, Finland, and Germany) with very substantial increases that amounted to a policy reversal.

On the other hand, half of the population aged 55–64 in employment seems like a modest goal, with a long way still to go towards activation. The critical issue that has generated conflict here is to what extent employment at this age is a free decision by the worker, and to what extent it is constrained by labor market conditions or health reasons. To the extent that elderly workers have become unfit for work or unable to find employment, a rising retirement age in pension schemes backed up by actuarially fair deductions for earlier exit will entail for them a drop in pension income beyond their own choice (also see Chapter 14).

Expanding Private Pension Provision

One other key area of reform has been the reconfiguration of the public–private mix in pension provision. Privatization was either direct or indirect and incremental through "layering" or "conversion" (Natali, 2008; Streeck & Thelen, 2005). The market portion of the pension mix expanded both in countries where it

Table 18.1 Typical reform trajectories in Europe (c. 1990–2010).

REFORM TYPE	TYPICAL REFORM TRAJECTORIES
Parametric reform	• Raising retirement ages (most countries, recently Czech Republic, Denmark, Germany, Greece, Hungary, Italy, Switzerland) • Increasing contribution years for entitlement (most countries, recently Czech Republic, France for public sector) • Eliminating or restricting early retirement options (most countries, recently Belgium, Denmark, Greece, Ireland for civil servants, Poland, France for public sector) • Introducing incentives for later retirement (Italy, France, UK, among others) • Changing indexation rules from wages to prices (most countries, recently Hungary, France for public sector) • Extending the working period for the calculation of benefits to the entire working life (most countries, recently Finland) • Adjusting benefits to changes in life expectancy (Germany, Finland, Portugal) • Adjusting eligibility conditions to changes in life expectancy (France, Denmark) Reducing transformation coefficients in NDC pensions, leading to pension cuts (Italy)
Structural reform	• Reconfiguration of the public PAYG pension scheme into a NDC system (Italy, Sweden, Latvia, Poland) • Shifting towards a mixed system with mandatory private individual accounts (Bulgaria, Croatia, Estonia, Hungary, Latvia, Lithuania, Poland, Slovak Republic)
Improving minimum protection, adequacy, and coverage	• Improving or extending coverage in the basic poverty-prevention pillar (Finland, Sweden, Italy, UK) • Increasing minimum benefits (Belgium, France, Spain) • Lowering earnings thresholds to cover low-income and part-time workers (Switzerland)
Multi-pillarization through "layering" and "conversion"	• Converting companies' severance pay into pension plans (Italy) • Adding new mandatory layers for individual savings (Denmark, Sweden, UK automatic enrolment to national pension savings scheme) • Encouraging voluntary individual pension savings and/or occupational pensions with tax incentives (France, Germany, Hungary, Poland, Portugal, among others) • Introducing minimum employer contributions to occupational pensions (Norway) Converting DB occupational pensions into DC (Sweden, UK, among others)

Source: Authors' elaboration based on OECD (2009) and national legislation.

had been virtually absent (most Bismarckian regimes) and in countries where it had already played a significant role (the Netherlands and Anglo-Saxon, and Scandinavian countries).

The most radical shift occurred in some Central-Eastern European and ex-Soviet Union countries, where public pension schemes were partly privatized following the "mixed" model already implemented in a number of Latin American countries (Müller, 2004). This model is the combination of a public "pay as you go" (PAYG) pillar that is sometimes means-tested and a second pillar of mandatory individual accounts, of varying size and importance. Contributions to the private pillar ranged from 10% in Latvia to 9% in Poland and Slovakia, 8% in Hungary, and between 2% and 5% in Bulgaria, Croatia, Estonia, and Lithuania, indicating that its size has indeed varied greatly across countries.

A growing role for private pensions can also be found in Western Europe, both in the mandatory

and voluntary systems. In the Italian case, traditionally characterized as a public pension monopoly, economic incentives were introduced to enhance the development of a private pension layer that could partly compensate for the projected fall in public pension benefits. Projections suggest that public benefits at retirement for dependent workers will fall from 79% of previous wages in 2004 to 64% in 2050, while the self-employed are expected to suffer still greater losses (European Commission, 2006). In 1992, the "Amato reform" (named after the then Prime Minister Giuliano Amato) created occupational ("closed") and personal ("open") pension funds financed through voluntary tax-deductible contributions (Ferrera & Jessoula, 2007), and in 2005 the contribution previously oriented to finance a severance pay started to be automatically directed to a supplementary pension pillar. Between 2006 and 2008, affiliation increased by 67%, reaching over two million workers in

Table 18.2 Employment rates of older workers (ages 55–64), 1997–2008 (percentages).

COUNTRY	1997	2001	2008
EU15	36.4	38.8	47.4
Denmark	51.7	58.0	57.0
Finland	35.6	45.7	56.5
Sweden	62.6	66.7	70.1
Ireland	40.4	46.8	53.6
United Kingdom	48.3	52.2	58.0
Austria	28.3	28.9	41.0
Belgium	22.1	25.1	34.5
Germany	38.1	37.9	53.8
France	29.0	31.9	38.2
Luxembourg	23.9	25.6	34.1
The Netherlands	32.0	39.6	53.0
Greece	41.0	38.2	42.8
Italy	27.9	28.0	34.4
Portugal	48.5	50.2	50.8
Spain	34.1	39.2	45.6

Source: European Commission (2010).

occupational pension funds, and by 81% in personal funds, reaching about 800 000 workers. By the end of 2008, private pension funds had accumulated assets of over 61 billion euros, or 3.9% of GDP (COVIP, 2009).

The expansion of private pensions has reached other countries in the Bismarckian family as well. In Germany, the "Riester reform" (named after the then Minister of Labor and Social Affairs) in 2002 boosted the development of private pensions, with the number of Riester contracts reaching over 11 million by March 2008 (Germany, 2008). Still, much of the small print of the Riester reform remained contentious, with the banks and insurers lobbying for fewer constraints in the regulation of the Riester funds in order to increase returns and thus attract more participants. In France, another typically single-pillar public system, voluntary salary-saving schemes with tax incentives were first established in 1997. The Raffarin government later created and developed new savings plans with wide-ranging impacts (Mandin & Palier, 2005). By December 2009, a funded occupational pension scheme financed through voluntary contributions by workers and employers (PERCO) had accumulated assets for 3 billion euro. Private pension development was also significant in Belgium, where about 45% of the employed population was covered in 2005 (European Commission, 2006).

In Sweden and Denmark, new mandatory funded layers were created on top of the existing public pension schemes as well as on top of the occupational schemes emerging from collective bargaining agreements. In the Anglo-Saxon countries, where the state has traditionally had a more limited role for social security, private pensions have always been important. In Ireland no public earnings-related pension exists, and in the United Kingdom the public earnings-related pension scheme (SERPS), finally implemented in 1978, had been designed in such a way as to avoid "crowding out" existing private provision. Changes after the 1980s further limited the state's role in income replacement and reinforced the development of the private pension market and the multi-pillar structure of British pension policy.

Towards Multi-Pillar Systems

Expanding private provision has reoriented pension arrangements in the direction of the multi-pillar model (Bonoli, 2003). This pension architecture is characterized by a number of pillars and layers that complement each other to meet different objectives in social security (from poverty prevention to income smoothing, insurance, and savings). Each pillar can be organized under a different mechanism of financing, administration, and benefit calculation. In general, the state keeps the functions of poverty-prevention and interpersonal redistribution, while income-smoothing over the life course is partly left to the private sector under mandatory or voluntary schemes with benefits linked to past earnings or contributions. Significant design variation exists among countries. In some cases, collective agreements promote non-statutory occupational pensions with wide coverage. Additional savings are often promoted through tax-deductible voluntary contributions to individual pension accounts in a third pillar.

In previously single-pillar schemes, like most Continental European ones, the development of occupational and private pensions has added new pillars. This has changed the structure of provision to a more complex interaction between state, occupational, and private pensions, similar to the one already found in some "latecomer" countries, most notably the United Kingdom, where repeated reforms modifying and adding new layers and pillars have constructed what is probably the most complex pension system in Europe.

From Defined Benefits to Defined Contributions

This reconfiguration has also usually included a shift from DB to DC systems, which have been promoted through the spread of notional defined contribution (NDC) schemes at the national level in countries such as Italy, Sweden, Latvia, and Poland (Holzmann & Palmer, 2006), as well as through the expansion of occupational pensions (typically DC) (Schulz & Borowski, 2006). NDC schemes are actuarially fair systems that do not accumulate funds (thus avoiding transition costs and risks of mismanagement and investment) but give only "notional" credits instead, as in Bismarckian PAYG schemes. To the extent that the latter offer benefits that are fully linked to the individual's contribution history and age of retirement and moreover comprise a link to the changing demographic conditions (as is the case for the German system after the reform of 2004), they in effect mimic an NDC system (Börsch-Supan, 2006). Some see NDC systems as representing the current wave of reforms. Moreover, they may turn out to be the point of convergence of the still-diverse systems of today.

In occupational pensions as well, DC systems have tended to replace existing DB arrangements (as has been the case in the US). In the UK, employers were allowed to convert their DB plans into DC in 1986, and many did in the years that followed. In the mid 1990s, over 60% of "contracted out" workers had joined a private DC pension. In Sweden, almost simultaneously to the reforms in the statutory pension system, non-statutory occupational

pensions were also modified following nationwide agreements between employers and trade unions. In 1998, the pension scheme for blue-collar workers started to move from DB to DC models (Palmer & Wadensjö, 2004), the scheme for local government personnel followed in 2000, and that for state workers in 2002. Although some schemes kept DB entitlements, the change has been significant.

Under both private and occupational DC and national NDC systems, the value of pensions depends on the amount of contributions paid as well as on life expectancy. A stronger link between contributions and benefits makes individual work histories matter more for future benefit levels (Arza, 2008). Periods outside the labor market, in unemployment or atypical work with no protection, will reduce benefits unless the scheme includes a special credit for them (as is the case, e.g., for childcare in Germany). Recent projections suggest that, by 2046, female workers who dedicate three years to childcare will have their net replacement rates cut by four percentage points in Latvia, Hungary, and the Netherlands, while workers who spend three years in unemployment will suffer cuts of six points in Slovakia and Finland, five points in Italy, and four points in Germany, Latvia, and Poland (European Commission, 2009). All these countries have recently adopted or reinforced DC systems either in public or private pension layers, or in both.

DC systems resemble savings schemes in that benefits closely reflect the distribution of income and work patterns prevailing over the course of one's working life. In a Post-Fordist world with more flexible labor markets, atypical employment, and non-traditional family structures, pension schemes that tighten the link between working lives and benefit levels can generate new gaps in old-age income protection.

Different Regimes, Similar Reform Trajectories?

The idea of "welfare regime" stresses that the various dimensions of welfare arrangements occur as packages where the parts depend on and complement each other, and that cross-country differences in these packages align themselves into a limited number of types or "families of nations" (Castles, 1993; Esping-Andersen, 1990; Ferrera, 1996). Regimes reflect the allocation of welfare roles among the state, the family, and the market, and the underlying principles that have guided policy choices. Once established, welfare regimes are thought to restrict the range of further choices in path-dependent ways. A similar idea has been offered by the Varieties of Capitalism approach, which focuses on the different ways in which capitalist economies are coordinated

(Hall & Soskice, 2001), and has been fruitfully applied to the articulation between pensions and the labor market (Ebbinghaus, 2006).

The wide-ranging reforms of the past two decades have put this idea to the test. If similar socioeconomic and demographic challenges are affecting European countries, do the pre-existing institutional structures specific to each regime orient pension reforms in diverging directions, thus deepening regime differentiation? Whether and how institutional structures influence the feasibility of alternative reform options has become a key concern in the analysis of the political economy of reform (for example, Myles & Pierson, 2001; Natali, 2008). Or, in contrast, do reform processes follow similar trajectories and thus wipe out the differences across regimes? Such convergence could take several forms: regimes may adopt some features of each other, they may all move towards one of the regimes (the most likely candidate being the Anglo-Saxon one, with its minimal public pillar and high share of funded private pensions), or they may follow the same new trajectory (such as towards NDC schemes).

The question can be framed in terms of the relative importance of the "push" of common reform objectives and the "pull" from institutions. In recent practice, there has been a bit of both: reforms have substantially modified the welfare architecture of previous systems but differences among states persist. Similar instruments and strategies were adopted in the service of similar goals across countries but policy-making encountered less resistance if it built on existing systems rather than radically transforming them. A common trajectory towards a multi-pillar architecture and an expansion of private DC pensions can be observed. There are no "pure" cases anymore; all of them have become hybrids. However, shared challenges and similar reform strategies have interacted with institutional structures and political processes, which vary across countries. As a result, there are still significant differences that tend to follow the conventional regime boundaries. To what extent this will remain so will depend on the sheer weight of the common challenges as well as on mutual policy learning and the evolution of a common policy framework in the EU.

THE POLITICS OF PENSION REFORM

Pensions as "Immovable Objects"

As mentioned above, the successful expansion of welfare states has created conditions that militate for their own continuity. Existing institutions are resistant to change, both in terms of general inertia and of the specific welfare regimes (path dependency).

In the literature of the 1990s, European pension systems were widely thought of as "immovable objects" (Pierson, 1998), as part of the "frozen landscapes" of welfare regimes (Esping-Andersen, 1996). This way of thinking had good reasons going for it. Welfare states had created their own constituencies; they had turned the citizenry or large parts of it into their "stakeholders," who would oppose dismantling or changing them. These interest-group networks produced lock-in effects that reinforced the status quo.

The empirical evidence on welfare state attitudes and preferences supports this view (Kohli, 2006). Many surveys have shown and still show that pensions are hugely popular – in fact the most popular part of the welfare state. This may reflect a perception that there is no moral hazard involved. Pensions and the life in retirement that they make possible are considered a well-deserved right; the elderly have been seen as unquestionably "worthy" benefit recipients. A large majority of respondents across all age groups and countries usually opt for maintaining or expanding pension benefits, even if the latter option is framed in such a way that respondents are made aware of the need to raise taxes or contributions for it. Raising the retirement age is almost unanimously opposed. In other words, European countries have developed a very successful and popular social security system to which citizens have become attached. Some generations saw these welfare rights expand over the course of their lives and participated in the political processes promoting this transformation. Social security has thus influenced the economic choices of workers and their families and their expectations on benefit rights from the state, the employers, and the market.

The early literature on the expansion of old-age security offered the demographic growth of the elderly population as a key explanation for this expansion: growing elderly populations create both a need for welfare spending and a political constituency to fight for it (Wilensky, 1975). This "gray power" thesis is still widely advocated today. In a formal model for Germany, Sinn and Uebelmesser (2002) have projected the median age of voters and the "indifference age" as the age of the cohort that is affected neither positively nor negatively by a pension reform. The assumption is that reform will be feasible if, and only if, the median voter favors it. The authors conclude that, until 2016, a reform can be democratically enforced because a majority of the voters will still be below the indifference age. Year 2016 is "Germany's last chance"; after that year, it will be a gerontocracy.

The reality of the two past decades has largely falsified the gray power thesis, however. Pension reforms involving cutbacks have broadly occurred, in spite of the growing number of elderly voters. The gray power thesis is also not a satisfactory explanation of the variation among welfare states with respect to their age orientation (Lynch, 2006). The failure of the gray power thesis is partly due to its erroneously mechanical model of voting preferences. Elderly voters do not only vote in their own narrow self-interest (Goerres, 2009). They are also interested in the well-being of their descendants and are net contributors in the intergenerational exchange with them (Kohli, 1999).

But while the gray power thesis is not borne out by the evidence, the broader popular dislike of all forms of pension retrenchment is amply documented. The argument that pensions are difficult, if not impossible, to scale back politically remains reasonable. How, therefore, have the large-scale pension reforms of the past decades been achieved? On this question there is a range of possible explanations, put forward to explain policy change in other domains as well (Streeck & Thelen, 2005). Many explanations focus on the dynamics of political institutions (Immergut & Anderson, 2007). There are also attempts at identifying the social-structural changes that underpin the making of new political coalitions in a post-industrial or post-Fordist context (Häusermann, 2009). Other explanations emphasize the political strategies and the ideas that facilitate retrenchment.

Political Strategies to Pass Unpopular Reforms

The shift from welfare state expansion to retrenchment has been coupled with a shift from the politics of "credit claiming" to those of "blame avoidance" (Pierson, 1994, 2001). It is hard to convince the voters that a government should get credit for cutting back welfare schemes. (The Schroeder government in Germany tried it but failed resoundingly because it was unable to frame the cutbacks as inevitable.) Attempts are made instead to avoid the blame, share it with the opposition, or redirect it altogether (the EU is often a handy scapegoat for this). In the politics of blame avoidance that characterize unpopular reforms, governments adopt strategies to minimize political costs and electoral punishment. People are more likely to accept pension cuts if they are not really visible or if they do not affect them directly. The first of these options leads to "obfuscation" strategies (Pierson, 1994) consisting of making reform outcomes too difficult to understand for a non-expert. Such strategies are typical of structural reforms, helped by the fact that even experts may lose sight of the key factors, as evidenced by the wide currency of myths in the evaluation and comparison of pension policy options (Barr, 2002). One way to obfuscate is to change the entire system at once so that it becomes difficult to compare pre- and post-reform conditions and identify winners and losers. Thus, paradoxically, path-breaking reforms may meet with less political resistance than incremental

(parametric) reforms, whose outcomes can more easily be calculated (Overbye, 2008).

The second option is to use long phasing-in periods for reforms to be implemented. This can reduce the opposition of workers close to retirement who are typically more concerned with pension issues and therefore more active defenders of their rights. It can also have a divisive effect on potential opponents as not everyone is affected in the same way. In Western Europe the phasing-in periods set by recent reforms have been particularly long. The full implementation of the French reform of 2003, for instance, will only take place in 2020; in Germany, the 1999 reform will be fully implemented around 2025, and the 2006 reform in 2029; the Italian structural reform, legislated in 1995, will be fully effective in 2035 (Bonoli & Palier 2007; and the recent rise in retirement ages in the UK, legislated in 2007, will be implemented between 2024 and 2046. Long phasing-in periods are also necessary to give individuals and families the time to adapt their life plans and choices to the new institutional context. However, they are not without costs. They obviously delay the onset of the budgetary easing that they are aimed at. Moreover, they may raise doubts among the population on the likelihood that costly reforms will be effectively implemented in the future, so that adaptation is stifled. They also pass the political costs of really applying controversial legislation on to the following governments, who may be tempted to renege on them. And finally, they may lag behind the evolution of the structural challenges they are supposed to respond to; e.g. if life expectancy increases more quickly than the phased-in increase in retirement age.

Another way is to divide potential opponents by introducing cutbacks or reducing generosity for one occupational group and not for others. Obviously, losers may also be acknowledged and compensated in other domains. Instead of direct cutbacks, a further key strategy of reform throughout Europe has been to operate via incentives: incentives to work, incentives to save, and incentives to retire later (Arza & Kohli, 2008a). Incentives are politically easier to apply than compulsion because, in principle, people can choose whether to take them or not. In practice (but less visible), reform via incentives has often included some indirect compulsion, such as when rejecting the "incentive" to work longer means receiving lower benefits, or when those who decide not to take an incentive cannot opt out of paying the fiscal costs for financing the incentives taken by others (e.g. tax deductions for private savings).

The Power of Ideas

Reforms are more likely to be accepted if they appear as "inevitable." This has been part of the "crisis" discourse that has spread across Europe, contributing to building the idea that cutbacks were necessary and unavoidable (Cox, 2001). Accounting for the power of ideas, and of the "epistemic communities" of experts that coin and carry them, has recently made a comeback in policy analysis (e.g. Béland, 2005; Taylor-Gooby, 2005). As Vivian A. Schmidt has observed, "no major and initially unpopular welfare-state reform could succeed in the medium term if it did not also succeed in changing the underlying definition of moral appropriateness" (Schmidt, 2000), and changing this definition requires the implementation of convincing ideas. As another example, reforms involving a stronger link between contributions and benefits may be more appealing than bare retrenchment because they have a claim on equity and fairness. In a process of retrenchment that necessarily entails a distribution of losses, an effective political strategy is to make these losses derive from widely shared principles of fairness, such as "to each what each has contributed." Thus, NDC or similar schemes may be more legitimate and easier to package in a discursive framework appealing to shared values and norms than other parametric reforms such as direct cuts on replacement rates or retirement-age increases.

Schmidt's (2008) concept of "discursive institutionalism" provides an approach to these issues. Overbye (2008), in a similar vein, speaks of attempts at "winning the defining-the-situation game" through appropriate framing. The international diffusion of policy models may also partly be attributed to the diffusion of guiding ideas. A key question here is whether diffusion reflects voluntary "policy learning" through convincingly superior ideas, or rather the power of those that propagate the ideas (Simmons et al., 2007). International actors such as the World Bank and the OECD fall into this second category (Orenstein, 2008); their power, while limited in Western Europe, has been considerable in Eastern Europe, where it was coupled with economic incentives and sanctions (Vukov, 2010).

This applies not least to the rhetoric of "reform" itself. Existing institutions can lose their legitimacy if they are successfully framed as obsolete and in need of reform or "modernization." A number of governments have been persuaded over the last decade to abolish PAYG pension schemes because they allegedly would be more vulnerable to demographic changes than funded schemes. This idea has been sponsored by many powerful actors and has gained wide currency even though, as Barr (2002), among others, has shown, it is economically mistaken. Both funding and PAYG are ways of organizing claims on future output, so they are both adversely affected by a fall in output. Among the ten "myths" that Barr aims to dispel, the myth that "funding resolves adverse demographics" is his number one. It remains to be seen whether such efforts at myth debunking will succeed in reversing the flow of ideas.

Many of the policy steps that currently go under the label of "reform" consist of retrenchment; in other words, of reducing entitlements or exposing them to market risk. More neutral terms for what is going on would be "change" or "transformation." The choice of terms is clearly not innocuous. Using the term "reform" for pension cutbacks or privatization is a specific way of framing. We follow this usage here because it has become the standard terminological currency. It also has some basic arguments going for it, in the sense that existing pension schemes need to be improved in order to live up to the challenges they face. But the translation of these challenges into specific institutional reform schemes owes much to the framing efforts of actors such as the World Bank and the OECD and, more generally, of the epistemic community of economics and finance with its basic conviction that markets perform better than governments. This should be kept in mind when speaking of "reform."

THE FUTURE OF PENSIONS

Contrary to widely held expectations about the political immobility of pension systems, they have been changed and scaled back considerably over the past two decades throughout Europe. Consequently, they have been made better equipped to deal with the challenges of demography and economic openness, with expenditure growth prospects having been contained. Whether this will be enough to keep pension costs within the limits that societies consider tolerable is an open question. Uncertainties loom large; the upward trends in longevity may overstretch the capacities for reform. Retirement ages have been raised in spite of broad opposition, but usually with long phasing-in periods. Many countries still lag behind, e.g. with retirement ages that are clearly unsustainable. This poses difficult issues of European-wide convergence and coordination. One recent example is the Greek financial crisis of 2010. Greek workers staged massive public protests against raising the retirement age to help solve public budget problems, while German workers opposed the idea that they should work longer in order to make Germany able to support the Greek budget so that Greek workers could retire earlier. On the other hand, the reforms already implemented in many countries have decreased future benefit levels to a point where adequate income protection for all pensioners will not be given any more. Pensions may still cost too much and achieve too little.

Pensions and Financial Market Risks

The 2007–2010 international financial crisis has shattered the belief that the risks of private pensions are fully under control. In OECD countries, pension funds lost an average of 23% of fund value in 2008. The impact on benefit entitlements across countries varies with the particular combination of pillars and layers that each country has. Workers in countries that rely heavily on private or occupational DC systems, where each individual saves for retirement in a personal pension account and the value of the benefit depends in large part on investment performance, have suffered most. The worst affected have been workers close to retirement, who will have no time to compensate current losses with better performance in the future. The crisis may also affect public pensions indirectly, through its impacts on employment and economic growth, two factors that are critical for resources and benefit levels; but here the losses are likely to be much smaller. As a result of these recent experiences, the crisis may also reduce the appeal of private pension reform ideas and discourse, and thus have an effect on future reform trajectories.

Falling Entitlements and New Life Course Risks

The thrust of most reforms has been to decrease future pension entitlements. Mean replacement rates of public schemes are projected to decrease considerably. This may increase again the risk of old-age poverty, which had been successfully tackled with the development of pensions over the second half of the twentieth century. Moreover, flexible labor markets and changing family patterns create new social risks that pose new challenges for pension policy. Obsolete skills and atypical jobs increase the risk of unemployment, forced early exit, and low wages, while having to care for children or frail relatives (a non-remunerated work usually performed by women) leads to interrupted labor market participation and part-time employment. Extended periods of education and training delay the entry into the labor market, and young cohorts of workers in some countries find it increasingly difficult to get a career job, shifting instead from one temporary low-wage job to another for some time. These new social risks negatively affect the capacities

of workers to build adequate pension entitlements. As pension reforms have strengthened the link between contribution history and benefits, the impact of working careers on future entitlements has become more salient. Future pensions will need to be adjusted to a context in which the life-long protected worker of the Fordist period is no longer predominant, which may lead to gaps in contributions and be another factor that increases the likelihood of old-age poverty.

Pensions in the Political Economy

The key theme of all this is that pensions cannot be addressed in isolation. They are embedded in the broader political economy and in the broader set of public policies. If pensions become part of a social policy shift towards what is variously called the "activation," "workfare," "investment," or "competition state," this needs to be backed up with appropriate policies that facilitate remaining active and competitive; e.g. policies that address the labor market for the elderly, the access to life-long (public or company-provided) education and retraining, and health prevention. In other words, the issues of income protection in old age cannot be solved by pension policy alone. The challenges for aging societies are not only about the elderly, but about the earlier life phases as well. The experience of the past decades seems to show that people can be persuaded to accept welfare cuts if they perceive the burden-sharing as fair. This implies political recognition of the full patterns of intergenerational exchange and of the whole life course.

ACKNOWLEDGMENTS

Parts of this chapter are based on our recent volume on pension reform in Europe (Arza & Kohli, 2008b). Martin Kohli acknowledges the help and inspiration of the MacArthur Foundation Aging Society Network.

REFERENCES

Abrahamson, P., & Wehner, C. (2003). *Pension reforms in Denmark.* Paper presented at Conference Pension Reform in Europe: Shared problems, sharing solutions? The LSE Hellenic Observatory, London, December 5, 2003.

Arza, C. (2008). Changing European welfare: The new distributional principles of pension policy. In C. Arza & M. Kohli (Eds.), *Pension reform in Europe: Politics, policies*

and outcomes (pp. 109–131). Abingdon: Routledge.

Arza, C., & Kohli, M. (2008a). Introduction: The political economy of pension reform. In C. Arza & M. Kohli (Eds.), *Pension reform in Europe: Politics, policies and outcomes* (pp. 1–21). London: Routledge.

Arza, C., & Kohli, M. (Eds.), (2008b). *Pension reform in Europe: Politics, policies and outcomes.* London: Routledge.

Barr, N. (2002). Reforming pensions: Myths, truths, and policy choices. *International Social Security Review,* 55, 3–36.

Béland, D. (2005). Ideas and social policy: An institutionalist perspective. *Social Policy and Administration,* 39, 1–18.

Beveridge, W. H. (1942). *Social insurance and allied services: Report.* London: HMSO.

Blackburn, R. (2008). The Anglo-American pension regime:

Failures of the divided welfare state. In C. Arza & M. Kohli (Eds.), *Pension reform in Europe: Politics, policies and outcomes* (pp. 155–174). Abingdon: Routledge.

Blossfeld, H. -P., Buchholz, S., & Hofäcker, D. (Eds.), (2006). *Globalization, uncertainty and late careers in society.* London: Routledge.

Bonoli, G. (2003). Two worlds of pension reform in Western Europe. *Comparative Politics, 35,* 399–416.

Bonoli, G., & Palier, B. (2007). When past reforms open new opportunities: Comparing old-age insurance reforms in Bismarckian welfare systems. *Social Policy & Administration, 41,* 555–573.

Börsch-Supan, A. (2006). What are NDC systems? What do they bring to reform strategies? In R. Holzmann & E. Palmer (Eds.), *Pension reform: Issues and prospects of non-financial defined contribution (NDC) schemes* (pp. 35–55). Washington, DC: The World Bank.

Brugiavini, A. (1997). *Social security and retirement in Italy.* Cambridge, MA: National Bureau of Economic Research.

Castles, F. G. (1993). Families of Nations: *Patterns of public policy in western democracies.* Aldershot: Dartmouth.

COVIP (2009). *Relazione annuale per l'anno 2008.* Roma: Commissione di Vigilanza sui Fondi Pensione.

Cox, R. H. (2001). The social construction of an imperative: Why welfare reform happened in Denmark and the Netherlands but not in Germany. *World Politics, 53,* 463–498.

Ebbinghaus, B. (2006). *Reforming early retirement in Europe, Japan and the USA.* Oxford: Oxford University Press.

Esping-Andersen, G. (1990). *The three worlds of welfare capitalism.* Cambridge: Polity.

Esping-Andersen, G. (1996). After the golden age? Welfare state dilemmas in a global economy. In G. Esping-Andersen (Ed.), *Welfare states in transition: National adaptations in global economies* (pp. 1–32). London: Sage.

European Commission (2006). *Adequate and sustainable pensions.*

Synthesis report 2006. Brussels: European Commission.

European Commission (2009). *Updates of current and prospective theoretical replacement rates, 2006–2046.* Brussels: Social Protection Committee.

European Commission (2010). Eurostat database. Retrieved April 9, 2010 from http://epp.eurostat. ec.europa.eu/portal/page/portal/ eurostat/home.

Ferrera, M. (1996). The 'southern model' of welfare in social Europe. *Journal of European Social Policy, 6,* 17–37.

Ferrera, M., & Jessoula, M. (2007). Italy: A narrow gate for path-shift. In K. Anderson, E. Immergut & I. Schulze (Eds.), *Handbook of West European pension politics* (pp. 396–454). Oxford: Oxford University Press.

Germany. (2008). *National strategy report. Social protection and social inclusion 2008–2010.* Report to the European Commission. Berlin, Germany.

Goerres, A. (2009). *The political participation of older people in Europe: The greying of our democracies.* Basingstoke: Palgrave Macmillan.

Hacker, J. (2002). *The divided welfare state: The battle over public and private social benefits in the United States.* Cambridge: Cambridge University Press.

Hall, P. A., & Soskice, D. (Eds.), (2001). *Varieties of capitalism: The institutional foundations of comparative advantage.* New York: Oxford University Press.

Häusermann, S. (2009). *What explains the "unfreezing" of Continental European welfare states? The US structural basis of the new politics of pension reform.* Florence: European University Institute.

Hinrichs, K. (2001). Elephants on the move: Patterns of public pension reform in the OECD countries. In S. Leibfried (Ed.), *Welfare state futures* (pp. 77–102). Cambridge: Cambridge University Press.

Holzmann, R., & Palmer, E. (Eds.), (2006). *Pension reform: Issues and prospects for non-financial defined contribution (NDC) schemes.* Washington, DC: World Bank.

Immergut, E., & Anderson, K. (2007). Editors' introduction: The

dynamics of pension politics. In E. Immergut, K. Anderson & I. Schulze (Eds.), *Handbook of West European pension politics* (pp. 1–45). Oxford: Oxford University Press.

Jessop, B. (2002). *The future of the capitalist state.* Cambridge: Polity Press.

Kohli, M. (1987). Retirement and the moral economy: An historical interpretation of the German case. *Journal of Aging Studies, 1,* 125–144.

Kohli, M. (1999). Private and public transfers between generations: Linking the family and the state. *European Societies, 1,* 81–104.

Kohli, M. (2000). Arbeit im Lebenslauf: Alte und neue Paradoxien. In J. Kocka & C. Offe (Eds.), *Geschichte und Zukunft der Arbeit* (pp. 362–382). Frankfurt/M: Campus.

Kohli, M. (2006). Aging and justice. In R. H. Binstock & L. K. George (Eds.), *Handbook of aging and the social sciences* (pp. 456–478) (6th ed.). San Diego: Academic Press.

Kohli, M., Rein, M., Guillemard, A-M., & van Gunsteren, H. (Eds.), (1991). *Time for retirement: Comparative studies of early exit from the labor force.* Cambridge: Cambridge University Press.

Lynch, J. (2006). *Age in the welfare state: The origins of social spending on pensioners, workers, and children.* Cambridge: Cambridge University Press

Mandin, C., & Palier, B. (2005). The politics of pension reform in France: The end of exceptionalism? In G. Bonoli & T. Shinkawa (Eds.), *Ageing and pension reform around the world* (pp. 74–93). Cheltenham: Edward Elgar.

Mayer, K. U. (2001). The paradox of global social change and national path dependencies: Life course patterns in advanced societies. In A. Woodward & M. Kohli (Eds.), *Inclusions and exclusions in European societies* (pp. 89–110). London: Routledge.

Müller, K. (2004). Latin American and East European pension reforms: Accounting for a paradigm shift. In M. Rein & W. Schmähl (Eds.), *Rethinking the welfare state* (pp. 372–391). Cheltenham: Edward Elgar.

Myles, J., & Pierson, P. (2001). The comparative political economy of pension reform. In P. Pierson (Ed.), *The new politics of the welfare state* (pp. 305–333). New York: Oxford University Press.

Myles, J., & Quadagno, J. (1996). Recent trends in public pension reform: A comparative view. In K. G. Banting & R. Boadway (Eds.), *Reform of retirement income policy: International and Canadian perspectives* (pp. 247–271). Kingston, ON: School of Policy Studies, Queen's University.

Myrskylä, M., Kohler, H.-P., & Billari, F. C. (2009). Advances in development reverse fertility declines. *Nature, 460*, 741–743.

Natali, D. (2008). *Pensions in Europe, European pensions: The evolution of pension policy at national and supranational level.* Brussels: PIE Peter Lang Editor.

OECD (2009). *Pensions at a glance. Retirement-income systems in OECD countries.* Paris: OECD.

OECD (2010). *Social expenditure database SOCX 1980–2005.* Retrieved April 9, 2010, from http://oecd.org/els/social/expenditure.

Oeppen, J., & Vaupel, J. W. (2002). Broken limits to life expectancy. *Science, 296*, 1029–1031.

Olsson, S. E. (1987). The people's old-age pension in Sweden: Past, present and future. *International Social Security Review, 40*, 361–372.

Orenstein, M. A. (2008). *Privatizing pensions: The transnational campaign for social security reform.* Princeton: Princeton University Press.

Overbye, E. (1992). *Public or private Pensions? Pensions and pension politics in the Nordic countries.* Berkeley: Institute of Industrial Relations, University of California.

Overbye, E. (2008). How do politicians get away with path-breaking pension reforms? The political psychology of pension reform in democracies. In C. Arza & M. Kohli (Eds.), *Pension reform in Europe: Politics, policies and outcomes* (pp. 70–86). Abingdon: Routledge.

Palmer, E., & Wadensjö, E. (2004). Public pension reform and contractual agreements in Sweden: From defined benefit to defined contribution. In M. Rein & W. Schmähl (Eds.), *Rethinking the welfare state* (pp. 226–248). Cheltenham: Edward Elgar.

Pierson, C. (2006). Beyond the welfare state? *The new political economy of welfare.* Cambridge: Polity Press.

Pierson, P. (1994). *Dismantling the welfare state? Reagan, Thatcher, and the politics of retrenchment.* Cambridge: Cambridge University Press.

Pierson, P. (1998). Irresistible forces, immovable objects: Post industrial welfare states confront permanent austerity. *Journal of European Public Policy, 5*, 539–560.

Pierson, P. (Ed.), (2001). *The new politics of the welfare state.* New York: Oxford University Press.

Ritter, G. (1991). *Der Sozialstaat: Entstehung und Entwicklung im internationalen Vergleich (2. Aufl.).* München: Oldenbourg.

Scharpf, F. W., & Schmidt, V. A. (Eds.), (2000). *Welfare and work in the open economy: From vulnerability to competitiveness.* New York: Oxford University Press.

Schmidt, V. A. (2000). Values and discourse in the politics of adjustment. In F. W. Scharpf & V. A. Schmidt (Eds.), *Welfare and work in the open economy: From vulnerability to competitiveness* (pp. 229–309). New York: Oxford University Press.

Schmidt, V. A. (2008). Discursive institutionalism: The explanatory power of ideas and discourse.

Annual Review of Political Science, 11, 303–326.

Schulz, J., & Borowski, A. (2006). Economic security in retirement: Reshaping the public–private pension mix. In R. Binstock & L. George (Eds.), *Handbook of aging and the social sciences* (pp. 360–379) (6th ed.). San Diego: Academic Press.

Simmons, B. A., Dobbin, F., & Garrett, G. (2007). The global diffusion of public policies: Social construction, coercion, competition, or learning? *Annual Review of Sociology, 33*, 449–472.

Sinn, H.-W., & Uebelmesser, S. (2002). Pensions and the path to gerontocracy in Germany. *European Journal of Political Economy, 19*, 153–158.

Streeck, W., & Thelen, K. (2005). Introduction: Institutional change in advanced political economies. In W. Streeck & K. Thelen (Eds.), *Beyond continuity: Institutional change in advanced political economies* (pp. 1–39). Oxford: Oxford University Press.

Taylor-Gooby, P. (Ed.), (2005). *Ideas and welfare state reform in Western Europe.* New York: Palgrave Macmillan.

United Nations Population Division (2000). *Replacement migration: Is it a solution to declining and ageing populations?* New York: UN.

Vis, B. (2007). States of welfare or states of workfare? Welfare state restructuring in 16 capitalist democracies, 1985-2002. *Policy and Politics, 35*, 105–122.

Vukov, V. (2010). *The rise of the competition state? Transnationalization and state policy in Eastern Europe.* Florence: European University Institute.

Wilensky, H. L. (1975). *The welfare state and equality: Structural and ideological roots of public expenditures.* Berkeley: University of California Press.

Chapter | 19 |

Politics and Aging in the United States

Andrea L. Campbell[1], Robert H. Binstock[2]

[1]*Department of Political Science, Massachusetts, Massachusetts Institute of Technology, Cambridge,* [2]*School of Arts and Sciences, Medicine, and Nursing, Case Western Reserve University, Cleveland, Ohio*

INTRODUCTION

As the proportions of their populations aged 65 and older have neared and exceeded 20% (Lutz et al., 2008), many developed nations throughout the world have already experienced the politics of reforming their old-age welfare states. Some of these international experiences in response to population aging are discussed elsewhere in this volume. Chapter 18 focuses on modern pension reform in Europe and Chapter 22 examines a variety of developments in long-term care financing and service delivery in nations throughout the world. This chapter, however, focuses on the politics of aging in the United States.

The United States is just beginning to experience the demographic transition that will rapidly increase the proportion of the population aged 65 and from 40 million in 2010 to 72 million in 2030; at that point one in five Americans will be aged 65 and older (US Census Bureau, 2008a). The aging of the 76 million US baby boomers will vastly increase the number of persons eligible for old-age benefits during the next two decades and beyond, and do so in the context of a large and growing national fiscal deficit and projected soaring costs of health care (see Chapter 25). Taken together, these pressures have put a greater spotlight than ever before on the politics of aging and issues of old-age welfare state reform in the US.

Another reason for focusing on the US is that it presents an interesting context for examining the politics of aging. For one thing, the US political system is highly fragmented, pluralist, and permeable, with an older population that is more organized than in other countries that have experienced rapid population aging (Walker & Naegele, 1999). Moreover, as noted by Danish sociologist Gøsta Esping-Andersen (1999) and many others, compared with the more social democratic political regimes in Europe, US politics has a strong strand of classical liberal ideology, which has been especially resurgent since the 1970s. This neoliberalism – termed 'conservatism' in everyday American political parlance – emphasizes the primacy of individuals and is suspicious of government intervention in the free market. Hence, the contemporary US politics of reforming old-age policies to deal with population aging includes efforts to "privatize" major elements of the old-age welfare state.

We begin the remainder of this chapter by examining the political behavior of older Americans. Then we analyze the impact that they and old-age-based

DOI: 10.1016/B978-0-12-380880-6.00019-8

organizations have had on public policy. We conclude by considering possible changes in the politics of aging in the US in the years ahead.

POLITICAL BEHAVIOR OF OLDER AMERICANS

Origins and Contemporary Patterns of Seniors' Political Participation

Sixty years ago, when political scientists first began gathering data on political participation by age group, we would have noted that senior citizens were the age group least likely to vote, make campaign contributions, work on campaigns, and engage in other political activities. But as Social Security became universal and more generous, and as Medicare was enacted as well, senior citizens became the most participant age group, outstripping non-seniors in the late 1970s and 1980s. By then, as Campbell (2003a) has documented, the political engagement of older persons became at least comparable to that of other age groups and in some cases greater.

Voting Participation

Figure 19.1 shows that, in the presidential election of 1972, the first year that all 18–20-year-olds in the nation were allowed to vote, the age group of 45–64-year-olds had the highest rate of participation (71%). However, since 1988, persons aged 65 and older have had the highest rates of participation (although not much higher than the rates for voters aged 45–64).

Why do older persons vote at a higher rate than younger persons? One contributing factor to comparatively high turnout rates in old age is sheer habit (Plutzer, 2002). Another factor is age group differences in voting *registration*, an essential precursor to voting. In the presidential elections from 1980 through 2008, the rate of registration among persons aged 65 and older was the highest among age groups, and substantially higher than the youngest group (US Census Bureau, 1981–2009; also see Goerres, 2009). A two-stage study of voter registration and turnout in national elections (Timpone, 1998) found that increased age (from ages 18 to 88) is monotonically related to being registered.

Other Forms of Political Participation

The political engagement of older Americans is hardly confined to election day. Campbell's (2003a) research on political participation by seniors, summarized below, documents their involvement in other arenas. Their participation rates in these various activities do not match their roughly 70% rate of voting. But their engagement is at least comparable to that of other age groups and is in some cases greater.

Elders make campaign contributions at higher rates than younger persons. In the 2000 presidential campaign, for instance, 13.7% of persons aged 65 and older contributed to a campaign; the percentage for 35–64-year-olds was 10.5, and for 18–34-year-olds it was less than 3%. As a consequence, seniors were 28% of all contributors. A much smaller proportion of seniors, just 2%, work in election campaigns; but this rate of participation is comparable to those in middle-aged and younger groups. In 2000, older persons were 12% of campaign workers.

Congressional staff members report anecdotes indicating that many older persons are not reticent about contacting their representatives regarding old-age policy issues. This is confirmed by Campbell's

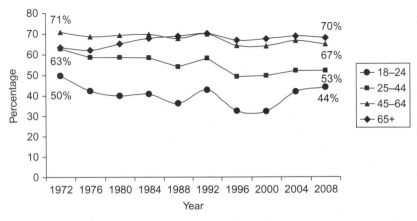

Figure 19.1 Voting turnout, by age groups in US presidential elections, 1972–2008.
Sources: *National exit polls & U.S. Census Bureau, Current Population Surveys.*

analysis of data from the Roper Social and Political Trends Archive, which covers the period from 1973 to 1993. Ten surveys were taken in 1993 that included the following sequence of statement and questions: "Here is a list of things some people do about government or politics. Have you happened to have done any of those things in the past year? Written your Congressman or Senator?" (Campbell, 2003a, p. 27). Responses indicated that older persons wrote letters to their senators and congressman at about the same rate as middle-aged persons (13% and 14%, respectively) and at about twice the rate of the youngest group (6%). However, as Campbell notes, the rate at which older persons contact their representatives can be much higher in response to specific policy events. In 1983, for example, the outlook for sustaining Social Security benefits looked bleak until remedial amendments to the program were enacted. During that year, the rate at which seniors contacted their representatives peaked at 20%.

Models featuring both "intrinsic" and "extrinsic" factors can help to explain seniors' relative rise in participation (Goerres, 2009). Individual-level models hold that political participation is a function of an individual's politically relevant resources such as money, free time, and engagement with politics as measured by political interest, political knowledge, efficacy, and strength of partisanship (Verba et al., 1995). Extrinsic factors such as Social Security and Medicare benefits enhance each of these participatory factors among seniors (Rosenstone & Hansen, 1993). These old-age entitlement programs give them steady incomes; contribute to their improved health; free their time by making retirement a reality; augment their interest in politics by tying their well-being so visibly to government policy; and boost their sense of political efficacy as elected politicians prove sensitive to their desires. The programs also create, from an otherwise disparate population, a group identity as benefit recipients, which in turn generates a basis for efforts by political parties and interest groups to mobilize seniors politically. With surges of participation they have been able to ward off threats to their programs, such as proposed cuts and changes to Social Security and Medicare (Campbell, 2003b). Senior citizens have become a prime example of government programs creating constituencies that in turn seek to shape subsequent policy outcomes (see Mettler & Soss, 2004 for an overview).

What also sets senior participation apart is its relatively egalitarian nature. Political participation in the US is marked by pronounced inequalities, with high-income and high-education individuals far more likely to vote, contribute, and contact, and even more likely to engage in activities – such as protests – that are supposedly more accessible to low-resource groups (Verba et al., 1995). But the participatory gradient is less steep among senior citizens, in part because lower-income seniors are mobilized at rates as high, if not higher than, their affluent counterparts and in part because lower-income seniors are more dependent on Social Security for income. For instance, Social Security accounts for 83% of income for seniors in the lowest income quintile, while it provides only 18% for those in the highest quintile (Federal Interagency Forum on Aging-Related Statistics, 2008). Thus, low-income seniors are more likely than the affluent to participate regarding Social Security concerns, which helps to democratize senior participation overall (Campbell, 2002; 2003a).

Seniors as Campaign Targets and Election-Day Voters

In an era when traditional mobilizing forces such as labor unions and well-organized local political party structures have waned, politicians and political consultants view seniors as a crucial "swing" group of voters, not heavily committed over the years to either Democrats or Republicans. Moreover, seniors are an easily identifiable constituency and one whose preferences politicians believe they know. Hence, politicians seeking to be elected and re-elected regard older voters as a tempting target in election campaigns and as a group to which they must be responsive in the policy processes of governing.

During election campaigns, especially presidential elections – the elections in which Social Security, Medicare, and other federal old-age benefit programs could be most salient – political consultants and journalists focus on older persons as an important voter demographic. A perennial journalistic cliché is, "Seniors are a key battleground in this election."

The fact that older voters participate in elections at a relatively high rate, as noted above, does not by itself account for the attention they receive. As Figure 19.2 indicates, older people are far from the largest age group in the electorate. In the 2008 presidential election, for example, Americans aged 45–64 cast 38% of the vote, and those aged 25–44 accounted for 36%, compared with only 16% by persons ages 65 and older.

Yet, older voters get substantial attention from journalists, campaign consultants and strategists, and candidates because in theory "the senior vote" may be swayed by campaign efforts focused on old-age-benefit issues. Presidential candidates have frequently addressed "senior issues" on the campaign trail, usually to portray themselves as champions for old-age-benefit programs and to make sure that their opponents don't best them in this strategy. Since John F. Kennedy's campaign for president in 1960, senior-citizen committees, "senior desks," and other types of special structures targeting older voters have been established within election campaigns (Binstock & Riemer, 1978; Pratt, 1976). Their aims are to register older voters, promulgate issue appeals to maintain and enhance the allegiance of these

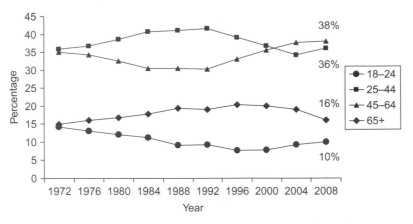

Figure 19.2 Percent of total vote cast by age groups in US presidential elections, 1972–2008.
Source: *National exit polls (1972–2008)*

voters, and then ensure that they turn out to vote. To do this, senior campaigns emphasize issues intended to appeal to older persons through methods commonly used to target other voting constituencies – robocalls, email blasts, direct mail, and television and radio ads; letters to the editor (vetted by higher echelons in the campaign); and appearances by the candidate or surrogates (members of Congress, state and local office holders, celebrities, and academics) before targeted audiences.

Such common efforts to reach out to particular groups of voters have some dimensions that are special in the case of seniors. One such dimension is that events featuring candidates and surrogates can be held in a great many venues where retired older voters can be easily targeted and, unlike voters who are still in the labor force, are available as audiences on weekdays. These venues include senior centers, congregate meal sites, retirement communities, public housing projects for the elderly, assisted-living facilities, nursing homes, AARP conferences, and the like. In June, 2010, for instance, with an eye to the upcoming fall elections, President Obama went to a senior center in Maryland to host a "tele-town-hall" meeting that was transmitted to 100 retirement communities and other senior venues throughout the nation in which he touted the fact that the federal government (in accordance with recent health care legislation) was about to send $250 checks to about four million Medicare beneficiaries to help them pay for their prescription drugs (Stolberg, 2010).

Another special dimension of campaigning for votes of seniors is that some swing states with large numbers of electoral votes also have higher proportions of older persons than the national average. Consequently, campaign efforts to capture the votes of seniors are potentially more rewarding there than elsewhere. For instance, Florida had 27 electoral votes

in 2008 and 25% of its voting-age population was aged 65 and older. In contrast, although 22% of West Virginia's voting-age population was aged 65 and over, that state had only 5 electoral votes.

These various strategies for targeting seniors during election campaigns are used because political consultants and parties know that seniors are a swing group that turns out to vote at a relatively high rate. At the same time, the fact that they have been contacted makes seniors more likely to vote (Campbell, 2005).

Despite election campaign efforts to target older voters with "senior issues" and special "senior campaign" structures, old age benefit issues do not have much impact on their electoral choices. As shown in Figure 19.3, in the last 10 presidential elections, all age groups except the youngest (ages 18–29) distributed their votes among candidates in roughly the same proportions. Old age is only one of many personal characteristics of older people with which they may identify; there is little reason to expect that a birth cohort – diverse in economic and social status, labor force participation, gender, race, ethnicity, religion, education, health status, family status, residential locale, political party attachments, and other characteristics in society – would suddenly become homogenized in self-interests and political behavior when it reaches old-age.

Candidates are on the ballot, not Social Security, Medicare, and other old-age policy issues. Older voters, like all voters, may be influenced by a variety of campaign issues (other than "elder issues") as well as candidates' traits such as their personalities, appearances, career and political backgrounds, performances, and even their religions, ethnicities, and races. For instance, race was clearly a factor in the 2008 election. As Table 19.1 shows, all age groups of whites aged 30 and older voted heavily in favor of John McCain, even as blacks and Latinos of all ages voted heavily for Obama.

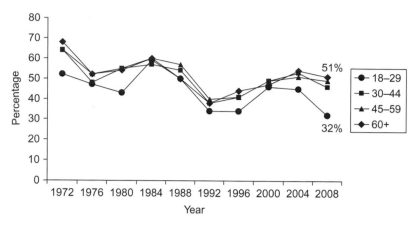

Figure 19.3 Percent voting for republican US presidential candidates, by age groups, 1972–2008.
Source: *National exit polls (1972–2008)*

Table 19.1 Nationwide percentage of votes for McCain for president, 2008, by age and race.

AGES	BLACKS	LATINOS	WHITES
All ages	4	31	55
65+	6	30	58
45–64	3	40	56
30–44	4	36	57
18–29	4	19	44

Source: Binstock, 2009.

Overall, there is little evidence to date that older Americans' electoral choices have been strongly influenced by their self-interest in old-age benefit programs (see Binstock, 2009; Campbell, 2005; Jacobs & Burns, 2005). However, if in the future seniors face distinct, clearly defined policy threats regarding their Social Security and Medicare benefits, they may vote in a more distinctive pattern. (For a fuller discussion of these and related matters involving the voting behavior of older Americans, see Schulz and Binstock [2008]; for a penetrating theoretical discussion of why voters may not vote for what seems to be in their economic self-interest, see Simon [1985]).

THE ELECTORAL BLUFF AND OLD-AGE-BASED ORGANIZATIONS

Despite their lack of significant impact on electoral outcomes to date, the image of older persons as bloc voters swayed by "senior issues" persists for several reasons. First, it helps political journalists to reduce the intricate complexities of politics down to something easy to write about: a tabloid symbol.

Second, and more important, politicians "share [the] widespread perception of a huge, monolithic, senior citizen army of voters" (Peterson & Somit, 1994, p. 178). This perception is reinforced because, as discussed above, older persons are generally quite active in making their views known to members of Congress, especially regarding old-age benefit programs. Hence, politicians are wary of "waking a sleeping giant" of angry older voters. For example, incumbents are continually concerned about how their actions in the governing process – such as votes in Congress and their proposals for legislation – can be portrayed to older voters in subsequent re-election campaigns. A classic example was the enactment and swift repeal of the Medicare Catastrophic Coverage Act (MCCA) of 1988. The legislation levied a progressive surtax on Medicare participants to finance catastrophic hospital costs not covered by Medicare, as well as additional new insurance benefits. But a vocal minority of seniors angrily protested the surtax – including a physical attack on the automobile driven by Congressman Dan Rostenkowski, Chairman of the House Ways and Means Committee, in his Chicago district – an attack that was widely photographed and publicized nationally. Subsequently, the MCCA was repealed in 1989 (see Himmelfarb, 1995).

Third, the image of a senior voting bloc is marketed by the leaders of dozens of old-age-based interest or advocacy groups, which are mostly based in Washington. These organizations have a strong incentive to inflate perceptions of the voting power of the constituency for which they purport to speak.

THE POLITICS OF OLD-AGE INTEREST GROUPS

Since the 1960s, old-age advocacy groups have proliferated in the US. Today there are dozens of interest groups that are more or less exclusively preoccupied with national policy issues related to aging, and many people believe that they are among the most powerful lobbies in Washington. This is especially true for AARP (formerly the American Association of Retired Persons), a mass-membership organization of over 40 million persons aged 50 and older. (None of the several other organizations based on older persons as members claim much more than 10 million members, and many have far fewer.)

The professed role of old-age interest groups as representatives of and advocates for "the elderly" has given them entrée into the policy process. Public officials are willing to listen to the views of such organizations and often find it useful to invite them to participate in policy activities. A brief meeting with the leaders of AARP and other old-age organizations enables an official to demonstrate that he or she has been "in touch" (symbolically) with tens of millions of older persons. In turn, this symbolic legitimacy of old-age organizations enables them to obtain platforms in the national media, congressional hearings, and other age-related policy forums.

Perhaps the most important form of power available to the old-age interest groups is what might be termed the "electoral bluff." Although these organizations have not demonstrated a capacity to swing a decisive bloc of older voters, they do attempt to mobilize their members when legislation affecting older persons is being contemplated. Thus, for these interest groups, the perception that they influence the votes of seniors is in itself a source of political influence. Incumbent members of Congress are hardly inclined to risk upsetting the existing distribution of votes that puts them into and keeps them in office.

Old-age interest groups have attempted to enhance their power by banding together in a 64-member Leadership Council of Aging Organizations (LCAO), a self-defined "coalition of national nonprofit organizations concerned with the well-being of America's older population and committed to representing their interests in the policy-making arena" (Leadership Council of Aging Organizations, 2010). The coalition sends letters to members of Congress and the Administration on a broad range of policy issues, conducts issue briefings and forums, holds press conferences, and comments on presidential and congressional budgets affecting older persons. However, the members of LCAO have been divided on a number of issues over the years, and this has limited their effectiveness.

There is considerable diversity among the 64 organizations in the LCAO. In this sense they parallel the dozens of arenas in which large clusters of organizations pursue their interests through American politics.

One group within the old-age arena consists of advocacy organizations that are highly focused on causes that affect selected categories of older persons. These include the Older Women's League and various organizations advocating for different ethnic and racial subgroups of older people, such as the National Caucus and Center on Black Aged, and Asociación Nacionale Personas Mayores.

Other organizations represent persons afflicted by specific illnesses that usually affect older people. For instance, the Alzheimer's Association lobbies Congress for greater funding for research on Alzheimer's disease, and for programs that facilitate better care of those afflicted with the disease and that support their caregivers (Binstock, 1998).

Another group of organizations in the LCAO coalition is trade associations involved in providing programs and services to older persons as clients and customers. These include, for example, the American Association of Homes and Services for the Aging, the National Association of Area Agencies on Aging (N4A), and the National Association of Nutrition and Aging Services Programs (NANASP). Such trade associations draw on state and local political connections, as well as on their clients, to protest possible cutbacks in the programs that sustain their operations.

There is also a cluster of professional organizations that focuses on promoting aging-related research, education, and favorable conditions for professional practice in the field of aging. This group includes the Gerontological Society of America and the American Geriatrics Society. These organizations have effectively lobbied Congress to fund programs to promote their professional activities, including a six-year effort by the Gerontological Society of America (from 1969 to 1974) that played a critical role in establishing the National Institute of Aging (NIA) at the National Institutes of Health (Binstock, 2010). Over thirty years later, the NIA has an annual budget of about $1 billion that funds research on aging.

The old-age interest groups that have the greatest potential for political power, of course, are those that have mass memberships of older persons because their members are part of the latent voting constituency of older voters that, in principle, might be influenced by their parent organizations in upcoming elections. Among these are the National Association of Retired Federal Employees (NARFE), the National Committee to Preserve Social Security and Medicare (NCPSSM), the Alliance for Retired Americans (ARA), and AARP. By far the most powerful of these is AARP, with huge financial and staff resources that are far larger than those of all the other old-age interest groups combined.

AARP's membership dues are nominal, currently $16 for a couple. The majority of its finances come from its extensive business operations. The organization offers a variety of commercial services: auto, health, prescription drug, and long-term-care insurance; mutual funds; credit cards; and support for travel (including hotel and automobile discounts). It reported assets of $99 million at the end of 2008 and operating revenues of $1.08 billion. The largest portion of this revenue – 60% ($653 million) – came from "royalties and service provider relationship management fees" on the many products it markets to its members, especially insurance policies (AARP, 2009). Other sources of revenue in 2008 were membership dues, advertising in its publications, grants, investments, program income, contributions, and "other."

Over 94% of AARP's $1.1 billion in operating expenditures in 2008 was for membership development, management, member programs, field services, publications, and other revenue-generating activities. However, the organization also spent $59 million on public policy research and legislative lobbying. This level of expenditure on aging policy activities, together with a membership of approximately 40 million, makes it dominant among old-age interest groups in framing age-related policy issues.

In the political arena, AARP's incentive system has long dictated that it should clearly establish a record that it is "fighting the good fight" with respect to policy proposals affecting old-age programs. However, as with all mass-membership organizations, there is always the danger that its political positions and tactics might jeopardize the stability of the organization's membership and, thereby, its financial resources. In AARP's case, the primary reasons that most individuals sign up for membership are material – the discounts, the products, and services – rather than advocacy for old-age benefit goals and other age-related causes.

From 1995 until 2003, AARP assumed a noticeably withdrawn public posture, in part due to two public policy advocacy episodes that antagonized some of its members and eroded some of its political standing in Washington. On both occasions a number of AARP members resigned. On the second occasion the president of AARP publicly acknowledged that his membership had widely divergent and strongly held views on the issue and that representing a diverse membership in public policy affairs is an ongoing struggle for the organization. (A membership of 40 million persons recruited on the basis of age – primarily through material incentives, compared with ideological or purposive incentives – will inevitably have large numbers of Democrats, Republicans, and independents.) Following these episodes, AARP became sufficiently cautious in its policy stances that a staff member for a Democrat in the House of Representatives observed,

"I've almost stopped thinking of them as a lobby. They have all kinds of valuable member services and do really good research work. But in terms of being a tough lobby, they're not what they used to be" (Holmes, 2001, D1). But all this changed in 2003. President Bush had promised to secure Medicare coverage of outpatient prescription drugs – a critical gap in the program – and Republicans in Congress were ready to act.

Three Case Studies of Senior Power

Three recent policymaking episodes help to illustrate the impact of older persons on public policy outcomes in the US: the Medicare Prescription Drug, Improvement, and Modernization Act (MMA) of 2003; the demise of efforts in 2005 to privatize Social Security; and public policy responses to the economic crisis that began in 2007. Each example documents the continuing responsiveness of elected politicians to the needs and preferences of older Americans up to now, as well as the political durability and economic importance for older persons of the major social insurance programs.

The Politics of the Medicare Modernization Act

The 2003 MMA legislation represented the largest Medicare benefit expansion since the program's inception in 1965. To Medicare's longstanding Parts A (hospital insurance) and B (insurance for doctors and various outpatient services), it added Part D, a new prescription drug benefit available through private insurance companies. It also modified and renamed Part C as Medicare Advantage, a plan under which senior citizens can leave the traditional fee-for-service Parts A and B Medicare and instead get all of their medical care through privately managed care (HMO or PPO) plans. As of 2009, about 40% of all seniors had enrolled in stand-alone Part D drug plans and one in five was enrolled in Medicare Advantage plans, which also provide prescription drug coverage (Kaiser Family Foundation, 2009).

The legislation had its origins in President Bill Clinton's 1999 State of the Union address, when he proposed adding a prescription drug benefit to Medicare. Many seniors at the time had prescription drug coverage, but it was deteriorating. Former employers were dropping drug benefits for their retirees, monthly premiums for so-called "medigap" supplemental insurance plans that covered prescription drugs were increasing rapidly, and the costs of prescription drugs were climbing dramatically. With most insurance plans for working-age people covering prescription drugs, Medicare's lack of coverage for retirees had become increasingly glaring. Moreover, the federal budget surplus that materialized during the late 1990s made a Medicare benefit expansion to cover drugs seem affordable.

Once Clinton let the prescription drug cat out of the bag, elected politicians were hard-pressed to ignore the issue. In the 2000 presidential election campaign, both George W. Bush and Al Gore promised to secure drug coverage (Toner, 2000). When the Republican Party achieved unified control of government with the 2000 election, conservatives sought to use the creation of a new drug benefit as an enticing carrot for liberals within a broader, major conservative effort to fundamentally reform Medicare into a more private-sector program – a goal that they had long desired. They wanted the new drug benefit to only be available to those seniors who enrolled in Medicare managed care plans. However, this early proposal faced flak from inside the Republican Party itself; senators and House members representing rural districts and states in which there were few or no managed care plans refused to go along.

The legislation for the new benefit was essentially financed with deficit spending. In order to keep the projected cost of the new legislation to $410 billion over 10 years, the drug benefit had an odd structure. It provided both excellent first-dollar coverage and catastrophic coverage, but it had a substantial "donut hole" coverage gap in between, in which seniors had to pay 100% of drug costs out of pocket.

During the legislative process, AARP withheld its endorsement until it secured greater subsidies for low-income seniors and for businesses to retain coverage for retirees. When AARP finally came through with an endorsement, it was criticized by some of its members and advocates on the left for failing to hold out for a more generous benefit. In fact, according to AARP's CEO at the time, some 45 000 of his members resigned in anger because of the organization's support for the MMA (Schulz & Binstock, 2008).

Nonetheless, by all accounts (e.g. Iglehart, 2004) AARP's ultimate endorsement of the bill gave politicians on Capitol Hill crucial political coverage to vote for it. Even so, the vote was the longest open roll call in Congressional history, as Republican leaders engaged in protracted arm-twisting to get enough co-partisans on board, including fiscal conservatives worried about having a hand in the creation of a costly new entitlement.

Thus, the influence of the senior constituency both made the enactment of a prescription drug benefit highly likely once it was on the table and thwarted Republican plans to confine the benefit to seniors in private plans. However, Republican framers of the law did succeed in several respects. First, the Part D prescription drug benefit was only available through private stand-alone prescription drug insurance plans, with no option available within traditional Medicare. Second, another portion of the MMA increased by 20% the subsidies that Part C managed care plans had obtained under the Balanced Budget Act (BBA) of 1997. The previous subsidies had proved untenable for many such plans, which subsequently withdrew from the Medicare market. With these new, much higher subsidies, managed care plans flocked back. Market logic underpinned both programs, with competition among Medicare Advantage and particularly Part D plans intended by Republicans to lead to lower costs and more value for enrollees.

The pharmaceutical and insurance industries were extremely nervous about this legislation but have fared better than they probably anticipated. The pharmaceutical industry succeeded in having the MMA explicitly prohibit both government price controls and the re-importation of drugs from Canada. The insurance industry has likewise fared well. No one knew whether Part D products would emerge, as this was an entirely new market; but more plans are available than anyone anticipated (although the plethora of choice appears to undermine senior welfare, as laboratory experiments show that the more choice people face, the less able they are to select the cost-minimizing plan, and seniors perform worse than non-seniors; Hanoch et al., 2009). Some insurers seem to be taking advantage of the stickiness in the market by raising premiums dramatically; while the average premium went up 35% between 2006 and 2009, the Humana Basic plan, which garnered the largest market share since it was initially the lowest cost plan in many areas, increased its premiums 400% over the same period (Hargrave et al., 2009).

As for older persons, the angry resignation of AARP members in 2003 has not been echoed by a political backlash against the MMA. To be sure, initial implementation of Part D was rocky, with considerable confusion among seniors. They had to choose whether to enroll in a prescription drug plan at all (or face a late enrollment penalty later on) and then, depending on their geographical location, had to select from among 27 to 52 plans (Kaiser Family Foundation, 2007). Dual eligibles (the low-income seniors who are eligible for both Medicare and Medicaid) had formerly received drug coverage through Medicaid, but now they were randomly assigned to a Part D plan and often faced different formularies or increased out-of-pocket expenses as a result. Pharmacists played a major role in assisting seniors who were confronting the complexities of choosing a plan, with rural and independent pharmacists bearing the brunt (Sussman, 2010).

By and large, however, seniors are happy with the new drug plans and with Medicare Advantage plans (Morgan & Campbell, forthcoming). Yet, many seniors are not enrolled in an optimal plan. Many are paying higher premiums than necessary (Kaiser Family Foundation, 2006). Further very few, only about 9%, switch plans from year to year (Neuman et al., 2007), even though research shows over

40% would benefit from doing so (Abaluck & Gruber, 2009).

In any event, the case of the MMA episode in many ways shows the influence of the senior constituency. Older persons were already the biggest beneficiaries of the American welfare state, but managed to secure the first major expansion of it in 40 years as well. They were also able to thwart conservatives' initial plans that would have more fundamentally changed the design of Medicare, although they are not as well served as they could be by the market-based design of Part D and Medicare Advantage plans.

The Case of Social Security Privatization

If conservatives who wished to remake the large entitlement programs to suit their preference for private sector mechanisms had some success with Medicare in 2003, they were thwarted in attempting to reshape Social Security in 2005. For years conservatives had sought to trim the public pension program, the biggest line item in the federal budget (see Williamson, 1997). Head-on attacks proved disastrous, as when Ronald Reagan proposed reducing Social Security benefits for early retirees in 1981 and meekly dropped the proposal after senior protests and exhortations from many quarters. Conservatives then adopted a cleverer, indirect approach by devising attractive private alternatives to the big entitlement programs (such as 401(k)s and individual retirement accounts) that would lure Americans away voluntarily. With these alternatives now widespread, conservatives could use them to "analogize" the private account idea (Teles & Derthick, 2009). It was proposed that a portion of a worker's Social Security payroll contributions could be funneled into an individual account that the worker would manage, selecting his or her own investments. The promise was that workers would gain control, could seek greater returns in equity markets than provided by the sleepy traditional program, and could pass the accumulated sum onto heirs upon death, unlike traditional Social Security.

With George W. Bush's election, private accounts finally had a proponent in the White House. The president had a long history of ideological distaste for Social Security. According to one of his professors at Harvard Business School in the mid-1970s, Bush denounced President Franklin Roosevelt in class as a socialist, and specifically identified Social Security as one of several New Deal programs that he opposed (Tsurumi, 2005). In spring 2001, he created a commission on Social Security reform consisting entirely of private account supporters. In his executive order to establish it (Bush, 2001), the president foreordained the commission's recommendations by stipulating that "modernization must include individually controlled, voluntary personal retirement accounts." Indeed, all three of the options included

in the commission's December 2001 report included individual accounts. But events related to the 9/11 terrorism attacks pushed the report into the background. However, Bush made privatization the centerpiece of his second-term domestic agenda, stating in his 2005 State of the Union address that the system was headed toward "bankruptcy." He ruled out an increase in payroll taxes and asserted that the "best way" to preserve the program for younger workers was to divert a portion of the Social Security payroll tax to create individual, private investment accounts. He spent the first half of 2005 barnstorming the country to sell his plan (see Schulz & Binstock, 2008).

Even with a president at the helm, however, Social Security privatization went nowhere. Seniors, the group for whom Social Security is most salient, were dead set against it. Majorities of younger people supported private accounts, but they paid far less attention to the issue than older persons (Campbell & King, 2010). Organized labor and AARP launched aggressive campaigns against privatization (Greenhouse, 2005; Pear, 2004). As joint trustees of huge pension assets, labor could threaten financial service companies and force them to withdraw support from lobbying groups backing individual accounts. For AARP, opposition to privatization provided a much-needed "easy issue." The organization had been burned by the MCCA episode, as well as by criticism that it had not held out for more in the MMA because it stood to make more money for its insurance plans from a drug program that did not have government price controls. But now, a fight against privatization of Social Security would allow AARP to have a strong clear message, without any allegations of conflict of interest. Moreover, its membership was nearly united in opposition to private accounts. It seemed to matter little that private account proponents promised that changes to Social Security would not affect current retirees; they are the citizens focused on the program and whose opinions on it matter to elected officials, and they opposed the program change despite these reassurances. Moreover, polls showed public support for individual accounts falling over time, most steeply among senior citizens (Campbell & King, 2010). So, privatization was an easy proposal for AARP to oppose.

AARP immediately countered the president's efforts with a nationwide campaign of television commercials and full-page color newspaper ads, raising strong objections to "privatization" of Social Security. In addition, it took out state and local ads to thank specific Democratic senators in swing states for holding the line against private accounts that take money out of Social Security.

In the face of senior opposition and a well-financed AARP media campaign, Republican support for privatization crumbled. Bush himself made some tactical errors, wasting valuable post-election momentum by traveling the country and delaying introduction of private account legislation, and presenting the idea as a presidential initiative and therefore denying congressional Republicans ownership (Calmes, 2005). With public support falling, especially among the crucial senior constituency, members of Congress had little incentive to go along with the president. The ideological desire to rein in the public pension program with individual accounts was trumped by electoral logic.

By 2005, AARP had revived its reputation as a powerful interest group and, in reality, had established itself as far more of a force in the politics of old-age policies than it had been in the past. AARP's willingness to spend millions of dollars of the organization's wealth on ads in nationwide and state media venues had a great deal to do with this reversal of image and the enhancement of power that imagery can confer.

Why did privatization make inroads in Medicare and not in Social Security? In both instances, conservatives offered a sweetener to encourage support for changing the program designs. But the Medicare offer was much sweeter: seniors got a new prescription drug benefit. All Social Security privatization proponents could offer was the promise of higher returns in the future, a risk that seniors, who embraced the familiar DB structure of the traditional program, did not want to take on. And, as it turned out, the risk of private investments as a source of retirement wealth became all too clear by the end of the decade.

The Great Recession and the Politics of Aging

A third episode – the economic crisis and recession that began in 2007 – demonstrates the importance both of the senior political constituency and of the major entitlement programs for the well-being of seniors and their families.

As indicated in Chapter 13, millions of older Americans are in poverty. And one of the factors accounting for the increased labor force participation of older persons in recent years (see Chapter 14) may be that existing provisions for retirement are falling short for many. However, thanks to Social Security and Medicare, and to other financial characteristics of the older population, on average, seniors have fared better than many younger Americans during the Great Recession. It is younger people who have faced the brunt of the recession, confronting high unemployment rates, reduced hours and pay, and receding health insurance coverage. In November 2009, the unemployment rate was 10.3% among those aged between 25 and 34, and 15.9% among those aged between 20 and 24 (US Bureau of Labor Statistics, 2010, Table A-10). Moreover, many without jobs are not eligible for unemployment insurance (UI) due to their occupation or the length of their joblessness.

Seniors did lose money when the value of most stocks dropped sharply. But they had the valuable Social Security annuity – which provides the majority of income for nearly two-thirds of persons aged 65 and older (Federal Interagency Forum on Aging-Related Statistics, 2008, p. 15) – and access to health care through Medicare and Medicaid. Seniors are also more likely to own their homes and to own them free and clear and they also hold less financial debt of all kinds, (US Census Bureau 2008a, 2008b, Table 17; US Census Bureau, 2009, Table 1134; US Department of Housing and Urban Development, 2008, p. 162). Although the personal bankruptcy filing rate of older persons has edged up in recent years, in 2007 it was still less than one-third that of 35–44-year-olds (Thorne et al., 2008, p. 5).

An April 2009 survey for *Time* magazine showed that senior citizens were far less likely than young and middle-aged adults to make lifestyle changes in the face of economic crisis. Respondents aged 65 and over were less likely to cut back on vacations or entertainment because of their cost (just 42% of seniors did so compared to 68% of those aged 18 to 64); to fail to pay a bill on time because of having the money (13% vs 32%); to borrow money from family or friends to make ends meet (6% vs 24%); or to avoid going to a doctor because of the cost (6% vs 27%). Older people were also far less likely to have suffered emotional distress, feel nervous or anxious (23% vs 44%), have trouble sleeping (17% vs 34%), get upset with someone for no apparent reason (6% vs 23%), or use alcohol, cigarettes, or food for comfort (authors' calculations from *Time* magazine, 2009).

Despite the fact that seniors have fared relatively well in the face of recession compared to younger people, it was seniors who received the largest individual income help from the federal government's February 2009 stimulus bill. Checks for $250 were mailed to Social Security recipients in May 2009; this was equivalent to about a 2% increase in Social Security benefits for the average recipient (Desjardins, 2009). These extra benefits came on the heels of a 5.8% cost-of-living adjustment (COLA) in January 2009, the largest since 1982, largely due to galloping energy prices the previous year (Ohlemacher, 2009). The political responsiveness to the old-age constituency was demonstrated again when the SSA announced in October 2009 that there would be no COLA for 2010 because inflation was negative in 2009. Shortly thereafter, President Obama called for a second round of $250 checks to Social Security recipients, a proposal widely criticized as political pandering (see Munnell & Biggs, 2010).

Although working-aged Americans have been hit hard by the recession, with no one sending them $250 checks, there is little evidence that intergenerational conflict is emerging. Indeed, the recession has highlighted the intergenerational and societal importance of the safety net. The non-elderly continue to be very supportive of the major entitlement programs. A July/August 2009 National Academy of Social Insurance/Rockefeller Foundation survey found that 45–48% of people aged 18–64 thought we do not spend enough on Social Security, compared to 37% of people aged 65 and older (Reno & Lavery, 2009, p. 8). The same poll found that large percentages of Americans said they did not "mind paying Social Security taxes," 72% because they knew they would be getting retirement benefits themselves; 76% because otherwise they would have to support family members financially; and 87% because the program provides "security and stability" to millions of retirees, disabled people, and survivors. More than three-quarters agreed that "it is critical that we preserve Social Security for future generations" even if it means increasing taxes.

WILL THE POLITICS OF AGING CHANGE?

In the mid-1990s, MIT economist Lester Thurow predicted that the aging of the baby boom generation would bring about substantial intergenerational conflict in US politics. As he saw it: "In the years ahead, class warfare is apt to be redefined as the young against the old, rather than the poor against the rich" (Thurow, 1996, p. 47). Will his prophecy come true?

As yet, there have been no signs of intergenerational political conflict in national elections and legislative processes. Older persons have not been an old-age-benefits voting bloc in national elections, the electoral arena that is most salient to those benefits. Further, AARP and other old-age advocacy groups have managed to conduct their lobbying on senior issues in a fashion that avoids any themes of intergenerational competition and conflict. Overall, the modern contexts of policy agendas regarding old-age benefits have yet to pit generations against each other.

On the other hand, there have been distinct signs recently that a changing context of policy agendas regarding old-age-benefits, within a broader context of political concerns about the nation's deficit spending, might conceivably lead to intergenerational political conflict during the next several decades.

Just prior to, and following, the enactment of the Patient Protection and Affordable Health Care Act of 2010, much attention in President Obama's administration, the Congress, the media, and various respected public policy and scientific sources turned to the general issue of reducing the long-run cumulative deficit of the federal government (which had already reached over $12 trillion and was projected to keep growing), and, in particular, to the relationship of old-age entitlement programs to that deficit. For instance the National Research Council and the National Academy of Public administration jointly issued a report titled "Choosing the Nation's Fiscal Future" (Committee on the Fiscal Future of the US, 2010) in which it singled out the Social Security, Medicare, and Medicaid programs as essential major targets for deficit reduction reforms, including restraints on their growth and greater taxes to support them. Ben Bernanke, Chairman of the Federal Reserve, persistently expressed this view in speeches (e.g. Chan & Hernandez, 2010) and congressional testimony (Chan, 2010). If the deficit is addressed through such reforms of entitlement programs, will intergenerational conflict be a likely consequence?

To deal with the issue of deficit reduction, President Obama established an 18-member National Commission on Fiscal Responsibility and Reform (White House, 2010), comprising six appointees by the president and six bipartisan appointees from each of the two houses of Congress. The Commission was charged with reporting its findings (if agreed to by at least 14 members) to Congress by December 1, 2010. It is a common assumption in Washington that the panel will focus on long-run ways to reduce spending on Social Security and Medicare in one way or another and perhaps ways to raise additional revenue for Social Security – although Republicans on the panel are likely to oppose new taxation for this purpose (see Calmes, 2010).

AARP publicly applauded the announcement of this commission, but at the same time anxiously anticipated that Social Security and Medicare would be the major deficit reduction targets of the Commission. In a newsletter to AARP members, the organization's CEO threw down the gauntlet in defense of Social Security and Medicare, saying that, if the benefits in these programs were reduced, "[M]illions of older Americans could not afford the necessities of life. We will do everything in our power to protect and strengthen these essential programs" (Rand, 2010, p. 26).

A number of relatively minor policy changes for reducing the costs of Social Security and raising more revenue for the program to bring it into long-run fiscal balance have been discussed over the years (e.g. Schulz & Binstock, 2008). There is no inherent reason that such reforms need engender intergenerational conflict, especially if they are carefully crafted through advance planning, enacted relatively soon, and implemented gradually, following the successful political model of the 1983 Social Security amendments. That legislation raised the age for full retirement benefits from 65 to 67, but structured the change to begin 20 years later, in 2003, and take an additional 24 years to be fully implemented in 2027. This policy elicited little outrage, unrest, or opposition either from voters (who paid little, if any, attention to it) or from vested interests such as employers responsible for paying Social Security payroll taxes.

Whatever approach Congress may take to reform Social Security, its members have no incentive, and definite disincentives, to frame legislation that would engender intergenerational conflict. Few of them have electoral constituencies that are more or less generationally monolithic that might reward them for such actions.

In the case of Medicare, the challenges of reducing its contributions to the long-run fiscal deficit and avoiding intergenerational conflict are far greater. Its costs grow quickly. Medicare was only 3.5% of the federal budget in 1990, but almost 16% in 2009 (Congressional Budget Office, 2009). By 2036, the proportion of GDP spent on Medicare is projected to more than triple to about 8% (Medicare Payment Advisory Commission, 2006) – one-twelfth of US national wealth, spent on one program.

The heart of the problem in spiraling Medicare costs is *not* the fact that the number of older people eligible for the program will double over the next 20 years. A number of studies have shown that population aging is a relatively minor factor in the growth of health care costs in the US and other industrialized nations (see Reinhardt, 2003). Rather, the problem is expense factors in the overall system, in which costs rise much faster than the general rate of inflation. The major sources of rising costs per patient in the health care sector are: a constant stream of new and costly technologies and procedures; high rates of utilization; huge administrative costs; and unnecessarily high comparative expenses and utilization in some regions and health centers as compared with others. The consensus among analysts of the growth in US healthcare costs is that the advance and application of medical technology is the single most important factor (Congressional Budget Office, 2007; Newhouse, 1992).

Consequently, efforts to contain Medicare costs – without limiting coverage for the health care of older patients – should in principle focus on reforming the health care system generally, not just Medicare. But as the recent politics of enacting the Patient Protection and Affordable Health Care Act of 2010 vividly demonstrated, there are substantial political barriers to major, sweeping health care reforms – especially because of the large financial stakes that the medical industrial complex has in current arrangements. Moreover, the larger healthcare arena is highly fragmented, so there is no entity "in charge" of it. In contrast, Medicare policies can be implemented more effectively because they can be centralized and carried out through concerted government policy actions. So, for the foreseeable future, attempts to contain health care costs are likely to continue focusing on limiting Medicare coverage.

If such reforms involve explicit near-term cuts in or withdrawal of Medicare coverage for selected procedures, and/or substantial more generalized cuts in Medicare reimbursements for physicians and hospitals, then a political backlash from older voters and old-age interest groups could very well emerge. To be sure, various forms of old-age-based health care rationing within the British National Health Service have been taking place for years (see Young, 2006) without causing a political uproar. But, as the politics of health care reform in the summer of 2009 illustrated, the response to such rationing phenomena within the US Medicare program might be much more politically volatile.

From the 2009 outset of his effort to reform healthcare, an overarching public message from President Obama was that the costs of reform would be substantially offset by *savings in the Medicare program* (see White House, 2009). Then, the theme of health care rationing for older Americans became especially prominent in the summer of 2009. A provision in the health care reform bill in the House of Representatives had expanded Medicare to cover the costs of a voluntary consultation with a physician, every five years, concerning end-of-life planning through living wills and health care durable power of attorney documents. A number of prominent Republican politicians and conservative broadcasters transformed these two themes – end-of life-planning and savings from Medicare – into the specters of "death panels" and efforts to "pull the plug on Granny." When members of Congress returned to their districts during the summer recess to hold town hall-style meetings, they faced rowdy crowds in which older persons expressed such concerns about rationing in the Medicare program (Blumenauer, 2009). Subsequently, AARP acknowledged that it faced a challenge in explaining to its members why it endorsed healthcare reform (Calmes, 2009).

The breadth and depth of concerns among older persons about death panels and other forms of old-age-based rationing and the political ramifications were unclear. To be sure, journalists opined that older persons would vote as a bloc in the 2010 Congressional elections against Democratic members of Congress who supported health care reform and various national polls during the summer were eager to issue reports that seniors were against health care reform; however, the headlines on these reports exaggerated their actual data (Gallup, 2009).

Perhaps the journalistic pundits will prove correct in their vision of a generational divide in the 2010 election, with seniors especially opposed to Democratic candidates because of the symbol of "death panels" and anticipated reductions in Medicare spending. But, based on decades of age-group electoral data, it is more likely that the distribution of older persons' votes in the 2010 election will closely resemble the distributions within other age groups, except for the youngest cohort of voters.

Fundamentally, the likelihood and intensity of intergenerational political conflict involving old-age-benefit programs will be shaped by the answers to two questions. First, will there be enough national wealth available to redistribute to older people? Second, will the prevailing US ideology in the decades ahead support a politics of collectively insuring against the risks of poverty and illness in old age? Popular support for Social Security and Medicare has been reasonably strong among all generations up to now (Campbell, 2009). According to a *New York Times*/CBS News Poll, even Tea Party members – who poll as more conservative than Republicans and are strongly anti-government – "think that Social Security and Medicare are worth the cost to taxpayers" (Zernike & Thee-Brenan, 2010, p. A1).

In the longer run, broad political support for old-age benefit programs – from all generations – will probably rely on the extent to which those programs are perceived as benefiting all generations, and

recognition that significant cutbacks in benefits could have considerable ramifications for the nature of family obligations and other familiar social institutions that are integral to the daily life of US citizens of all ages. Older people are not hermetically sealed from their families, communities, and society. Neither are old-age benefits hermetically sealed from other age groups within families and society at large. If this multigenerational perspective prevails, the probability of a politics of intergenerational conflict will remain low.

ACKNOWLEDGMENTS

Andrea Campbell would like to thank Ryan King, Kimberly Morgan, and Mike Sances. Robert Binstock wishes to acknowledge the intellectual stimulation and support of the MacArthur Foundation's Research Network on an Aging Society.

REFERENCES

AARP. (2009). *AARP consolidated financial statements. December 31, 2008 and December 31, 2007.* Retrieved June 12, 2010 from http://www.assets.aarp.org_TopicAreas/annual_reports/assets/AARPConsolidatedFinancialStatements.pdf.

Abaluck, J. T., & Gruber, J. (2009). Choice inconsistencies among the elderly: Evidence from plan choice in the Medicare Part D program. *NBER Working Paper 14759*, February. Retrieved May 13, 2010 from http://www.nber.org/papers/w14759.

Binstock, R. H. (1998). *Public policy and voluntary health agencies.* Washington, DC: National Health Council.

Binstock, R. H. (2009). Older voters and the 2008 election. *Gerontologist, 49*, 697–701.

Binstock, R. H., & Riemer, Y. (1978). Campaigning for "the senior vote": A case study of Carter's 1976 campaign. *Gerontologist, 8*, 517–524.

Binstock, R. H. (2010). 1974: GSA play major role in NIA's development. *Gernotology News, 38*(3), 7.

Blumenauer, E. (2009). My near death panel experience. *New York Times*, November 15, 12wk.

Bush, G. W. (2001). President's Commission to strengthen Social Security. *Executive Order 13201*, May 2, 2001. Retrieved June 22, 2010 from www.presidency.ucsb.edu/ws/index.php?pid=61491.

Calmes, J. (2005). Lost appeal: How a victorious Bush fumbled plan to revamp Social Security. *Wall Street Journal*, October 20, A1.

Calmes, J. (2009). AARP says its chore is educating members on bill's benefits. *New York Times*, October 14. Retrieved October 14, 2009 from http://prescriptions.blogs.nytimes.com/2009/1014/aarp-says-its-chore-is-educating-elderly-on-bills-benefits/

Calmes, J. (2010). Next big issue? Social Security pops up again. *The New York Times*, March 22, p. 1.

Campbell, A. L. (2002). Self-interest, Social Security, and the distinctive participation patterns of senior citizens. *American Political Science Review, 96*, 565–574.

Campbell, A. L. (2003a). *How policies make citizens: Senior citizen activism and the American welfare state.* Princeton: Princeton University Press.

Campbell, A. L. (2003b). Participatory reactions to policy threats: Senior

citizens and the defense of Social Security and Medicare. *Political Behavior, 55*, 29–49.

Campbell, A. L. (2005). The non-distinctiveness of senior voters in the 2004 election. *Public Policy and Aging Report, 15*(2), 1 & 3–6.

Campbell, A. L. (2009). Is the economic crisis driving wedges between young and old? Rich and poor? *Generations, 33*(3), 47–53.

Campbell, A. L., & King, R. (2010). Social Security: Political resilience in the face of conservative strides. In R. H. Hudson (Ed.), *The new politics of old-age policy* (pp. 223–253) (2nd ed.). Baltimore: Johns Hopkins University Press.

Chan, S. (2010). Bernanke says a plan to address the U.S. deficit could keep rates down. *New York Times*, April 15, B8.

Chan, S., & Hernandez, J.C. (2010). Bernanke says nation must take action soon to shape fiscal future. Retrieved April 8, 2010, from http://www.nytimes.com/2010/04/08/business/economy/08fed.html

Committee on the Fiscal Future of the United States (2010). *Choosing the nation's fiscal future.*

Washington, DC: National Academies Press.

Congressional Budget Office. (2007). *The long-term outlook for health care spending*. Washington, DC: United States Government Printing Office, November.

Congressional Budget Office. (2009). *The budget and economic outlook: An update*. Washington, DC: CBO.

Desjardins, L. (2009.) $250 checks going to millions of seniors Thursday. Retrieved on May 7, 2009, from www.cnn.com/2009/POLITICS/05/07/seniors.stimulus/index.html.

Esping-Andersen, G. (1999). *Social foundations of postindustrial economies*. New York: Oxford University Press.

Federal Interagency Forum on Aging-Related Statistics (2008). *Older Americans 2008: Key indicators of well-being*. Washington, DC: US Government Printing Office.

Gallup. (2009). Seniors most skeptical of healthcare reform. Most seniors think reform law would be harmful, not beneficial, to them. Retrieved, April 12, 2010, from http://www.gallup.com/poll/121982/seniors-skeptical-healthcare-reform.aspx

Goerres, A. (2009). *The political participation of older people in Europe: The greying of our democracies*. London: Palgrave MacMillan.

Greenhouse, S. (2005). Labor unions enter Social Security debate. *New York Times*, March 17, C2.

Hanoch, Y., Rice, T., Cummings, J., & Wood, S. (2009). How much choice is too much? The case of the Medicare prescription drug benefit. *Health Services Research*, 44, 1157–1168.

Hargrave, E., Hoadley, J., Cubanski, J., & Neuman, P. (2009). Medicare prescription drug plans in 2009 and key changes since 2006. Kaiser Family Foundation publication number 7917. Retrieved June 10, 2010 from www.kff.org/medicare/upload/7917.pdf.

Himmelfarb, R. (1995). *Catastrophic politics: The rise and fall of the Medicare Catastrophic Coverage Act of 1988*. University Park, PA:

Pennsylvania State University Press.

Holmes, S.A. (2001). The world according to AARP. *New York Times*, March 21, E1.

Iglehart, J. K. (2004). The new Medicare prescription-drug benefit – A pure power play. *New England Journal of Medicine*, 350, 826–833.

Jacobs, L., & Burns, M. (2005). Don't lump seniors. *Public Policy and Aging Report*, 15(1), 7–9.

Kaiser Family Foundation. (2006). Seniors' early experiences with the Medicare prescription drug benefit. Retrieved, June 10, 2010 from www.kff.org/kaiserpolls/upload/7502.pdf.

Kaiser Family Foundation. (2007). Medicare Part D plan characteristics, 2007. Publication number 7426-02. Retrieved June 10, 2010 from www.kff.org/medicare/upload/7426-02.pdf.

Kaiser Family Foundation. (2009). The Medicare prescription drug benefit. Publication Number 7044-10. November. Retrieved June 10, 2010 from http://www.kff.org/medicare/upload/7044-10.pdf.

Leadership Council of Aging Organizations. (2010). Our mission. Retrieved June 11, 2010 from http://www.lcao.org/our_mission.htm

Lutz, W., Mamolo, M., Potancoková, M., Scherbov, S., & Sobotka, T. (2008). *European Demographic Data Sheet: 2008*. Vienna: Austrian Academy of Sciences, and Washington, DC: Population Reference Bureau.

Medicare Payment Advisory Commission (2006). *Report to the Congress: Medicare payment policy*. Washington, DC: US Government Printing Office.

Mettler, S., & Soss, J. (2004). The consequences of public policy for democratic citizenship: Bridging policy studies and mass politics. *Perspectives on Politics*, 2, 55–73.

Morgan, K. J., & Campbell, A. L. (forthcoming). *The delegated welfare state: Medicare, markets, and the governance of social policy*. New York: Oxford University Press.

Munnell, A. H., & Biggs, A. G. (2010). Adjusting to reality. *New York Times*, March 8, A19.

Newhouse, J. (1992). Medical care costs: How much welfare loss? *Journal of Economic Perspectives*, 6(3), 3–21.

Neuman, P., Strollos, M. K., Guterman, S., Roger, W. H., Li, A., Rodday, A. M. C., & Safran, D. G. (2007). Medicare prescription drug benefit progress report: Findings from a 2006 national survey of seniors. *Health Affairs*, 26(5), W630–W643.

Ohlemacher, S. (2009). Obama calls for $250 to seniors. *Associated Press*. Retrieved October 14, 2009 from apnews.myway.com/article/20091015/D9BB77S00.html.

Pear, R. (2004). In ads, AARP criticizes plan on privatizing. *New York Times*, December 30, A16.

Peterson, S. A., & Somit, A. (1994). *Political behavior of older americans*. New York: Garland.

Plutzer, E. (2002). Becoming a habitual voter: Inertia, resources, and growth in young adulthood. *American Political Science Review*, 96, 41–56.

Pratt, H. J. (1976). *The gray lobby*. Chicago: University of Chicago Press.

Rand, A.B. (2010). Where we stand: Attacking the deficit. *AARP Bulletin*, June, p. 26.

Reinhardt, U. E. (2003). Does the aging of the population really drive the demand for health care? *Health Affairs*, 22(6), 27–39.

Reno, V.P., & Lavery, J. (2009). *Economic crisis fuels support for Social Security: Americans' views on Social Security*. Washington, DC: National Academy of Social Insurance.

Rosenstone, S., & Hansen, J. M. (1993). *Mobilization, participation, and democracy in America*. New York: MacMillan.

Schulz, J. H., & Binstock, R. H. (2008). *Aging nation: The economics and politics of growing older in America*. Baltimore: Johns Hopkins University Press.

Simon, H. A. (1985). Human nature in politics: The dialogue of psychology with political science. *American Political Science Review*, 79, 293–304.

Stolberg, S.G. (2010). Obama lobbies elderly on benefits of health law. *New York Times*, June 9, A-16.

Sussman, T. (2010). Pharmacists' prescriptions for Medicare Part D. PhD dissertation. Cambridge, MA: Harvard University.

Teles, S. M., & Derthick, M. (2009). Social Security from 1980 to the present: From third rail to presidential commitment – and back? In B. J. Glenn & S. M. Teles (Eds.), *Conservatism and American political development* (pp. 261–290). New York: Oxford University Press.

Thorne, D., Warren, E., & Sullivan, T.A. (2008). *Generations of struggle*. AARP Public Policy Institute #2008-11. June. Washington, DC: AARP.

Thurow, L. C. (1996). The birth of a revolutionary class. *New York Times Magazine*, May 19, 46–47.

Time magazine. (2009). *Economic downturn poll #2009-4666*, April 1–5. Retrieved July 15, 2009 from http://www.ropercenter.uconn. edu.libproxy.mit.edu/.

Timpone, R. J. (1998). Structure, behavior, and voter turnout in the United States. *American Political Science Review, 92*, 145–158.

Toner, R. (2000). Basic differences in rival proposals on drug coverage. *New York Times*, October 1, A1.

Tsurumi, Y. (2005). Hail to the robber baron? *The Harvard Crimson*, April 6, 2005. Retrieved April 8, 2005 from http:///www. thecrimson.com/printerfriendly. aspx?ref=506836.

US Bureau of Labor Statistics. (2010). *Labor force statistics from the Current Population Survey*. Retrieved June 28, 2010 from http://www.bls.gov/web/empsit/ cpseea10.pdf

US Census Bureau. (2008a). *National population projections. Projections of the population by selected age groups and sex for the United States: 2010– 2050*. Retrieved January 11, 2010 from http://www.census.gov/ population/www/projections/ summarytables.html

US Census Bureau. (2008b). *Housing vacancies and homeownership survey*. Retrieved June 28, 2010 from www. census.gov/hhes/www/housing/ hvs/annual08/ann08t17.xls. Washington, DC.

US Census Bureau (2009). *Statistical abstract of the United States*. Washington, DC: US Government Printing Office.

US Department of Housing and Urban Development (2008). *American housing survey for the United States: 2007*. Washington, DC: US Government Printing Office.

Verba, S., Schlozman, K. L., & Brady, H. E. (1995). *Voice and equality: Civic voluntarism in American politics*. Cambridge, MA: Harvard University Press.

Walker, A., & Naegele, G. (Eds.), (1999). *The politics of old age in Europe*. Philadelphia: Open University Press.

White House. (2009). *America's seniors and health insurance reform: Protecting coverage and strengthening Medicare*. Retrieved December 18, 2009 from http:// www.healthreform.gov/reports/ seniors/index.htm

White House. (2010). *President Obama establishes bipartisan National Commission on Fiscal Responsibility and Reform*. Retrieved March 20, 2010, from http://www. whitehouse.gov/the-ress-office/ president-obama-establishes- bipartisan-national-commission- fiscal-responsibility-an

Williamson, J. B. (1997). A critique of the case for privatizing Social Security. *The Gerontologist, 37*, 561–571.

Young, J. (2006). Ageism in services for transient ischemic attack and stroke. *British Medical Journal, 333*, 508–509.

Zernike, K., & Thee-Brenan, M. (2010). Discontent's demography: Who backs the Tea Party. *New York Times*, April 15, A1.

Chapter | 20 |

The Future of Retirement Security

John B. Williamson

Department of Sociology, Boston College, Chestnut Hill, Massachusetts

INTRODUCTION

The focus of this chapter is on recent developments relevant to the future of retirement security, particularly public pension policy. Recent trends in the US are discussed, as are developments in several other countries, some of which have potential relevance for future pension policy debates in the US. A focus throughout is on efforts to privatize pension programs in the US and in other countries, which often turn out to be part of a more general effort aimed at welfare state retrenchment (Harrington Meyer & Herd, 2007).

SOCIAL SECURITY IN THE US

Social Security is important to any discussion of the future of retirement security in the US because so many people depend on this program for a substantial fraction of their retirement income. See Chapter 13 for a thorough account of the importance of Social Security to the income of older persons. Social Security is generally referred to as a pay-as-you-go-defined benefit (PAYG-DB) scheme. It is less common, but more precise, to describe it as a "partial reserve" scheme (Schulz, 2001). This is because the Social Security trust funds always hold at least modest (and currently quite substantial) reserves

DOI: 10.1016/B978-0-12-380880-6.00020-4

designed to make it possible to pay benefits during periods when the payroll tax revenues being collected fall below benefits promised under current statutes. It is a PAYG scheme because benefits to current pensioners are paid for via payroll taxes on current workers and their employers. It is a DB scheme because benefits are based on a wage-indexed average of past covered wages and the number of years as a contributor.

A recent projection is that the Social Security trust funds will be exhausted in 2037 unless some legislative changes are made (Board of Trustees, 2009). In recent decades, conservative commentators have made extensive use of the term "crisis," and some have even described Social Security as a pyramid scheme (Borden, 1995; Peterson, 1999). In contrast, liberal analysts have tended to use a different and much less sensationalistic rhetoric designed to convey the idea that there is a problem that needs to be addressed, but one that can be dealt with using a combination of modest adjustments – sometimes referred to as "parametric" reforms (Diamond & Orszag, 2004; Kingson & Williamson, 2001).

Efforts to Partially Privatize Social Security in the US

The idea of partially privatizing Social Security emerged during the early 1980s. Several of the early proponents were associated with the Cato Institute, a Washington-based libertarian think tank (Ferrara, 1985). Throughout the late 1980s and early 1990s, a small number of analysts and commentators associated with conservative think tanks continued the call to at least partially privatize Social Security, but it was not viewed as politically feasible by mainstream policy analysts. However, due to the relentless call from commentators on the right promoting the idea that Social Security would soon "go bankrupt," the concept of privatization eventually gained traction. Many Americans became fearful that the funds would not be available to pay their pensions; but, despite this loss of confidence, support for the program remained strong (Reno & Friedland, 1997).

Starting in the mid-1990s, the idea of partially privatizing Social Security moved into the mainstream of pension policy discourse with the creation of a number of highly visible national commissions. During this period, many conservative commentators were calling for partial privatization, and some viewed full privatization of Social Security as the eventual goal (Ferrara & Tanner, 1998; Peterson, 1999). Liberals generally opposed all proposals calling for the diversion of payroll taxes currently used to finance Social Security into funded individual retirement savings accounts (Kingson & Williamson, 1999).

In 2001 the Bush administration created a "bipartisan" committee called the President's Commission to Strengthen Social Security (2001). To be on the committee, one had to be a proponent of some sort of plan based on individual accounts. Three proposals emerged from the commission, all calling for the introduction of individual accounts. When it became clear that along with the individual accounts would come substantial cuts in the traditional DB component of Social Security, the proposed reforms looked a lot less attractive to many Americans. With the terrorists attacks of September 11, 2001 and the sharp drop in the stock market between 2000 and 2002, calls for the partial privatization of Social Security became much less frequent (Béland, 2005).

But President George W. Bush was not ready to give up. Soon after he won re-election in 2004, he began a full-court press to sell the American public on the idea of adding funded individual accounts as part of Social Security reform. He highlighted this proposal in his 2005 State of the Union Address and then traveled around the country for about six months trying to get the American public behind the idea. In an effort to undercut support for Social Security as it is currently structured, he argued that the Social Security Trust Fund was nothing but a bunch of IOUs – his term for the US government bonds held by the SSA (Hardy & Hazelrigg, 2007). In the end, this argument and his effort to sell partial privatization fell flat; the more the American public learned about the specifics of what would be involved with the partial privatization of Social Security, the less they liked the idea. In the 2006 midterm elections and in the 2008 presidential election, many Republicans who were up for re-election went out of their way to avoid discussion of Social Security reform and particularly proposals to partially privatize Social Security (Williamson & Watts-Roy, 2009).

Social Security "Parametric" Reform Proposals

There is general agreement by analysts on both the right and the left that changes in US Social Security policy must soon be made to balance projected revenues and pension spending. The list below briefly summarizes some of the parametric proposals likely to be under consideration:

(1) a shift to a less generous COLA;
(2) a shift to a less generous formula for determining benefits;
(3) an increase in the age of eligibility for full retirement benefits;
(4) an increase in the cap on earnings subject to payroll taxation;
(5) a flat across-the-board cut in benefits;
(6) the introduction of "progressive price indexing";

(7) an increase in the number of years of lifetime covered employment used to compute benefits; and/or

(8) an increase in the payroll tax rate.

For more detailed discussions of these and other proposals, see Favreault & Michelmore (2009), Sass et al. (2009), Shelton (2008), Social Security Administration (2008a) and US Department of the Treasury (2008).

EMPLOYER-SPONSORED PENSIONS IN THE US

The Rapid Move from DB Pensions to DC Pensions

There are two broad categories of employer-sponsored pensions: DB pensions and DC pensions (O'Rand et al., 2009; Schulz & Borowski, 2006). Pensions based on the DB model typically provide eligible employees with a highly predictable lifetime pension based on a formula taking into consideration years of service and earnings. Often the size of the benefit is entirely or largely based on earnings during the last few years of employment, and the benefit is sometimes adjusted or partially adjusted for inflation during the payout years. Typically, contributions to these DB plans are only made by the employer. In contrast, DC pension plans only specify the amount contributed (by the employee, employer, or both) to the employee's retirement account, not the size of the eventual pension to be paid. The eventual pension benefit is largely a function of the amount contributed and market trends over the years.

Over the past 25 years or so, the fraction of the private sector wage and salary labor force covered by an employer-based pension scheme has been relatively steady at just under 50%, but the shift from those based on the DB model to those based on the DC model has been dramatic (O'Rand et al., 2009). While coverage by DB schemes has not been declining among public sector workers, the story is quite different in the private sector. In 1980, among private sector workers who were covered by some sort of employer-sponsored pension plan, 60% were covered by DB plans alone, 17% by DC plans alone, and 23% by both. By 2006 only 8% were covered by DB plans alone, while 70% were covered by DC plans alone and 22% by both (Munnell et al., 2008). In the discussion that follows, the focus will be on DC schemes because the trend from DB to DC schemes in the private sector is the major arena in which the partial privatization of retirement security is currently taking place in the US.

The Emergence and Future of 401(k) Pensions

The most pervasive employer-sponsored DC pension schemes are the 401(k) plans, first introduced in 1981 (VanDerhei et al., 2008). Initially, these plans were viewed as savings plans or supplements to employer-sponsored DB plans (Munnell et al., 2009); that is, as part of the third leg of the proverbial three-legged stool needed to assure adequate retirement income, the other two being occupational pensions (often DB plans) and Social Security. However, the 401(k) plans have generally replaced those DB plans. Relative to DB plans, the 401(k) plans have a number of benefits for employers, but for employees the picture is more a mixture of pros and cons.

Pros and Cons of 401(k) Plans

One of the most important consequences of the shift from DB plans to 401(k) plans has been a dramatically reduced level of retirement income security for many workers because: (1) enrolment in 401(k) plans is voluntary and many workers (particularly young workers) elect not to participate (Munnell et al., 2009); (2) many workers "cash-out" when they move between employers; (3) many do not contribute enough to assure an adequate pension at retirement; (4) many do not sufficiently diversify their portfolio, or make unwise asset allocation choices or invest too heavily in their company's stock (Munnell et al., 2009); and (5) their holdings are vulnerable to sharp corrections in financial markets just prior to the time of planned retirement.

There are, however, some benefits of 401(k) plans for employees. In comparison with DB plans: (1) it is easier for the employee to keep track of the account balance in a DC scheme; (2) it is also easier to transfer the account balance when moving to a new employer; (3) 401(k) plans allow those employees who want to actively manage their pension assets to do so, although this turns out to be a mixed blessing because many of those who actively manage their accounts do a poor job of it (Munnell & Sundén, 2004); and (4) the pension assets are better protected than with many company DB schemes. The assets are administered by an independent third party, such as a mutual fund company, and as a result they are much less likely to be appropriated in connection with bankruptcy or a merger.

For employers, among the most important benefits of shifting to DC schemes are: (1) 401(k) plans reduce the cost of administering the pension system and the burdensome bureaucratic obligations associated with the 1974 Employee Retirement Income Security Act (ERISA) regulations and requirements (Schulz & Borowski, 2006), a particularly important consideration for small businesses; (2) the risks associated with pension fund financing are shifted from the employer to the employee (Hacker, 2006), including market risks as well as risks associated with increased longevity (of retired workers), corporate downsizing, and pension fund under-funding; and (3) unlike company DB plans, most 401(k) plans are largely employee-funded, with employers often contributing much less than they did to prior DB schemes.

The Problem of Major Market Corrections

Important lessons were learned from the two recent deep stock market corrections, the first between 2000 and 2002 and the second, even deeper, between late 2007 and early 2009. Both were associated with dramatic reductions in 401(k) retirement account assets, and it has become clear to many analysts that pension plans based on the 401(k) model are often less than adequate substitutes for traditional DB schemes with respect to the predictability and adequacy of the eventual pension. Market risk is only one of many reasons that the 401(k) model is not living up to expectations. In response to increasing evidence concerning the limitations of the 401(k) model, a number of proposals for reforms have been made.

The Implicit Assumption of Financial Literacy

The 401(k) model shifts much of the decision-making about asset allocation and how much to contribute from the employer to the employee. Although some workers like the idea of being in control of these decisions, the reality is that financial literacy among many workers is quite low (Schulz & Borowski, 2006). The financial information needed to make well-informed decisions can be hard to find even for those who are interested. More problematic is the evidence suggesting that many workers are unable or unwilling to take the time to acquire the level of financial literacy called for to protect against bad investment decisions. In an effort to deal with this lack of adequate information, a number of recent reforms in 401(k) plans have been proposed that are designed to help protect workers with low levels of financial literacy.

Recent 401(k) Reform Proposals

It is not mandatory that employees join a 401(k) provided by an employer. Research shows that whether they do and their investing approaches are both strongly influenced by the default action set up by the employer. Recent 401(k) reform proposals focus on these default options (items 1–4 following) and include:

(1) automatically enrolling employees in the plan (i.e. requiring employees to take specific opt-out action if they do not want to start a plan);

(2) making it the default option to invest contributions in a mix of highly diversified mutual funds (e.g. index stock and bond funds) pegged to the approximate year the employee is projected to retire, with adjustments in the mix of funds in the investment portfolio increasingly conservative as the worker gets older and closer to retirement (D'Antona, 2009);

(3) adding a default provision that automatically increases the employee's contribution rates over the years – starting at, for example, 3% and then gradually increasing to 6% or 9% – substantially increasing the size of the accounts at retirement (D'Antona, 2009);

(4) making it the default option to pay the 401(k) retirement benefit as a lifetime annuity rather than as a lump sum, with the aim of reducing the number of retirees who currently take the assets as a lump sum and use them up very quickly (Harris & Walker, 2009);

(5) requiring employees to roll over 401(k) assets rather than allowing them to cash out when changing jobs; and

(6) replacing the current tax deduction for contributions with a tax credit.

INTERNATIONAL DEVELOPMENTS IN RETIREMENT SECURITY POLICY

The most important international public pension policy trend in recent years is the shift toward less dependence on PAYG-DB schemes and greater dependence on multi-pillar schemes that include a funded defined contribution (FDC) pillar. Typically, the FDC pillar is funded by a mandatory tax paid by employees (sometimes supplemented by employer contributions). Each employee has an individual account that is invested by a private sector money management organization in financial markets. The value of the assets in these accounts is a function of the amount contributed, the fees charged to manage this money, and trends in financial markets. Because most schemes that include an FDC pillar also include a publicly financed PAYG-DB pillar, it is common to refer to such multi-pillar schemes as being partially privatized. Given this trend and the extent to which the issue has been debated in the US, it is of interest to discuss how well partial privatization is working in other countries.

The Trend Toward Partial Privatization

By the early 1980s, many nations around the world with maturing PAYG-DB pension schemes in place were running deficits. In 1981, Chile became the first of these nations to confront this problem by replacing its PAYG-DB scheme with a FDC scheme. By the 1990s, many nations around the world had begun to introduce reforms influenced by the Chilean model. Today, approximately thirty countries have at least partially privatized their public pension schemes by adding a mandatory FDC pillar managed by private sector organizations, subject to a variety of government regulations and controls (James, 2005).

Although many factors have contributed to the spread of reforms involving reductions in commitments to existing public PAYG-DB pillars in favor of privately managed FDC pillars, among the most important has been the influence of the World Bank and the International Monetary Fund (IMF). The World Bank has provided experts willing to help set up FDC pillars and has often offered economic incentives as well. The impact of the World Bank has been largely as a purveyor of reform policies based on the neo-liberal ideology that has been reshaping welfare-state-related social policies around the world (Madrid, 2005). Of particular note was an influential World Bank (1994) publication, *Averting the Old Age Crisis*. It called for a "three-pillar pension scheme" – with the first pillar being a modest publicly financed demogrant or means-tested benefit focusing on poverty reduction and redistribution, the second being a mandatory privately managed and fully funded FDC pillar designed to promote preretirement income replacement, and the third being a voluntary private individual savings pillar (World Bank, 1994).

In recent years, the original three-pillar World Bank model came under criticism from policy analysts both outside (Kay & Sinha, 2008) and inside the World Bank. This led to a revised five-pillar version of the model (Holzmann et al., 2008). The "zero pillar" is typically a noncontributory social pension (or social assistance plan) financed by the local or national government. Its focus is on provision of a minimum pension aimed at poverty alleviation among the elderly poor. The "first pillar" is a mandatory PAYG-DB government scheme financed largely by an earnings-related tax. Its focus is on preretirement income replacement. The "second pillar" is a mandatory individual savings account often taking the form of a FDC pillar financed by a tax on employees. The "third pillar" is made up of one or more voluntary individual savings plans. It can take many forms including individual retirement accounts (IRA)-type plans, employer-sponsored DB plans, and 401(k)-type plans. The "fourth pillar" is described as a non-financial pillar. It includes informal support and various government social programs, such as those providing health or housing benefits (Holzman et al., 2008).

In the discussion below the focus is on pension schemes in four countries, each of which has introduced an FDC pillar as an optional or a mandatory pillar. These cases have been selected to illustrate some of the issues and potential outcomes with which pension analysts are dealing.

Chile: A Very Influential Move from the PAYG-DB to the FDC Model

One reason that the Chilean FDC scheme has been so influential is that it was the first country to shift from a PAYG-DB model to the FDC model (Kritzer, 2008). Although more accurately described as a partially privatized, than a fully privatized, scheme, it is one of the most privatized pension programs in the world. In addition, it has been in place for almost 30 years, substantially longer than the FDC schemes introduced in other countries. Another reason the Chilean scheme has received much attention is that reports on it, particularly during the first 15 years or so, were very favorable and seemed to point to far higher "returns" for covered workers than seemed possible with comparable payroll taxes associated with existing PAYG-DB schemes in other countries (Williamson, 2005). During the 1990s it was common for proponents of partial privatization in the US to point to what was described as a very successful privatized pension scheme in Chile (Borden, 1995). For years, pension policy experts from around the world came to Chile to study its pension system, and many left as enthusiastic supporters of what they saw.

However, over time, some of the limitations of the model, as originally implemented, have emerged. This has led to a moderation of the enthusiasm for the model both within and outside of Chile (Gill et al., 2005; Holzmann & Stiglitz, 2001). Recent reforms in Chile have focused on improving the FDC pillar by increasing coverage and reducing administrative costs. At the same time there has been more government involvement, increasing attention to poverty reduction and reducing exposure to market risk (Bertranou et al., 2009).

The Chilean scheme seems to have worked quite well for affluent workers, particularly men with many years of full-time covered employment. It also seems to have contributed to the development of the financial sector in Chile and to the strength of the economy more generally. However, it has also become evident that the scheme has not been working as well for low-wage workers, women, rural workers, and those in the informal sector (those who work off-the-books, domestics, day labor, and the like) (Kritzer, 2008; Williamson, 2005). In addition, due to the structure of the Chilean economy, with many workers in temporary jobs and frequent periods of unemployment between covered jobs, the requirement that workers contribute for at least 20 years has excluded many workers from a very important benefit, the government-subsidized minimum pension. A major reason is that the requirement is actually for 240 months, which adds up to 20 years only for those who are employed for every month for 20 years, but can stretch to 40 years or more for workers with frequent periods of unemployment (Williamson, 2005).

In recent years, a number of major reforms have been made in the original "privatized" Chilean pension scheme, representing an effort to better provide for those falling through the cracks in the scheme as structured in the early 2000s (Kritzer, 2008). It had been possible to retire early and many did so, but often the result was that workers ended up with very low pensions. Changes made in 2007 limit early retirement to those with much larger retirement accounts, thus ensuring that they have more adequate pension benefits. A number of major reforms were also introduced in 2008 (Barr & Diamond, 2008). The prior minimum pension guarantee was merged with the prior social assistance program to create a new program with two types of pension benefits. One is a noncontributory pension benefit that will be paid to the poorest 60% of the elderly population. The other is a new pension top-up for workers who meet the standard pension eligibility criteria but have low levels of assets in their FDC accounts. As of 2009, mandatory insurance premiums for disability and survivorship that had been paid by employees are now paid for by employers. In addition, over the next seven years a new requirement that the self-employed participate is being phased in. This set of reforms is expected to substantially increase coverage and the adequacy of benefits for women, low-wage workers, rural workers, and those working in the informal sector of the economy more generally (Bertranou et al., 2009).

Argentina: A Less Successful Latin American Experiment with Partial Privatization

During the 1970s and 1980s the Argentine PAYG-DB public pension system expanded rapidly. By the end of the 1980s it was running huge deficits, leading to lawsuits over unpaid benefits and to a major restructuring in 1993 (Arza, 2008). The pension system, which was much influenced by the Chilean scheme, includes a mandatory PAYG-DB first pillar financed by employers. The mandatory second pillar was financed by employees themselves and offered two options: either (1) a second government-administered PAYG-DB plan or (2) a privately managed FDC plan (Baker & Weisbrot, 2002).

The introduction of the FDC option was motivated by several goals, such as shifting risk from the government to workers, augmenting returns on tax contributions, and reinforcing ownership rights by reducing the political risk that the government would cut previously promised benefits. Unfortunately, the diversion of tax contributions, previously available to pay pensions to current retirees, into the new FDC accounts reduced government revenues far more than anticipated, making it impossible to pay the full pensions to current retirees. According to some analysts, the introduction of these new FDC accounts significantly contributed to Argentina's financial meltdown in 2001 (Arza, 2008). The FDC accounts were US dollar-denominated and at the time the peso was pegged to the US dollar. In an effort to deal with its fiscal crisis the government required that these accounts be shifted from US dollars to pesos. These assets soon lost 60–70% of their value when the peso was allowed to float (Bertranou et al., 2003). In addition, the government was forced to cut benefits from the DB component of the public pension system by 13%, a cut that according to some analysts was more drastic than would have been necessary absent the introduction of the FDC account option (Baker & Weisbrot, 2002).

One of the goals of the FDC accounts was to protect pension tax contributions from the political risks of benefit cuts during periods of fiscal crisis, a goal that clearly was not realized in connection with the 2001 crisis. Yet another example of failure in connection with this goal was the reform in 2008, which required many workers who had previously opted for the FDC second pillar to shift to the government-administered DB option for the second pillar. The assets in their individual accounts were nationalized. At retirement, workers who had been contributing to these FDC accounts are to be given "credit" for the years contributing to the now defunct FDC second pillar (Social Security Administration, 2008b). It is not clear that they will ever be fully compensated for the appropriation of the funds in these accounts (Rofman et al., 2008). Given the Argentine experience, there is reason to question the argument by many FDC advocates that such accounts will be safe from government appropriation because they will be viewed as private property (Kay, 2009).

China: Funded Accounts for Both Urban and Rural Areas?

Old-age pensions for the general (urban) population were introduced in 1951, very soon after the founding of the People's Republic of China in 1949. The original pensions for the PAYG-DB schemes covered only the urban population working in state-owned enterprises and urban collectives. By the 1980s it had become clear that with the move toward a market economy the traditional PAYG-DB pension schemes, which were administered and financed by the large state-owned enterprises, were not going to be sustainable. During the 1990s, China began to experiment with schemes that included both a PAYG-DB pillar and an individual FDC pillar (Williamson & Deitelbaum, 2005). The current scheme for the urban population is based primarily on two pillars. The first is a PAYG-DB pillar financed by a 20% payroll tax on employers. The second is an FDC pillar financed by an 8% payroll tax on employees (OECD, 2009).

There is some good news and some bad news with respect to how well the current urban system is working. The good news is that the income replacement rates are high for China across a range of income levels, with a 68% replacement rate for those with average earnings; this compares favorably with an average of 58% for the OECD nations (OECD, 2009). The bad news is that, in about 75% of China's 31 provinces, for most workers the 8% payroll contribution designated to fund their individual accounts is being diverted to pay pensions to those who are currently retired. A record is being kept of those tax contributions with a promise to repay workers (with interest) at some later point in time (Williamson et al., 2009). For this reason the FDC component of the current Chinese urban scheme is arguably a variant of the NDC model, to be discussed below.

Prior to 2009, no more than 10% of rural old people were receiving pensions from any sort of scheme, but, in 2009, China started to implement a new voluntary contributory pension scheme for rural residents that includes contributions from workers and from the government (Shen & Williamson, 2010). The government's goal is to offer the program in 10% of the counties in each province by the end of 2009, increasing to 100% of counties by 2020. The number of workers actually participating will be lower in poor areas and higher in more affluent areas, such as the suburbs of Beijing, where it is already about 80% (Shen & Williamson, 2010). The program, called New Rural Social Pension Insurance, began as an experimental program in 2007 and 2008 in selected areas (HelpAge International, 2008). There are two components of the pension. One is the basic pension; it is based on contributions from both the national and local (provincial and county) governments. In poor counties, benefits from this pension are set at a level close to the poverty level. In more affluent counties, there is a greater contribution from the local government and the benefits can be much higher. The second is a funded component based on the amount the worker contributes over the years. For those who elect to participate, there is a minimum contribution that varies from one county to another and tends to range between 4% and 8% of the average wage; but, if workers contribute more, they are promised higher pension benefits when they become age-eligible (60 for men, 55 for women) and have contributed for at least 15 years.

This new pension plan is a great improvement for those living in rural areas, but it is unlikely to meet the needs of the poorest of the poor because participation is voluntary and many of them will not be able to afford to pay the necessary premiums (HelpAge International, 2008). There is also the issue of how well the money in the FDC accounts will be managed by the county-level officials responsible for overseeing the funds generated from the contributions made by participating workers.

UK: An Industrial Nation Shifting Toward Greater Emphasis on the FDC Model

In 1975, legislation was enacted that created a second-tier earnings-related plan in the UK called the State Earnings Related Pension System (SERPS), but also allowed employers to opt out of that scheme in favor of their own occupational schemes (Williamson, 2002). In 2002, SERPS was replaced by the State Second Pensions (S2P) plan. The new scheme made some changes that favored low-wage workers.

More relevant to the debate over the proposed partial privatization of Social Security in the US was the legislation enacted by Thatcher's government in 1986, creating incentives for workers to opt out of SERPS (or out of their employer-sponsored occupation pension plans) in favor of individually directed DC schemes called "approved personal pensions" (hereafter, personal pensions) with freedom to choose from among many privately managed plans (Schulz & Borowski, 2006). These pensions were in many ways similar to IRAs in the US. While popular at first, within a few years public support for the personal pensions started to weaken. One reason was that workers became more aware of the high fees when buying into or transferring between providers. The high annual management charges were also a concern. The net effect of these fees was poor returns for many workers, particularly those with smaller accounts (Waine, 2009). Another problem was the loss of confidence in the scheme due to the misleading financial advice given to potential clients by sales staff working for some of the organizations managing the personal pension plans (Blake, 2000).

An effort was made by the Blair government to respond to some of these problems with the introduction in 2001 of a new scheme call stakeholder pensions. These pensions worked in much the same way as the personal pensions, but they were designed to better serve lower-income employees (Schulz & Borowski, 2006). Employers that did not offer their own occupational pensions were required to offer stakeholder pensions to their workers. The stakeholder pensions were in many ways an improvement over the personal pensions. For example, they reduced the fees that made the personal pensions particularly bad investments for those with small personal accounts and they eliminated the fees associated with moving from one provider to another (House of Commons Treasury Committee, 2006; Walker & Foster, 2006). But the changes made were not enough to solve the problem of "undersaving" as relatively few workers signed up for the new stakeholder pensions (Waine, 2009).

In 2002, a government-appointed Pensions Commission was charged with making a thorough review of the British pension system. It concluded that it was not working well (Pensions Commission, 2005). It was described as the most complex pension system in the world, as contributing to increasing inequality, as failing to provide adequate incentives to save, and as having very high administrative costs (Schulz & Binstock, 2008).

More recently, based largely on recommendations from the Pensions Commission, the Pensions Act of 2008 introduced yet another program designed to deal with what the government calls the problem of undersaving on the part of British workers (Waine, 2009). This legislation mandates that, as of 2012, every new employee over age 22 and earning over a specified income threshold must be automatically enrolled in either the employer's occupational pension plan or in a new plan called "personal accounts" (DWP, 2009). This new scheme will by 2016 require a contribution of 8% per year split among the employee (4%), the employer (3%), and the government (1%). Employees will still have the ability to opt-out of either of these alternatives, but through a series of incentives the government is attempting to make the personal accounts plans affordable and appealing so that many employees will continue participating (Curry, 2008).

The new personal accounts scheme does have potential problems, some of which it shares with the prior stakeholder pensions and personal pensions. It still puts workers at risk of potentially large declines in fund assets due to adverse swings in the stock market during the period just prior to planned retirement. It also puts the worker at annuity risk due to the substantial differences in the value of the annuity depending on interest rate fluctuations just prior to retirement. In addition, the model still assumes much more by way of financial literacy than most workers have or are willing to acquire. Some British analysts argue that the long-term real returns for low-wage workers contributing to personal account schemes may be positive, but are more likely to be negative. Others emphasize that low returns are particularly likely for women (Price, 2007; Waine, 2009). These problems and the tendency to foster increased economic inequality are all problems that are common to the FDC component of partial privatization schemes in the UK and in the other countries that we have considered as well.

Are there Viable Alternatives to Partial Privatization?

When partial privatization has been introduced in transition nations such as China, the diversion of payroll tax contributions into funded accounts can put a major strain on the capacity of a nation to finance pensions for those currently retired. This fiscal stress can, as in the case of Argentina, contribute to a financial meltdown of the national economy. In some developing economies such as Chile and Argentina, partial privatization has been associated with a decrease in pension coverage and an incentive to shift to jobs in the grey economy. But not all of the consequences of partial privatization are bad. There is evidence from Chile and several other countries that partial privatization does promote the development of capital markets, which in the long run is likely to foster economic development (Williamson, 2005). It has also proven useful as a way to reduce government pension spending, which in an era of population aging is a high government priority in many nations.

Around the world, PAYG-DB pension systems are being reformed and partial privatization is the new model getting the most attention. However, there are two others that have also been attracting attention in recent years, the NDC plans and social pensions. Both can be viewed as alternatives to partial privatization.

The Notional Defined Contribution (NDC) Model

The NDC model combines elements of the PAYG-DB model with elements of the FDC model. It incorporates DC provisions into PAYG pension schemes designed to assure a tighter actuarial link between payroll tax contributions made and benefits paid than is the case with most PAYG-DB schemes. It does this in part by creating notional (unfunded) individual accounts that are "annunitized" at retirement. NDC schemes are typically one pillar in a multi-pillar scheme. Between 1995 and 2002, NDC schemes were introduced in Italy, Latvia, Sweden, Poland, Russia, the Kyrgyz Republic, and Mongolia (Holzmann & Palmer, 2006; Williamson, 2004; Williamson et al., 2006). In addition, both Brazil and China have added quasi-NDC pillars (Lindeman et al., 2006).

Pension policymakers generally turn to the NDC model when confronted with serious budgetary pressure linked to unsustainable PAYG-DB pension schemes (Holzman & Palmer, 2006). This is the same context in which many nations have turned to the FDC model. The NDC model can look particularly attractive when a nation cannot afford the startup costs associated with the transition from a mature and relatively generous PAYG-DB scheme to an FDC scheme. That transition often calls for the diversion of at least a portion of current payroll tax contributions into funded individual accounts; but, if payment of current pensions under the existing scheme is a major fiscal burden, a new scheme calling for the diversion of a portion of current revenues into individual accounts can be very problematic. The NDC model, however, being unfunded, does not require the diversion of payroll tax revenues to get started as all tax contributions continue to be used to pay benefits to current pensioners.

Each of the existing NDC schemes has its unique provisions, but the following are characteristics that all or most of them share. First, each worker has an individual notional (unfunded) account that records notional credit based on the payroll tax contributions made by the worker and any matching contributions made by the employer. Second, the tax contributions made are not used to purchase financial securities and for this reason the notional assets are not vulnerable to a dramatic decrease in value due to a sharp drop in financial markets during the period just prior to retirement. Third, the notional assets (credit) in the account are indexed each year based on changes in wage levels, price levels, the "wage-sum," or the gross domestic product (GDP). The wage-sum is based on the number of workers contributing (and thus changes in the size of the workforce) and the average wage level. Fourth, with an NDC scheme, the link between payroll tax contributions and the eventual pension paid is more transparent and actuarially fair in the eyes of many workers than is the case with typical PAYG-DB schemes. Fifth, NDC schemes have a specified minimum number of years of contributing and a minimum age for eligibility (which may vary by gender). Sixth, there is an annuity formula, which varies in details from one country to another, for converting the notional credit into a pension at retirement. Typically, this formula factors in the unisex life expectancy for the person's age cohort at the time of retirement. Seventh, many NDC schemes have automatic stabilizer provisions that help bring the schemes into fiscal balance when pension costs start to exceed revenues. For example, such provisions may call for lower pensions or a reduction in the annual amount credited to the accounts. Eighth, some countries give notional credit for time covered by a prior PAYG-DB scheme; others credit periods when the person is not contributing to the scheme for certain designated reasons such as time spent at home caring for a young child (Williamson, 2004).

How well do the NDC schemes seem to be working out? In many countries they have been in place for 10 years or less, so any conclusions must be viewed as tentative. The cases of Sweden and Italy illustrate that outcomes for different industrial nations vary. In general, reports from Sweden are positive (Palmer, 2007; Sundén, 2009). Sweden has a multi-pillar scheme and there have not been problems with the NDC pillar, but the FDC pillar has not lived up to expectations. In Italy the new NDC pillar has been problematic (OECD, 2009). There have been problems linked to overly generous formulas used to calculate pension entitlements and problems due to the slow rate of transition from the prior PAYG-DB scheme to the new NDC-based scheme.

The NDC model has also been used in a number of transitional economies including Latvia, Russia, Poland, the Kyrgyz Republic, and Mongolia. Latvia implemented its scheme in 1996 and during the early years there were a lot of problems, particularly with how to deal with those who were retired or near retirement under the prior, very-generous, PAYG-DB schemes inherited from the Soviet era. The government felt obligated to make ad hoc adjustments to deal with the high poverty levels among those already retired or trying to retire in connection with the new scheme. The pension records were poor, and the new nation did not have an administrative structure in place that was fully up to the task of managing the scheme (Fultz, 2006; Vanovska, 2006).

The Latvian model adjusts notional assets based on the wage-sum, and this provision turned out to introduce much more volatility than had been anticipated. In 2009, Latvia made several adjustments, including substantial cuts in benefits to current pensioners, designed to balance payroll tax revenues and pension expenditures. Of particular note is a recent decision to substantially increase the size of tax contributions to the NDC pillar while at the same time reducing tax contributions to the FDC pillar, reflecting a preference for the NDC pillar during periods of fiscal stress (Social Security Administration, 2009).

The NDC model has some potential benefits relative to the PAYG-DB alternative and other benefits relative to the FDC alternative, but like any pension model it has its own limitations as well. Among the most frequently mentioned limitations are the following. First, it requires the capacity to keep accurate long-term records of tax contributions and the annual adjustments added to those contributions. This will not be a problem in industrial nations, but could be a problem in some transitional nations and very likely will be a problem in many poor nations. The administrative structure requirements make it inappropriate for poor nations or for the large poor rural populations in some middle-income nations such as Brazil. Brazil has a pension system for its urban population that draws on some NDC principles, but no effort is currently being made to extend the NDC model to its poor rural population to supplement or replace the current rural social pension. Second, without some sort of social assistance, minimum pension, or social pension pillar, there will be problems of pension adequacy for low-wage workers. An NDC pillar is generally not redistributive and has no way to provide pension benefits for workers who spend much of their lives working in the informal sector of the economy. Third, being wage-based and not being redistributive, the NDC model is not going to work as well for women as for men. This is in part due to patterns of lower wages, lower rates of attachments to the formal sector of the economy, and more irregular work histories among women. However, there are some countries, such as Sweden, in which notional credit is given, up to specified limits, for time spent out of the labor force taking care of young children. This benefit helps to reduce, but does not eliminate, the gender gap. Fourth, while the notional assets in an NDC scheme are protected from the fluctuations in financial markets that FDC schemes are vulnerable to, the NDC schemes do need indexing and the various forms of indexing that are used (wage changes, price changes, wage-sum changes, and GDP changes) are also potential sources of risk.

Do Social Pensions Make Sense for Rural Areas of Developing Nations?

Social pension schemes (also referred to as social assistance) are noncontributory universal or means-tested pensions that focus on poverty alleviation. Such a scheme may serve as the only public pension, as in Namibia, or as a supplementary pillar, often a safety net for those not covered by contributory schemes, as with the schemes for the rural population in Brazil (Palacios & Sluchynsky, 2006). A recent World Bank report calls for the inclusion of a "zero pillar" (social pension) funded from general government revenues (Holzmann & Hinz, 2005; Willmore, 2007). This pillar may be particularly useful in rural areas of developing countries, venues that often lack the administrative infrastructures needed to support contributory pension schemes (Palacios & Sluchynsky, 2006). Social pensions are sometimes combined with PAYG-DB schemes, FDC schemes, or NDC schemes, but they are typically designed to cover workers, often rural workers, not covered by contributory pension schemes (Johnson & Williamson, 2006).

Any assessment of the appropriateness of the social pension model for a particular country calls for consideration of the relative economic position of the older population; the more impoverished the older population is relative to other age groups, the stronger the case for such schemes. However, if the differences are not large, some analysts will argue there may be better ways for the government to spend that money to meet the needs of the poor (Palacios &

Sluchynsky, 2006). Some point to potential adverse consequences of social pensions, such as reduced familial assistance to the elderly and the substantial fiscal cost (Palacios & Sluchynsky, 2006). However, many countries that have adopted these schemes experience not only reductions in poverty among the elderly, but also other indirect benefits, such as increased investment in children's education and increased local investment (Johnson & Williamson, 2006; Lloyd-Sherlock, 2006).

Namibia has a universal social pension as its primary old-age security scheme for both the rural and the urban population. There is no mandated contributory pension scheme. The social pension is financed by the central government from general revenues. It is a very low flat-rate pension, and participation is high (Stewart & Yermo, 2009). To qualify for this pension a resident must be 60 years old and a citizen; there is no means-testing involved. The impact of the pension benefit often extends beyond the recipients themselves because pensioners spend on average only 28% of the benefit on their own expenses, with the rest going to meet other family needs (Palacios & Sluchynsky, 2006).

During the early years there were serious problems with fraud (e.g. efforts to collect benefits on behalf of those who were long dead) and armed robbery of those responsible for disbursing the payments. These have been largely overcome, through outsourcing administration to private contractors who since 1996 have used armored cars, armed guards, and a sophisticated pensioner identification system based on fingerprint checks and electronic ID cards. All this has substantially increased administrative costs (Willmore, 2007). Although the benefits of the program are far reaching, there is some concern about the long-term future of the scheme as the population of Namibia ages. The proportion of people who are aged 60 and over in Namibia is projected to increase from 6% to 21% within a few decades. This has led to discussions about the need to add a mandatory contributory pension pillar to the current social pension scheme in the not-too-distant future (Stewart & Yermo, 2009).

In 1988, Brazil introduced a social pension called the Previdência Rural to reduce rural poverty (Barrientos, 2002). To become eligible for this pension, one must be at least 60 years old, be a rural resident, and have proof of being a rural worker. The Previdência Rural substitutes years of rural work for the years of contribution associated with the urban contributory scheme. There is also a 2.2% contribution to the program made by the purchaser of rurally produced goods, but these tax revenues alone are insufficient to entirely fund the program. The gap is filled by the diversion of a portion of the revenues from the urban contributory scheme (Schwarzer &

Querino, 2002). For 80–90% of rural pensioners, their social pension benefits are set at a level close to the minimum wage and this typically provides at least half of the household income. The benefits of this rural pension extend beyond poverty alleviation as it also fosters agricultural development, trade union financing, and support for the local economy (Schwarzer & Querino, 2002). However, for a variety of reasons, this program does not reach the entire rural poor older population. Many of the poorest of the poor in both rural and urban areas are covered by a separate means-tested social assistance program. This program requires that per capita household income not exceed a quarter of the minimum wage and that the beneficiary be at least 65 years old. It also requires that no other social insurance program benefits are received and re-certification of eligibility every two years (Barrientos, 2002; SSA & ISSA, 2008).

CONCLUSION: THE FUTURE OF RETIREMENT SECURITY

In the US much of the debate over the future of retirement security has in recent years focused on proposals to divert a portion of the Social Security payroll tax into funded individual accounts. This effort has been part of a more general push for welfare state retrenchment and, most recently, federal budget deficit reduction. Although it is unlikely that we will soon see the introduction of mandatory individual accounts, it is likely that we will see a number of parametric reforms enacted, some of which will have important distributional consequences. There will be both winners and losers.

While the debate over the partial privatization of Social Security via the introduction of FDC accounts is currently off the table in the US, this is not true with respect to the partial privatization of retirement security. The dramatic shift from employer-sponsored DB schemes to 401(k) and similar FDC schemes represents an increase in dependence on the FDC model for retirement security that has not been given the attention that it deserves. The question is not whether the US should consider the partial privatization of retirement security based on the FDC model, as this has already taken place. The discussion now is how to reform the 401(k) model to better protect the millions of American workers who will have an increasing share of their retirement assets invested in and retirement security linked to these accounts.

To date, relatively few nations have extensive experience with the partial privatization of social security

based on the inclusion of FDC pillars as part of multi-pillar schemes. The evidence from the 30 or so countries that have introduced such schemes is mixed, as is illustrated by the experience of the countries considered here. Many of these countries, including Chile, are making changes designed to remedy some of the problems that have emerged in connection with the original versions of their FDC schemes. In the years ahead, these reformed schemes may turn out to work well, and the models could end up having a significant impact on future debates over Social Security reform in the US. It is also possible that, in the vast majority of countries, privatization will turn out to work well only for the most affluent workers, an outcome that may also influence future debates in the US.

Is the international experience with the NDC model likely to influence future debates over Social Security reform in the US? Reforms need to be made and an NDC pillar could be used to help realize some of the goals reformers will be considering. It would offer a way to help balance revenues and pension costs. It would also add a way to share the burden of balancing pension revenues and expenditures between retirees and workers. It would strengthen the link between tax contributions and eventual pension benefits without making workers vulnerable to swings in financial markets. It would also help avoid several other sources of risk that would increase were we to add an FDC pillar (Hacker, 2006). The experience of Sweden suggests that the NDC model can work well in an advanced industrial country. But the NDC model would represent a radical structural change in Social Security, a scheme that can be brought into balance financially by a combination of far less radical changes, referred to as parametric reforms. An NDC pillar could be used and would be useful if introduced, but it is not needed and probably would not be politically popular in the US at this point in time. NDCs make more sense for nations with PAYG-DB pension schemes that are much more seriously out of balance.

ACKNOWLEDGMENTS

The author thanks the following for their comments on preliminary drafts and other forms of help in connection with the preparation of this chapter: Robert Binstock, Yung-Ping (Bing) Chen, Andrew Eschtruth, Elaine Fultz, Karen Glenn, Shari Grove, Elizabeth Johnson, Anna Rhodes, Sara Rix, Steven Sass, James Schulz, Ce Shen, and Barbara Waine.

REFERENCES

Arza, C. (2008). The limits of pension privatization: Lessons from Argentine experience. *World Development*, 35(12), 2696–2712.

Baker, D., & Weisbrot, M. (2002). *The role of social security privatization in Argentina's economic crisis*. Washington, DC: Center for Economic and Policy Research. Retrieved August 27, 2009 from http://www.cepr.net/documents/publications/argentina_2002_04.pdf

Barr, N., & Diamond, P. (2008). *Reforming pensions: Principles and policy choices*. New York: Oxford University Press.

Barrientos, A. (2002). *Comparing pension schemes in Chile, Singapore, Brazil and South Africa*. (Discussion Paper No. 67). Manchester, UK: Institute for Development Policy and Management, University of Manchester.

Béland, D. (2005). *Social Security: History and politics from the new deal to the privatization debate*. Lawrence, KS: University of Kansas Press.

Bertranou, F. M., Rofman, R., & Grushka, C. O. (2003). From reform to crisis: Argentina's pension system. *International Social Security Review, 56*(2), 103–114.

Bertranou, F., Calvo, E., & Bertranou, E. (2009). Is Latin America retreating from individual retirement accounts? (Issue Brief No. 9-14). Chestnut Hill, MA: Center for Retirement Research at Boston College.

Blake, D. (2000). Two decades of pension reform in the UK: What are the implications for occupational pension schemes? *Employee Relations, 22*(3), 222–245.

Board of Trustees. (2009). *Annual report of the Board of Trustees of the Federal Old-Age and Survivors Insurance and Federal Disability Insurance Trust Funds*. Washington, DC: Social Security Administration.

Borden, K. J. (1995). *Dismantling the pyramid: The how & why of privatizing Social Security*. (Social Security Choice Paper No. 1). Washington, DC: Cato Institute.

Curry, C. (2008). The introduction of auto-enrolment and personal accounts to the UK in 2012. *Pensions, 13*(4), 237–245.

D'Antona, J., Jr. (2009). A future full of change. *Pensions & Investments, 37*(3), 12–16.

Diamond, P. A., & Orszag, P. R. (2004). *Saving Social Security: A balanced approach*. Washington, DC: Brookings Institution Press.

DWP. (2009). *Pensions reform*. London: Department for Work and Pensions. Retrieved July 16, 2009 from http://www.dwp.gov.uk/pensionsreform/

EPI. (2004). Social Security and income. *Economic Snapshot* (November 18). Washington, DC: Economic Policy Institute.

Favreault, M., & Michelmore, K. (2009). *How could we revitalize Social Security?* Washington, DC: Urban Institute. Retrieved June 15, 2009 from http://www.urban.org/retirement_policy/reform.cfm

Ferrara, P. J. (Ed.), (1985). *Social Security: Prospects of real reform*. Washington, DC: Cato Institute.

Ferrara, P. J., & Tanner, M. (1998). *A new deal for Social Security*. Washington, DC: Cato Institute.

Fultz, E. (2006). Discussion of NDC pension schemes in middle- and low-income countries. In R. Holzmann & E. Palmer (Eds.), *Pension reform: Issues and prospects for non-financial defined contribution (NDC) schemes* (pp. 323–324). Washington, DC: The World Bank.

Gill, I. S., Packard, T., & Yermo, J. (2005). *Keeping the promise of Social Security in Latin America*. Washington, DC: The World Bank.

Hacker, J. (2006). *The great risk shift: The assault on American jobs, families, health care, and retirement and how you can fight back*. New York: Oxford University Press.

Hardy, M., & Hazelrigg, L. (2007). *Pension puzzles: Social Security and the great debate*. New York: Russell Sage Foundation.

Harrington Meyer, M., & Herd, P. (2007). *Market friendly or family friendly? The State and gender inequality in old age*. New York: Russell Sage Foundation.

Harris, B. H., & Walker, L. (2009). Beyond the storm: New reforms for 401(k) plans. *Tax Notes, 123*, 1131–1136.

HelpAge International (2008). *The new rural social pension insurance programme of Baoji City*. Retrieved July 22, 2009 from http://www.helpage.org/Resources/Briefings#MWN5

Holzmann, R., & Hinz, R. (2005). *Old-age income support in the 21st century: An international perspective on pension systems and reform*. Washington, DC: The World Bank.

Holzmann, R., & Palmer, E. (2006). The status of the NDC discussion: Introduction and overview. In R. Holzmann & E. Palmer (Eds.), *Pension Reform: Issues for non-financial defined contribution (NDC) schemes* (pp. 1–15). Washington, DC: The World Bank.

Holzmann, R., & Stiglitz, J. E. (Eds.), (2001). *New ideas about old age security: Toward sustainable pension systems in the 21st century*. Washington, DC: The World Bank.

Holzmann, R., Hinz, R. P., & Dorfman, M. (2008). *Pension systems and reform conceptual framework*. (SP Discussion Paper No. 0824). Washington, DC: The World Bank.

House of Commons Treasury Committee. (2006). *The design of the national pensions savings scheme and the role of financial services regulation* (Fifth Special Report of Session 2005-06, HC 1068-1). London: The Stationery Office.

James, E. (2005). *Reforming social security: Lessons from thirty countries*. (NCPA Policy Report No. 277). Dallas, TX: National Center for Policy Analysis.

Johnson, J. K. M., & Williamson, J. B. (2006). Do universal non-contributory old-age pensions make sense for rural areas in low-income countries? *International Social Security Review, 59*(4), 47–65.

Kay, S. J. (2009). Political risk and pension privatization: The case of Argentina (1994–2008). *International Social Security Review, 62*(3), 1–21.

Kay, S. J., & Sinha, T. (Eds.), (2008). *Lessons from pension reform in the Americas.* New York: Oxford University Press.

Kingson, E. R., & Williamson, J. B. (1999). Why privatizing Social Security is a bad idea. In J. B. Williamson, D. M. Watts-Roy & E. R. Kingson (Eds.), *The generational equity debate* (pp. 204–219). New York: Columbia University Press.

Kingson, E. R., & Williamson, J. B. (2001). Economic security policies. In R. H. Binstock & L. K. George (Eds.), *Handbook of aging and the social sciences* (pp. 369–386) (5th ed.). San Diego: Academic Press.

Kritzer, B. E. (2008). Chile's next generation pension reform. *Social Security Bulletin, 68*(2), 69–84.

Lindeman, D., Rablino, D., & Rutkowski, M. (2006). Pension schemes in middle- and low-income countries. In R. Holzman & E. Palmer (Eds.), *Pension reform: Issues and prospects for non-financial defined contribution (NDC) schemes* (pp. 293–320). Washington, DC: The World Bank.

Lloyd-Sherlock, P. (2006). Simple transfers, complex outcomes: The impacts of pensions on poor households in Brazil. *Development and Change, 37*(5), 969–995.

Madrid, R. L. (2005). Ideas, economic pressures, and pension privatization. *Latin American Politics and Society, 47*(2), 23–50.

Munnell, A. H., Aubry, J.-P., & Muldoon, D. (2008). *The financial crisis and private defined benefit plans* (Issue Brief No. 8-18). Chestnut Hill, MA: Center for Retirement Research at Boston College.

Munnell, A. H., Golub-Sass, F., & Muldoon, D. (2009). *An update on 401(k) plans: Insights from the 2007 SCF.* (Issue Brief No. 95). Chestnut Hill, MA: Center for Retirement Research at Boston College.

Munnell, A. H., & Sundén, A. (2004). *Coming up short: The challenge of 401(k) plans.* Washington, DC: Brookings Institution Press.

OECD. (2009). *Italy: Highlights from OECD pensions at a glance 2009.* Washington, DC: Organization of Economic Co-operation and Development.

O'Rand, A. M., Ebel, D., & Isaccs, K. (2009). Private pensions in international perspective. In P. Uhlenberg (Ed.), *International handbook of population aging* (pp. 429–443). New York: Springer.

Palacios, R., & Sluchynsky, O. (2006). *Social pensions part I: Their role in the overall pension system.* (Discussion Paper No. 0601). Washington, DC: Social Protection, The World Bank.

Palmer, E. (2007). *Sweden's move to defined contribution pensions.* (Issue Paper No. 2007-16). Washington, DC: AARP.

Pensions Commission (2005). *A new pension settlement for the twenty-first century: Second report of the Pensions Commission.* London: The Stationery Office.

Peterson, P. J. (1999). How will America pay for the retirement of the baby boom generation? In J. B. Williamson, D. M. Watts-Roy & E. R. Kingson (Eds.), *The generational equity debate* (pp. 41–59). New York: Columbia University Press.

President's Commission to Strengthen Social Security. (2001). *Strengthening Social Security and creating personal wealth for all Americans: Final report of the President's Commission.* Washington, DC: President's Commission to Strengthen Social Security.

Price, D. (2007). Closing the gender gap in retirement income: What difference will recent UK pensions reforms make? *Journal of Social Policy, 34*(3), 561–584.

Reno, V. P., & Friedland, R. B. (1997). Strong support but low confidence: What explains the contradiction? In E. R. Kingson & J. H. Schulz (Eds.), *Social Security in the 21st Century* (pp. 178–194). New York: Oxford University Press.

Rofman, R., Fajnzylber, E., & Herrera, G. (2008). *Reforming the pension reforms: The recent initiatives and actions on pensions in Argentina and Chile.* (SP Discussion Paper No. 0831). Washington, DC: Social Protection & Labor, The World Bank.

Sass, S., Munnell, A. H., & Eschtruth, A. (2009). *The Social Security fix-it book* (Rev. ed). Chestnut Hill, MA: Center for Retirement Research at Boston College.

Schulz, J. H. (2001). *The economics of aging* (7th ed.). Westport, CT: Auburn House.

Schulz, J. H., & Binstock, R. H. (2008). *Aging nation: The economics and politics of growing older in America.* Baltimore, MD: Johns Hopkins University Press.

Schulz, J. H., & Borowski, A. (2006). Economic security in retirement: Reshaping the public-private pension mix. In R. H. Binstock & L. K. George (Eds.), *Handbook of aging and the social sciences* (pp. 360–379) (6th ed.). San Diego: Academic Press.

Schwarzer, H., & Querino, A. C. (2002). *Non-contributory pensions in Brazil: The impact on poverty reduction.* (ESS Working Paper No. 11). Geneva: Social Security Policy and Development Branch, International Labour Office.

Shelton, A. (2008). *Reform options for Social Security.* Washington, DC: Public Policy Institute, AARP. Retrieved August 27, 2009 from http://www.aarp.org/ppi

Shen, C., & Williamson, J. B. (2010, in press). China's new rural pension scheme: Can it be improved? *International Journal of Sociology and Social Policy, 30.*

Social Security Administration (2008a). *Provisions that could change the Social Security program.* Washington, DC: Office of the Chief Actuary. Retrieved June 15, 2009 from http://www.ssa.gov/OACT/solvency/provisions/index.html

Social Security Administration. (2008b). *Argentina. International Update*, December, pp. 1–2. Retrieved October 14, 2009 from http://www.socialsecurity.gov/policy/docs/progdesc/intl_update/2008-12/index.html

Social Security Administration. (2009). *Latvia. International Update*, May, p. 1. Retrieved August 25, 2009 from http://www.socialsecurity.gov/policy/docs/progdesc/intl_update/2009-05/index.html

SSA & ISSA (2008). *Social security programs throughout the world: The Americas.* Geneva: Social Security Administration & International Social Security Association.

Stewart, F., & Yermo, J. (2009). *Pensions in Africa.* (Working Paper No. 30). Paris, France: Organisation for Economic Co-Operation and Development.

Sundén, A. (2009). *The Swedish pension system and the economic crisis.* (Issue Brief No. 9-25). Chestnut Hill, MA: Center for Retirement Research at Boston College.

US Department of the Treasury. (2008). *Social Security reform: Strategies for progressive benefit adjustments.* (Issue Brief No. 5). Washington, DC: US Department of the Treasury.

VanDerhei, J., Holden, S., Alonso, L., & Copeland, C. (2008). *401(k) plan asset allocation, account balances, and loan activity in 2007.* (Issue Brief No. 324). Washington, DC: Employee Benefit Research Institute.

Vanovska, I. (2006). Pension reform in Latvia. In E. Fultz (Ed.), *Pension reform in the Baltic States* (pp. 143–265). Budapest: International Labour Office.

Waine, B. (2009). New Labour and pension reform: Security in retirement? *Social Policy and Administration, 43*(7), 754–771.

Walker, A., & Foster, L. (2006). Caught between virtue and ideological necessity: A century of pension policies in the UK. *Review of Political Economy, 18*(3), 427–448.

Williamson, J. B. (2002). Privatization of social security in the United Kingdom: warning or exemplar? *Journal of Aging Studies, 16*(4), 415–430.

Williamson, J. B. (2004). Assessing the pension reform potential of a notional defined contribution pillar. *International Social Security Review, 57*(1), 47–64.

Williamson, J. B. (2005). *An update on Chile's experience with partial privatization and individual accounts.* (Issue Paper No. 2005-19). Washington, DC: AARP.

Williamson, J. B., & Deitelbaum, C. (2005). Social security reform: Does partial privatization make sense for China? *Journal of Aging Studies, 19*(2), 257–271.

Williamson, J. B., Howling, S. A., & Maroto, M. (2006). The political economy of pension reform in Russia: Why partial privatization? *Journal of Aging Studies, 20*(2), 165–175.

Williamson, J. B., Shen, C., & Yang, Y. (2009). Which pension model holds the most promise for China: A funded defined contribution scheme, a notional defined contribution scheme, or a universal social pension? *Benefits: The Journal of Poverty and Social Justice, 17*(2), 101–111.

Williamson, J. B., & Watts-Roy, D. M. (2009). Aging boomers, generational equity, and framing the debate over Social Security. In R. B. Hudson (Ed.), *Boomer bust? Economic and political issues of the graying society, Vol. 1. Perspectives on the boomers* (pp. 153–169). Westport, CT: Praeger.

Willmore, L. (2007). Universal pensions for developing countries. *World Development, 35*(1), 24–51.

World Bank (1994). *Averting the old age crisis: Policies to protect and promote growth.* New York: Oxford University Press.

Chapter | 21 |

Organization and Financing of Health Care

Marilyn Moon
American Institutes for Research, Silver Spring, Maryland

INTRODUCTION

Older Americans receive a substantial share of their health care coverage from government programs, especially Medicare and Medicaid, setting seniors apart from the population as a whole. It is important to continue to examine the effectiveness of these programs in meeting the needs of older Americans and to contrast them with the rest of the health care system. And, as the aging baby boom generation begins to move into these programs, the population served by them will grow each year as a share of all Americans.

Enacted in 1965 as additions to the Social Security Act, Medicare and Medicaid offer important resources that individuals can rely upon in old age. Without these protections, few Americans could afford to retire, given the costs of health care and the barriers in the private sector to obtaining reasonably priced coverage. But Medicare and Medicaid do not cover all the health care needs of the population aged over 65, despite high levels of federal and state expenditures, leaving gaps that have increased risks for low- and moderate-income retirees. Further, declines in retiree health benefits from former employers place higher-income retirees at risk as well. These pressures indicate a need for expanding, not contracting, levels of protection. Nonetheless, Medicare and Medicaid will continue to come under scrutiny and perhaps face further major changes in the future because their share of federal and state spending make them targets in an era of continuing skepticism about government programs. As such changes take place, these programs need to be viewed in the context of both meeting health care needs and offering financial protections to older Americans.

Medicare is a federal health insurance program that serves over 97% of persons aged 65 and older in the US (and over six million younger disabled persons), providing basic protection for their acute-care needs. Medicaid, which offers help for the aged and other specifically designated categories of low-income and low-wealth Americans, is also important for older persons because it fills in crucial gaps in Medicare coverage for this group. Medicaid, which is a joint federal/state program, supplements Medicare coverage for about one in every seven seniors – approximately 8.8 million people (Coughlin et al., 2009). For elderly dually eligible beneficiaries, Medicare spent $42.2 billion, while Medicaid spent $54.4 billion, in 2003. Medicaid is the only public program that helps cover the long-term care costs of older Americans, accounting for about two-thirds of its spending on the population aged over 65. In addition, a complicated arrangement of private supplemental insurance has also evolved over time to fill in Medicare's gaps

DOI: 10.1016/B978-0-12-380880-6.00021-6

for many beneficiaries. Because of the complexities of the health system for older Americans, this chapter does not attempt to take an international perspective, but rather focuses on experiences only in the US. (See Chapter 22 for an international perspective on long-term care.)

Although in many ways Medicare has been one of the most successful federal programs, it has also faced criticism as a result of its rapid expansion. Medicare spending in 2008 stood at $462 billion (Board of Trustees, 2009). From the late 1970s until 2003, Medicare was a frequent target in efforts to reduce federal spending. These efforts peaked in 1997 when the Balanced Budget Act (BBA) set in motion a broad range of changes expected to slow Medicare's growth. In contrast, in 2003, the addition of a new prescription drug benefit represented a major expansion in the program.

Growth in the costs of Medicare and Medicaid is attributable to the same factors generating rising costs in the rest of the health care system. To be sure, the size of Medicare and Medicaid means that changes in payment levels or decisions about medical necessity will have some impact on all of health care spending. But these public programs are far from the main drivers of health care spending. The constant development of new technologies and procedures, increasing rates of utilization, and a high rate of inflation in the overall health care arena have much greater effects. In the first decade of the twenty-first century, costs rose rapidly in all sectors of health care, particularly for hospital care and prescription drugs, although they are showing some signs of slowing by 2008 (Hartman et al., 2010). Consequently, it is not only difficult but inappropriate to treat these programs as separable from the rest of the system.

A BRIEF HISTORY OF MEDICARE AND MEDICAID

Medicare was established by legislation in 1965 as Title XVIII of the Social Security Act and first went into effect on July 1, 1966. The overriding goal was to provide mainstream acute health care – hospital, physician, and related services – for persons aged 65 and over. This age group had been under-served by the health care system, largely because many older persons could not afford insurance. Retiree insurance benefits were relatively rare, and insurance companies were reluctant to offer coverage even to those older persons who could afford it.

Consequently, Medicare has contributed substantially to the well-being of America's oldest citizens. It is the major source of insurance for the elderly (and, since 1972, for individuals who receive federal disability insurance benefits and those with end-stage renal disease). One of Medicare's important

accomplishments is that the very old and the very sick have access to the same basic benefits as younger, healthier beneficiaries. While there is certainly room for improvement, Medicare is insurance that is never rescinded because of the poor health of the individual.

When Medicare was implemented in 1966, it revolutionized health care coverage for persons aged 65 and older. It almost immediately doubled the proportion of seniors with health insurance as only about half of people in this age group had insurance before Medicare (Andersen et al., 1976). By 1970, 97% of older Americans were covered, and that proportion has remained about the same ever since (Moon, 1996). Anyone aged 65 or over who is eligible for any type of Social Security benefit (e.g. as a worker or a dependent), receives Part A, hospital insurance (HI). Part A covers hospital, skilled nursing, and hospice care and is funded by payroll tax contributions from workers and employers that are earmarked for an HI trust fund. Supplementary medical insurance (Part B) is available to persons aged 65 and over on a voluntary basis. It covers physician services, hospital outpatient services, and other ambulatory care and is funded by a combination of general revenues and beneficiary premiums. Home health care benefits are covered by both Parts A and B.

When Medicare began, it was dominated by inpatient hospital care, which accounted for about two-thirds of all spending. Indeed, most of the focus of debate before Medicare's passage was on Part A (HI). But, as care has moved out of the inpatient setting, Part B (supplementary medical insurance) has become a much larger share of the program. Care in hospital outpatient departments and in physicians' offices now replaces many surgeries and treatments formerly performed in inpatient settings. In addition, skilled nursing facility care and home health services – referred to as post-acute care – have also increased in importance over time as hospital stays have been shortened. When individuals leave a hospital after only a few days, post-acute care is often needed as a transition, either in a nursing facility or at home with visits from nurses or other skilled technicians such as rehabilitation therapists. The financial incentives established by payment to health providers and by coverage of benefits have affected the mix of services used.

One original promise of the program was that it would not interfere with the practice of medicine. Payments were designed to be like standard insurance policies then in place. But costs for the program rose rapidly almost from the beginning, and, in the late 1970s, the government sought to slow spending growth in Medicare, and chose to do so largely through application of new payment policies. These policies both affected how much would be paid and moved payments away from per unit pricing. Such cost containment efforts remain a major challenge facing the program.

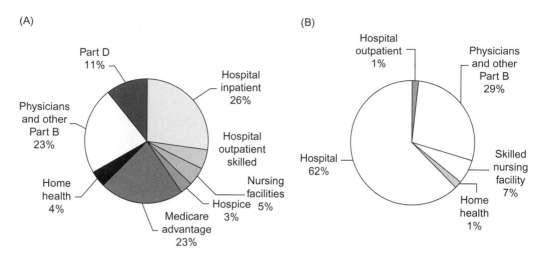

Figure 21.1 (a) Medicare expenditures by type of service, 2009. (b) Medicare expenditures by type of service, 1967. **Source:** Health Care Financing Administration (2000) and Medicare Payment Advisory Commission.

Payments for hospital services – the biggest component of Medicare – were modified in the early 1980s to pay on the basis of the patient's primary diagnosis, regardless of length of stay in a hospital or the actual costs of a particular case. This new system encouraged hospitals to be more efficient, although it also resulted in some premature discharges. Over time, however, this payment system has been judged to be relatively successful (Moon, 1996). It has helped to encourage movement away from long inpatient stays and to more care being delivered outside of hospitals for patients of all ages. In general, Medicare deserves credit for helping to improve the efficiency of US hospitals.

Physician reform came later and established payments on the basis of a relative value scale, initially limiting payments to specialists and increasing them for basic primary care (Physician Payment Review Commission, 1987). Many other health care insurers now use Medicare's so-called physician relative value payment system. Both hospital and physician payments require periodic updating, and Medicare is sometimes criticized for falling behind in making adjustments in response to new medical procedures. In particular, the flawed system for updating payments to physicians has come under heavy criticism, generating requirements for cutting fees each year; because of the expense of fixing that flaw, only ad hoc adjustments have been made to date (Medicare Payment Advisory Commission (MedPAC), 2009).

Nevertheless, the program has been a major player affecting the delivery of care. Overall, Medicare has served as a leader in changing the way that providers of care are paid, and these payment reforms have fundamentally changed the way that hospitals and doctors are paid in the US regardless of payer. The financial incentives created by the payment reforms helped to reduce the length of hospital stays, and, at least initially, to raise payments for primary care physicians relative to specialists.

In 1983, a private plan option was added to Medicare, first as a demonstration but soon thereafter as a standard option. This option allows beneficiaries to choose to get all of their care from an insurer, paid a monthly fee from Medicare to meet the needs of those who enroll. Initially, these were managed care plans – health maintenance organizations (HMOs) – that were touted as the future for health care delivery. Over the years, the option has expanded and contracted as the levels of payments offered and the enthusiasm of the Congress for such options have gone up and down. In 2009, nearly one quarter of Medicare beneficiaries signed up for such plans, largely because of extra benefits offered to enrollees. Extra benefits – usually lower premiums, vision and dental care, and more recently more comprehensive drug benefits – were made possible by 2003 legislation, which also provided for subsidies to these plans to encourage both plans and beneficiaries to participate. In 2009, that subsidy was about 14% above what it costs traditional fee-for-service Medicare to provide similar care (MedPAC, 2009). The 2010 health reform legislation will reduce those subsidies (Kaiser Family Foundation, 2010).

Figure 21.1 contrasts the program at two points in time. In 1967, hospital care (and hence Part A) dominated spending. By 2009, several major changes were notable. Inpatient hospital services declined as a share of the traditional part of the program, and Medicare Advantage – the private option portion – accounted for more than a fifth of all spending.

The situation for Medicaid is quite different because its implementation is controlled by the states, which have considerable latitude in establishing eligibility and coverage. Hence, approaches to holding the line on Medicaid spending can vary substantially across the nation. In general, however, states have relied both on keeping payments to providers very low and on requiring beneficiaries to go into managed care plans. Low payments have sometimes led to access problems when providers of services decide not to take on Medicaid patients. This effectively reduces government costs both through the lower payments and through the reduced volume of services available, although it creates substantial issues for those qualified to receive Medicaid. For example, for persons dually eligible for Medicare and Medicaid, a number of states decline to use the federally authorized option of having Medicaid pay for Medicare copayments to physicians, thereby effectively lowering the payments doctors receive. Further, nursing home access is sometimes a problem for Medicaid patients.

THE PRESSURES ON THE MEDICARE PROGRAM

Although Medicare has performed well relative to total health care costs since the 1980s, the program nonetheless is often portrayed as a runaway item in the federal budget. The evidence cited for this is the higher overall growth in spending on Medicare as compared to the rest of the budget. Both Medicare and Medicaid have grown as a share of the federal budget and of the GDP – the output of all goods and services produced in the US. Medicare, however, has not grown faster than the costs of private health insurance (Boccuti & Moon, 2003; Levit et al., 2004). Moreover, contrary to the belief of some policymakers and journalists, it is largely a myth that the senior lobby has been mainly responsible for this growth in Medicare (Binstock & Quadagno, 2001). In fact, at various points in time, it has been politically feasible to adopt regulatory and legislative changes that have held down program growth.

Nonetheless, since these public programs are funded with tax dollars in an era of anti-tax sentiment, they get more scrutiny than health expenditures paid for by individuals or by businesses. In the early 1970s, Medicare was only 3.5% of the federal budget and by 1990 accounted for 8.6%. The percentage has grown steadily such that Medicare's share totaled nearly 16% of the 2009 federal budget (Congressional Budget Office, 2009).

As a result of Medicare's growth, some policymakers believe that it may be crowding out expenditures on other domestic programs. Critics often argue that Americans will only accept a certain level of overall public spending, so, if Medicare grows rapidly, it hurts other spending even if it has its own revenue sources. In this argument, Medicare gets most of the attention because of the near-term increases in spending that the aging of the baby boomers will foster. Already,

the number of beneficiaries has grown faster than the population as a whole, reflecting longer life expectancies for the elderly. Looking out over the next decade, Medicare is expected to rise from $468 billion in 2008 to nearly double that – $927 billion – in 2018 if there is no change in policy (Board of Trustees, 2009).

A second fiscal pressure on Medicare arises from the status of the Part A, HI, trust fund. Current law provides a fixed source of funding, the Federal Insurance Contributions Act payroll tax, for HI. These revenues typically have not grown as fast as spending, creating periodic crises when the date of trust fund exhaustion is close at hand. So far, that day of reckoning has been postponed several times by major cost-cutting efforts and an increase in the wage and salary base subject to taxation (Figure 21.2). For instance, a strong economy and the slow growth in Medicare spending in 1998 and 1999 pushed that date to 2029, based on the 2002 report of the Medicare trustees. But in 2009, the date of exhaustion of the Part A trust fund was projected to occur in 2017 until the 2010 health reform legislation pushed the date back another 12 years (Kaiser Family Foundation, 2010).

In addition to pressures on financing, it is important to note that the program has key gaps in coverage that could be addressed by policy reforms. When Medicare and its benefit package were created in 1965, medical care needs and insurance looked very different from how they do today. For example, many workers had only hospital coverage, in part because health care spending as a share of income was much smaller, and services such as physician care were not inordinately expensive. Today, most good private plans for workers cover almost all aspects of acute care, including generous drug coverage. Yet the basic package for Medicare remained largely unchanged until December 2003, when a new drug benefit option was enacted as part of the Medicare Prescription Drug, Improvement, and Modernization Act (MMA) of 2003.

In January of 2006, the drug program financed by a combination of beneficiary premiums (covering about 25% of costs) and general revenues (paying the other 75%) began. This benefit requires anyone who wishes to obtain a drug benefit to enroll in a private plan. As a result, individuals are confronted with difficult decisions as many types of private plans are available. This requires that people deal with a large number of plan differences – including variations in the formulary that will be used (i.e. what drugs are covered), the type and amount of cost sharing, and what pharmacies participate in each plan. Moreover, in 2009, premiums varied from $10 per month to $100 per month (Hoadley et al., 2008). For those who remain in traditional Medicare, this private plan operates as a separate supplemental benefit.

On average, this new drug benefit covers about half of all drug costs for those who enroll. There is a large gap in coverage, referred to as the "donut hole," which represents a period in which insurance temporarily ends (in 2010, after the first $2830 in spending has occurred) and does not begin again until a catastrophic benefit is triggered after spending reaches $6440 – that is, there is a gap of $3610 for which an individual is fully responsible for the costs of prescription drugs. In 2007, 26% of Medicare Part D enrollees reached the coverage gap and hence had at least some drug expenditures that were not covered by insurance (Hoadley et al., 2008). This gap resulted from the competing goals of offering generous initial coverage to encourage people to sign up for the voluntary benefit, offering catastrophic protection for those with high expenditures, and meeting limits on how much the Congress was willing to contribute toward these costs. The health reform legislation will, over time, close this gap (Kaiser Family Foundation, 2010).

The other crucial gaps in Medicare coverage arise because of the high deductibles and copayments required for covered services. For example, in 2010, the hospital deductible was $1100 for each admission in a spell of illness, no matter how short the stay. Further, coverage of physician and other ambulatory services is limited to 80% of allowed charges, with no upper limit on copayments as is often found in insurance coverage for working families. Mental health benefits are also quite limited. Consequently, coverage still lags behind what younger, well-insured families have for insurance. In 2007, the average benefit value of Medicare was only about 87% as generous as the typical large employer plan, largely because of Medicare's higher cost-sharing requirements (Yamamoto et al., 2008).

Finally, Medicare does not cover long-term care costs, such as nursing home and supportive home benefits, for those with needs for help in daily living. Medicare coverage is limited to acute care needs so that even services that provide some supportive benefits (skilled nursing care and home health benefits) are limited, and the beneficiary must be making progress in recovering in order to stay eligible. While long-term care is not generally part of insurance for younger families either, it is something that many older Americans need when disabilities and long-term health problems make it difficult to survive independently. The costs of nursing home care can be very high, averaging about $80 000 a year in 2009 (MetLife, 2009). For financial support in this area, seniors must turn to the Medicaid program, which is limited to those with very low incomes (or who have depleted their assets to the point where they cannot pay all of the costs of essential long-term care) They then become eligible for Medicaid support to pay costs beyond what a person's income will cover.

The current financing pressures make it unlikely that Medicare will expand in the near future in a manner sufficient to fill in the important gaps in coverage. At present, these are filled in part by supplemental benefits from the public and private sources described below.

SUPPLEMENTING MEDICARE WITH MEDICAID AND OTHER INSURANCE

Because of Medicare's limited benefits, private and public supplemental plans have developed to meet older persons' additional needs for health insurance. Four kinds of supplemental policies have evolved. As described above, Medicaid, a means-tested public benefit established at the same time as Medicare, subsidizes many poor older persons through several different arrangements. Employer-based retiree insurance and individual supplemental coverage policies (termed Medigap) are provided by private insurers. These three sources of coverage normally are associated with beneficiaries enrolled in the traditional part of the program. The fourth option is Medicare Advantage (MA), in which private health plans that contract with Medicare to provide Medicare-covered services also offer at least some additional supplemental benefits. (Some beneficiaries in MA plans also participate in other supplemental policies, but less is known about those arrangements.) These supplemental coverages vary in quality, beneficiaries' ability to access them, and the degree to which they relieve financial burdens. Understanding how these supplemental plans operate and the contributions they make is essential for any analysis of the health care system for older Americans. Figure 21.3 shows the extent and type of supplemental coverage for Medicare beneficiaries. It is broken into two elements, distinguishing first between those who go into MA plans and then what supplemental benefits are received by those in traditional Medicare.

Medicaid

Medicaid offers generous fill-in benefits for persons with low incomes and assets. However, because states have latitude in establishing eligibility and coverage, there is considerable variation in the quality and quantity of services provided across the states. For example, Medicaid spending in 2005 on persons aged 65 and above ranged from $6157 in Maine to $26 429 per person in Pennsylvania (Holahan et al., 2009). Today, two separate programs provide some benefits under the Medicaid umbrella. Basic Medicaid coverage is limited to those with the lowest incomes, generally well below the federal poverty level. In addition to paying the Part B premium and relieving beneficiaries of the responsibility for copayments and deductibles in the Medicare program (even if Medicaid fails to compensate providers

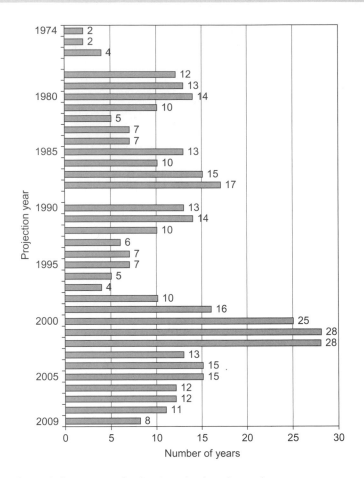

Figure 21.2 Number of years before H1 trust fund projected to be exhausted.
Source: O'Sullivan (1995) and Board of Trustees (2009).

for these costs), these state-based programs all offer long-term care coverage.

Beginning in 1988 and varying by income, several other benefits under Medicaid provide relief for low-income Medicare beneficiaries. Together, these are termed the Medicare Savings Programs. The Qualified Medicare Beneficiary Program (QMB) covers full Part B premiums, deductibles, and co-insurance for those whose incomes fall below 100% of the poverty level (about $11 000 in 2008 for a single person). The Specified Low Income Medicare Beneficiary (SLMB) program provides Part B premium subsidies for those with incomes between 100% and 120% of the poverty level. Finally, the 1997 Balanced Budget Act created the Qualified Individuals (QI) program to cover only the premium costs for people with incomes between 120% and 135% poverty (Moon et al., 1998).

In 2007, similar protections were contained in the prescription drug benefit legislation, with protection that extends up to 150% of the poverty line. This is referred to as the low income subsidy (LIS). The 2007 legislation removed Medicaid from providing prescription drug coverage to Medicare beneficiaries. While states can offer some further supplements, they have not chosen to do so in this fiscally constrained climate. Many critics of the Medicare drug benefit have argued that low-income beneficiaries have been treated less well by the drug benefit than the benefits that had been available under many state Medicaid plans.

In practice, all of these programs cover only some of the people who qualify for them. Participation rates remain low because of individuals' reluctance to seek help from a "welfare program," substantial barriers to enrollment, burdensome reporting requirements, and sometimes lack of awareness of potential eligibility. Fewer than half of all elderly persons below the poverty line participate in the basic Medicaid program. Moreover, in 1996, only 55% of those eligible participated in QMB, and just 16% of those eligible participated in SLMB (Barents Group, 1999). Thus,

Medicaid is only partially successful in assuring comprehensive coverage to low-income seniors. But the LIS program for the drug benefit, with outreach sponsored by the SSA, has also had its problems, resulting in disappointing rates of participation as well.

In addition, the asset test for determining Medicaid eligibility, which is even more stringent than the income test, results in a number of individuals who would qualify on the basis of income being excluded (Moon et al., 2002). Although income limits have been increased over time, most states have asset tests that have been in place since 1987, often restricting benefits to persons with assets below $2000 or $4000 and couples with assets below $3000 or $6000. A key policy issue here is how to balance the desire to target benefits to those most in need with the goal of encouraging older Americans to save for their future needs.

The financing issues facing Medicaid are also complicated. The concern about crowding out within state budgets can be made for this program as well, especially because the constitutions of almost all states require them to balance their budgets. Moreover, states vary in the shares of their programs going to different Medicaid-eligible subgroups – and by amounts greater than would be suggested by population differences alone. Thus, states can decide when to favor the old over the young, or vice versa, within the Medicaid program. The response to hard economic times by states is generally to reduce payments to providers of care rather than cutting benefits or eligibility directly, although these changes can still certainly affect access to care. The federal government can and has supplemented Medicaid to reduce the effects of recessions. The most recent of these occurred in the fiscal stimulus legislation of 2009, the American Recovery and Reinvestment Act (ARRA), and has been credited with softening the blow of the serious economic downturn of 2008–2009. Recovery has been slow, however, and Medicaid took some substantial hits in a number of states in 2010.

Employer-Sponsored Plans

Employer-based retiree health plans normally offer comprehensive supplemental insurance. Employers usually subsidize retiree premiums and establish benefits comparable to what their working population receives by filling in gaps left by Medicare. A large proportion of these plans, for example, cover prescription drugs. Thus, these plans both reduce out-of-pocket expenses and increase access to services, often without limiting provider choice. Beneficiaries in these plans have among the lowest out-of-pocket costs (Medicare Payment Advisory Commission, 2002), even though they are heavy users of care. They are thus among the best protected of all seniors.

But such plans are limited to workers and dependents whose former employer offers generous retiree benefits. Among current Medicare beneficiaries in the traditional part of the program, about 40% have such employer-sponsored retiree health plans (MedPAC, 2009). And, these benefits accrue disproportionately to high-income retirees. This privileged group does not need improvements in Medicare to assure them access to care as they are covered very well at present.

The strength of resistance to change by those with retiree insurance may decline in the future, however, because employers are beginning to cut back benefits in order to control costs. They are placing more controls on the use of care, raising retiree contributions in the form of premiums or cost sharing, and even changing the benefit package (Kaiser Family Foundation and Health Research and Educational Trust, 2006). Concern that the addition of the Part D benefit would cause employers to cut benefits at a greater pace than they had been has thus far been unfounded, however. In fact, participation by employers has remained higher than what initial estimates assumed (Moon, in press).

A number of studies have tracked changes in employer behavior, each showing the same downward trend. For example, a study of large firms (with 200 or more workers, the firms most likely to offer such benefits) found that the percentage offering retiree health benefits declined from 66% in 1988 to 33% in 2007 (Kaiser Family Foundation and Health Research and Educational Trust, 2007). Another approach to reducing employer financial liabilities is to raise the requirements for qualifying for coverage; for example, by adding more years of employment as a condition of participation. This trend has also been on the upswing (Kaiser Family Foundation and Health Research and Education Trust, 2006).

Medigap Insurance

A traditional form of private supplemental coverage, commonly referred to as Medigap, does not lower overall out-of-pocket burdens because the premium is fully paid by the beneficiary and includes substantial administrative and marketing charges, and, often, profits for the insurer (US General Accounting Office, 1998). Thus, many beneficiaries have higher, not lower, financial burdens when they buy Medigap. Medigap is most useful for reducing potential catastrophic expenses for those who have high costs in a particular year. The ten standardized plans that insurance companies are allowed to offer under federal law cover a basic package of Medicare's required cost sharing and in some cases include a limited prescription drug benefit. This form of supplemental insurance provides the least protection for beneficiaries, yet it remains popular with beneficiaries seeking to keep their out-of-pocket costs from being high in any one year.

Another issue is that Medigap premiums rose dramatically over the 1990s. Between 1992 and 1996, premium rates in Arizona, Virginia, and Ohio rose

18%, 19%, and 41% respectively, though the majority of those rate increases took place between 1995 and 1996 (Alecxih et al., 1997). National estimates for rate increases in 1999–2000, according to insurance experts, were 8–10% (Medicare Payment Advisory Commission, 2000). There have been no recent major studies in this area. However, anecdotal evidence suggests continued rapid increases over the last decade.

Over time, Medigap plans have changed the way they price policies, also contributing to access problems. Medigap providers can sell policies that are community-rated, attained age-rated, or rated according to the purchaser's age at time of issue. Companies have moved away from "community-rated" plans where the premium is the same for everyone, regardless of age. Most providers have moved to an attained age structure in which policies increase in cost rapidly as people age. This puts greater burdens on beneficiaries just as their incomes are declining. For the unwary buyer at age 65, these plans appear less costly than community-rated options (Alecxih et al., 1997). But, because most beneficiaries cannot change their minds after a six-month open enrollment period at age 65, they may lock themselves into a very bad deal over time. These high premiums reduce some of the advantages of traditional Medicare – which does an excellent job of pooling risks across a large group – and also raise issues about access to care.

Private Plan Options

As noted above, beneficiaries also can obtain additional benefits to supplement Medicare's basic package by enrolling in private health plans, termed "Medicare Advantage" in the MMA of 2003. In such a case, enrollees agree to get all their coverage from the private plan, rather than from a combination of traditional reimbursements for services from Medicare and private supplemental coverage. For many years in the 1980s and 1990s, private plans that participated in Medicare were mainly HMOs, which restrict enrollees to a specific network of doctors and hospitals. Cost sharing was usually lower than for traditional Medicare and some additional benefits were offered for less than the price of a Medigap plan.

After legislative changes in 1997, however, these plans became more expensive for consumers through higher premiums and cost sharing, and many plans withdrew from Medicare altogether. The number of beneficiaries enrolled in these private plans reached as high as 16% in 1999 followed by a decline to about 12% in 2003 (Board of Trustees, 2009). To counter this retrenchment in private plan participation, the 2003 MMA legislation increased payments from the federal government to plans to encourage them to stay or return to offering coverage. Once again, there was a rapid increase in Medicare Advantage plans, growing faster than during the last expansionary period.

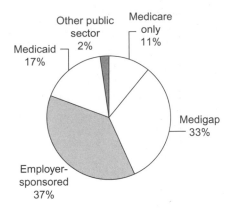

Figure 21.3 Sources of supplemental coverage among fee-for-service beneficiaries, 2005.
Source: Medicare Payment Advisory Commission (2009): MedPAC analysis of Medicare Current Beneficiary Survey, Cost and Use files.

This popularity was due not only to additional payments to plans that allowed them to offer enriched benefits, but also to the rapid rise of private fee-for-service plans and preferred provider plans under Medicare Advantage that carry fewer restrictions (as compared with the HMO-style plans) concerning which doctors or other providers of care can be used by patients. Together, these changes have led to nearly one in four Medicare beneficiaries being enrolled in Medicare Advantage in 2009, up from 14% in 2005, including a large number of low- and moderate-income beneficiaries who would otherwise do without supplemental coverage.

In 2009, it was estimated that these private plans were still paid, on average, about 14% more than it would cost to provide benefits to the same individuals through the traditional program (MedPac, 2009). But, in that same year, additional restrictions were added to these plans, which, along with modest reductions in the growth of payments, suggests that plan participation is likely to remain stable or grow slowly. Further, more stringent changes enacted as part of 2010 reform legislation will again potentially usher in a decline in participation. These boom and bust cycles have been disruptive to Medicare beneficiaries in the past and may well be so in the early part of this decade. The policy changes that have led to these expansions and contractions reflect an active debate over the desirability of relying on the private market as opposed to the traditional Medicare program.

No Coverage

Finally, some beneficiaries cannot afford any supplemental policy. As shown in Figure 21.3, 11% of Medicare beneficiaries in traditional Medicare had no extra policy to cover what Medicare's benefit package does not. In addition, some of those in Medicare Advantage plans, especially the private fee-for-service options, also continue to face considerable out-of-pocket costs, although data are not available on how much these plans reduce out-of-pocket spending as compared to the traditional benefit package.

Lack of supplemental coverage is associated with problems of access to care. Those who have no supplemental coverage, for example, are less likely to see a doctor in any given year, less likely to have a usual source of care, and more likely to postpone getting care in a timely fashion. For example, 21% of beneficiaries who relied on traditional Medicare alone reported delaying care due to its cost while only 5% of beneficiaries with private supplemental coverage reported delaying care (Gluck & Hanson, 2001).

FUTURE CHALLENGES AND CHANGES

The financing of the Medicare program is likely to face key challenges in moving forward. The health care reform legislation of 2010 generated substantial Medicare cuts to help to offer up savings coverage for fund the population aged under 65 (Kaiser Family Foundation, 2010). Reluctance to raise taxes for both Medicare and broader health reform suggest little in the way of new resources for Medicare and only modest improvement in the portion of Medicaid that serves older Americans. In fact, Medicare will still be a target for deficit reduction efforts going forward. This will likely mean that, in the near future, cost containment efforts will again begin to dominate legislative activities. And proposals to improve Medicare are barely on the horizon.

The future of Medicare remains a controversial political issue mainly because this is a large and popular public program that faces projections of rapid growth. As a government program, either new revenues will have to be added to support Medicare or its growth will have to be curtailed. Some of the problem is driven by the expected increase in the number of persons eligible for Medicare, from 45 million in 2009 to 78 million in 2030 as the baby boom generation becomes eligible for benefits (Board of Trustees, 2009). Enrollment in the program will grow from one in every eight Americans to more than one in every five. But more important is the issue of growth in the overall costs of care. That issue is best tackled by dealing with US health care on a universal basis because this is not just a Medicare or Medicaid problem.

Making changes to Medicare that can improve its viability both in terms of its costs and in how well it serves older and disabled beneficiaries should certainly be pursued. But the challenge remains to contrast what seems like a "simple" solution of turning over Medicare to the private sector, with a set of changes that would need to be done to the program through the usual legislative process. The flux and complexity of our healthcare system will necessitate continuing attention to this program.

A Private Plan Approach

Medicare could be modified so that beneficiaries choose from an array of private plans (perhaps including the traditional program as one among many options). The standard proposal would be to have the federal government provide oversight of plans and subsidize the premium up to some average level, usually starting at an amount comparable to the current level of per capita spending on the program (now in the range of $12 000 annually). This approach has often been referred to as "premium support." Individuals wishing to buy more comprehensive coverage would have to pay the difference between the federal contribution and the premium charged by a particular plan.

This restructuring approach could profoundly affect Medicare's future. In particular, the traditional Medicare program could be priced beyond the means of many beneficiaries, leaving only private plan options from which to choose. Further, if plans begin to sort into two groups of higher cost and lower cost, the likely result would be to segregate beneficiaries in plans on the basis of their ability to pay. This would be quite different from today, where the basic program treats all beneficiaries alike. The details of a private sector approach would be very important in determining the impacts on both federal savings and beneficiaries.

Some supporters of a private approach assume that private plans inherently offer advantages that traditional Medicare cannot achieve. But there is no magic bullet to holding the line on growth of costs. Per capita spending rises because of the higher use of services, higher prices, or a combination of the two. Medicare's price clout is well known and documented, so it is difficult for private plans to do better in that area. So what about managed care's ability to control use of services? Studies of managed care have concluded that, in the past, most such plans saved money by obtaining price discounts for services and not by changing the practice of health care (Strunk et al., 2001). Controlling use of services represents a major challenge for both private insurance and Medicare.

A private approach has the *potential* to allow greater flexibility for innovation and change in coverage of benefits. This allows private insurers to respond more quickly than a large government program can to adopt new innovations and to intervene where insurers believe too much care is being delivered (Butler & Moffit, 1995). But what looks like cost-effectiveness activities from an insurer's perspective may be seen by a beneficiary as the loss of potentially essential care. Further, there are too few examples of truly innovative new techniques, organizational strategies, and other contributions from private plan competition. Some managed care plans, for example, do not even have the data or administrative mechanisms to undertake care coordination (Strunk et al., 2001). Further, private plans, which must compete to attract a strong patient base, may be reluctant to be perceived as overly restrictive.

Under the traditional Medicare program, beneficiaries do not need to fear loss of coverage when they develop health problems. On the other hand, private insurers are interested in satisfying their own customers and generating profits for stockholders. When the financial incentives they face are very broad (such as receiving fixed monthly payments for providing all care), private insurers respond as good business entities should. They seek the easiest ways of holding down costs in the provision of services. Even though many private insurers are willing and able to care for Medicare patients, the easiest way to stay in business as an insurer is to seek out the healthy enrollees and avoid the sick. Under the current Medicare Advantage program, risk adjustment has improved substantially but has not totally eliminated the incentives to attract healthier patients. For example, special needs plans under Medicare, which were explicitly established to focus on the sick, remain only a very small share of private offerings (MedPAC, 2009).

Finally, private insurers will almost surely have higher administrative overhead costs than does Medicare. Private insurance, for example, tends to have administrative costs in the range of 15% (Levit et al., 2004). Insurers need to advertise and promote their plans. They face smaller risk pools than traditional Medicare, requiring them to make more conservative decisions regarding reserves and other protections against losses over time. Private plans expect to return a profit to shareholders. These factors cumulate and work against the likelihood that private companies can perform better than Medicare, which has administrative costs totaling about 2% of program spending (Board of Trustees, 2009).

Reform options stressing competition seek savings by relying not only on private plans but also on competition among those plans. Often this includes allowing premiums paid by beneficiaries to vary, with premiums being higher for the more expensive plans, even if benefits remain the same. The theory is that beneficiaries will become more price conscious and choose the lower-cost plans, rewarding those that are more efficient. But the experiences in Medicare lend considerable doubt to the notion that the theory will prove true in practice for the Medicare population (US General Accounting Office, 2000). Studies on retirees show less willingness to change doctors and learn new insurance rules in order to save a few dollars each month, particularly for those who have health problems.

Further, new approaches to the delivery of health care under Medicare may generate a whole new set of problems, including problems in areas where Medicare is now working well. For example, shifting among plans is not necessarily good for patients; it is not only disruptive, but can also raise costs of care. Studies have shown that having one physician over a long period of time reduces costs of care (e.g. Weiss & Blustein, 1996). And, if it is only the healthier beneficiaries who choose to switch plans, the sickest and most vulnerable beneficiaries may end up being concentrated in plans that become increasingly expensive over time (Buchmueller, 2000).

Will reforms that lead to a greater reliance on the market still retain the emphasis on equal access to care and plans? For example, differential premiums could undermine some of the redistributive nature of the program, which assures even low-income beneficiaries access to high-quality care and responsive providers. Support for a market approach that moves away from a "one-size-fits-all" type is a prescription for risk selection problems. If plans have flexibility in tailoring their offerings, they can, for example, raise cost sharing on benefits such as home health care, which are disproportionately used by older, sicker beneficiaries. About one in every three Medicare beneficiaries has severe mental or physical health problems. What are the tradeoffs from attempts to increase the role of private plans in serving Medicare beneficiaries? Any modest gains in lower costs that might come from some increased competition and from the flexibility that the private sector enjoys could be more than offset by increased discrepancies in access to care between the healthy and the sick or the wealthy and the poor.

More Incremental Approaches

A more realistic approach would be to emphasize improvements in *both* the existing private plan options and the traditional Medicare program, basically retaining the current structure in which traditional Medicare is the primary option. The emphasis could thus be placed on innovations necessary for improvements in health care delivery regardless of setting. This would require, for example, that the traditional Medicare program be offered with expanded benefits to avoid the problem of generating a complex, jerry-rigged system of government and supplemental plans. It also means changing some of the financial incentives in the fee-for-service system (such as encouraging patients to use primary care physicians instead of relying as much on specialists, or on bundling certain groups of services) without going all the way to a capitated (that is, a system that puts everyone in a more formal managed care environment) program.

In addition, better norms and standards of care are needed if we are to provide quality of care protections to all Americans. Investment in outcomes and effectiveness research, disease management, and other techniques that could lead to improvements in treatment of patients will require a substantial public commitment. This cannot be done as well in a proprietary, for-profit environment where dissemination of innovative ways of coordinating care may not be shared. Further, innovations in treatment and coordination of care should focus on those with substantial health problems – exactly the population that many private plans avoid. Reform needs to focus on enhancing the effectiveness of private plans by rewarding innovation.

A good area to begin improvements in knowledge about the effectiveness of medical care would be with prescription drugs. The Medicare prescription drug benefit will require major efforts to hold down costs over time. Part of that effort needs to be based on evidence of the comparative effectiveness and safety of various drugs. Establishing rules for coverage of drugs should reflect good medical evidence so that, for example, higher co-payments could be reserved for less effective drugs or for brand-name drugs when equivalent generics are available. Too often, differential co-payments are established instead on the basis of the price of the drug or depending upon which manufacturer offers the best discounts. Undertaking these studies and evaluations represents a public good and needs to be funded on that basis. As of 2009, the ARRA has been funding some work in this area, but it is not linked directly to health coverage or benefit deliberations. Private plans and others are reluctant to do this on their own. Finally, resources also need to be devoted to disseminating that information and educating consumers on what it means to adopt an evidence-based approach to health care delivery.

Within the fee-for-service environment, it would be helpful to energize both patients and physicians in helping to coordinate care. Patients need information and support as well as incentives to become involved. Many caring physicians, who have often resented the low pay in fee-for-service and the lack of control in managed care, would likely welcome the ability to spend more time with their patients. It has now become popular to talk about a "medical home" in which individuals would rely upon a primary care physician (or team) to help with coordination of care and managing health needs in general. One way to do this would be to give beneficiaries a certificate that spells out the care consultation benefits to which they are entitled and allow them to designate a physician to provide those services. Such care would likely reduce confusion and unnecessary duplication of services that go on in a fee-for-service environment. This change should be just one of many in seeking to improve care coordination.

Additional flexibility to the Centers for Medicare and Medicaid Services (CMS) in its management and development of payment initiatives using competition also could result in long-term cost savings and serve patients well. In the areas of durable medical equipment and perhaps even for some testing and laboratory services, competitively bid contracts could be used to obtain better prices (although efforts in this area have been ineffectual to date). Better-funded demonstrations and studies on new payment approaches are also worthy investments. These are but a few of the options that ought to be considered.

The Issues of Financing Medicare and Medicaid

More resources will be needed to finance Medicare over time (Gluck & Moon, 2000). This means asking beneficiaries to pay more or taxpayers to increase their contributions to Medicare or a combination of the two. It is simply not feasible to absorb a doubling of the Medicare population over the next 30 years without dealing with the financing issue. In fact, avoiding discussions of higher taxpayer revenues has already led to cost shifting onto beneficiaries – which implicitly represents a financing decision.

A wide range of mechanisms can be used to explicitly or implicitly require beneficiaries to contribute more to the costs of their care. For example, increased premiums or cost-sharing requirements can be and have been applied over time to shift costs onto those who use the program. The MMA included not only an increased across-the-board Part B deductible in 2005, but also provided for phasing in a higher premium for persons with annual incomes above $80 000, beginning in 2007. However, the 2010 reform legislation will result in better coverage for those aged under 65 than for medicare beneficiaries. (Kaiser Family Foundation, 2010).

Efforts to raise the age of eligibility for the program to 67 also implicitly mean cost shifting to beneficiaries. If individuals must then seek coverage through the private insurance market until they reach the new age of eligibility, they will quickly find that coverage is very expensive or even unavailable (Pollitz et al., 2001). Once some of the recently legislated changes to reform insurance go into effect, this option will become more feasible (Kaiser Family Foundation, 2010). Because Medicare would be eliminating eligibility for its younger, least expensive older patients on average, the approximately 5% of people disenfranchised if eligibility age goes to 67 would only save Medicare about 2% of its costs (Waidmann, 1998).

In terms of Medicaid, it is not feasible to ask beneficiaries – who are by definition on lower incomes – to bear a greater share of the costs of their care. Indeed, the way that Medicaid works for long-term care services is to require that individuals devote most of their incomes to the costs of institutionalization; for example, with the government then only filling in the gaps. This program will also be important to retirees who need long-term care in the next several decades. The new CLASS Act that was part of the reform in 2010 will provide some new opportunities over time. But the financing crisis will come later, when the baby boom generation is in its eighties and nineties and hits Medicaid. So, although less attention is currently focused on Medicaid, it too will need additional financial support over time. It is not known how well states will do in financing future needs.

What then about the costs of financing relying on greater contributions from taxpayers? Technically, new revenues would not have to be raised for a number of years. However, doing so soon would likely increase taxes most on baby boomers, who will be drawing heavily on Medicare and Medicaid in the future. If broader revenue sources are tapped, they will affect different groups of the population depending upon which sources are used. For example, payroll taxes remain relatively popular with the general public, likely because they know where the revenues raised are supposed to go. But economists criticize these taxes as raising the costs of workers to employers, discouraging employment. General revenues, the other major source of income for Medicare, are more progressive – asking higher income persons to pay more – and require that older persons as well as the young contribute. Other taxes, such as those on alcohol and tobacco, often do not bring in enough revenue to resolve the financing issues. Whatever choices are made, raising taxes is likely to be a last resort approach given the political costs often associated with such measures.

Nonetheless, someone will need to pay more to provide care for an aging population. Issues of fairness raise important considerations about how much beneficiaries can be asked to pay and how much should be required from others. The key issue will be how to share that burden, not whether it will increase over time, because it surely will.

REFERENCES

Alecxih, L. M. B., Lutzky, S., Sevak, P., & Claxton, G. (1997). *Key issues affecting accessibility to medigap insurance*. New York: The Commonwealth Fund.

Andersen, R., Lion, J., & Anderson, O. W. (1976). *Two decades of health services: Social survey trends in use and expenditure*. Cambridge, MA: Ballinger Publishing Company.

Barents Group LLC. (1999). A profile of QMB-eligible and SLMB-eligible Medicare beneficiaries. Report prepared for Health Care Financing Administration, Washington, DC.

Binstock, R. H., & Quadagno, J. (2001). Aging and politics. In R. H. Binstock & L. K. George (Eds.), *Handbook of aging and the social sciences* (pp. 333–351) (5th Edn). San Diego: Academic Press.

Board of Trustees. (2009). *2009 annual report of the Boards of Trustees of the Federal Hospital Insurance and Federal Supplementary Medical Insurance Trust Funds*. Washington, DC: U.S. Government Printing Office.

Boccuti, C., & Moon, M. (2003). Comparing Medicare and private insurance: Growth rates in spending over three decades. *Health Affairs, 22*, 230–237.

Buchmueller, T. (2000). The health plan choices of retirees under managed competition. *Health Affairs, 35*, 949–976.

Butler, S., & Moffit, R. (1995). The FEHBP as a model for a new Medicare program. *Health Affairs, 14*, 8–30.

Congressional Budget Office (2009). *The budget and economic outlook: An update*. Washington, DC: CBO.

Coughlin, T., Waidmann, T., & O'Malley-Watts, M. (2009). Where does the burden lie? Medicaid and Medicare spending for dual eligible beneficiaries. Issue Paper. Washington, DC: Kaiser Commission on Medicaid and the Uninsured, April.

Gluck, M., & Moon, M. (2000). *Financing Medicare's future: Final report of the study panel on Medicare's long term care financing*. Washington, DC: National Academy of Social Insurance.

Gluck, M., & Hanson, K. (2001). *Medicare chartbook*. Washington, DC: The Henry J. Kaiser Family Foundation.

Hartman, M., Martin, A., Nuccio, O., & Catlin, A. The National Health Expenditure Accounts Team (2010). Health spending growth at a historic low in 2008. *Health Affairs, 29*, 147–155.

Health Care Financing Administration (2000). *Health care financing review. Medicare and Medicaid statistical supplement*. Baltimore, MD: US Department of Health and Human Services.

Hoadley, J., Thompson, J., Hargrave, E., Cubanski, J., & Neuman, T. (2008). *Medicare Part D 2009 data spotlight: Premiums*. Menlo Park, CA and Washington, DC: The Henry J. Kaiser Family Foundation.

Holahan, J., Miller, D., & Rousseau, D. (2009.) Dual Eligibles: Medicaid enrollment and spending for Medicare beneficiaries in 2005. Issue Brief. Washington, DC: Kaiser Commission on Medicaid and the Uninsured, February.

Kaiser Family Foundation and Health Research and Educational Trust. (2006). *Retiree health benefits examined*. Menlo Park, CA: Kaiser Family Foundation.

Kaiser Family Foundation and Health Research and Educational Trust. (2007). *Employer health benefits 2007 annual survey*. Menlo Park, CA: Kaiser Family Foundation.

Kaiser Family Foundation. (2010). Summary of key changes to Medicare in 2010 health reform law. Focus on health reform. Retrieved from http://www.kff.org/healthreform/upload/7948-02.pdf.

Levit, K., Smith, C., Cowan, C., Sensenig, A., Catlin, A., & Health

Accounts Team. (2004). Health spending rebound continues in 2002. *Health Affairs, 23,* 147–159.

Medicare Payment Advisory Commission (MedPac) (2000). *Report to congress: Medicare payment policy.* Washington, DC: MedPac.

Medicare Payment Advisory Commission (MedPac) (2002). *Report to congress: Assessing medicare benefits.* Washington, DC: MedPac.

Medicare Payment Advisory Commission. (2009). *A data book: Healthcare spending and the Medicare program.* Washington, DC: MedPAC.

Medicare Payment Advisory Commission (MedPac) (2009). *Report to congress: New approaches in medicare.* Washington, DC: Medpac.

MetLife (2009). *The 2009 MetLife market survey of nursing home, assisted living, adult day services and home care costs.* New York: Mature Market Institute.

Moon, M. (1996). *Medicare now and in the future* (2nd Edn.). Washington, DC: Urban Institute Press.

Moon, M. (in press). *Medicare: A policy primer* (2nd Edn.). Washington, DC: Urban Institute Press.

Moon, M., Brennan, N., & Segal, M. (1998). Options for aiding low-income Medicare beneficiaries. *Inquiry, 35,* 346–356.

Moon, M., Freidland, R., & Shirey, L. (2002). *Medicare beneficiaries and their assets: Implications for low-income programs.* Menlo Park, CA: Henry J. Kaiser Family Foundation.

O'Sullivan, J. (1995). *Medicare: History of part a trust fund insolvency projections.* Washington, DC: Congressional Research Service.

Physician Payment Review Commission. (1987). *Medicare physician payment: An agenda for reform.* Washington, DC: US Government Printing Office.

Pollitz, K., Sorian, R., & Thomas, K. (2001). *How accessible is individual health insurance for consumers in less-than-perfect health?* Menlo Park, CA: The Henry J. Kaiser Family Foundation.

Strunk, B. C., Ginsburg, P. B., & Gabel, J. R. (2001). Tracking health care costs. *Health Affairs, Web Exclusive,* W39–W50.

US General Accounting Office. (1998). *Medigap insurance: Compliance with federal standards has increased,* GAL/HEHS-98-66, Washington, DC: US General Accounting Office.

US General Accounting Office. (2000). *Medicare+Choice: Payments exceed cost of fee-for-service benefits, adding billions to spending* (Rep. No. GAO/HEHS-00-161). Washington, DC: US General Accounting Office.

Yamamoto, D., Neuman, T., & Kitchman Strollo, M. (2008). *How does the benefit value of medicare compare to the benefit value of typical large employer plans?* Menlo Park, CA: Kaiser Family Foundation.

Waidmann, T. (1998). Potential effects of raising Medicare's eligibility age. *Health Affairs, 17,* 156–164.

Weiss, L., & Blustein, J. (1996). Faithful patients: The effect of long-term physician-patient relationships on the costs and use of health care by older Americans. *American Journal of Public Health, 86,* 1742–1747.

Chapter | 22 |

Long-Term Care Financing, Service Delivery, and Quality Assurance: The International Experience

Joshua M. Wiener
RTI International, Washington, DC

(Johnson et al., 2007). The US is not unique in this regard; most of the world will face a growing need for long-term care services, and issues regarding financing, service delivery, and quality of care will gain increasing policy prominence. In particular, the strong role of government financing makes long-term care a public policy issue in almost all high-income countries, including those in Europe and in Japan, Canada, Australia, and New Zealand (Organisation for Economic Co-operation and Development (OECD), 2005, 2006).

Although many of the fundamental issues are the same, compared with the US, other countries have a wide diversity of systems of financing and organizing long-term care and of ensuring quality of care. Unlike medical care, however, for which the US is an extreme outlier in terms of coverage and costs, the US is well within the normal range of variation among high-income countries for long-term care financing, service delivery, and quality assurance.

This chapter provides an overview of long-term care in other countries, with an emphasis on the United Kingdom, Germany, and Japan. After a brief discussion of international population aging, the chapter discusses financing, service delivery, and quality assurance. The chapter concludes with some reflections on the utility of comparative international research.

INTRODUCTION

The US is aging, and the number of older people with disabilities is sure to grow substantially. According to one estimate, the number of older people with disabilities will approximately double between 2000 and 2030

POPULATION AGING

Although disability affects people of all ages, disability rates increase with age (Steinmetz, 2006). As a result, an increase in the number of older people, especially persons aged 85 and older, is associated

DOI: 10.1016/B978-0-12-380880-6.00022-8

Table 22.1 Population aged 85 and older as a percentage of total population, selected high-income and middle-income countries, 2010 and 2050.

HIGH-INCOME COUNTRIES	2010	2050
Australia	1.9	4.8
Germany	2.4	7.5
Ireland	1.3	4.3
Netherlands	1.8	5.9
Spain	2.5	7.2
Sweden	2.7	5.9
United Kingdom	2.3	5.7
US	1.9	4.3
MIDDLE-INCOME COUNTRIES	**2010**	**2040**
Brazil	0.4	2.6
China	0.5	4.0
India	0.2	1.3
Mexico	0.6	3.0
Russia	1.0	5.0

Source: US Census Bureau (2009).

with an increased need for long-term care. In much of Europe, the proportion of the population aged 85 and older is higher than in the US (see Table 22.1). For example, in 2010, 1.9% of the US population was aged 85 and older, compared with 2.3% of the population in the United Kingdom, 2.4% of the population in Germany, and 2.7% of the population in Sweden. Moreover, although the figures vary across countries, in developed countries the proportion of the population aged 85 and older is likely to more than double between 2010 and 2050.

The aging of the population in the developed countries is well known; much less appreciated is that the population in middle-income countries is also aging rapidly. Indeed, the proportion of the population aged 85 and older in Brazil, China, India, Mexico, and Russia will more than quadruple between 2010 and 2050, bringing them to at least the 2010 level of the US or higher (US Census Bureau, 2009). Thus, increasingly, these countries will have to face the issues of long-term care, which are currently low on their policy agendas.

FINANCING

Long-term care financing differs among high-income countries across several dimensions. These

characteristics include how much of the economy is spent on long-term care, the extent to which care is publicly or privately financed, whether public programs are means-tested or provide universal coverage, whether responsibility for long-term care is a national or state and local government responsibility, and how the relationship between medical and long-term care is defined.

Background

Total long-term care expenditures are a modest portion of the economy, especially compared with overall health expenditures. Public and private long-term care expenditures for older people in many developed countries ranged from about 1.0% to 1.5% of GDP in 2000 (see Table 22.2). Sweden, at almost 3.0% of the GDP, was a high outlier. Although the US spends more on medical care overall than any other country, for long-term care it was about average among developed countries (about 1.29% of GDP in 2000).

Public or Private Financing

Whereas private spending for long-term care plays a role in long-term care financing in all high-income countries, public spending dominates expenditures. Not surprisingly, public spending plays a

Table 22.2 Total, public, and private long-term care expenditures for older people as a percentage of gross domestic product (GDP), selected high-income countries, 2000.

COUNTRY	PUBLIC	PRIVATE	TOTAL
Australia	0.86	0.33	1.19
Germany	0.95	0.40	1.35
Ireland	0.52	0.10	0.62
Netherlands	1.31	0.13	1.44
Spain	0.16	0.44	0.61
Sweden	2.74	0.14	2.89
United Kingdom	0.89	0.48	1.37
US	0.74	0.54	1.29

Source: Organisation for Economic Co-operation and Development (2005).

Table 22.3 Public long-term care expenditures as a percentage of GDP, selected high-income countries, 2005 and 2050 (low and high projections).

COUNTRY	2005	2050 – LOW	2050 – HIGH
Australia	0.9	2.0	2.5
Germany	1.0	2.2	2.9
Ireland	0.7	3.2	4.6
Netherlands	1.7	2.9	3.7
Spain	0.2	1.9	2.6
Sweden	3.3	3.4	4.3
United Kingdom	1.1	2.1	3.0
US	0.9	1.8	2.7

Source: Organisation for Economic Co-operation and Development (2006).

bigger proportional role in countries with public long-term care insurance or public provision, such as Sweden and the Netherlands, and less in countries with means-tested systems of financing, such as the United Kingdom and the US. Some countries, such as Germany, straddle the division between the public and private sector by relying on quasigovernmental insurance organizations that are technically private, nonprofit organizations, but that are very highly regulated and are financed through mandatory premium contributions (Cuellar & Wiener, 2000; Gibson & Redfoot, 2007). Recent projections suggest that the aging of the population and other factors will push up public spending for long-term care by an additional average 1.0–2.0% of the GDP between 2005 and 2050

in the OECD countries (including the US), which is a doubling or tripling of current public expenditures (see Table 22.3).

Private-sector financing for long-term care is almost entirely direct out-of-pocket payments or cost sharing for government-financed services rather than private long-term care insurance, although a modest market for private long-term care insurance exists in Germany and France (Cuellar & Wiener, 2000; Kessler, 2008). In Germany, about 11% of the population has private long-term care insurance, which higher-income individuals can choose as an alternative to the sickness fund system, but all Germans must be insured (German Federal Ministry of Health, 2009). Barriers to purchase of private long-term care insurance include the high cost, modest incomes of retired persons, and the reticence of the insurance industry to participate in what is thought to be a highly risky product.

Means Testing or Universal Coverage of Public Programs

Within public-sector programs, some countries have means-tested approaches whereas other countries have universal coverage programs. The philosophical premise in some countries is that the primary responsibility for care of older people and younger persons with disabilities belongs with individuals and their families and that government should act only as a payer of last resort for those unable to provide for themselves. Countries holding this view operate means-tested programs that limit public benefits to people who are poor or who become poor because of the high costs of medical and long-term care. The long-term care financing systems of the United Kingdom, New Zealand, and the US largely reflect this view (OECD, 2005).

In England, for example, primary funding for social care is through means-tested programs operated by local authorities. These programs operate as appropriated programs rather than as insurance or entitlement programs. Local authorities have substantial discretion over who is eligible, what type of cost sharing beneficiaries must pay, what services beneficiaries receive, and how providers are paid. In 2006, a single individual in a nursing home with about $41 600 (£21 000) in assets was eligible for government aid, but that figure included the person's house (Gleckman, 2009). In contrast, in the US, to be covered by the means-tested Medicaid program, a single individual residing in a nursing home generally cannot retain more than $2000 in financial assets, but the value of the person's house is usually excluded (Bruen et al., 2003). However, states are supposed to recover the costs of Medicaid long-term care spending from the estate of the beneficiary after death. Individuals in residential care homes in England must contribute all of their income, except for a personal needs allowance, towards the cost of care. In the US, Medicaid works similarly, except that the personal needs allowance is smaller.

The opposite philosophical approach is that the government should take the lead in ensuring that all people with disabilities, regardless of financial status, should be eligible for the long-term care services they need. In this type of system, social solidarity is highly valued and the right to long-term care is viewed similarly to the right to medical care. The long-term care financing systems of Germany, Japan, France, the Netherlands, and Sweden reflect this view (OECD, 2005).

In Germany, for example, the primary source of financing is through a universal social insurance program for long-term care (*Soziale Pfgeversicherung*) that provides nursing home and home care benefits for people of all ages who have disabilities (Campbell et al., 2010; Cuellar & Wiener, 2000; Gibson & Redfoot, 2007; Wiener & Cuellar, 1999). The insurance program is administered by sickness funds for 70 million Germans and, as noted above, by private health insurers for 10 million, mostly upper-income, individuals.

Unlike acute care insurance, in which contribution rates vary by insurer, long-term care insurance has one uniform contribution rate set in law: 1.95% of salary up to a fairly low maximum. The contribution rate is split equally by employers and employees. In a unique provision required by the courts, individuals without children pay a higher contribution rate because of their higher risk of using paid services due to their relative lack of access to informal care. Retirees pay the full contribution rate. As with Medicare in the US, the rate is set in law and does not automatically increase to match changes in costs. Because the premium is a percentage of salary, higher-income people pay more than lower-income people, but the premium is not technically progressive because the premium percentage is the same for all salary levels and the income subject to the premium is capped. Although the program has not had an explosion of costs since its implementation in 1994, expenditures have increased faster than revenues in recent years, due to relatively slow growth in revenues and a modest shift toward more expensive services (German Federal Ministry of Health, 2009; Gibson & Redfoot, 2007).

Eligibility for the insurance program is limited to persons with fairly severe functional disabilities and is determined by the medical offices of the sickness funds (Cuellar & Wiener, 2000). In 2007, about 30% of applicants were denied (Campbell et al., 2010). All individuals who meet the disability threshold are entitled to benefits; the benefit amounts vary by three levels of disability and by the location of care (in the community or in an institution). Although the program is geared toward older people, 21% of beneficiaries are under age 65. Persons choosing home and community-based services have an option of accepting cash instead of in-kind services; the amount of the cash benefit is half the maximum service benefit or less. In 2009, cash benefit levels varied from $250 to $794 per month, whereas the home and community-based service benefit was between $490 and $1730 per month. Cash benefits are lower than service benefits because there is no administrative overhead to pay and because the cash payment is meant primarily to be used as support for informal caregivers rather than to purchase services. No copayment is required for home and community-based services. The cost of the institutional benefit varied from $1200 to $1730 per month, not including room and board (German Federal Ministry of Health, 2009). From the program's inception in 1995 until 2008, the maximum expenditure level for each disability level was unchanged in nominal terms, which resulted in a substantial deterioration of the inflation-adjusted value of the benefit. For those for whom the benefit is not adequate to cover their needs, *laender* (state)-operated, means-tested, social assistance programs fill in the gaps.

In Japan, the primary source of financing is the government-operated long-term care insurance, *Kaigo Hoken* (Campbell & Ikegami, 2000, 2003; Campbell et al., 2010). The program pays for benefits for people who have disabilities and who are aged 65 or older, as well as for persons who are aged 40 or older and have an "aging-related" condition (such as early-onset Alzheimer's disease), a group added partly to justify charging premiums to the younger, working population. Younger people with disabilities, such as people with spinal cord injuries, are not covered by the insurance program. As a result of these restrictions, only about 3% of beneficiaries are under age 65 (Campbell et al., 2010). The insurance program is administered by the municipalities.

Financing for the Japanese long-term care insurance program is a mixture of general tax revenues and premiums. Half of the financing comes from general tax revenues from the national, prefecture, and municipal governments. The remaining financing is from mandatory insurance premiums. Persons aged 40 to 64 pay 1% of income, split between employees and employers, up to a ceiling. In addition, older people pay a smaller premium, which varies by income and is deducted from their government pension. The program is administered by the municipalities, who also act as the insurance carriers, although most policy decisions are made at the national level. The premiums for persons aged 40 to 64 are pooled at the national level and distributed to the municipalities on a formula basis related to demographics and income. As with Germany, expenditures have increased somewhat faster than revenues, which led to some trimming of program benefits in 2006 (Campbell et al., 2010).

Also as with Germany, the level of benefits varies by disability level, but Japan assigns beneficiaries to one of seven levels: two for a preventive care program and five for the regular long-term care insurance program (Campbell et al., 2010). All services are subject to a 10% coinsurance level, which is reduced to 3% for lower-income older people. In 2009, depending on the category, the maximum benefits varied from $430 to $950 per month for preventive services and from $1440 to $3400 per month for home and community-based services. The benefits for institutional care vary from $1680 to $3670 per month. On average, Japanese beneficiaries use about half the maximum benefit. The many case managers play an important role in helping to arrange services; they are viewed as providing services to beneficiaries rather than acting as gatekeepers for the program. To restrain rising costs – mostly related to a greater-than-expected number of people in the lowest disability categories – recent reforms transferred beneficiaries in the lower categories to a new, less expensive, preventive caregiving program with lower benefit ceilings and programming geared toward health and wellness.

Public or Private Provision

Although financing of long-term care is overwhelmingly by the public sector, service providers include a mix of government-run, nonprofit, and for-profit organizations. The issue of the "purchaser–provider split" is a major one in countries in which the public provision of services is important. In the US, about two-thirds of nursing homes are operated for profit, about one-quarter are nonprofit, and only about one-twentieth are government-owned (American Health Care Association, 2009). In contrast, in the so-called Scandinavian model, such as in Sweden, most providers are government agencies and institutions, although there has been movement toward privatization (Andersson & Karlberg, 2000; Swedish Ministry of Health and Social Affairs, 2007). The goal of government ownership is to provide care without consideration of whether an activity is profitable. In England, local authorities traditionally ran care homes, but the number of private for-profit facilities exploded during the 1980s and 1990s, leaving government facilities with fewer than 10% of all care homes (United Kingdom Commission for Social Care Inspection, 2009). The theory motivating this privatization is that competing organizations will provide more choice to consumers at lower cost, with more flexibility, and with greater consumer orientation.

Devolution or National Programs

A key issue in the design of long-term care systems is the level of government responsible for financing and delivery. Many developed countries, including the US, the United Kingdom, Sweden, the Netherlands, and Canada, rely heavily on subnational governments to design and administer their long-term care systems, albeit often with substantial policy guidance from the national government. For example, Sweden devolves virtually all responsibility for the financing, organization, and administration of long-term care to 289 municipalities, even though it is a small country with fewer than 10 million people (Swedish Ministry of Health and Social Affairs, 2007).

Advocates for devolution make three arguments in favor of assigning responsibility for long-term care to smaller geographic governmental units (Wiener, 1996a). First, states, provinces, and municipalities are heavily involved with a variety of social services in many countries. Thus, a local approach can establish needed linkages between long-term care and other services often needed by people with disabilities. Second, long-term care is an intensely personal issue involving decisions about how consumers want to live their lives. Thus, the planning and delivery of services can be influenced by local circumstances, norms, and values as well as by the local preferences of the disabled population, their caregivers, and providers. And, finally, because subnational governments are less driven to routinize their decision making process and because individual cases loom larger in the policy process, locally administered programs are arguably less rigid and bureaucratic than centrally run programs.

At the other end of the continuum are countries such as Germany and Japan, which have a more nationalized and centralized approach to long-term care, although subnational governmental entities are often still involved. For example, under the long-term care insurance program in Japan, 2895 municipal governments or alliances of municipalities are the insurers; they have a generalized responsibility to provide adequate services (Campbell & Ikegami, 2000, 2003; Ikegami & Campbell, 2008). However, because almost all aspects of the program – eligibility, most benefits, and reimbursement rates – are fixed at the national level, the ability of the municipalities to shape the program is strictly limited. Thus, although premiums are set at the municipal level, almost all parameters of the financing are set at the national level.

Two main arguments favor consolidation at the national level (Wiener, 1996a). First, a uniform national program helps to guarantee horizontal equity across geographic areas. In other words, national rules help ensure that similarly situated individuals in different geographic areas are treated similarly. In England, for example, which relies on subnational governmental units, beneficiaries often complain of a "postcode lottery," in which persons with similar needs and financial status are treated very differently because they are subject to different local authorities (Wiener & Cuellar, 1999). Uniform national programs minimize the undesirable variations in access to services that exist with more decentralized programs. In countries with insurance approaches, such as Germany, regional variations are thought to be unfair and efforts are made to eliminate them (Cuellar & Wiener, 2000). Second, developing a single national program may involve less administrative expense because program rules and systems need to be developed only once; each subnational governmental unit need not reinvent the wheel.

Relationship to Medical the Care System

Across almost all countries, individuals with disabilities have fragmented financing and delivery systems

that separate medical and long-term care services. In the US, for example, acute care for older and disabled persons is primarily the responsibility of the federal government and the Medicare program, whereas long-term care is primarily the domain of states and the Medicaid program for the poor (Wiener, 1996b). On the one hand, fragmentation makes integrating acute and long-term care difficult; on the other hand, a separate long-term care program helps to protect funding for these services and militates against the unnecessary medicalization of long-term care.

As in the US, in the Netherlands, Japan, Germany, Sweden, and the United Kingdom, long-term care is financed and organized apart from acute care. In many countries, including Belgium, France, Italy, Portugal, Spain, and the United Kingdom, the "medical" component of home care is part of the health care system; the "social" component is part of the social service system (WHO, 2008).

In the United Kingdom, for example, medical care services are provided through the National Health Service, a tax-financed system of private physicians and public hospitals. The National Health Service is also responsible for paying for skilled nursing services in nursing homes. In contrast, long-term care is financed and managed through local authorities, which are subnational governmental units, often roughly equivalent to counties in size. Whereas services are available from the National Health Service free at the point of use, long-term care services are means-tested. Without the administrative structures of managed care organizations through which a single entity can receive funds for both health and long-term care services for an enrolled individual, integration initiatives have focused on joint commissioning between the National Health Service and local authorities' social services departments (Goodwin, 2007).

Japan also separates its long-term care insurance from its acute care insurance, but provides some medical care in its long-term care benefits and continues to provide a substantial amount of institutional long-term care through its medical care insurance (Campbell et al., 2010). Several medical services are included in the list of covered services under long-term care insurance, including visiting nurses and rehabilitation. The long-term care insurance program also covers physician supervision, but the benefit is not very widely used, in part because no natural relationship exists between family doctors and care managers.

Before the introduction of the long-term care insurance program, hospitals were major providers of institutional care, in part because older people paid little in out-of-pocket costs for these services. A major goal of the insurance program is to convert hospitals that functioned primarily as nursing homes to long-term care beds. This conversion has been slower than expected, partially because it is more prestigious to be a hospital than a nursing home.

Sweden places responsibility for acute care at the county level and that for long-term care at the municipal level (Swedish Ministry of Health and Social Affairs, 2007). The reduction of backlogs in hospitals was the major impetus for the Adel reforms of 1992 (*Ädelreformen*), which consolidated responsibilities for long-term care and for older people in hospitals who no longer need a hospital level of care at the municipal level. Backlogged hospital patients were primarily people waiting for nursing home care, home care, or rehabilitation. The reforms reduced the number of people backlogged in hospitals by providing a strong financial incentive for municipalities to use their long-term care resources to find lower-cost placements for patients unnecessarily waiting in hospitals.

SERVICE DELIVERY

As in the US, most high-income countries are pursuing policies to increase the role played by home and community-based services and reduce the role played by institutions. Most countries have declared their intention to help older people "age in place"; that is, to help them to the extent possible to remain in their own homes if they become disabled or at least to live in residential settings that are not institutional in character (OECD, 2005; WHO, 2008). For example, in England the goal is "care at home, not care in a home," and in Germany the main principle of reform is "priority of care in the home over institutional care" (Wiener & Cuellar, 1999).

The rationale for this policy direction has at least four components (WHO, 2008). First, people with

disabilities prefer home and community-based services to institutional care. Second, people with disabilities living in the community have substantial unmet needs for personal care and other home and community-based services. Third, the quality of home and community-based services is believed to be superior to that of nursing home care. Fourth, and most controversially, home and community-based services are believed to be less costly than institutional care (Grabowski, 2006; Kaye et al., 2009).

Distribution of Expenditures between Home and Community-Based Services and Nursing Homes

Countries vary in the proportion of their long-term care expenditures for older people that are directed to home and community-based services (see Table 22.4). In 2000, home care accounted for more than 30% of public spending on long-term care in many countries in the OECD. Notably, Sweden and the Netherlands, which spend more of their GDP on home care than any other country, also spend very substantial amounts on institutional care. Thus, a direct tradeoff between institutional and noninstitutional care does not always exist.

Some countries seek to change the balance between institutional and noninstitutional care by spending more on community care (e.g. Germany and Japan), whereas other countries are more focused on reallocating funds from nursing homes to home care. As a way of emphasizing the tradeoffs between the two types of care, one of the goals of the Community Care Act of 1990 in England was to make one governmental entity

Table 22.4 Total, home care, and institutional care expenditures for older people as a percentage of GDP, selected high-income countries, 2000.

COUNTRY	HOME CARE	INSTITUTIONS	TOTAL
Australia	0.38	0.81	1.19
Germany	0.47	0.88	1.35
Ireland	0.19	0.43	0.62
Netherlands	0.60	0.83	1.44
Spain	0.23	0.37	0.61
Sweden	0.82	2.07	2.89
United Kingdom	0.41	0.96	1.37
US	0.33	0.96	1.29

Source: Organisation for Economic Co-operation and Development (2005).

(i.e. the local authorities) responsible for both institutional and community-based services (Wiener & Cuellar, 1999).

A number of countries have taken steps to make more intensive home care available as an alternative to nursing home care. In the US, home care funding is increasingly through Medicaid home and community-based services waivers, which are limited to people who need nursing home level of care (Wiener & Anderson, 2009). Similarly, Australia provides "aged care packages" and an Extended Aged Care at Home program as a community alternative for older people needing institutional care (OECD, 2005). Sweden and the United Kingdom have also developed a more targeted approach, providing more hours of care to a more limited number of people.

Despite government policy to emphasize home and community-based services, changes in financing sometimes work in the opposite direction. For example, use of nursing homes increased in Germany after introduction of the long-term care insurance program and would have increased in Japan were it not for capital controls that limited the supply of nursing homes (Campbell et al., 2010). Although older people resist using nursing homes, such facilities in these two countries appear to be "normal goods" in that use goes up when out-of-pocket prices go down.

Consumer Direction

A key issue in the design of home and community services programs is the extent to which clients control their services. Traditional public home care programs rely on public or private agencies that are responsible for hiring and firing home care workers, scheduling and directing services, monitoring quality of care, disciplining workers if necessary, and paying workers and applicable taxes. In the agency-directed model, clients can express preferences for services or workers but have no formal control over them.

A major innovation in long-term care in the US and Europe is the development of consumer-directed home care (Lundsgaard, 2005; Wiener et al., 2003). These programs represent the other end of the management continuum; they give consumers, rather than home care agencies, control over who provides services, when they are provided, and how they are delivered. Typically, consumer-directed programs allow the consumer to hire, train, supervise, and fire the home care worker. In some programs, beneficiaries receive cash payments enabling them to purchase the services they want. In the US, consumer-directed care is strongly supported by the national government's CMS, but adoption of this approach is up to the states (O'Keeffe et al., 2009).

Consumers in an increasing number of countries, including the Netherlands, Norway, Sweden, the United Kingdom, Germany, and Luxembourg, have a choice between agency-directed and consumer-directed home care (Lundsgaard, 2005). In Austria, all home and community-based services are funded through a cash allowances for care program (*Pflegegeld*). Of these countries, only in Germany, Austria, and Luxembourg do a substantial proportion of home care beneficiaries receive consumer-directed care, although its use is growing. In England, local authorities must explicitly offer consumer-directed care as an option to consumers. In Germany, the overwhelming majority of noninstitutional beneficiaries opt for consumer-directed care. In Germany in 2008, 62% of home care expenditures – and 79% of home care beneficiaries – were for the cash allowance rather than in-kind services (German Federal Ministry of Health, 2009). In the Netherlands, about 20% of older people and younger persons with physical disabilities receiving home care used consumer-directed care for at least part of their needs in 2008 (Netherlands Ministry of Health, Welfare and Sport, 2009). Especially in the Netherlands, consumer-directed home care (and the use of family caregivers) has grown, in part as a frustrated response to the waiting lists for agency-provided care.

The countries differ in how they structure their consumer-directed options (Wiener et al., 2003). In the Netherlands and England, clients are provided funds ("personal budgets" in the Netherlands and "direct payments" in England) that they must use for home and community services. In Germany, clients receive uniform levels of cash payments, based on their level of disability, which they may spend on anything they like. The cash payments are mostly used to support informal caregivers, and few formal services are purchased.

Contrary to the expectations of some observers, consumer-directed home care in these three countries is used by older as well as younger persons with disabilities (although less so in England) and by people with severe as well as mild disabilities. Indeed, all three countries allow some cognitively impaired persons to participate in these programs, relying on surrogates to make the decisions for the consumers when necessary.

Despite concern by some observers about the capability of people with disabilities to handle the management tasks, England, Germany, and the Netherlands provide only modest help to clients to cope with the administrative tasks inherent in consumer direction, leaving clients mostly to find their own way. The Netherlands and England provide the most help with handling social insurance and other taxes and paying the worker; because few people are formally "hired" in the German system, very little formal assistance is provided.

Although much of the policy interest in consumer-directed home care derives from a desire to empower people with disabilities and give them more control over their lives, this approach is also attractive to governments because of its lower per-person costs. Payment rates for consumer-directed care are much lower than for agency care, partly because the cost of administrative overhead, which can be substantial for agencies, is little or nothing. However, the increase in use for consumer-directed care may offset the per-person savings.

Despite the potential for savings, many issues remain. Labor force issues are a major component of the dynamics of consumer-directed home care. Reflecting the more developed social protections in European countries, consumer-directed home care workers have higher wages and far better fringe benefits than similar workers in the US. Moreover, while independent workers in these countries are compensated better than American workers, they tend to do less well financially than at least a significant segment of agency workers in other countries. Fringe benefits for home care workers improve their lives but add significantly to the cost of services.

In the Netherlands and Germany, a substantial portion of paid caregivers in consumer-directed care are family members. In England, payments cannot normally be used to pay for services from a spouse, partner, or close relative (or their spouse or partner) living in the household (Disability Alliance, 2009). Japan consciously chose not to offer consumer-directed care because they did not want to create incentives to further burden informal caregivers by having them provide paid care (Campbell & Ikegami, 2000, 2003).

Probably the most contentious issue surrounding consumer-directed programs in the US is whether quality of care is adequate and how services are monitored. Compared with agency-directed care, consumer-directed services lack the standard quality assurance structures of training of paraprofessionals, supervision by professionals, and provision of technical services by professionals. Despite some concerns about quality of services, England, Germany, and the Netherlands take minimalist approaches to monitoring quality. In place of formal quality assurance mechanisms, consumer-directed programs generally rely on the ability of clients to fire unsatisfactory workers and to hire replacements to ensure quality – in other words, the market. In addition, at least in Germany and the Netherlands, they rely on the strength of family ties and the notion that relatives are much more likely than strangers to provide high-quality care. The adage that "blood is thicker than water" may account for some of the countries' relatively laissez-faire approach to program management.

The use of informal caregivers also illustrates the conflict between equity and efficiency. For example, Germany's cash payments can be justified on an equity basis in that they make family caregivers better off. On moral grounds, policymakers want to reward informal caregivers for their sacrifices. But, from an efficiency perspective, the sickness funds are spending a great deal of money without causing a large change in behavior. Extensive informal care is being provided now in Germany – just as it was before the cash benefit was introduced. For people receiving the cash benefit, it is not clear that much has changed in terms of care arrangements.

Support for Informal Caregivers

Informal care – unpaid care by relatives and friends – is the dominant form of care of disabled persons throughout the world, despite the considerable burdens that it places on those who do it (Wiener, 2003). Paid services, either at home or in institutions, play a relatively small role, except in a few countries. Yet, modern society – especially with its trend toward smaller families, greater longevity, separate and more independent living situations for older people, greater freedom for women, and workplaces that are separate from home – places strain on the traditional mechanisms of providing unpaid care. Because of the potential fiscal and care implications of a decline in the supply of informal care, public policymakers want to ensure that this resource is maintained.

Support for informal caregivers takes many forms. In the US, public support for family caregivers is fairly modest. The National Family Caregiver Support Program, funded by the Older Americans Act, provides very limited funding for services. Consumer-directed home care programs in the US almost always allow beneficiaries to hire family members as paid caregivers, except for spouses and parents of minor children. And, finally, workers in larger firms are entitled to up to 12 weeks of unpaid family leave to care for a family member with a serious health condition. In Belgium and the Netherlands, employees may take a break from work to care for relatives, during which time they receive a limited stipend (Pilj, 2003).

Aside from consumer-directed home care, countries have adopted a variety of strategies to support informal caregivers (OECD, 2005). A few countries, such as the United Kingdom, provide an assessment of need to "carers" as well as to persons with disabilities, although local authorities are not required to provide any services as a result of that assessment. Some countries, including Germany and the United Kingdom, give public pension credits to partially compensate people who leave their jobs because of caregiving responsibilities. For example, in Germany, if a family member provides at least 14 hours of care a week, long-term care insurance covers their social security premiums (Gibson & Redfoot, 2007). In the United Kingdom, a "carer's allowance" provides modest government financial support for low-income informal caregivers who provide at least 35 hours a week of caregiving. One aim of these provisions is to make the role of primary caregiver less financially burdensome.

Finally, in many countries, formal respite care is one of the available services, although it is often $$ whether these services serve primarily the person with disabilities or the informal caregiver. In Germany, informal caregivers who provide a lot of care are entitled to respite care for a vacation.

QUALITY ASSURANCE

Concern about poor quality of care by nursing homes in the US is longstanding (US Government Accountability Office, 2007, 2009; Wiener et al., 2007a). In addition, one of the key policy rationales for expanding home and community-based services is that the quality of life for beneficiaries is better than in nursing homes. However, little is actually known about the quality of home and community services, even though increasing numbers of people are receiving paid care in those settings. The US is not alone in its unease about inadequate care for people with disabilities (OECD, 2005).

In general, the American quality assurance system is dominated by an adversarial, regulatory system (Wiener et al., 2007a). To receive Medicare and Medicaid reimbursement, nursing homes and home health agencies must meet federal quality standards. Nursing homes are also licensed by the states, as are home health agencies in some states. Inspections of nursing homes and home health agencies are performed about once a year by the states on behalf of the federal government. Enforcement options include suspending admissions and decertifying from participation in the Medicare and Medicaid program, but the most common remedy is for the facility to devise a "plan of correction." Quality regulation for nonmedical home care and residential care facilities, such as assisted living facilities, is the responsibility of the states. In general, these services are more lightly regulated than nursing homes. Over the past 10 years, however, regulation of residential care facilities, such as assisted living, has increased (Mollica et al., 2008).

To make the market work better, the federal government promotes nonregulatory approaches to quality assurance. The US collects a great deal of resident-specific health and functional data on nursing home residents and home health patients, which the government uses to create quantitative quality measures that are posted on the Internet for each facility or agency. Importantly, no other country has invested in a similar effort to collect such detailed resident- and patient-specific data to develop quantitative measures of quality for nursing homes and home health agencies. Similar data are not available for nonmedical home and community services. In addition, although not actively promoted by the government, quality initiatives that change the organizational culture of nursing homes to make them more homelike are popular among consumer advocates and some providers (Koren, 2010).

Quality assurance systems in England, Australia, Germany, and Japan differ in philosophy and approach (see Wiener et al., 2007b; Table 22.5). In England, regulation of publicly funded services is a philosophically important component of New Labor's "third way." Regulation seeks to enhance the "steering" rather than the "rowing" capacity of the central government (Osborne & Gaebler, 1992). Regulation provides a way of controlling the quality of long-term care without having to directly operate the services. Thus, it stands between unbridled laissez-faire markets and direct public ownership. England is probably most like the US in its emphasis on regulation to force compliance with national standards for nursing homes while allowing localities to impose additional quality standards. The regulatory agency, which is a quasigovernmental organization, is aggressively reforming the inspection process with the goal of making the system more client- and outcome-oriented. The placement of the regulatory agency at the national level and outside of the Department of Health is a conscious decision to "long-arm" the relationship between payers and quality regulators. Both residential care homes and home care are regulated and regularly inspected; results are posted on the Internet according to a star-rating system that predates the one in the US. In addition, England has an explicit national strategy for regulating and improving the workforce in all long-term care settings and for disseminating best practices.

In contrast to the English and American approach of regulation as policing, the Australian system for quality assurance relies heavily on consultation and collaboration between the industry, governmental, and quasi-governmental officials. This collaborative approach is made easier by the fact that about two-thirds of nursing homes and hostels and virtually all home care agencies are nonprofit or government-owned. Inspections of residential care are carried out by a quasigovernmental accrediting agency, but approving providers to receive public funds and enforcing quality standards remains a fully governmental responsibility. The Australian quality standards for institutional care are very broad and nonspecific to allow providers considerable latitude in demonstrating how they achieve quality goals. Although detailed resident-assessment data are collected, the information is used for payment purposes and not for quality monitoring. Quality assurance for home and community-based care is more decentralized and has been implemented only recently.

Although German states (*laender*) regulate nursing homes, Germany's quality assurance approach increasingly relies on the national sickness funds to negotiate quality standards as part of contracts with providers. These contracts articulate general expectations of provider quality as well as of the structures and processes that providers should have to monitor and improve quality. Thus, in principle, quality assurance is increasingly about enforcing contracts rather

Table 22.5 Overview of long-term care quality assurance systems in England, Australia, Germany, Japan, and the United States.

	ENGLAND	AUSTRALIA	GERMANY	JAPAN	UNITED STATES
Extent to which quality is perceived as a problem	High	Low	Medium	Low	High for nursing homes, low for HCBS
Overall approach	Regulation (under-going reform)	Consultation and collaboration	Enforcement of contracts and consultation	Regulation, group processes, and workforce training	Regulation (and consumer information)
National or subnational responsibility for quality assurance	National	National for institutions, shared national and state/territories for HCBS	Sickness funds dominate, but Laender (states) license nursing homes	National standards for nursing homes; prefectures perform inspections	National standards for nursing homes and home health with state inspections; state standards and inspections for HCBS
Separation of quality assurance from payers	Yes	Yes for institutions, no for HCBS	No	No	No requirement, but health departments, which inspect nursing homes and home health agencies, are typically separate from Medicaid
Use of private third-party evaluation	No	No	Voluntary accreditation used by small percentage of nursing homes	Third-party evaluation required for group home for dementia care	Voluntary accreditation used by small percentage of nursing homes and assisted-living residences
Use of quasigovernmental agencies	Yes	Yes	No	No	No
Institutions					
Inspection frequency	Varies by quality, at least once every three years	Varies by quality, most once every three years	Varies by sickness funds, some not yet inspected	Annually, but on-site inspection only every other year	Annually
Detail of standards	Medium	Low	Varies	High	High
Use of strong enforcement, such as freezing admissions	Infrequent	Infrequent	Infrequent	Infrequent	Infrequent
Home care regulation	Recent, but same framework as institutions; consumer-directed care and assisted living excluded	Recent, but regular	Low priority for sickness funds	Almost nonexistent for home care; regulation for assisted living and Alzheimer's group homes	Varies by state, but much less than nursing homes
Alternative strategies to ensure quality	Regulation of workforce; dissemination of best practices; inspection results on Internet	Education of providers; inspection results on Internet but not consumer-friendly	Development of protocols; workforce training, demonstrations; no data on Internet	Care managers; workforce training and focus; some information on Internet	Inspection results and resident/patient quality indicators on Internet for nursing homes and home health agencies
Detailed health and functional data collected and used for quality indicators	No	Data collected for reimbursement of institutions but not used for quality indicators	No	No	Yes for nursing home residents and home health patients; limited data for HCBS users

Source: Wiener et al., 2007b.
HCBS = home and community-based services.

than assessing whether providers meet some minimum regulatory standard. Home care is not regulated very much. Developing a consensus between providers and payers is important to this contractual process, but consumers are not much involved.

Japan's implementation of its public long-term care insurance program in 2000 provided additional resources to improve the quality of institutional and home care services, as opposed to simply policing providers. Although formal quality assurance mechanisms are now more prominent, the Japanese system relies heavily on training and certification to develop the skills of long-term care workers, on regular communications from the government and among providers to motivate and disseminate best practices, and on care managers to help clients and ensure quality. In addition, new competition among providers, especially home and community-based services agencies, gives consumers a voice in quality assurance through greater choice in providers. In principle, the same mechanisms should also apply to institutional care, but in practice the long waiting lists for nursing homes limit competition.

THE UTILITY OF LOOKING BEYOND OUR BORDERS

As the population ages, long-term care is an issue of worldwide concern, now and for the future, in both high-income, developed countries and middle-income, developing countries. On the basis of their historical backgrounds, cultural traditions, and governmental structures, countries vary in their approaches to financing and organizing long-term care and to ensuring adequate quality.

Although debate over American social policy tends to ignore the experience of other countries because of the belief in American exceptionalism, several advantages can be realized by examining the experiences of other countries. First, an analysis of other long-term care systems emphasizes the commonality of problems across societies, stressing that we are not alone in coping with the challenges of long-term care. Second, although the problems are similar, other countries come to problems with a different set of assumptions about how they should be solved. Thus, analysis of how other countries address common issues provides an opportunity to think creatively and to identify new approaches that could be tried in the US. Third, some initiatives that have been only proposed and debated in the US have actually been implemented in other countries. Other countries, then, offer some insight as to what might happen if these programs and policies were implemented here. And, fourth, comparative analysis can highlight unique and important characteristics of the US system in comparison with other countries. The debate on the future of long-term care in the US would be enriched with more understanding of how the rest of the world addresses the problems of long-term care.

REFERENCES

American Health Care Association (2009). *Nursing facility ownership: CMS-OSCAR data current surveys, December 2009*. Washington, DC: American Health Care Association.

Andersson, G., & Karlberg, I. (2000). Integrated care for the elderly: The background and effects of the reform of Swedish care of the elderly. *International Journal of Integrated Care, 1*(October–December).

Bruen, B., Wiener, J. M., & Thomas, S. (2003). *In brief: Medicaid eligibility for aged, blind and disabled beneficiaries*. Washington, DC: AARP.

Campbell, J. C., & Ikegami, N. (2000). Long-term care insurance comes to Japan. *Health Affairs, 19*(3), 26–39.

Campbell, J. C., & Ikegami, N. (2003). Japan's radical reform of long-term care. *Social Policy & Administration, 37*, 21–34.

Campbell, J. C., Ikegami, N., & Gibson, M. J. (2010). Lessons from public long-term care insurance in Germany and Japan. *Health Affairs, 29*, 87–95.

Cuellar, A. E., & Wiener, J. M. (2000). Can social insurance for long-term care work? The case of Germany. *Health Affairs, 19*(3), 8–25.

Disability Alliance. (2009). Community care direct payments factsheet. Retrieved January 18, 2010, from http://www.disabilityalliance.org/f5.htm

German Federal Ministry of Health. (2009). Selected facts and figures on long-term care insurance (7/09). Retrieved January 18, 2010, from http://www.bmg.bund.de/SharedDocs/Downloads/EN/Long-term-care-insurance/pdf-Selected-Facts-and-Figures--07-2009-pdf,templateId=raw, property=publicationFile.pdf/pdf-Selected-Facts-and-Figures--07-2009-pdf.pdf

Gibson, M. J., & Redfoot, D. L. (2007). *Comparing long-term care in Germany and the United States: What can we learn from each other?* (Report No. 2007-19). Washington, DC: AARP Public Policy Institute.

Gleckman, H. (2009). *Caring for our parents: Inspiring stories of families seeking new solutions to America's most urgent health crisis*. New York: St. Martin's Press.

Goodwin, N. (2007). Developing effective joint commissioning between health and social care: Prospects for the future based on lessons from the past. *Journal of Care Services Management, 1,* 279–293.

Grabowski, D. C. (2006). The cost-effectiveness of noninstitutional long-term care services: Review and synthesis of the most recent evidence. *Medical Care Research and Review, 63*(1), 3–28.

Ikegami, N., & Campbell, J. C. (2008). Dealing with the medical axis-of-power: The case of Japan. *Health Economics, Policy and Law, 3,* 107–113.

Johnson, R. W., Toohey, D., & Wiener, J. M. (2007). *Meeting the long-term care needs of the baby boomers: How changing families will affect paid helpers and institutions.* Washington, DC: The Urban Institute.

Kaye, H. S., LaPlante, M. P., & Harrington, C. (2009). Do noninstitutional long-term care services reduce Medicaid spending? *Health Affairs, 28*(1), 262–272.

Kessler, D. (2008). The long-term care insurance market. *The Geneva Papers on Risk and Insurance—Issues and Practice, 33,* 33–40.

Koren, M. J. (2010). Person-centered care for nursing home residents: The culture change movement. *Health Affairs.* Retrieved January 23, 2010, from http://content. healthaffairs.org/cgi/reprint/ hlthaff.2009.0966v1 doi:10.1377/ hlthaff.2009.0966

Lundsgaard, J. (2005, May). *Consumer direction and choice in long-term care for older persons, including payments for informal care: How can it help improve care outcomes, employment and fiscal sustainability?* (OECD Health Working Papers No. 20). Paris: Organisation for Economic Co-operation and Development. Retrieved January 18, 2010, from http://www.oecd.org/ dataoecd/53/62/34897775.pdf

Mollica, R., Sims-Kastelein, K., & O'Keeffe, J. (2008). *Residential care and assisted living compendium: 2007.* Washington, DC: US Department of Health and Human Services, Office of the Assistant Secretary for Planning and Evaluation, Office of Disability, Aging and Long-Term Care Policy. Retrieved January 10, 2010, from

http://aspe.hhs.gov/daltcp/ reports/2007/07alcom.htm.

Netherlands Ministry of Health, Welfare and Sport. (2009, February). *Host country report: Long-term care in the Netherlands: The Exceptional Medical Expenses Act.* Utrecht: Netherlands Ministry of Health, Welfare and Sport. Retrieved January 19, 2010, from http://www.minvws.nl/en/folders/ lz/2009/host-country-report.asp

O'Keeffe, J., Harahan, M. F., O'Keeffe, C., & Anderson, W. L. (2009). *Real choice systems change grant program: FY 2001 to FY 2004 Systems change grants: Summary final report.* Research Triangle Park, NC: RTI International. Retrieved January 18, 2010, from http://www.hcbs. org/moreInfo.php/source/151/ doc/2706/Real_Choice_Systems_ Change_Grant_Program_-_ FY_2001

Organisation for Economic Co-operation and Development (2005). *Long-term care for older people.* Paris: Organisation for Economic Co-operation and Development.

Organisation for Economic Co-operation and Development (2006). *Projecting OECD health and long-term care expenditures: What are the main drivers?* (OECD Economics Department Working Papers No. 477). Paris: Organisation for Economic Co-operation and Development. Retrieved January 20, 2010, from http://titania. sourceoecd.org/vl=19312462/ cl=22/nw=1/rpsv/cgi-bin/ wppdf?file=5l9x36wg1cxs.pdf

Osborne, D., & Gaebler, T. (1992). *Reinventing government: How the entrepreneurial spirit is transforming the public sector.* Boston: Addison-Wesley.

Pilj, M. (2003). The support of carers and their organizations in some northern and western European countries: The role of informal support in long-term care. In J. Brodsky, J. Habib & M. J. Hirschfeld (Eds.), *Key policy issues in long-term care* (pp. 25–60). Geneva, Switzerland: World Health Organization.

Steinmetz, E. (2006). *Americans with disabilities: 2002* (Current Population Reports No. P70-107). Washington, DC: US Department

of Commerce, Economics and Statistics Administration, US Census Bureau.

Swedish Ministry of Health and Social Affairs. (2007). Care of the elderly in Sweden. Stockholm: Swedish Ministry of Health and Social Affairs. Retrieved January 23, 2010, from http:// www.sweden.gov.se/content/1/ c6/08/76/73/a43fc24d.pdf

United Kingdom Commission for Social Care Inspection. (2009). *The state of social care in England.* London, UK: United Kingdom Commission for Social Care Inspection. Retrieved January 26, 2010, from http:// www.dhcarenetworks.org. uk/_library/Resources/Housing/ Support_materials/Other_reports_ and_guidance/The_state_of_social_ care_in_England_2007-08.pdf.

US Census Bureau. (2009). *International data base.* Washington, DC: US Census Bureau. Retrieved January 19, 2010, from http://www.census. gov/ipc/www/idb/index.php

US Government Accountability Office. (2007). *Nursing homes: Efforts to strengthen federal enforcement have not deterred some homes from repeatedly harming residents* (Report No. GAO-07-241). Washington, DC: US Government Accountability Office.

US Government Accountability Office. (2009). *Nursing homes: Opportunities exist to facilitate the use of the temporary management sanction* (Report No. GAO-10-37R). Washington, DC: US Government Accountability Office.

Wiener, J. M. (1996a). Long-term care reform: An international perspective. In *Health Care Reform: The will to change* (pp. 67–79). Health Policy Studies No. 8. Paris: Organisation for Economic Cooperation and Development.

Wiener, J. M. (1996b). Managed care and long-term care: The integration of services and financing. *Generations, 20*(2), 47–52.

Wiener, J. M. (2003). The role of informal support in long-term care. In J. Brodsky, J. Habib & M. J. Hirschfeld (Eds.), *Key policy issues in long-term care* (pp. 3–24). Geneva: World Health Organization.

Wiener, J. M., & Anderson, W. L. (2009). *Follow the money: Financing home and community-based services*. Pittsburgh, PA: University of Pittsburgh.

Wiener, J. M., & Cuellar, A. E. (1999). Public and private responsibilities: Home and community-based services in the United Kingdom and Germany. *Journal of Aging and Health, 11*, 417–444.

Wiener, J. M., Freiman, M. P., & Brown, D. (2007a). *Strategies for improving the quality of long-term care*. Washington, DC: National Commission for Quality Long-Term Care.

Wiener, J. M., Tilly, J., & Cuellar, A. E. (2003). *Consumer-directed home care in the Netherlands, Germany, and England*. Washington, DC: AARP.

Wiener, J. M., Tilly, J., Cuellar, A. E., Howe, A., Doyle, C., Campbell, J., et al. (2007b). *Quality assurance for long-term care: The experiences of England, Australia, Germany, and Japan*. Washington, DC: AARP Public Policy Institute.

World Health Organization (2008). *The solid facts: Home care in Europe*. Geneva, Switzerland: World Health Organization.

Chapter | 23 |

Gender, Aging, and Social Policy

Madonna Harrington Meyer[1], Wendy M. Parker[2]

[1]*Center for Policy Research, Syracuse University, Syracuse, New York,* [2]*Albany College of Pharmacy and Health Sciences, Albany, New York*

INTRODUCTION

Are gender differences in old age disappearing in the US? At times it seems they might. For example, in 2008, political representation of women in the US Congress reached an all-time high, with 74 of the 435 members of the House of Representatives, and 17 of the 100 senators, being women (Frantz, 2008; US Senate, 2009). Increasing visibility of women in high-status and high-powered positions demonstrates just how far women have come. But the fact that women comprise 52% of the voting age population, and only 17% of the House and Senate representatives, suggests just how far women still have to go.

Despite dramatic social, economic, and political changes, one point remains constant: being an older woman is a fundamentally different experience from being an older man. The US has undergone substantial social and demographic changes over the last several decades, and many of the gender gaps have narrowed. Nonetheless, increasing numbers of women are raising children outside of marriage, women continue to perform a disproportionate share of unpaid care work at home, and women continue to receive lower rates of pay in the labor force. Women reach old age with fewer resources and more health problems. They also live significantly longer than men; thus, they are more likely to experience many of the difficulties associated with aging. While government old age income and health programs provide important resources, they may not sufficiently address some of the key concerns of older women.

This chapter reviews the theoretical, empirical, and policy-related research on gender differences in old age in the US. After laying out various theoretical perspectives, we summarize two key socio-demographic trends – changes in marriage and care work – that shape gender differences in old age. We then examine gender differences in income and health, and explore the degree to which these are, or are not, addressed by current old age policies in the US. Finally, we evaluate some policy solutions that could reduce gender inequality in old age.

THEORETICAL PERSPECTIVES

When analyzing gender inequality, old age scholars tend to highlight how social and economic factors

DOI: 10.1016/B978-0-12-380880-6.00023-X

constrain individual actions across the life course. An emphasis on life course highlights the cumulative effects of various choices, opportunities, policies, and programs at different stages of life (Moen & Spencer, 2006; Settersten, 2003). For example, when women take time out from work to raise children, an immediate consequence is loss of salary, but long-term consequences include reduced access to, or lower pay outs from, public pensions, private pensions, and savings. A cumulative (dis)advantage perspective points out that advantages and disadvantages accumulate across the life course, generating even greater inequalities in old age. These advantages and disadvantages are not randomly distributed; they are linked to gender, race, class, and marital status (Acker, 2006; Baca Zinn & Thornton Dill, 2005; Dannefer, 2003; Lorber, 2005; Settersten, 2003). The impact of cumulative disadvantage is especially evident among older, single, black, and Hispanic women, whose poverty rates approach 40% and whose health outcomes are significantly lower than for any other age group (National Center for Health Statistics, 2007; US Census Bureau, 2006).

Theorists and policy analysts alike debate how government programs and policies might best be used to reduce the resulting inequalities. Some favor dismantling the existing programs and relying on families and markets to provide for the elderly. Supporters of market-friendly policies emphasize individual rather than collective responsibility. Their aim is to reduce government spending on, and involvement in, old age policies. Some want to privatize old-age provision by reducing government supports and increasing private market options for older people and their families (Becker, 2005; Estes & Associates, 2001; Hacker, 2002; Quadagno, 2005). Others, notably many liberal or gender-equity feminists, generally oppose government programs that would help women juggle work and family, such as paid parental leave, because they further entrench the gendered division of labor at home and tend to concentrate women in part-time and lower-paying traditionally female occupations (Jacobs & Gerson, 2004; Mandel & Semyonov, 2006; Padavic & Reskin, 2002). By contrast, supporters of family-friendly policies favor collective responsibility and tend to support public policies that help women and men balance work and family (Harrington Meyer & Herd, 2007; Korpi & Palme, 1998). For example, socialist, or gender-accommodative, feminists support public policies that help women and men balance work and family across the life course, arguing that policies such as paid parental leave are needed to offset the unequal amounts of unpaid work that women continue to perform (Herd, 2005). They point out that, thus far, privatization has not reduced costs but has introduced new insecurities in old age (Lorber, 2005; Mandel & Semyonov, 2006; O'Rand & Henretta, 1999). Moreover, they point out that these programs are needed by single mothers raising children on their own. These different theoretical approaches have very different implications for gender inequality in old age.

CHANGING GENDER DYNAMICS

While some gender inequalities are diminishing, others are persisting or even increasing. Two key factors, increases in single parenting and the increasing intensity of unpaid care work, continue to shape gender inequality across the life course and well into old age. They are redefining inequality between men and women, and among women along the lines of race, class, and marital status (Harrington Meyer & Herd, 2007; Moen & Spencer, 2006).

Gender and Marital Status

The US has experienced a retreat from marriage and a dramatic rise in single-parent families. Between 1960 and 2005, the percentage of women married dropped from 67% to 54%, the percentage of women divorced rose from 3% to 11%, and the percentage of families headed by single mothers rose from 8% to 23% (US Census Bureau, 2008). During the same time period the percentage of married-couple households declined from 69% to 53% (Spraggins, 2005). These trends vary significantly by race and ethnicity. In 2005 over half of white and Hispanic women were married, but only about one-third of black women were married (US Census Bureau, 2008). In 2006, 39% of all US births were to unmarried women. Notably, 51% of Latino and 72% of black babies were born to single mothers (Hamilton et al., 2009; US Census Bureau, 2008).

The rise in single parenting is particularly problematic for women across the life course. In 2005, 80% of single parents were women (US Census Bureau, 2008). Single parenting is linked to poverty in part because many children have little contact with their non-custodial fathers, and many mothers receive little child support (Carlson, 2006; Sorensen & Zibman, 2000). About one-quarter of single mothers are not receiving child support payments to which they are legally entitled, and another one-third are not receiving the full award (Sorensen & Hill, 2004; Sorensen & Zibman, 2000). Among families with a child under age 18, 7% of all married couples, compared to 36% of female-headed households, are poor (US Census Bureau, 2006). The economics of single parenting are especially difficult for black and Hispanic mothers; 45% of Hispanic and 42% of black single mothers live in poverty (US Census Bureau, 2006). Many of these single mothers will reach old age with incomes at or near the federal poverty line.

At all ages, women are less likely than men to be married, and the gender gap in marital rates grows with age in part because women outlive men by an average of five years. As Figure 23.1 shows, among those aged 65 and older, 72% of the men and only 42% of the women are married (US Census Bureau, 2008). Among those aged 85 and older, 54% of the men and only 14% of the women are married. There is a strong link between being unmarried and poverty in old age. Older people who live alone do not enjoy the economies of scale afforded to those who live together. Indeed, among those aged 65 and older, married couples have poverty rates of five percent (He et al., 2005). But, as Figure 23.2 shows, single black and Hispanic women have poverty rates of 40%. Because they are more likely to live longer, and to live alone, the next section shows that women are more likely than older men both to need a caregiver and to be a caregiver (National Alliance for Caregiving and AARP, 2009).

Gender and Care Work

At every point in the life course, women are more likely than men to provide care. Gender differences among younger families are not as pronounced as they were in the 1960s and 1970s, but women continue to spend about twice as much time as men caring for children and doing housework such as cooking and cleaning (Bianchi et al., 2006; Krantz-Kent, 2009). Childcare and homemaking responsibilities lead many women to reduce or eliminate employment and education, with lifelong implications for financial security. Even though there has been some closing of the care work gap, qualitative life course research by Pamela Stone (2007) shows just how firmly held traditional expectations about women's responsibilities for raising children and running the household continue to be for many. In her investigation of 50 high-status, high-paid married women who had left their jobs after bearing

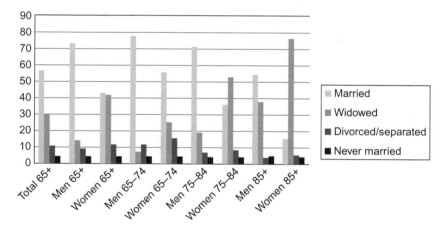

Figure 23.1 Percentage in each marital category by gender and age, 2008.
Source: US Census Bureau (2008).

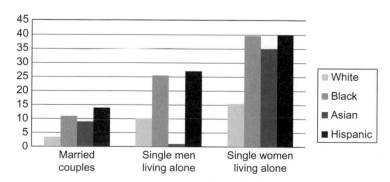

Figure 23.2 Percentage aged 65 and older, below poverty line, by gender, race, and living arrangements, 2003.
Source: US Census Bureau (2006).

children, she found that, following the arrival of children the men tended to devote themselves to their careers and reduce or eliminate their contributions to the housework and child care. Additionally, at least for the middle and upper class, the definition of a good mother has shifted from a supervisory role to an intensive form of mothering that includes hands-on assistance with a multitude of activities including homework, music lessons, clubs, sports, and summer camps (Stone, 2007). Moreover, there is no division of labor for the growing legions of women who are heading households on their own.

The gender gap in providing care to frail older relatives has also eased, but women continue to perform about twice as much care work as men. Overall, families are providing close to 80% of all long-term care (Brody, 2004). The majority of family caregivers are on call seven days a week for at least three hours a day (National Alliance for Caregiving & AARP, 2004; Navaie-Waliser et al., 2002). Care work includes cooking, cleaning, helping with finances, running errands, and assisting with eating, bathing, dressing, and mobility. Not only are women more likely to provide care; they spend more time doing it than men. Seventy percent of spousal caregivers are wives, and 60% to 80% of children who care for their older parents are daughters. On average, daughters do significantly more care work than sons (National Alliance for Caregiving and AARP, 2004; Navaie-Waliser et al., 2002). Black and Hispanic women report higher levels of care work than do whites. Given that they have lower incomes and worse health, these additional duties add up to an even greater burden (National Alliance for Caregiving and AARP, 2009; Wolf et al., 1997).

The nature and scope of care work has intensified since 1984 when Medicare and later Medicaid altered the reimbursement structures in ways that gave healthcare providers financial incentives to shorten stays and release patients earlier (Estes & Associates, 2001). With little training, families, mainly wives and daughters, were expected to take on highly technical work including chemotherapy, apnea monitoring, phototherapy, oxygen tents, tubal feedings, dressing changes, and more. Estes (1989) calculated that, in the first five years of the prospective payment system, more than 21 million days of care work had been transferred from hospitals to families. In recent decades, Medicare and Medicaid coverage of community-based long-term care has shrunk considerably. Since 1997, the Medicare budget devoted to home care has dropped by 50% and the number of recipients and the number of home visits have dropped significantly (Harrington Meyer & Herd, 2007). Stone (2000) estimates that there are 40 unpaid informal care workers for every paid formal care worker. The total value of annual care work is now estimated to be over $50 billion (Holtz-Eakin, 2005; National Alliance for Caregiving & AARP, 2004).

While care work can be rewarding, it can also lead to caregiver burden and stress. Some caregivers report higher rates of physical and psychological distress, anxiety, depression, loneliness, family tension, sleeplessness, exhaustion, inadequate exercise, increases in chronic conditions, and drug misuse (Brody, 2004; National Alliance for Caregiving & AARP, 2009; Pavalko & Woodbury, 2000; Stone, 2000). The longer individuals provide care, the more it weakens the immune systems, increases psychological distress, and accelerates aging (Epel et al., 2004; Pavalko & Woodbury, 2000). The impact of care work on women's work and wages is mixed. Some women add unpaid care work to their paid responsibilities, while others tend to reduce or eliminate paid work. Women whose jobs do not provide flexible hours, unpaid family leave, or paid sick leave are more likely to leave employment, reducing financial security for their own old age (Pavalko & Henderson, 2006).

GENDER AND ECONOMIC INEQUALITY IN OLD AGE

Throughout their lives, women tend to work fewer hours and receive lower wages, in part because of their greater responsibilities for care work. In old age, they have less income from all three major streams: Social Security, private pensions, and private savings. As a result, women over age 65 are almost twice as likely as older men to be poor (He et al., 2005). Older black and Hispanic women are particularly likely to be poor. The US CB reports that 10% of white women aged 65 and older are poor, compared to 16% of Asian, 22% of Hispanic, and 27% of black women (He et al., 2005).

Gender and Income

Over the past several decades the gender gap in employment and in wages has narrowed. Nonetheless, women continue to work fewer hours for lower pay. Despite an enormous increase in women's labor force participation, women are more likely than men to work part-time, less likely to work year-round, and more likely to have entire years out of the labor force (Rose & Hartmann, 2004). Nearly 60% of all women aged 16 and older work in the US; 75% of them work full time and 25% work part time. By contrast, 70% of all adult men work; and nearly 90% of them work full time, and only 10% part time (US Department of Labor, 2005, 2008). Overall, only about 45% of women work full time, year round. The gender gap in wages among full-time year-round workers has narrowed. In 1979, women's average earnings were just 62% of men's; by 2008 they were nearly 80%

(Institute for Women's Policy Research, 2006; US Department of Labor, 2008).

Although most discussions of the gender gap in wages focus on annual differences, the cumulative wage gap, which adds wages over many years, may be more revealing. Rose and Hartmann (2004) analyzed data from 1983 to 1998 and found that, for all women aged 26–59 with at least one year of earnings, women earned just 38% of what men earned. They also traced a cohort of college-educated women and men who were aged 25 to 29 in 1984. By 2004, the women were $440 000 behind the men in cumulative wages. It is interesting to note that the women fell further behind the men with each passing year. When they were in their twenties, women's average annual full-time year-round earnings were about 75% of men's; by their late forties, 62%. These data exclude women who were not working full-time, year-round; if those women were included, these cumulative wage differentials among college graduates would have been even more pronounced. Lower cumulative wages translate into smaller savings and investments, smaller private pensions, and smaller public pensions in old age.

The gender gap in wages continues into old age. Relatively few older people are in the labor force. Among those aged 65 and older in 2007, just 20% of men and 12% of women were employed (US Department of Labor, 2008). Employment is highest among those who are in the younger years of this age group. Among people aged 65 to 69, 33% of men and 23% of women are employed (He et al., 2005). Though the gap has narrowed in recent decades, older women are still only 57% as likely as older men to be employed. When employed, they work fewer hours and accrue smaller earnings (He et al., 2005; Social Security Administration, 2009; Wu, 2008). Given the recent economic downturn, some older men and women are increasing hours of employment and the gap between them may narrow further (Gendell, 2008). While earnings in old age are important, they account for only 22% of all income for persons aged 65 and older. The other main sources are Social Security and private pensions.

Social Security

Social Security is the most important source of income for the elderly and this is particularly true for older women, blacks, and Hispanics. Because on average they live longer, women comprise 57% of Social Security beneficiaries. Social Security provides 42% of income for all people aged 65 and older and 60% of income for all older women. Notably, Social Security contributes 100% of income for one in five women aged 65 and older (Furman, 2005; Social Security Administration, 2009). Social Security is even more important for black and Hispanic older

people; half of Hispanics and African Americans aged 65 and older rely on Social Security for 90% or more of their income (Torres-Gil et al., 2005; Wu, 2004). For black and Hispanic women over age 65, Social Security comprises almost 80% of income.

Several programmatic features make Social Security particularly useful for older women. First, older people may make claims either as retired workers or as spouses and widows. Those making claims as spouses or widows must either still be married or, if divorced, have been married at least 10 years. Although the rules are gender-neutral, 97% of spouse beneficiaries are women (Harrington Meyer & Herd, 2007; Social Security Administration, 2009). Wives aged 62 and older may receive spouse benefits equal to 50% of their husband's benefits. Widows aged 60 and older may receive widow benefits equal to 100% of their deceased husband's benefits. Spouse and widow benefits are not available to the growing numbers of both homosexual and heterosexual couples that cohabitate without marriage. Currently, about 60% of older women receive benefits as wives and widows, rather than as workers, because the benefits they would receive as workers would be smaller. (The SSA describes dually eligible spouses as receiving their own retired worker benefit, and then an additional spouse or widow benefit. This wording suggests that older women are receiving two Social Security benefits, but in fact spouse and widow beneficiaries are receiving one benefit, equal to half or all of their husband's benefits.) Despite advances in the labor force, the majority of women are expected to rely on spouse and widow benefits for the next several cohorts as they reach old age (Levine et al., 2000; Social Security Administration, 2009).

Second, the benefit formula for calculating the worker benefit is redistributive in that it is designed to provide a higher return on contributions to lower earners, many of them women. Thus, the progressive benefit formula serves to reduce the size of the hit women take for lower and more disrupted earnings. Third, Social Security provides actuarial advantages for women. Even though they live longer than men, and therefore can be expected to draw benefits for an average of five additional years, the program does not give women lower benefits (Harrington Meyer & Herd, 2007).

One recent policy change that may affect women adversely is the increase in age for full eligibility. Since 2003, the age of eligibility for full Social Security benefits has been gradually increasing from age 65 to age 67, where it will be in 2027. The age for early retirement remains 62, but the penalty for taking early benefits, which most men and nearly all women take, has increased from 20% to 30% (Social Security Administration, 2009). Hardest hit are those who retire before eligible for full benefits due to poor health, unemployment, or retirement of a spouse.

This group is predominantly made up of women and blacks and Hispanics (Gendell, 2008; Moon with Herd, 2002).

Recent debates about Social Security have focused on privatizing the program. Indeed, after he was re-elected in 2004, President George Bush made the privatization of Social Security his top domestic priority (Schulz & Binstock, 2008). The plan most often discussed would have allowed those under age 55 to divert as much as 4% of their 6.2% Social Security contribution to private accounts (Herd & Kingson, 2005; President's Commission to Strengthen Social Security, 2001). Supporters of privatization argued that the existing program would soon be fiscally unsustainable and proposed individual accounts that would maximize each person's choice and responsibility. Opponents pointed out that the kind of privatization being proposed would make the fiscal situation worse, while increasing program costs and exposure to risk for older people and their families. Moreover, many of the features that make the existing program advantageous for older women – such as the spouse and widow benefits, the redistributive benefit formula, and the actuarial advantage – would most likely disappear or be reduced under privatization (Harrington Meyer & Herd, 2007).

Many scholars note that Social Security does not effectively compensate women for time spent out of the labor force caring for family members. Benefits calculations for all workers exclude the five lowest years of earnings within the system, but many women spend more than five years out of the labor force and in lower-paying jobs while they are performing unpaid care work (Harrington Meyer & Herd, 2007; Social Security Administration, 2009). Historically, the spouse or widow benefit provided benefits for women with low wages or interrupted labor, but access to these noncontributory benefits is linked to marital status, and there is both a retreat from marriage and a growing race gap in marriage. By the time women born in the 1960s reach old age, 80% of white and Hispanic women, compared to only 50% of black women, will be eligible to receive benefits on the basis of their marital status (Harrington Meyer et al., 2006). This means that older black women, who already have fewer economic resources and higher poverty rates, may be especially vulnerable in old age in future cohorts.

One proposed solution to address such gender and race differences would be to create a new type of minimum benefit. US Social Security had a significant minimum benefit, but it was terminated in the early 1980s. Today, Social Security has a special minimum benefit, but few qualify and the benefits are meager (Harrington Meyer & Herd, 2007; Social Security Administration, 2009). Numerous proposals attempt to address this concern. Some policy analysts favor a plan that functions a lot like the EITC, so that each year, when older people with lower incomes file their taxes, they receive additional Social Security benefits. This benefit would be income-tested and would encourage employment. Other policy analysts prefer a plan in which the minimum benefit slides up with the number of years contributing to the system and, as in the European tradition, care credits are provided to offset time out of the labor market (Favreault & Steuerle, 2007; Herd, 2005). While some of these plans accommodate gender differences in responsibility for care work, they tend to be complex and to reward mostly those who are already faring better under Social Security. The simplest proposed plan would provide a minimum benefit to all who are eligible for Social Security. Implementation of a minimum set near the federal poverty line could significantly reduce poverty and inequality in old age (Harrington Meyer & Herd, 2007; Herd, 2005). It would also reduce claims for spouse benefits or SSI and thereby help pay for the benefit expansion. As with any proposed revisions to Social Security, such plans would be controversial.

Supplemental Security Income

SSI has provided monthly cash benefits to the aged, blind, and disabled poor since it was created in 1972. Because women live longer and are more likely to be poor, nearly two-thirds of SSI recipients aged 65 and older are women (Social Security Administration, 2009). SSI use among the elderly has dropped from 10% in 1975 to an all-time low of 3% in 2006 (Social Security Administration, 2009). Some of the decline is due to expansion of Social Security and a decrease in old age poverty over this period of time. But some of the decline is due to features of the SSI program itself (Harrington Meyer & Herd, 2007). Some older people who are eligible for SSI do not apply because they are either unaware of the benefits, overwhelmed by the cumbersome eligibility forms, or discouraged by strict earnings and asset tests that have not been updated in decades. Unlike Social Security, SSI considers all earned and unearned income in calculating benefits. Under federal guidelines, the first $65 in earned income, along with an additional $20, is disregarded each month. Any additional earnings decrease benefits by $1 for every $2 earned. Assets, excluding a house, car, and burial funds under certain conditions, must be below $2000 for individuals and $3000 for couples. SSI's modest income disregards have been in place since 1981; the asset maximums have been in place since 1989 (Social Security Administration, 2009). Neither has been linked to cost of living and neither can be raised except by congressional legislation. When poverty-based programs are left to languish in this way, older women who rely on them disproportionately face even more difficult financial circumstances.

Private Pensions and Private Savings

Private pensions are the third largest income stream for older people, accounting for 18% of all old age income. They are funded in part by government tax subsidies to businesses that total over $100 billion a year (Employee Benefit Research Institute, 2005; Hacker, 2006). Despite these subsidies, many individuals do not receive private pensions. Among those aged 65 and older in the top earnings quartile, 63% have private pensions, and, among those in the lowest earnings quartile, only 20% do (Employee Benefit Research Institute, 2005). Older women are only 60% as likely as older men to receive a private pension, and those pensions are only one-half as large (Employee Benefit Research Institute, 2005; McDonnell, 2005). The gender gap in private pensions is expected to shrink in the future because, among younger workers, women are 76% as likely as men to have private pension coverage. The race gap in pension coverage, however, is not expected to improve. Among those aged 65 and older, 57% of white and 44% of black women have pension coverage, and, among women age 33 to 42, 64% of white and only 49% of black women have pension coverage (Verma, 2003).

The value of private pension coverage is fading as benefits shift from DB to DC. As described in Chapter 20, instead of promising a specific benefit amount that rises with hours, salaries, and years of service, most employers now promise only to contribute a specific amount to workers' pension accounts (Employee Benefit Research Institute, 2005). The eventual value of those benefits will be determined by employer contributions, employee contributions, and investment decisions. DC plans shift investment responsibilities, costs, and risks from employers to employees. Because they are not as compulsory or as automatic as DB plans, DC-plan employees are more readily able to opt out, reduce their contributions, or withdraw money before retirement. Women are more likely than men to do all three (Munnell & Sundén, 2004; Shuey & O'Rand, 2006). And, because they concentrate rather than spread the risk of unfortunate investment strategies, DC plans create shortfalls that are much harder for those with lower incomes to absorb (Harrington Meyer & Herd, 2007). Studies show that employers are contributing less and less to these plans, making employees even more responsible for their own pension accumulations (Munnell & Sundén, 2004; Shuey & O'Rand, 2006). So, while the gender gap in private pension coverage is shrinking, the risks and shortfalls associated with DC plans are growing. The overall effect is increasing economic instability for many women as they age.

Personal savings and assets have also been declining in recent years, especially for older women who were ever single mothers (Zeller, 2007). Gender differences are hard to untangle among married couples. But, among Americans aged 65 and older who are not married, older men's assets are 30% higher than older women's (Levine et al., 2000). Women aged 65 to 75 who were single mothers for at least 10 years report asset income equal to just one-third of that for women who were married mothers (Yamokoski & Keister, 2006). Women generally, and single mothers in particular, average much lower assets in old age, and as a result they are financially less secure.

HEALTH AND HEALTH CARE

Older women live longer than older men, and at every age they are more likely to be sick. Gender differences in health, and in access to various types of health benefits, vary significantly across the life course. For a variety of socio-demographic reasons, women are less likely to receive health insurance through their own jobs, more likely to be burdened by Medicare's meager coverage of long-term care, and more likely to rely on a poverty-based Medicaid program that reimburses providers at well below market rates.

Gender and Health

Older people are living longer and healthier lives. Generally, older men, whites, and those with greater income and education have better health and functional mobility (Halfon & Hochstein, 2002). Older women live on average five years longer. Among those born in 2004, men are projected to live an average of 75 years while women will live an average of 80 years (National Center for Health Statistics, 2007). At every age, men are more likely than women to die of fatal conditions such as heart disease, stroke, cancer, flu, cirrhosis, diabetes, HIV, unintended injuries, suicide, and homicide (He et al., 2005; National Center for Health Statistics, 2007). At every age, women tend to report higher rates of chronic conditions such as anemia, thyroid conditions, migraines, arthritis, hypertension, urinary incontinence, osteoporosis, gall bladder conditions, colitis, eczema, and depression (National Center for Health Statistics, 2007). Older women are also significantly more likely to report having two or more limitations in both ADLs and IADLs and cognitive impairment (Kaiser Family Foundation, 2009). Generally, black, Hispanic, and Native American women have shorter life expectancies and report significantly more health problems and health limitations than do white and Asian women (He et al., 2005; National Center for Health Statistics, 2007). Health advantages and disadvantages accumulate over the life course. Women and other disadvantaged groups have higher levels of stress and strain, which may translate into higher rates of morbidity (House, 2002; Link et al., 2000).

Before age 65, the majority of Americans rely on employment-based health insurance coverage. Employers and employees receive tax incentives aimed at encouraging the provision of health insurance through jobs. The distribution of these benefits, subsidized through tax expenditures of over $100 billion a year, is far from equal (Hacker, 2006; Selden & Gray, 2006). Whites, men, full-time, and higher-paid workers are most likely to have health insurance while blacks and Hispanics, women, part-time, and low-waged workers are more likely to be uninsured or rely on poverty-based programs (Employee Benefit Research Institute, 2009). Health insurance coverage by employers has declined steadily for three decades. Between 1979 and 2004, the proportion of working men with insurance through their own jobs declined from 65% to 51%, while the proportion of women declined from 47% to 39% (Employee Benefit Research Institute, 2009). Women are twice as likely as men to be insured through a spouse's job. In 2004, 26% of women and only 13% of men had insurance through their spouse's job. While dependent coverage helps to offset the paucity of coverage women have through their own jobs, they are at risk of losing that coverage should their partners lose their jobs or the marriages end through death or divorce (Harrington Meyer & Pavalko, 1996). Obtaining health insurance through a spouse's job is not an option for growing numbers of single women.

Medicare

Medicare, which is addressed more fully in Chapter 21, is the main source of health care for those aged 65 and older, and 56% of the beneficiaries are women. Among those aged 85 and older, who make the majority of Medicare claims, 70% are women (Kaiser Family Foundation, 2009). Medicare expenditures have risen dramatically over the years and recent policy initiatives have shifted costs in ways that have especially affected older women. Moreover, while Medicare provides extensive coverage of acute health care such as doctor and hospital visits, some types of health care that women are more likely to need, most notably long-term care, remain virtually uncovered.

Costs began rising dramatically from the moment Medicare was created in 1965. By 2008, Medicare expenditures were $428 billion, or $10 500 per beneficiary (MedPac, 2008). Medicare has contained costs by shifting some of them to older persons. Some estimate that Medicare covers only about 45%

of old age health care costs (Moody, 2002). Four decades into the Medicare and Medicaid programs, the costs of health care for the aged are, in fact, a greater burden for older persons than before the programs began. This is in part due to the rising costs of health care for all people in the US. Out-of-pocket expenses for the elderly rose from 15% of annual income in 1965 to 22% in 1998. By 2025, out-of-pocket health care expenses are expected to reach 30% of personal income (Moon with Herd, 2002). Given that women live longer and have lower incomes, they shoulder the expense of Medicare cost shifting disproportionately.

As demonstrated earlier, Medicare has also contained costs by shifting care work to families, more often women (Estes & Associates, 2001; Moon with Herd, 2002). In the end, women are both more likely to need, and to provide, care work. Thus Medicare's spotty coverage of long-term care is particularly problematic for women across the life course (Kaiser Family Foundation, 2009; National Alliance for Caregiving & AARP, 2004). Older women's out-of-pocket lifetime health care expenses are higher than men's, almost entirely due to their tendency to have greater long-term care costs; further, their incomes are lower than men's in part due to their greater tendency to provide long-term care services to others. Thus, a policy proposal that would ease the financial, social, and health burdens on women would be to expand Medicare to provide national, universal, compulsory coverage of long-term care in the community and in nursing homes (Kaiser Family Foundation, 2009; Harrington Meyer & Herd, 2007). Comprehensive coverage of community and institutional long-term care would reduce the amount of care work women perform, reduce out-of-pocket expenses, and ensure that those with the lowest incomes receive needed care.

One Medicare policy that would be difficult for many older women, and older blacks and Hispanics, to absorb is the proposal to raise the age of eligibility from 65 to 67. Given that they are less likely to be employed, less likely to have retiree health insurance, and more likely to have chronic conditions, delaying eligibility for Medicare might make older women much more likely to be uninsured or do without needed care. Raising the age is usually justified as a cost-cutting mechanism, but, because those between 65 and 67 are the healthiest of older people, it would have little measurable impact on Medicare expenditures but a sizable impact on the amount of risk faced by those approaching retirement age (Harrington Meyer & Herd, 2007; Medpac, 2008).

Retiree and Medigap Supplemental Insurance

Retiree receipt of employment-based health insurance has dropped significantly in recent years. Even among large employers, the proportion offering retiree health benefits has dropped from 66% in 1988 to just 36% in 2004 (MedPac, 2008). The gender gap in coverage has narrowed, and, by 2006, 37% of men and 33% of women aged 65 and older had an employer-sponsored plan (Kaiser Family Foundation, 2009). Moreover, employers who still offer retiree coverage are pushing more of the costs onto retirees by tightening eligibility requirements, capping benefits, and increasing cost sharing (Employment Benefit Research Institute, 2005).

Because Medicare leaves many costs uncovered, many older persons also purchase private Medigap or supplemental policies that cover out-of-pocket expenses such as Medicare premiums, co-pays, deductibles, and exclusions such as long-term care, eye exams, and hearing aids (Kaiser Family Foundation, 2009). But access to these policies is shrinking. Supplemental insurance premiums have risen significantly and navigating the market can be difficult because many private Medigap insurers deny, duplicate, or sever coverage (Moon with Herd, 2002). Reliance on private supplemental policies shifts responsibility for the aged out of both the government and the employment-based benefit sectors into the private market. Those with fewer resources and poorer health, mainly older women and blacks and Hispanics, are less likely to be able to obtain and retain private insurance (Harrington Meyer & Herd, 2007).

Medicaid

Since 1965, Medicaid has provided free and comprehensive coverage of health care for many of the poor aged and disabled. Because they live longer and have fewer resources, over 70% of persons aged 65 and older who are eligible for Medicaid are women (Kaiser Family Foundation, 2009; Social Security Administration, 2009). The proportion of older people relying on Medicaid has been dropping, now just 13%, both because poverty among the elderly is now below 10% and because Medicaid eligibility criteria are strict. The federal maximum allowable income for eligibility is set below 78% of the federal poverty line and the federal asset maximum has been frozen for decades at just $2000 per individual and $3000 per couple (Commonwealth Fund, 2005; Kaiser Family Foundation, 2009; Social Security Administration, 2009). Only one-half of those who are potentially eligible actually receive Medicaid, in part because the process of applying is difficult and stigmatizing and the rules of participation are restrictive (Kaiser Family Foundation, 2009; Moon with Herd, 2002). A subset of dual Medicare and Medicaid enrollees receive limited coverage under new rules that relax eligibility guidelines. For those in these special programs, out-of-pocket costs are reduced to 13% of total annual incomes (Kaiser Family Foundation, 2003). But the application procedures and eligibility criteria for the expanded program are also quite onerous; thus, only a fraction of those who qualify actually participate (Moon with Herd, 2002; MedPac, 2008).

For Medicare beneficiaries who are also receiving Medicaid, 70% of whom are women, Medicaid provides tremendous economic relief from health care costs. Medicaid covers costs Medicare does not, including the Medicare Part B premiums, nursing home care, and nearly all Medicare co-pays and deductibles (Harrington Meyer, 2000; Kaiser Family Foundation, 2009; Social Security Administration, 2009). Because coverage is comprehensive for these enrollees, and because health care providers are generally prohibited from charging costs above the allowable rates to Medicaid recipients, full Medicaid coverage with Medicare coverage reduces out-of-pocket expenses from over 20% to about 5% of annual income (Kaiser Family Foundation, 2009; Ku & Broaddus, 2005).

Although Medicaid coverage is quite comprehensive, older Americans who rely on Medicaid sometimes find that access to health care is problematic. Medicaid reimbursement rates to providers are well below market rates, leading many doctors, clinics, labs, hospitals, and nursing homes to refuse to treat, or cap the number of, Medicaid patients (Commonwealth Fund, 2005; Harrington Meyer, 2000). Thus, among primary care physicians in the US in 2002, 85% were accepting new private payers, 83% were accepting new Medicare recipients, and only 66% were accepting new Medicaid patients (MedPac, 2008). Because they are more likely to be on Medicaid, older women, blacks and Hispanics, and unmarried persons are more likely to face denial of, or delays in, treatment and admission.

FUTURE RESEARCH

Given the life course and cumulative (dis)advantage approaches that dominate old age research, scholars are well aware that much of the inequality that shapes old age has its origins in the younger years. Women's disproportionate responsibility for unpaid child care and house work tends to interfere with their earnings. Further, the paucity of government programs to help young families juggle work and family weighs more heavily on women, particularly single mothers. US old age policies, coupled with employment-based benefits, provide important economic and health benefits that generally reduce inequality in old age. But cost shifting, care shifting, and general neglect of long-term care benefits leave many women, particularly if they are single, vulnerable in old age.

In the years ahead, old age scholars will continue to analyze how the recent emphasis on cutting costs and on privatizing public benefits has overshadowed policy proposals that have the potential to make our existing programs more responsive to changing social and demographic trends. How can we implement policies that will help younger families juggle work and family responsibilities without leaving older women so economically vulnerable in old age? How can policies be reshaped to better accommodate single mothers and cohabiters, whether gay or straight? How can poverty-based programs such as Supplemental Security Income and Medicaid, whose asset tests have been neglected for decades, be made less strict? How might we reorganize or replace Social Security spouse and widow benefits to respond to the growing race gap in marriage and to reduce poverty among single older women? And how can Medicare policy best be reshaped to expand coverage of old age health care benefits generally, and long term care benefits specifically, and ease the burden on caregivers?

Public policies in other nations provide models for more comprehensive and responsive benefits across the life course, as discussed in Chapter 22. How might policies such as paid maternity leaves, universal or subsidized child care, mandatory paid sick leave, and more generous vacation time, all of which are widespread in many European countries,

be implemented to better shore up women's financial and health security at younger ages in the US? For example, the US Family and Medical Leave Act only provides up to 12 weeks of unpaid leave – and only for those who work in a company with more than 50 employees, have been employed for at least 12 months with that employer, and average at least 24 hours of work per week. By contrast, many European countries offer between 3 and 12 months of fully or partially paid leave (Bond & Galinsky, 2006; Gornick & Meyers, 2003). In addition, long-term care policies in Europe and Asia have helped to reduce some of the burden that women predominately face (see Chapter 22). Policies that allow women to juggle work and family by strengthening their links to the labor force have the potential to increase women's earnings, savings, and public and private pensions, leaving them less vulnerable in old age.

Ironically, many policymakers have been working to reduce old age support at a time when the vast majority of Americans think we are already doing too little for the elderly. Between 70% and 90% of poll respondents report that they would be willing to pay higher taxes to keep universal old age benefits and that they favor universal health insurance for all ages (AARP, 2005; Public Agenda, 2005; Street & Cossman, 2006). The next few years will offer a great deal of insight into the future direction of US old age policy and gender inequalities in old age.

REFERENCES

AARP (2005). *Public attitudes toward social security and private accounts*. Washington, DC: AARP Knowledge Movement.

Acker, J. (2006). *Class questions: Feminist answers*. Lanham, MD: Rowman & Littlefield Publishers.

Baca Zinn, M., & Thornton Dill, B. (2005). What is multiracial feminism? In J. Lorber (Ed.), *Gender inequality: Feminist theories and politics* (pp. 271–285) (3rd Edn). Los Angeles: Roxbury Publishing.

Becker, G. S. (2005). A political case for social security reform. *Wall Street Journal*, February 15, A-18.

Bianchi, S. M., Robinson, J. P., & Milkie, M. A. (2006). *Changing rhythms of American family life*. New York: Russell Sage Foundation.

Bond, J. T., & Galinsky, E. (2006). What workplace flexibility is

available to entry-level, hourly employees? *Families and Work Institute*, Research Brief No 3.

Brody, E. M. (2004). *Women in the middle: Their parent care years* (2nd Edn.). New York: Springer Publishing Company.

Carlson, M. J. (2006). Family structure, father involvement, and adolescent behavioral outcomes. *Journal of Marriage and the Family*, 68(1), 137–154.

Commonwealth Fund (2005). *The long-term budget outlook*. Washington, DC: Congressional Budget Office.

Dannefer, D. (2003). Cumulative advantage/disadvantage and the life course: Cross-fertilizing age and social science theory. *The Journals of Gerontology Series B: Psychological Sciences and Social Sciences*, 58, S327–S337.

Employee Benefit Research Institute. (2005). *EBRI databook on employee*

benefits (Chapter 4: Table 1: Participation in employee benefit programs). Retrieved December 10, 2009, from www.ebri.org/ publications/books/index. cfm?fa=databook.

Employee Benefit Research Institute. (2009). *Sources of health insurance and characteristics of the uninsured: Issue Brief 334*. Retrieved December 10, 2009, from www. ebri.org/publications/ib/index. cfm?fa=ibDisp&content_ id=4366.

Epel, E. S., Blackburn, E. H., Lin, J., Dhabhar, F. S., Adler, N. E., Morrow, J. D., & Cawthon, R. M. (2004). Accelerated telomere shortening in response to life stress. *Proceedings of the National Academy of Sciences of the United States of America*, 101(49), 17312–17315.

Estes, C. (1989). Aging, health and social policy. Crisis and crossroads. *Journal of Aging and Social Policy*, 1, 17–32.

Estes, C., & Associates (2001). *Social policy and aging: A critical perspective*. Thousand Oaks: Sage Publications.

Favreault, M., & Steuerle, E. (2007). *Social security and spouse and survivor benefits for the modern family*. Retrieved December 10, 2009, from www.urban.org/UploadedPDF/311436_Social_Security.pdf

Frantz, A. (2008). Women gaining political power. *CNN*, November 13. Retrieved December 10, 2009, from http://www.cnn.com/2008/POLITICS/11/13/women.in.politics/

Furman, J. (2005). *Policy basics: Top ten facts on Social Security's 70th anniversary*. Washington, DC: Center on Budget and Policy Priorities. Retrieved January 14, 2010 from www.cbpp.org/cms/index.cfm?fa=view&id=531

Gendell, M. (2008). Older workers increasing their labor force participation and hours of work. *Monthly Labor Review*, 41, 41–54.

Gornick, J. C., & Meyers, M. (2003). *Families that work: Policies for reconciling parenthood and employment*. New York: Russell Sage Foundation.

Hacker, J. S. (2002). *The divided welfare state: The battle over public and private social benefits in the United States*. New York: Cambridge University Press.

Hacker, J. S. (2006). *The great risk shift: The assault on American jobs, families, health care, and retirement and how you can fight back*. New York: Oxford University Press.

Halfon, N., & Hochstein, M. (2002). Life course health development: An integrated framework for developing health, policy, and research. *Milbank Quarterly*, 80(3), 433–479.

Hamilton B. E., Martin, J. A., & Ventura, S. J. (2009). Births: Preliminary data for 2007. *National Vital Statistics Reports*, Web release; 57(12), March 18. Hyattsville, MD: National Center for Health Statistics.

Harrington Meyer, M. (Ed.), (2000). *Care work: Gender, labor, and the welfare state*. New York: Routledge Press.

Harrington Meyer, M., & Herd, P. (2007). *Market friendly or family friendly? The state and gender inequality in old age*. New York: Russell Sage.

Harrington Meyer, M., & Pavalko, E. (1996). Family, work, and access to health insurance among mature women. *Journal of Health and Social Behavior*, 37(4), 311–325.

Harrington Meyer, M., Wolf, D., & Himes, C. (2006). Declining eligibility for social security spouse and widow benefits in the United States? *Research on Aging*, 28(2), 240–260.

He, W., Sangupta, M., Velkoff, V. A., & Debaros, K. A. (2005). 65+ in the United States. *Current Population Reports, Special Studies Series P23*, no. 209. Washington, DC: US Census Bureau.

Herd, P. (2005). Reforming a breadwinner welfare state: Gender, race, class and social security reform. *Social Forces*, 83(4), 1365–1394.

Herd, P., & Kingson, E. R. (2005). Reframing social security: Cures worse than the disease. In R. B. Hudson (Ed.), *The new politics of old age policy*. Baltimore: Johns Hopkins University Press.

Holtz-Eakin, D. (2005). The cost and financing of long-term care services. Statement of Douglas Holtz-Eakin, Director, before the Subcommittee on Health Committee on Ways and Means, US House of Representatives. April 27. Washington, DC: Congressional Budget Office.

House, J. S. (2002). Understanding social factors and inequalities in health: 20th century progress and 21st century prospects. *Journal of Health and Social Behavior*, 43(2), 125–253.

Institute for Women's Policy Research. (2006). Memo to John Roberts: The gender wage gap is real. IWPS #C362. Retrieved December 10, 2009, from www.iwpr.org/pdf/C362.pdf.

Jacobs, J. A., & Gerson, K. (2004). *The time divide: Work, family, and gender inequality*. Cambridge, MA: Harvard University Press.

Kaiser Family Foundation. (2003). Dual enrollees: Medicaid's role for low-income Medicare beneficiaries. Kaiser Commission

on Medicaid and the uninsured, February. Washington, DC: KFF.

Kaiser Family Foundation. (2009). Medicare's role for women. Fact Sheet, June. Washington, DC. Retrieved December 10, 2009, from www.kff.org/womenshealth/upload/7913.pdf

Korpi, W., & Palme, J. (1998). The paradox of redistribution and strategies of equality: Welfare state institutions, inequality, and poverty in the western countries. *American Sociological Review*, 63, 661–687.

Krantz-Kent, R. (2009). Measuring time spent in unpaid household work: Results from the American time use survey. *Monthly Labor Review*, July, 46–59.

Ku, L., & Broaddus, M. (2005). *Out-of-pocket medical expenses for medicaid beneficiaries are substantial and growing*. Washington, DC: Center on Budget and Policy Priorities.

Levine, P. B., Mitchell, O. S., & Phillips, J. W. R. (2000). Benefit of one's own: Older women's entitlement to social security retirement. *Social Security Bulletin*, 63(2), 47–53.

Link, B., Phelan, J. C., & Fremont, A. M. (2000). Evaluating the fundamental cause explanation for social disparities in health. In C. E. Bird & P. Conrad (Eds.), *Handbook of medical sociology* (pp. 33–46) (5th Edn). Upper Saddle River, NJ: Prentice Hall.

Lorber, J. (2005). *Gender inequality: Feminist theories and politic* (3rd Edn.). Los Angeles: Roxbury Publishing.

Mandel, H., & Semyonov, M. (2006). A welfare state paradox: State interventions and women's employment opportunities in 22 countries. *American Journal of Sociology*, 111(6), 1910–1949.

McDonnell, K. (2005). Retirement annuity and employment-based pension income. *EBRI Notes*, 26(2), 7–14.

MedPac (2008). *A data book: Health care spending and the medicare program*. Washington, DC: Medicare Payment Advisory Commission.

Moen, P., & Spencer, D. (2006). Converging divergences in age, gender, health, and well-being: Strategic selection in the third age.

In R. H. Binstock & L. K. George (Eds.), *Handbook of aging and the social sciences* (pp. 129–145) (6th Edn). San Diego: Academic Press.

Moody, H. R. (2002). *Aging: Concepts and controversies*. Newbury Park: Pine Forge Press.

Moon, M., with Herd, P. (2002). *A place at the table: Women's needs and medicare reform*. New York: The Century Foundation.

Munnell, A. H., & Sundén, A. (2004). *Coming up short: The challenge of 401(k) plans*. Washington, DC: Brookings Institution Press.

National Alliance for Caregiving & AARP. (2004). Caregiving in the US. Washington, DC: National Alliance for Caregiving and AARP.

National Alliance for Caregiving, & AARP. (2009). *Caregiving in the U.S. 2009*. Washington, DC: National Alliance for Caregiving and AARP.

National Center for Health Statistics (NCHS). (2007). Health, United States, 2007 with chartbook on trends in the health of Americans. Washington, DC: US Government Printing Office.

Navaie-Waliser, M., Spriggs, A., & Feldman, P. H. (2002). Informal caregiving – differential experiences by gender. *Medical Care*, 40(12), 1249–1259.

O'Rand, A. M., & Henretta, J. C. (1999). *Age and inequality: Diverse pathways through later life*. Boulder, CO: Westview Press.

Padavic, I., & Reskin, B. F. (2002). *Women and men at work* (2nd Edn.). Newbury Park: Pine Forge Press.

Pavalko, E., & Henderson, K. (2006). Combining care work and paid work: Do workplace policies make a difference? *Research on Aging*, 28(3), 359–374.

Pavalko, EK., & Woodbury, S. (2000). Social roles as process: Caregiving careers and women's health. *Journal of Health and Social Behavior*, 41(1), 91–105.

President's Commission to Strengthen Social Security. (2001). Strengthening social security and creating personal wealth for all Americans. Final Report. December 21, 2001. Washington, DC: President's Commission to Strengthen Social Security.

Public Agenda. (2005). Medicare: Results of survey question re federal budget. PublicAgenda.org Issue Guides. April 18–22.

Quadagno, J. S. (2005). *One nation uninsured: Why the U.S. has no national health insurance*. New York: Oxford University Press.

Rose, S., & Hartmann, H. (2004). *Still a man's labor market: The long term earning's gap*. Washington, DC: The Institute for Women's Policy Research.

Schulz, J. H., & Binstock, R. H. (2008). *Aging nation: The economics and politics of growing old in America*. Baltimore, MD: Johns Hopkins University Press.

Selden, T., & Gray, B. (2006). Tax subsidies for employment based health insurance, estimates for 2006. *Health Affairs*, 25(6), 1568–1579.

Settersten, R. A. (2003). Introduction. In R. A. Settersten (Ed.), *Invitation to the life course: Toward new understandings of later life* (pp. 1–14). Amityville, NY: Baywood Publishing.

Shuey, K. M., & O'Rand, A. M. (2006). Changing demographics and new pension risks. *Research on Aging*, 28(3), 317–340.

Social Security Administration (SSA). (2009). Annual statistical supplement 2008. Social Security Bulletin. Washington, DC: Department of Health and Human Services.

Sorensen, E., & Hill, A. (2004). Single mothers and their child-support receipt: How well is child-support enforcement doing? *Journal of Human Resources*, 39(1), 135–154.

Sorensen, E., & Zibman, C. (2000). Child support offers some protection against poverty. New federalism: National survey of America's families. March 15, B-10. Washington, DC: Urban Institute.

Spraggins, R. E. (2005). We the people: Men and women in the United States. Census 2000 Special Reports, CENSR-20. Washington, DC: U.S. Census Bureau.

Stone, P. (2007). *Opting out: Why women really quit careers and head home*. Berkeley and Los Angeles, CA; London, England: University of California Press.

Stone, R. I. (2000). *Long-term care for the elderly with disabilities: Current policy, emerging trends, and implications for the twenty-first century*. Washington, DC: Milbank Memorial Fund.

Street, D., & Cossman, J. S. (2006). Greatest generation or greedy geezers? Social spending preferences and the elderly. *Social Problems*, 53(1), 75–96.

Torres-Gil, F., Greenstein, R., & Kamin, D. (2005). Hispanics' large stake in the social security debate. June 28. Washington, DC: Center on Budget and Policy Priorities.

US Census Bureau. (2006). Poverty status by type of family, presence of related children, race and hispanic origin; Historical poverty tables. Retrieved December 10, 2009, from www.census.gov/hhes/www/poverty/histpov/famindex.html

US Census Bureau. (2008). Table MS-1. Marital status of the population 15 years old and over, by sex and race: 1950 to present and table FM-1. Families by presence of own children under 18: 1950 to present. Retrieved December 10, 2009, from www.census.gov/population/www/socdemo/hh-fam.html#ht

US Department of Labor. (2005). Women in the labor force: A databook. Report 985. US Bureau of Labor Statistics Table 2. Employment status of the civilian noninstitutional population 16 years and over by sex, 1970–2004 annual averages. Washington, DC. Retrieved December 10, 2009, from www.bls.gov/cps/wlf-databook2005.htm.

US Department of Labor. (2008). Highlights of women's earnings in 2008. Report 1017. Retrieved December 10, 2009, from http://stats.bls.gov/cps/cpswom2008.pdf

US Senate. 2009. Senators of the 111th Congress. www.senate.gov/general/contact_information/senators_cfm.cfm. Retrieved January 11, 2010.

Verma, S. (2003). Retirement coverage of women and minorities: Analysis from SIPP 1998 data. Report DD92, October. Washington, DC: AARP

Public Policy Institute. Retrieved December 10, 2009, from www.aarp.org/research/ppi/econ-sec/pensions/articles/aresearch-import-350-DD92.html.

Wolf, D. A., Freedman, V., & Soldo, B. J. (1997). Division of family labor: Care for elderly parents. *Journals of Gerontology: Psychological and Social Sciences*, *52B*(Special Issue), 102–109.

Wu, K. B. (2004). African Americans age 65 and older: Their sources of income. Fact Sheet 100. Washington, DC: AARP Public Policy Institute.

Wu, K. B. (2008). Sources of income for older persons, 2006. Fact Sheet 143. Washington, DC: AARP Public Policy Institute. Retrieved December 10, 2009, from www.aarp.org/research/ppi/econ-sec/income/articles/income_sources.html

Yamokoski, A., & Keister, L. (2006). The wealth of single women: Marital status and parenthood in the asset accumulation of young baby boomers in the United States. *Feminist Economics*, *12*(1–2), 167–194.

Zeller T., Jr. (2007). Savings rate at depression-era lows…does it matter? *New York Times*, February 1.

Chapter | 24 |

Aging and Social Intervention: Life Course Perspectives

Lisa F. Berkman, Karen A. Ertel, Maria M. Glymour

Department of Society, Human Development, and Health, Harvard School of Public Health, Cambridge, Massachusetts

DOI: 10.1016/B978-0-12-380880-6.00024-1

INTRODUCTION: CONTRASTING OBSERVATIONAL AND EXPERIMENTAL STUDIES OF HEALTHY AGING

Observational studies of aging indicate that there are a number of social conditions that impact health outcomes in older men and women from functioning to morbidity to mortality. Socioeconomic conditions, social isolation and exclusion, and lack of social participation and engagement all have been linked in numerous longitudinal studies to poorer health, worse physical and cognitive functioning, and higher mortality risk. There are, however, many fewer studies showing that we can successfully intervene in these social processes to improve health and well being at older ages.

There are only a few types of established explanations for the discrepancy between the findings from the observational studies, which almost uniformly show strong ties between these exposures and health outcomes, and the results of the randomized control trials, which show much weaker results. The first explanation is that the interventions fail to change the exposure, or, to be more specific, do not change the exposure sufficiently or during the correct etiologic period. By correct etiologic period, we mean the time at which the exposure causes the disease process to develop or progress. The second explanation is that the exposure is causally related to the outcomes and the intervention changes the exposure, but there were heterogeneous treatment effects; that is, the intervention was efficacious in some groups and not in others. The third is that the exposures are not causally related to the outcomes and the observational findings are the result of confounding by some unmeasured variable or reverse causation. The contrasts between findings from observational studies and randomized clinical trials are growing and discrepancies in findings have been observed for a number of recent interventions. Of particular importance is the fact that observational studies rarely help us identify the etiologic period clearly enough to know when to intervene. In this chapter we argue that there are multiple ways of interpreting the differences we find between observational studies and experimental ones. We focus here particularly on contrasting the findings between observational and intervention studies related to social networks and social support as an example of what we might learn with the adoption of life course approaches to improving the health of middle-aged and older adults.

A LIFE COURSE APPROACH TO UNDERSTANDING SOCIAL DISPARITIES IN HEALTH

Some social circumstances take their tolls on health throughout the life course, so that, while they are often expressed in later life, they emerge from a long set of experiences, often poorly measured. We also hypothesize that most of our interventions to improve the health of older populations come too late in the evolution of disease and disabling processes. Thus, the aim of this chapter is to bring life course perspectives more fully into our understanding of the dynamic interplay between social and psychological situations and health and aging. Life course epidemiology can inform the development of appropriate and effective interventions to change social conditions in order to achieve the greatest benefit with respect to health outcomes in the elderly. In this chapter, we are particularly interested in cardiovascular disease and cognitive function. Although much life course research has emphasized early, critical developmental periods, it is important to explore a range of models that try to identify periods across the life course that influence health outcomes.

The core premise of life course epidemiology, that current health reflects the effects of a lifetime of past exposures, is now firmly established; however, the results from this body of research have not been fully integrated into the design and implementation of health interventions. In part, this is because only recently has enough evidence accumulated, at least in some areas, to provide useful guidance regarding the etiologic periods of significance. Specifically, the life course perspective can inform several fundamental considerations in intervention development, such as when the exposure can be changed, when the disease process begins and the most sensitive time points to

interrupt its progression, and, in combination, the optimal timing to effect change in both.

To begin the discussion, we will first outline alternative etiologic models frequently considered in life course epidemiology. Life course models are important to identify and three distinct trajectories have been linked with each of the most common life course models (Ben-Shlomo & Kuh, 2002; Hertzman & Power, 2003). The first life course model that has been dominant in developmental studies is related to critical or sensitive periods in which early childhood or even prenatal exposures shape subsequent outcomes, which may or may not be evident for years. In this model, early exposures shape subsequent outcomes independently of later experiences or changes in exposure. The exposure may not lead to obvious outcomes until later life due to some latency period. In the second life course model, exposures throughout life have a cumulative effect. In such cases, there do not appear to be sensitive periods but, rather, it is the exposures over years and years that have the larger impacts. In the final life course model, early exposures may shape opportunities or barriers to critical exposures in later life that are themselves the critical exposure linked to disease outcomes. This latter model is often called a social trajectory. In the next section, each of these three models is discussed in greater depth (all three models are shown in Figure 24.1).

Sensitive Periods and Latency: Childhood Origins of Adult Health

Developmentalists interested in early development and childhood have focused for decades on the importance of early life exposures in shaping cognition and brain function (Shonkoff, 2003). Over the last decades, epidemiologists have come to understand the "early origins of diseases," often focusing on fetal origins, which evidence suggests shape patterns of metabolic function related to diabetes and other health outcomes (Barker et al., 1989, 2001). The causal pathway invoked in this trajectory can be seen in the top diagram of Figure 24.1. According to this causal diagram, early life conditions (in this case social conditions of interest) become embodied immediately and may go on to influence either adult social conditions or adult health outcomes. In this model, there is only a causal link between early exposure and subsequent adult disease, with no pathway leading from adult social conditions to adult health. In this case of "early embodiment," intervention in adulthood cannot offset the harm incurred in childhood.

What are the types of exposures and outcomes linked to this trajectory? There are many examples related to cognitive and brain development in both animals

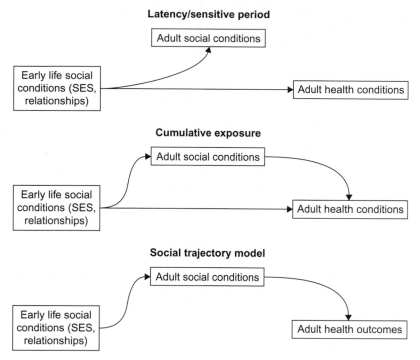

Figure 24.1 Three life course models of disease: latency, cumulative exposures, and social trajectories.
Source: Berkman (2009).

and humans. Of interest to us, however, are exposures related to both social experiences and health outcomes. For instance, with regard to cognitive function in old age, Meaney has a host of studies related to nurturing experiences in early post-natal life in rats (Bredy et al., 2003; Cameron et al., 2008; Champagne & Meaney, 2006; Meaney et al., 1985; Menard et al., 2004; Zhang et al., 2006). In these experiments, rats were randomized to handling and not handling post-natally. Rats randomized to both groups were very similar to each other at earlier ages but, by midlife and at older ages, the non-handled rats developed significant cognitive impairment and simultaneously had higher levels of corticosterone. More recent studies by Meaney and Francis et al. show differences in epigenetic processes also leading to behavioral outcomes (Francis et al., 1999, 2003; Meaney, 2001).

Cumulative Exposure Over the Life Course

Many epidemiologists interested in life course issues hypothesize that the majority of adult disease is not likely to be the result of early childhood or prenatal exposure but rather of a lifetime of accumulated exposures (Lynch & Smith, 2005; Lynch et al., 1997). Such a model can relate to early exposures and simultaneously to adult exposures because it is the impact of cumulative exposures across the life course that takes a toll at older ages. Early experiences may retain some independent impact on outcomes, but that is not the central issue in this model. In this model, the etiologic period is long and covers decades of an individual's life, starting either in early childhood or in adulthood. In this model, we see that, even if early experiences set people up for adult experiences, it is the cumulative impact that is critical. Of central importance to the development of effective interventions is the understanding that intervention in adulthood can offset some of the harm related to the exposures. This is illustrated in the middle diagram of Figure 24.1, in which causal arrows go from the adult experience/exposure to the health outcome even though there is also a causal arrow directly from the early exposure to adult health outcomes. Ben-Shlomo and Kuh (2002) as well as Lynch and Smith (2005) offer fuller reviews of life course models in epidemiology. They point out that in risk models of accumulative exposure there can be both independent and uncorrelated insults as well as correlated insults with risk clustering or chains of risk.

One of the risk factors we know the most about is tobacco consumption. It is interesting to put tobacco consumption into this life course model so that we can understand effective points of intervention. For instance, almost all smokers start to smoke as adolescents. If we had a goal of preventing tobacco consumption, our goal would most likely be to stop adolescents from starting to smoke because quitting is very difficult. Once people start smoking, we have come to understand that the effects on specific disease outcomes are varied. Quitting after the diagnosis of lung cancer does not change the prognosis related to lung cancer, because it is the cumulative impact that has already taken its toll to produce disease. However, quitting after a diagnosis of heart disease can alter prognosis, because there is an immediate effect of quitting that soon alters cardiovascular function. In these two cases there are different etiologic periods, and, because epidemiologists have studied tobacco exposure so well for so long, there is a good understanding of the differential impacts that exposures have on specific disease outcomes. Unfortunately, data on social exposures is much more limited.

Social Trajectories of Risk

In a social trajectory model of health and disease, early life exposures impact adult exposures, which in turn directly influence disease risk. In the bottom diagram of Figure 24.1, the causal pathways indicate that early life exposures do not directly affect adult health. They influence adult social conditions which, in turn, affect adult health. In this case, intervention in adulthood can completely offset harm incurred in childhood.

A clear example of such causal patterns relates to occupational exposures. One can imagine that early life experiences, education, and training in young adulthood place people on a trajectory to obtain certain jobs. Certain occupations, however, carry with them risks related to the physical environment (toxic exposures to chemicals or ergonomic risks) as well as to challenging and stressful jobs. These job exposures are well known to have risks related to a multitude of poor health outcomes related to cardiovascular, musculoskeletal, and cancer disease. In this model, altering the job exposure will completely offset the risk to the individual. Even though specific social or other experiences in childhood may place people at risk for having certain occupations, risks can be substantially reduced by interventions aimed at adult exposures, especially at the level of the worksite. Parallel findings may be related to other adult exposures related to neighborhood exposures or other adult contexts.

Evidence for Continued Neuroplasticity in Adulthood: An Example of Change After Early Childhood Development

Although there is tremendous emphasis on the special importance of early childhood for cognitive development, it is also manifest that humans maintain neurologic plasticity throughout their lives. Not only do humans continue to learn, acquire new memories, and master new skills throughout adulthood, but adult brains can be shown to remodel in response to environmental demands or insults. The extent and biological basis of adult neuroplasticity is an area of intense and expanding research. It now seems that we have long underestimated the possibility of dramatic changes, underwritten by both synaptic/ network remodeling and neurogenesis, that can be achieved in the adult brain.

Much of the most compelling research on the biological plausibility of neurologic changes in response to environmental complexity comes from animal research. For example, recent evidence indicates that spatial memory deficits induced by focal neuronal injury in adult mice can be offset by environmental enrichment. In this model, the mice actually recovered memories that had been lost due to the neuronal injury (Fischer et al., 2007).

Many of the research techniques used to demonstrate plasticity in animals cannot be applied directly to humans. Nonetheless, recent evidence from imaging studies indicates that adult humans also have extensive brain plasticity and many of the animal results are likely to extend to humans. For example, Maguire et al. (2000) found that the posterior hippocampus – an area of the brain responsible for spatial representation and thus navigation – is larger in London taxi drivers compared to controls. Remarkably, dedicated attention to navigation may have costs in terms of other cognitive skills. For example, taxi drivers performed worse than bus drivers (who follow fixed routes) on various visuospatial tests (Maguire et al., 2006). Bilinguals have greater gray matter density in the left inferior parietal cortex compared to monolinguals. This density is greater for early bilinguals than those who acquired a second language later in life and is positively correlated with performance in the second language (Mechelli et al., 2004). Studies that incorporate a longitudinal design following interventions are especially compelling. Training for juggling induced localized gray matter enlargements, and subsequent neglect of juggling was associated with loss of the new volume (Draganski et al., 2004). Adults who receive cochlear implants have been shown to recruit new brain areas (outside the typical language processing regions) to make sense of sounds (Giraud et al., 2001). Stroke recovery is mediated by such plasticity (Cramer, 1999; Cramer et al., 2000). Among blind individuals who learn Braille, areas of the brain typically devoted to visual interpretation are recruited to assist with tactile information processing (Hamilton & Pascual-Leone, 1998).

Epidemiologic evidence also suggests that leisure activities and/or complexity of activities protect against cognitive decline in humans (Scarmeas et al., 2001; Schooler & Mulatu, 2001). Patients with Alzheimer's disease (AD), for instance, show less diversity and intensity of intellectual activities in midlife compared to those without AD (Friedland et al., 2001). The association may occur because cognitive stimulation protects against AD or because a disease process that reduces activity levels may already be operating prior to midlife.

Because of the strong influence of early life educational experiences on subsequent cognitive exposures (via, for example, occupational stratification, social norms about leisure time, financial conditions), observed associations between education and cognitive changes in old age provide incomplete information about whether and how the timing of exposures matters. There is biological evidence for neural plasticity in early life, but adult exposure extending through old age may also affect reserve and resilience.

EFFECTS OF SOCIAL INTEGRATION ON CARDIOVASCULAR RISK AND COGNITIVE AGING: RESULTS FROM OBSERVATIONAL STUDIES

Various aspects of social contacts have been considered in health research, including both structural features of social networks and the content or substance of relationships. Integrating life course models into our thinking about social contacts and aging seems especially timely. First, recent intervention efforts focused on improving social support after stroke or myocardial infarction (MI) most often had null or weak effects (see later discussion). One explanation for why the interventions did not work is that it was not possible to change important features of social context at the targeted moment. Following extreme illness, the individuals and their families had too many other demands to respond to psychosocial interventions. An alternative explanation is that the effects of social support documented in observational research reflect the accumulated benefits of a lifetime of connections, and short-term changes offer little benefit. Both explanations may be partially true.

A key reason to focus on social connections, however, is that the demographic changes that will occur in the next few decades will necessarily entail some level of reorganization in core domains that determine social contacts, such as housing arrangements, residential stability, retirement patterns, and involvement in non-paid work. In thinking about how best to organize such reorganizing decisions, it would be invaluable to understand how social integration affects health.

We use the term "social integration" to broadly refer to aspects of the social environment that have to do with social relationships from intimate ties to more extended community ties and social participation. Under this umbrella, we are interested in social networks, social engagement, and social support. Social networks typically refer to structural aspects of social relationships, such as the size and diversity of the network. Social engagement refers to participation in social or productive activities, such as getting together with friends or participating in an organized group (Barnes et al., 2004; Berkman & Kawachi, 2000). Social support can be seen as the substance of these relationships and activities. At the outset, we use the term social integration very broadly, trying to focus on timing questions rather than the specific domains or characteristics of social ties that matter most. This may ultimately be untenable, because various features of social connections may have different etiologic periods. For example, social contacts may be most relevant for setting behavioral norms during adolescence but most relevant for providing emotional support and meaning during old age. Further, there is evidence that specific aspects of social relations have different associations with health outcomes. In fact, there is some evidence that aspects of networks relate differentially to our two major outcomes: cardiovascular health and cognition. Our intent here, however, is to focus on aspects of timing and be clear about which dimensions of social integration we are examining.

For decades, scientists have reported that the loss of a spouse is related to mortality from coronary heart disease (Ben-Shlomo et al., 1993; Elwert & Christakis, 2008; Martikainen & Valkonen, 1996).

As research in this area developed, investigators came to understand that social isolation, not just loss of an intimate partner, was related to risk. By the 1980s, research on social integration suggested that both men and women without social ties in terms of relationships with partners, friends and family, and voluntary and religious organizations, had an increased risk of dying from cardiovascular-related causes (Berkman & Syme, 1979; Blazer, 1982; House et al., 1982). These studies were conducted in random samples of adult men and women who were middle-aged and older. Often, investigators reported that people who were socially isolated had from two to three times the mortality risk of those with many sources of ties. After this initial wave of studies, scientists confirmed these results in a number of other countries (Sweden, France, Japan, Denmark, Spain) (Berkman et al., 2004; Ikeda et al., 2008; Kaplan et al., 1988; Orth-Gomer et al., 1993, 1998; Rosengren et al., 2004).

A review of the evidence linking social ties and social support to cardiovascular disease reported consistent findings between social isolation and CVD (CVD) morbidity and mortality, low social support, and negative cardiovascular outcomes (Everson-Rose & Lewis, 2005). In another review article, nine out of ten studies found a positive association between social support or social networks and course of disease after initial cardiac event (Hemingway & Marmot, 1999).

The vast majority of studies have examined outcomes that are late in the disease process, such as death or MI. Associations between psychosocial risk factors and CHD endpoints could reflect an effect on initial stages of disease, pace of progression, precipitation of manifestations of CHD among individuals with advanced disease, or some combination. Studies conducted among younger individuals and those without clinical disease offer an opportunity for insight into when psychosocial factors may first exert their influence on cardiovascular function and anatomy. Several review articles describe the evidence linking social factors with the development of atherosclerosis, autonomic dysregulations, and impaired immune function (Knox & Uvnäs-Moberg, 1998; Uchino, 2006; Uchino et al., 1996). For instance, in studies across age groups and among individuals with and without hypertension, social support has been shown to be inversely associated with high blood pressure and directly associated with more favorable blood pressure response to stressors (for a review see Uchino et al., 1996). Among healthy women aged 30–65 years, social isolation and low social support were cross-sectionally associated with decreased heart rate variability (Horsten et al., 1999), a predictor of developing CHD and a predictor of mortality after an MI. Social contact may buffer against psychological stress (Christenfeld & Gerin, 2000; Gerin et al., 1995), which is associated with atherosclerosis (Kop, 1999). Additionally, there is emerging evidence that social networks and social integration are inversely associated with some inflammatory markers in men (Ford et al., 2006; Loucks et al., 2006a, 2006b).

In addition to direct physiological changes induced by the social environment, social factors impact behavioral patterns that are implicated in cardiac health. Behavioral patterns related to smoking, diet, and physical activities have profound effects on cardiovascular health. Such behaviors are importantly affected by peer group and social networks starting in adolescence and continuing into adulthood. In all of these cases, we have some clue that the social environment may begin to exert its effect on cardiovascular health early in the life cycle and, importantly, before the presence of clinical disease.

EXPERIMENTAL STUDIES LINKING SOCIAL INTEGRATION TO CVD

There are two classes of experimental studies that inform us about the nature of social relationships and the effect modifications of these relationships may have on health outcomes. The first class is fairly classical experimental work in social psychology where subjects (animals or humans) are randomized to control conditions or support interventions. The second is large-scale randomized clinical trials in which subjects are given an intervention aimed at improving their social support or social networks and the effect is tested in terms of their reduced risk of major clinical outcomes including re-infarction, mortality, and disability.

Social Psychology Experiments in Humans and Animals

Randomized laboratory studies that manipulate social support in humans (typically with either the presence of a friend or with the supportive behavior of a confederate) have demonstrated quite consistent results. Subjects who receive social support during a stressful task show blunted cardiovascular responses to that task compared to subjects who do not receive social support (for a review see Christenfeld & Gerin, 2000). Whilst supportive behavior of a stranger dampens cardiovascular reactivity, supportive behavior from a friend is even more protective, at least for some cardiovascular measures (Christenfeld et al., 1997). Further, the mere presence of a friend (even one who is not displaying supportive behaviors) (Kamarck et al., 1990) and the mental activation of supportive relationships (Smith et al., 2004) may reduce cardiovascular reactivity to stressful tasks. These findings provide important insight into the possible mechanism through which social integration may reduce poor cardiovascular outcomes.

These human studies are supported by more intensive animal studies that manipulate maternal behavior or social contacts more generally (typically through isolation or status in the hierarchy). For example, in cynomolgus monkeys, social isolation was associated with increased heart rates among those who were moved from social housing to individual housing (Watson et al., 1998). In rats, social isolation has been shown to disturb the functioning of the hypothalamo-pituitary-adrenocortical axis (HPA) (Mar Sánchez et al.,

1995). Also in rats, differences in maternal behavior, such as licking, are associated with stress reactivity in offspring (Caldji et al., 2000; Meaney, 2001), demonstrating the role of the social environment in early life on life-long physiology.

Randomized Clinical Trials to Reduce Recurrent Events, Disability, and Mortality

With a substantial number of observational studies suggesting that social isolation and/or support are linked to cardiovascular-related mortality and two meta-analyses that reported a reduction in mortality and cardiac morbidity with psychosocial interventions among coronary heart disease patients (Dusseldorp et al., 1999; Linden et al., 1996), two large-scale trials were undertaken to assess whether modifying social support would improve clinical outcomes in patients with substantial CVD. In the late 1990s, the Montreal Heart Attack Readjustment Trial (M-HART) was started with the aim of reducing mortality from cardiac causes during the first year after MI. The intervention was aimed at reducing psychosocial distress via monthly telephone monitoring and in-home visits by nurses to patients exhibiting high distress. However, at one year post-MI, the intervention and control groups did not differ on distress. The survival results of the trial were null and there was some hint that women in the intervention arm of the trial had poorer outcomes than women in the control arm of the trial (Frasure-Smith et al., 1997). After M-HART was underway, the Enhancing Recovery in Coronary Heart Disease Patients (ENRICHD)

trial was launched with the aim of reducing depression and increasing social support among patients with a recent MI. The intervention for ENRICHD was cognitive behavioral therapy delivered by a trained psychologist or social worker to alter both depressive symptoms and perceived lack of social support. While the treatment group showed less depression and higher perceived social support, this did not translate into a difference in event-free survival between the treatment groups at an average of 29 months follow-up (Berkman et al., 2003).

The Families in Recovery from Stroke Trial (FIRST) used a psychosocial intervention after stroke with the aim of enhancing recovery. The intervention consisted of up to 16 in-home sessions, conducted by a psychologist or social worker, with the patient's support network, with the aims of increasing self-efficacy and problem-solving as well as optimizing social support and social cohesion (Glass et al., 2004). The intervention, however, was not effective at enhancing functional recovery from stroke (assessed by the Barthel Index), nor did it alter the hypothesized mediator of social support (Glass et al., 2004). For several outcomes (including functional recovery, IADLs, physical performance, and general cognition), the FIRST intervention showed heterogenous treatment effects, with the healthier subgroups showing some improvement with the intervention, but some less-healthy subgroups showing possible harmful effects of intervention compared to usual care (Ertel et al., 2007; Glass et al., 2004) (see Figure 24.2).

Thus, while there is some evidence for the beneficial effects of psychosocial interventions, there have been several disappointments in this arena. It is possible that these trials did not affect cardiac and other

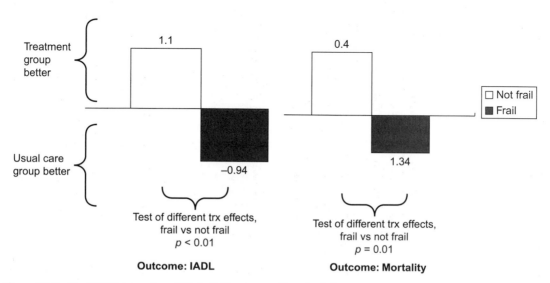

Figure 24.2 The FIRST intervention: differential treatment effects by frailty.
Source: Ertel et al. (2008).

endpoints because they did not alter social conditions enough. It is also possible that they did not show results because the exposure was not altered at the appropriate etiologic period. Other possible reasons include heterogeneous treatment effects (for which secondary analyses provided some support) and that the true causal agent was not targeted (and the results of observational studies linking social integration with cardiovascular health were due to confounding or reverse causation). At this point, we have very little information to help us tease out these alternative explanations, but these questions point to an important area of research to further our understanding of these links and to inform future intervention development.

In summary, there is strong and consistent evidence from observational studies that social factors play an important role in cardiovascular health. Evidence from social psychology experiments in humans and animals is compelling, but human epidemiologic evidence from intervention trials is mixed. To better understand these relationships, we need studies that examine social integration at various points throughout the life course (with adequate assessments of social integration, which may include age-appropriate indices as well as multiple domains of integration, such as network size *and* social support). Integration of these measures with our expanding understanding of cardiovascular aging and growing use of indicators of preclinical disease may provide insight into the time points when social factors produce important changes.

Currently, there is evidence for (1) immediate effects of social support on mortality rates – witness increases in mortality after grievous losses such as widowhood; (2) indirect effects of social connections across the life course on CVD risk, mediated by behavioral patterns such as smoking; (3) accumulation of repeated short-term stressors to cause cardiovascular damage via allostatic load/HPA axis dysregulation, and evidence that social support is likely to offset the consequences of these multiple short experiences; and (4) a possible period of truly special biological vulnerability to social interactions in early infancy, as suggested by rat model studies. This early life stage is a period of very quick physiological changes, and, although the evidence suggests epigenetic changes can occur later in life, there appears to be much more activity early in development. The human analogue of rat licking and grooming of their infants is not clear.

Thus, we can make an argument for several alternative causal models, but emphasizing different pathways. This should be incorporated when thinking about interventions. It may be too hard, for instance, to change social support in the aftermath of a major health event, but easier to change specific health behaviors.

EFFECTS OF SOCIAL INTEGRATION ON COGNITIVE OUTCOMES: RESULTS OF OBSERVATIONAL STUDIES

A number of studies have now shown that features of the social environment, especially those related to social engagement and social networks, are important predictors of cognitive outcomes among the elderly (for a review, see Fratiglioni et al., 2004). For example, Fratiglioni and colleagues reported that limited social networks were associated with increased risk of incident dementia (Fratiglioni et al., 2000). Barnes and colleagues found that high social networks and high social engagement reduced the rate of cognitive decline (Barnes et al., 2004). Bassuk et al. reported that individuals with many social ties were at decreased risk for incident cognitive decline compared to individuals with few social ties (Bassuk et al., 1999). Zunzunegui et al.'s results indicated that older persons with few social ties, poor social integration, and social disengagement were at greater risk of cognitive decline (Zunzunegui et al., 2003). Similarly, we report that, in a sample representative of US elderly individuals, higher levels of social integration (assessed according to marital status, engaging in volunteer activities, and frequency of contact with parents, children, and neighbors) predicted a reduced rate of memory decline over six years; comparison of the most integrated to the least integrated revealed a twofold difference in the rate of memory decline during the follow-up period (Ertel et al., 2008). These studies provide very strong evidence from sound observational studies on the link between social engagement and cognitive outcomes. Although questions have been raised about the possibility of reverse causation, many of these studies have attempted to test the causal pathways from cognitive decline to social disengagement and found limited evidence for this.

Most studies in this area assessed social integration only once and only in elderly individuals, but there are notable exceptions. Although not all studies with repeated assessments found an association between social activities and cognitive change (Hultsch et al., 1999), there is evidence to support a causal and perhaps reciprocal relationship between social engagement and cognitive functioning in the elderly. The Honolulu-Asian Aging Study assessed social engagement among men in midlife (average of 27.5 years before dementia diagnosis) and late-life (average of 4.6 years before dementia diagnosis). In fully adjusted models that included both mid- and late-life social engagement, only low late-life social engagement showed a statistically significant association with increased risk of dementia (Saczynski et al., 2006). When modeling changes in social engagement, the authors found that, compared to those with high social engagement at both time points, individuals whose social engagement decreased from mid- to late life had increased risk of dementia. Similar, although not statistically significant, results were seen for those with low social engagement at both time points. The authors interpret this as possible evidence that prodromal dementia may have influenced social engagement in late life. Similarly, Bosma and colleagues found a reciprocal relationship between social activities and a range of cognitive tests over a three-year period in elderly individuals in the Netherlands (Bosma et al., 2002).

Marital status is a component of most social integration measures, but it has also been examined as a single element, perhaps measuring social integration or social support. Helmer and colleagues (1999) reported that, among elderly individuals (over age 65) in France, the risk of incident Alzheimer's disease over five years was more than two-fold for never-married individuals compared to those married or cohabitating at baseline. Similar results held in a longitudinal study in Sweden with dementia as the outcome (Fratiglioni et al., 2000). Assessing the effect of a change in marital status over five years in elderly men in the FINE Study, Van Gelder and colleagues reported that 10-year cognitive decline was the lowest in men who remained married compared to those who remained unmarried and those who became unmarried (Van Gelder et al., 2006).

As mentioned earlier, a concern in all of these observational studies is the extent to which one can be confident in assigning a causal relationship from social integration to cognitive outcomes. Social withdrawal and apathy are common symptoms in dementia (Galynker et al., 1995; Reichman & Negron, 2001), and even subtle cognitive declines might result in withdrawal from social or community networks. Further, compelling evidence suggests that people who ultimately develop dementia exhibit cognitive differences decades before dementia is diagnosed (Elias et al., 2000; Snowdon et al., 1996). No matter how long the time lag between measured social ties and measured cognitive outcomes, there is always a concern that both were influenced by prior cognitive function. Several studies have made concerted efforts to examine this issue – see, for example, Bassuk et al. (1999) and Ertel et al. (2008) – but observational studies cannot definitely rule out, and in some cases support, reciprocal or reverse causation models.

In summary, we have evidence from observational studies that social integration in older persons is associated with cognitive outcomes. It is not clear to what extent the social engagement measured during an elder's years serves as an indicator of their social engagement across their life course, although, as reviewed earlier, many aspects of social integration show significant stability across adulthood and into old age for many individuals. Interestingly, in the one study that we know of that examined it, there is some evidence that late-life engagement may be as, or more important, than midlife engagement for cognitive outcomes.

INTERVENTION STUDIES LINKING SOCIAL INTEGRATION TO COGNITIVE OUTCOMES

To our knowledge, there are few intervention studies exploring the possible protective effect of social integration on cognitive outcomes in late life. Several interventions have aimed to change the social environment (family functioning, social support, etc.) after stroke, but these studies have typically not focused on cognitive outcomes (for example Clark et al., 2003; Dennis et al., 1997). As discussed earlier, one study that included cognitive outcomes was the FIRST. This study enrolled patients soon after a stroke and randomized them to control or intervention. The intervention consisted of up to 16 in-home sessions, conducted by a psychologist or social worker, with the patient's support network, with the aims of increasing self-efficacy and problem-solving as well as optimizing social support and social cohesion (Glass et al., 2004). The intervention, however, was not effective at enhancing global cognitive functioning (assessed via 10 cognitive tests), nor did it alter the hypothesized mediator of social support (Ertel et al., 2007; Glass et al., 2004). The Experience Corps Model recruits older men and women to work with young children in schools. It has had success in changing some factors (Fried et al., 2004). We know of no other intervention studies of social integration and cognitive outcomes among adult or elderly non-patient samples.

There is, however, suggestive evidence that intervening in the social environment in early childhood can alter cognitive outcomes in young children. The Bucharest Early Intervention Project randomly assigned children in Romanian orphanages to continued institutional care or placement in a foster family (Nelson et al., 2007). The 187 children were less than 31 months of age at randomization and cognitive testing was conducted at 42 and 54 months of age. Children who were moved from institutional care to foster care had, on average, higher scores on the Bayley Scales of Infant Development at 42 months (mean difference = 0.62 SD) and the Weschsler Preschool Primary Scale of Intelligence at 54 months (mean difference = 0.47 SD). These intervention findings are supported by observational findings that children in foster care have higher cognitive scores compared to children in institutional settings (Miller et al., 2005).

Difficulties arise in assigning the effect of foster vs institutional care to the social environment because it is likely that all aspects of the environment, including those important to cognitive development, such as material resources, were different between foster and institutional care. However, the data are suggestive that strong attachments and relationships with caregivers in early childhood confer cognitive benefits. These ideas have received strong theoretical support and have been demonstrated in animal models (Kaffman & Meaney, 2007).

There is also evidence from some animal studies, for example showing that recovery from experimentally induced stroke is improved in group-housed animals compared to isolated animals (Craft et al., 2005). Environmental enrichment studies that have tried to identify the important components of enrichment suggest social interactions are crucial (Risedal et al., 2002).

In summary, the observational evidence linking social integration with cognitive outcomes is quite strong, though few intervention studies exist that would either bolster or refute the observational evidence. In terms of the relevant timing of social factors and cognitive health, we also have very little information to guide our thinking. Similarly to the possible avenues for better understanding the relationship between social integration and cardiovascular health to better understand the relationship with cognitive health, we need studies that examine social integration at various points throughout the life course (with adequate assessments of social integration, which may include age-appropriate indices as well as multiple domains of integration, such as network size *and* social support).

CAN WE CHANGE SOCIAL INTEGRATION? WHEN HAVE INTERVENTIONS BEEN SUCCESSFUL?

There are several good reviews of interventions aimed at changing some aspect of the social environment, for example Glass (2000) and Hogan et al. (2002). Here we will highlight findings that provide some clues about what types of interventions may be successful and which aspects of social integration may be amenable to change. However, definitive conclusions cannot be made because many of these studies had small sample sizes and it is difficult to compare results across the range of populations studied.

Self-help groups have shown some success in changing friendship networks (Humphreys & Noke, 1997;

Humphreys et al., 1999), which may be particularly important for reducing problem behaviors, such as substance abuse. Some interventions have succeeded in producing enhanced social support for specific behaviors; for example, Wing and Jeffery (1999), in which social support for healthy eating was enhanced with the intervention. These studies, however, have not randomly allocated group membership, so it could be that these groups are only helpful for individuals who seek them out themselves (Hogan et al., 2002). Interventions that have targeted social skills have shown mixed success at increasing the participants' social environment, such as perceived social support (Brand et al., 1995) and increased social networks (Lovell & Hawkins, 1988), although others have not produced changes (Hogan et al., 2002). Studies among older people have shown mixed success, with one small study offering the possibility of enhancing the social environment of elders (Bogat & Jason, 1983). However, a telephone-based intervention was not successful at enhancing social support (Heller et al., 1991), nor was an intervention aimed at increasing social contacts (Baumgarten et al., 1988).

In light of the purposes of this chapter, there are three important limitations in this literature and, more generally, in our understanding of social integration interventions. First, it appears that most studies have focused on method of delivery (such as self-help group or individual counseling with a psychologist), instead of timing of delivery (whether it be timing according to age of recipient: young, middle, or old age) or timing with respect to course of disease (initial stages of development of disease, during treatment for disease, etc.). Second, most studies of social support interventions have been among patient groups, instead of a broader-based community sample. It may be the case that different interventions are more successful for different patient groups, but, if our goal is prevention, focus on community samples of healthy individuals should be a priority. There are many programs that may increase social integration, such as Big Brother, Big Sister, and other volunteer activities that may benefit both volunteer and recipient of services. However, such programs have rarely been studied for their effect on social factors, although it seems likely that they impact social engagement, networks, and support. This is a potential avenue for future research, in addition to linking involvement in these programs with health outcomes. Third, studies have tended to examine physical or mental outcomes, with less focus on whether the proposed mediator, some aspect of social integration, was changed. Indeed, in a review of 100 social support interventions, Hogan and colleagues (2002) concluded that, "the most salient problem is that *most* studies examining efficacy of support interventions failed to include a measure of social support" (p. 425).

The notion of intervening in complex social relationships and structures is inherently difficult and complicated. Given this complexity, along with the state of the science and the limitations discussed above, it seems that we have a lot of work before us to figure out how and when to best intervene to enhance the social environment.

IMPLICATIONS FOR SOCIAL INTERVENTION

How do we use our current understanding of risk factors across the lifespan to promote healthy aging?

Much of the research reported here inevitably focuses on small, manipulative exposures in order to demonstrate causal etiological relationships between social conditions and health. In contrast, when thinking about the translation of these results to best improve population health, individual-level interventions are likely to be only a small component of a successful response. The broad-sweeping secular changes in the past 50 years demonstrate that contextual factors can entirely reshape the population distribution of socioeconomic conditions, including financial and educational opportunities, and the context of social connections. For example, key social trends reflected in current elderly cohorts include dramatic differences in the levels and content of education; changing family structure due to declines in fertility and increases in divorce; changes in experiences of poverty and the gender patterns of financial insecurity; and reshaping of residential patterns due to migration of children away from natal communities and general population movements away from rural and rust-belt areas. These changes illustrate that nothing about the social world is inevitable. Macro-level forces, such as economic change and policy initiatives, can rewrite the lives of individuals not only with respect to socioeconomic position but even in very personal domains such as the structure of social networks and engagement.

The first implication of life course epidemiology is that what we do now can pay off for elderly people 80 years from now, and for many such investments the payoffs will be greater if investments are made in early childhood. We are now very likely reaping the health benefits of major social investments made in earlier decades of the twentieth century, when we put high school within reach of the majority of adolescents, implemented much stronger social safety nets for working adults, and improved occupational conditions. The evidence in support of early childhood investments is large. Cost–benefit analyses of such investments should probably consider the benefits of reduced burden of illness as those cohorts age (Knudsen et al., 2006), but this does not imply that investments in older people are useless.

In addition to these implications regarding investments in children for later health benefits, we think life course epidemiology has implications for social policies that specifically affect currently elderly individuals:

(1) Cognitive plasticity remains into adulthood, and the absence of environmental demands and educational opportunities in the daily lives of older persons is likely to have negative consequences for their cognitive health. Retirement policies, housing policies, and the organization and targeting of public education systems should be considered in light of these concerns. Do these institutions serve elderly people or do they foster isolation, environmental constraints and simplification, and loss of social roles for older individuals? In this sense, many policies maintain and stabilize lifelong trajectories of disadvantage, in which individuals deprived of schooling in childhood also have limited access to workplace training or environmental stimulation, and ultimately are most likely to be isolated from cognitive challenges and engagement in old age.

(2) People continue to want and need close relationships in old age, and during young-old age they are reasonably good at maintaining such relationships. However, it is not just family contacts overall that influence health; friendship contacts probably also matter and these are threatened in old age. If the old-old have special challenges in establishing new friend relationships, due to physical frailty and mobility restrictions, the surviving relationships can come to be dominated by non-beneficial exchanges (e.g. receiving help instead of exchanging support). The intervention results should make us worry, if nothing else, that interrupting social connections and introducing sources of psychosocial stress might be harmful, especially for women and for the frailest. Housing policies and health care distribution systems that force older persons to relocate away from longstanding networks of friends are likely to have undesirable consequences if they occur at moments in the life course when these networks are hard to replace. We should recognize the differences between young-old and old-old and help the young-old prepare to be old-old, for example with respect to social relationships and residential location.

ACKNOWLEDGMENTS

We would like to acknowledge the support of the MacArthur Foundation Network on the Aging

Society for their support of this work. In addition, the Harvard Program on the Demography of Aging has provided support for this work (NIA#: P30 AG024409-05).

Parts of the chapter have been taken from: Ertel KA, Glymour M, Berkman LF. Social networks and Health: A life course perspective integrating observational and experimental evidence. *JSPR* 2009:26 (1): 73–92 and Berkman LF. Social Epidemiology: Social Determinants of Health in the US: Are we losing ground? *Annu Rev Public Health* 2009 Apr 29; 30:27–41.

REFERENCES

Barker, D. J., Winter, P. D., Osmond, C., Margetts, B., & Simmonds, S. J. (1989). Weight in infancy and death from ischaemic heart disease. *Lancet, 2*(8663), 577–580.

Barker, D. J., Forsen, T., Uutela, A., Osmond, C., & Eriksson, J. G. (2001). Size at birth and resilience to effects of poor living conditions in adult life: Longitudinal study. *British Medical Journal, 323*(7324), 1273–1276.

Barnes, L. L., Mendes de Leon, C. F., Wilson, R. S., Bienias, J. L., & Evans, D. A. (2004). Social resources and cognitive decline in a population of older African Americans and whites. *Neurology, 63*(12), 2322–2326.

Bassuk, S. S., Glass, T. A., & Berkman, L. F. (1999). Social disengagement and incident cognitive decline in community-dwelling elderly persons. *Annals of Internal Medicine, 131*(3), 165–173.

Baumgarten, M., Thomas, D., de Courval, L. P., & Infante-Rivard, C. (1988). Evaluation of a mutual help network for the elderly residents of planned housing. *Psychology and Aging, 3*(4), 393–398.

Ben-Shlomo, Y., & Kuh, D. (2002). A life course approach to chronic disease epidemiology: Conceptual models, empirical challenges and interdisciplinary perspectives. *International Journal of Epidemiology, 31*(2), 285–293.

Ben-Shlomo, Y., Smith, G. D., Shipley, M., & Marmot, M. G. (1993). Magnitude and causes of mortality differences between married and unmarried men. *Journal of Epidemiology and Community Health, 47*, 200–205.

Berkman, L. F., & Kawachi, I. (2000). *Social epidemiology.* New York: Oxford University Press.

Berkman, L. F., & Syme, S. L. (1979). Social networks, host resistance and mortality: A nine year follow-up study of Alameda County residents. *American Journal of Epidemiology, 117*, 1003–1009.

Berkman, L. F., Blumenthal, J., Burg, M., Carney, R. M., Catellier, D., Cowan, M. J., et al. (2003). Effects of treating depression and low perceived social support on clinical events after myocardial infarction: The enhancing recovery in coronary heart disease patients (ENRICHD) randomized trial. *Journal of American Medical Association, 289*(23), 3106–3116.

Berkman, L. F., Melchior, M., Chastang, J. F., Niedhammer, I., Leclerc, A., & Goldberg, M. (2004). Social integration and mortality: A prospective study of French employees of Electricity of France-Gas of France: the GAZEL cohort. *American Journal Epidemiology, 259*(2), 167–174.

Berkman, L. F. (2009). Social epidemiology: Social determinants of health in the United States: Are we losing ground?. *Annual Review of Public Health, 30*, 27–41.

Blazer, D. G. (1982). Social support and mortality in an elderly community population. *American Journal of Epidemiology, 115*, 684–694.

Bogat, G. A., & Jason, L. A. (1983). An evaluation of two visiting programs for elderly community residents. *International Journal of Aging and Human Development, 17*, 267–279.

Bosma, H., van Boxtel, M. P., Ponds, R. W., Jelicic, M., Houx, P., Metsemakers, J., et al. (2002). Engaged lifestyle and cognitive function in middle and old-aged, non-demented persons: A reciprocal association? *Zeitschrift fur Gerontologie und Geriatrie, 35*(6), 575–581.

Brand, E. F., Lakey, B., & Berman, S. (1995). A preventive, psychoeducational approach to increase perceived social support. *American Journal of Community Psychology, 23*(1), 117–135.

Bredy, T. W., Grant, R. J., Champagne, D. L., & Meaney, M. J. (2003). Maternal care influences neuronal survival in the hippocampus of the rat. *European Journal of Neuroscience, 18*(10), 2903–2909.

Caldji, C., Diorio, J., & Meaney, M. J. (2000). Variations in maternal care in infancy regulate the development of stress reactivity. *Biological Psychiatry, 48*(12), 1164–1174.

Cameron, N., Del Corpo, A., Diorio, J., McAllister, K., Sharma, S., & Meaney, M. J. (2008). Maternal programming of sexual behavior and hypothalamic-pituitary-gonadal function in the female rat. *PLoS ONE, 3*(5), e2210.

Champagne, F. A., & Meaney, M. J. (2006). Stress during gestation alters postpartum maternal care and the development of the offspring in a rodent model. *Biological Psychiatry, 59*(12), 1227–1235.

Christenfeld, N., & Gerin, W. (2000). Social support and cardiovascular reactivity. *Biomedicine & Pharmacotherapy, 54*(5), 251–257.

Christenfeld, N., Gerin, W., Linden, W., Sanders, M., Mathur, J., Deich, J. D., et al. (1997). Social support effects on cardiovascular reactivity: Is a stranger as effective as a friend? *Psychosomatic Medicine, 59*(4), 388–398.

Clark, M., Rubenach, S., & Winsor, A. (2003). A randomized controlled trial of an education and counseling intervention for families after stroke. *Clinical Rehabilitation, 17*, 703–712.

Craft, T. K. S., Glasper, E. R., McCullough, L., Zhang, N.,

Sugo, N., Otsuka, T., et al. (2005). Social interaction improves experimental stroke outcome. *American Heart Association, l,* 2006–2011.

Cramer, S. C. (1999). Stroke recovery. Lessons from functional MR imaging and other methods of human brain mapping. *Physical Medicine & Rehabilitation Clinics of North America, 10*(4), 875–886, ix.

Cramer, S. C., Moore, C. I., Finklestein, S. P., & Rosen, B. R. (2000). A pilot study of somatotopic mapping after cortical infarct. *Stroke, 31*(3), 668–671.

Dennis, M., O'Rourke, S., Slattery, J., Staniforth, T., & Warlow, C. (1997). Evaluation of a stroke family care worker: Results of a randomised controlled trial. *British Medical Journal, 12*(7087), 1071–1076.

Draganski, B., Gaser, C., Busch, V., Schuierer, G., & Bogdahn, U. (2004). Neuroplasticity: Changes in grey matter induced by training. *Nature, 427,* 311–312.

Dusseldorp, E., van Elderen, T., Maes, S., Meulman, J., & Kraaij, V. (1999). A meta-analysis of psychoeducational programs for coronary heart disease patients. *Health Psychology, 18*(5), 506–519.

Elias, M. F., Beiser, A., Wolf, P. A., Au, R., White, R. F., & D'Agostino, R. B. (2000). The preclinical phase of alzheimer disease: A 22-year prospective study of the Framingham Cohort. *Archives of Neurology, 57*(6), 808–813.

Elwert, F., & Christakis, N. A. (2008). The effect of widowhood on mortality by the causes of death of both spouses. *American Journal of Public Health, 98*(7), 2092–2098.

Ertel, K. A., Glymour, M. M., & Berkman, L. F. (2008). Effects of social integration on preserving memory function in a nationally representative US elderly population. *American Journal of Public Health, 98*(7), 1215–1220.

Ertel, K. A., Glymour, M. M., Glass, T. A., & Berkman, L. F. (2007). Frailty modifies effectiveness of psychosocial intervention in recovery from stroke. *Clinical Rehabilitation, 21*(6), 511–522.

Everson-Rose, S. A., & Lewis, T. T. (2005). Psychosocial factors and cardiovascular diseases. *Annual Review of Public Health, 26*(1), 469–500.

Fischer, A., Sananbenesi, F., Wang, X. Y., Dobbin, M., & Tsai, L. H. (2007). Recovery of learning and memory is associated with chromatin remodeling. *Nature, 447*(7141), 178–182.

Ford, E. S., Loucks, E. B., & Berkman, L. F. (2006). Social integration and concentrations of C-Reactive Protein among US adults. *Annals of Epidemiology, 16*(2), 78–84.

Francis, D. D., Caldji, C., Champagne, F., Plotsky, P. M., & Meaney, M. J. (1999). The role of corticotropin-releasing factor–norepinephrine systems in mediating the effects of early experience on the development of behavioral and endocrine responses to stress. *Biological Psychiatry, 46*(9), 1153–1166.

Francis, D. D., Szegda, K., Campbell, G., Martin, W. D., & Insel, T. R. (2003). Epigenetic sources of behavioral differences in mice. *Nature Neuroscience, 6*(5), 445–446.

Frasure-Smith, N., Lesperance, F., Prince, R. H., Verrier, P., Garber, R. A., Juneau, M., et al. (1997). Randomised trial of home-based psychosocial nursing intervention for patients recovering from myocardial infarction. *Lancet, 350,* 473–479.

Fratiglioni, L., Paillard-Borg, S., & Winblad, B. (2004). An active and socially integrated lifestyle in late life might protect against dementia. *The Lancet Neurology, 3*(6), 343–353.

Fratiglioni, L., Wang, H. -X., Ericsson, K., Maytan, M., & Winblad, B. (2000). Influence of social network on occurrence of dementia: A community-based longitudinal study. *Lancet, 355,* 1315–1319.

Fried, L. P., Carlson, M. C., Freedman, M., Frick, K. D., Glass, T. A., Hill, J., et al. (2004). A social model for health promotion for an aging population: Initial evidence on the experience corps model. *Journal of Urban Health-Bulletin of the New York Academy of Medicine, 81*(1), 64–78.

Friedland, R. P., Fritsch, T., Smyth, K. A., Koss, E., Lerner, A. J., Chen, C. H., et al. (2001). Patients with Alzheimer's disease have reduced activities in midlife compared with healthy control-group members. *Proceedings of the National Academy of Sciences of the United States of America, 98*(6), 3440–3445.

Galynker, I. I., Roane, D. M., Miner, C. R., Feinberg, T. E., & Watts, P. (1995). Negative symptoms in patients with Alzheimers disease. *American Journal of Geriatric Psychiatry, 3*(1), 52–59.

Gerin, W., Milner, D., Chawla, S., & Pickering, T. G. (1995). Social support as a moderator of cardiovascular reactivity in women: A test of the direct effects and buffering hypotheses. *Psychosomatic Medicine, 57*(1), 16–22.

Giraud, A. L., Price, C. J., Graham, J. M., & Frackowiak, R. S. (2001). Functional plasticity of language-related brain areas after cochlear implantation. *Brain, 124*(pt7), 1307–1316.

Glass, T. (2000). Psychosocial intervention. In L. Berkman & I. Kawachi (Eds.), *Social epidemiology* (pp. 267–305). New York: Oxford University Press.

Glass, T. A., Berkman, L. F., Hiltunen, E. F., Furie, K., Glymour, M. M., Fay, M. E., et al. (2004). The families in recovery from stroke trial (FIRST): Primary study results. *Psychosomatic Medicine, 66*(6), 889–897.

Hamilton, R. H., & Pascual-Leone, A. (1998). Cortical plasticity associated with Braille learning. *Trends in Cognitive Sciences, 2*(5), 168–174.

Heller, K., Thompson, M. G., Trueba, P. E., Hogg, J. R., Vlachos-Weber, I. (1991). Peer support telephone dyads for elderly women: Was this the wrong intervention? *American Journal of Community Psychology, 19*(1), 53–74.

Helmer, C., Damon, D., Letenneur, L., Fabrigoule, C., Barberger-Gateau, P., Lafont, S., et al. (1999). Marital status and risk of Alzheimer's disease: A French population-based cohort study. *Neurology, 53*(9), 1953–1958.

Hemingway, H., & Marmot, M. (1999). Evidence based cardiology: Psychosocial factors in the aetiology and prognosis of coronary heart disease: Systematic review of prospective cohort studies. *British Medical Journal, 318*(7196), 1460–1467.

Hertzman, C., & Power, C. (2003). Health and human development: Understandings from life-course research. *Developmental Neuropsychology, 24*(2–3), 719–744.

Hogan, B. E., Linden, W., & Najarian, B. (2002). Social support interventions. Do they work? *Clinical Psychology Review, 22,* 381–440.

Horsten, M., Ericson, M., Perski, A., Wamala, S. P., Schenck-Gustafsson, K., & Orth-Gomer, K. (1999). Psychosocial factors and heart rate variability in healthy women. *Psychosomatic Medicine, 61*(1), 49–57.

House, J. S., Robbins, C., & Metzner, H. L. (1982). The association of social relationships and activities with mortality: Prospective evidence from the Tecumseh community health study. *American Journal of Epidemiology, 116,* 123–140.

Hultsch, D. F., Hertzog, C., Small, B. J., & Dixon, R. A. (1999). Use it or lose it: Engaged lifestyle as a buffer of cognitive decline in aging? *Psychology and Aging, 14*(2), 245–263.

Humphreys, K., Mankowski, E. S., Moos, R. H., & Finney, J. W. (1999). Do enhanced friendship networks and active coping mediate the effect of self-help groups on substance abuse? *Annals of Behavioral Medicine, 21*(1), 54–60.

Humphreys, K., & Noke, J. M. (1997). The influence of posttreatment mutual help group participation on the friendship networks of substance abuse patients. *American Journal of Community Psychology, 25*(1), 1–16.

Ikeda, A., Iso, H., Kawachi, I., Yamagishi, K., Inoue, M., Tsugane, S., et al. (2008). Social support and stroke and coronary heart disease: The JPHC Study Cohorts II. *Stroke, 39*(3), 768–775.

Kaffman, A., & Meaney, M. J. (2007). Neurodevelopmental sequelae of postnatal maternal care in rodents: Clinical and research implications of molecular insights. *Journal of Child Psychology and Psychiatry, 48*(3–4), 224–244.

Kamarck, T. W., Manuck, S. B., & Jennings, J. R. (1990). Social support reduces cardiovascular reactivity to psychological challenge: A laboratory model. *Psychosomatic Medicine, 52*(1), 42–58.

Kaplan, G. A., Salonen, J. T., Cohen, R. D., Brand, R. J., Syme, S. L., & Puska, P. (1988). Social connections and mortality from all causes and from cardiovascular disease: Prospective evidence from eastern Finland. *American Journal of Epidemiology, 128,* 370–380.

Knox, S. S., & Uvnäs-Moberg, K. (1998). Social isolation and cardiovascular disease: An atherosclerotic pathway? *Psychoneuroendocrinology, 23*(8), 877–890.

Knudsen, E. I., Heckman, J. J., Cameron, J. L., & Shonkoff, J. P. (2006). Economic, neurobiological, and behavioral perspectives on building America's future workforce. *Proceedings from National Academy of Sciences U.S.A, 103,* 10155–10162.

Kop, W. J. (1999). Chronic and acute psychological risk factors for clinical manifestations of coronary artery disease. *Psychosomatic Medicine, 61*(4), 476–487.

Linden, W., Stossell, C., & Maurice, J. (1996). Psychosocial interventions for patients with coronary artery disease: A meta-analysis. *Archives of Internal Medicine, 156*(7), 745–752.

Loucks, E. B., Berkman, L. F., Gruenewald, T. L., & Seeman, T. E. (2006a). Relation of social integration to inflammatory marker concentrations in men and women 70 to 79 years. *American Journal of Cardiology, 97*(7), 1010–1016.

Loucks, E. B., Sullivan, L. M., D'Agostino, R. B. S., Larson, M. G., Berkman, L. F., & Benjamin, E. J. (2006b). Social networks and inflammatory markers in the Framingham Heart Study. *Journal of Biosocial Science, 38*(6), 835–842.

Lovell, M., & Hawkins, J. D. (1988). An evaluation of a group intervention to increase the personal social networks of abusive mothers. *Children and Youth Services Review, 10,* 175–188.

Lynch, J., & Smith, G. D. (2005). A life course approach to chronic disease epidemiology. *Annual Review of Public Health, 26,* 1–35.

Lynch, J. W., Kaplan, G. A., & Shema, S. J. (1997). Cumulative impact of sustained economic hardship on physical, cognitive, psychological, and social functioning. *New England Journal of Medicine, 337*(26), 1889–1895.

Maguire, E. A., Gadian, D. G., Johnsrude, I. S., Good, C. D., Ashburner, J., Frackowiak, R. S., et al. (2000). Navigation-related structural change in the hippocampi of taxi drivers. *Proceedings of the National Academy of Sciences of the United States of America, 97*(8), 4398–4403.

Maguire, E. A., Woollett, K., & Spiers, H. J. (2006). London taxi drivers and bus drivers: A structural MRI and neuropsychological analysis. *Hippocampus, 16*(12), 1091–1101.

Mar Sánchez, M., Aguado, F., Sánchez-Toscano, F., & Saphier, D. (1995). Effects of prolonged social isolation on responses of neurons in the bed nucleus of the stria terminalis, preoptic area, and hypothalamic paraventricular nucleus to stimulation of the medial amygdala. *Psychoneuroendocrinology, 20*(5), 525–541.

Martikainen, P., & Valkonen, T. (1996). Mortality after the death of a spouse: Rates and causes of death in a large Finnish cohort. *American Journal of Public Health, 86,* 1087–1093.

Meaney, M. J. (2001). Maternal care, gene expression, and the transmission of individual differences in stress reactivity across generations. *Annual Review of Neuroscience, 24*(1), 1161–1192.

Meaney, M. J., Aitken, D. H., Bodnoff, S. R., Iny, L. J., & Sapolsky, R. M. (1985). The effects of postnatal handling on the development of the glucocorticoid receptor systems and stress recovery in the rat. *Progress in Neuro-Psychopharmacology and Biological Psychiatry, 9*(5–6), 731–734.

Mechelli, A., Crinion, J. T., Noppeney, U., O'Doherty, J., Ashburner, J., Frackowiak, R. S., et al. (2004). Neurolinguistics: Structural plasticity in the bilingual brain. *Nature, 431*(7010), 757.

Menard, J. L., Champagne, D. L., & Meaney, M. J. (2004). Variations of maternal care differentially influence 'fear' reactivity and regional patterns of cFos immunoreactivity in response to the shock-probe burying test. *Neuroscience, 129*(2), 297–308.

Miller, L., Chan, W., Comfort, K., & Tirella, L. (2005). Health of children adopted from Guatemala: Comparison of orphanage and foster care. *Pediatrics, 115*(6), e710–e717.

Nelson, C. A., III, Zeanah, C. H., Fox, N. A., Marshall, P. J., Smyke, A. T., & Guthrie, D. (2007). Cognitive recovery in socially deprived young children: The Bucharest early intervention project. *Science, 318*(5858), 1937–1940.

Orth-Gomer, K., Horsten, M., Wamala, S. P., Mittleman, M. A., Kirkeeide, R., Svane, B., et al. (1998). Social relations and extent and severity of coronary artery disease: The Stockholm female coronary risk study. *European Heart Journal, 19*(11), 1648–1656.

Orth-Gomer, K., Rosengren, A, & Wilhelmsen, L. (1993). Lack of social support and incidence of coronary heart disease in middle-aged Swedish men. *Psychosomatic Medicine, 55*(1), 37–43.

Reichman, W. E., & Negron, A. (2001). Negative symptoms in the elderly patient with dementia. *International Journal of Geriatric Psychiatry, 16*, S7–S11.

Risedal, A., Mattsson, B., Dahlqvist, P., Nordborg, C., Olsson, T., & Johansson, B. (2002). Environmental influences on functional outcome after a cortical infarct in the rat. *Brain Research Bulletin, 58*(3), 315–321.

Rosengren, A., Wilhelmsen, L., & Orth-Gomer, K. (2004). Coronary disease in relation to social support and social class in Swedish men: A 15 year follow-up in the study of men born in 1933. *European Heart Journal, 25*(1), 56–63.

Saczynski, J. S., Pfeifer, L. A., Masaki, K., Korf, E. S. C., Laurin, D., White, L., et al. (2006). The effect of social engagement on incident dementia: The Honolulu-Asia aging study. *American Journal of Epidemiology, 163*(5), 433–440.

Scarmeas, N., Levy, G., Tang, M. X., Manly, J., & Stern, Y. (2001). Influence of leisure activity on the incidence of Alzheimer's disease. *Neurology, 57*(2), 2236–2242.

Schooler, C., & Mulatu, M. S. (2001). The reciprocal effects of leisure time activities and intellectual functioning in older people: A longitudinal analysis. *Psychology and Aging, 16*(3), 466–482.

Shonkoff, J. P. (2003). From neurons to neighborhoods: Old and new challenges for developmental and behavioral pediatrics. *Journal of Development & Behavioral Pediatrics, 24*(1), 70–76.

Smith, T. W., Ruiz, J. M., & Uchino, B. N. (2004). Mental activation of supportive ties, hostility, and cardiovascular reactivity to laboratory stress in young men and women. *Health Psychology, 23*(5), 476–485.

Snowdon, D. A., Kemper, S. J., Mortimer, J. A., Greiner, L. H., Wekstein, D. R., & Markesbery,, W. R. (1996). Linguistic ability in early life and cognitive function and Alzheimer's disease in late life. Findings from the Nun Study. *Journal of the American Medical Association, 275*(7), 528–532.

Uchino, B. N. (2006). Social support and health: A review of physiological processes potentially underlying links to disease outcomes. *Journal of Behavioral Medicine, 29*(4), 377–387.

Uchino, B. N., Cacioppo, J. T., & Kiecolt-Glaser, J. K. (1996). The relationship between social support and physiological processes: A review with emphasis on underlying mechanisms and implications for health. *Psychological Bulletin, 119*(3), 488–531.

Van Gelder, B. M., Tijhuis, M., Kalmijn, S., Giampaoli, S., Nissinen, A., & Kromhout, D. (2006). Marital status and living situation during a 5-year period are associated with a subsequent 10-year cognitive decline in older men: The FINE study. *Journal of Gerontology: Psychological Sciences, 61*(4), 213–219.

Watson, S. L., Shively, C. A., Kaplan, J. R., & Line, S. W. (1998). Effects of chronic social separation on cardiovascular disease risk factors in female cynomolgus monkeys. *Atherosclerosis, 137*(2), 259–266.

Wing, R. R., & Jeffery, R. W. (1999). Benefits of recruiting participants with friends and increasing social support for weight loss and maintenance. *Journal of Consulting and Clinical Psychology, 67*(1), 132–138.

Zhang, T. Y., Bagot, R., Parent, C., Nesbitt, C., Bredy, T. W., Caldji, C., et al. (2006). Maternal programming of defensive responses through sustained effects on gene expression. *Biological Psychology, 73*(1), 72–89.

Zunzunegui, M. -V., Alvarado, B. E., Del Ser, T., & Otero, A. (2003). Social networks, social integration, and social engagement determine cognitive decline in community-dwelling Spanish older adults. *Journal of Gerontology: Social Sciences, 58*(2), S93–100.

Chapter | 25 |

Fiscal Implications of Population Aging

John Gist
The George Washington University, Washington, DC

CHAPTER CONTENTS

INTRODUCTION

The aging of the US and world populations has caused grave concern among experts about the ability of our nation, and other developed nations, to afford the programs that benefit the retired population, especially public pensions and health insurance. The costs of Social Security, Medicare, and the federal share of Medicaid are projected by the Congressional Budget Office (CBO) to double by mid-century to 18% of GDP – a figure well below that projected for most of the European Community (European Commission, 2006) but equal to the average total annual revenue collected by the federal government for the past 50 years (CBO, 2009a), which leaves no room for other spending. This poses the daunting challenge of how to afford the rest of government and benefits for aging populations too.

The fiscal dilemma posed by the three largest "entitlement" programs has been complicated by the economic and financial meltdown that triggered the Great Recession of 2008–09 in the US and around the world. In the US, recession-induced automatic spending increases and revenue contraction, coupled with strong stimulative actions by the President, the Congress, the US Treasury, and the Federal Reserve created unprecedented peacetime deficits and sharply increased the federal debt. Further complicating the policy problem, most economists agree that fiscal actions that would normally be appropriate and necessary to address long-term deficits are ill-advised in a severely weakened economy.

RECENT HISTORY AND NEAR-TERM OUTLOOK

Our current dismal fiscal picture is a sharp turnabout from a decade ago. At the beginning of this century, the US federal budget outlook was rosy in the short term with some important but manageable demographic challenges in the long term. Four consecutive budget surpluses and robust revenue growth allowed the CBO to project in its January 2001 *Budget Outlook* that "off-budget surpluses (i.e. excluding Social Security) alone would be sufficient to eliminate the debt available for redemption by 2006" (CBO, 2001). In other words, *not counting* the substantial accumulating Social Security surpluses, which would ordinarily be lent to the Treasury to finance deficits, the public debt could have been eliminated by now.

DOI: 10.1016/B978-0-12-380880-6.00025-3

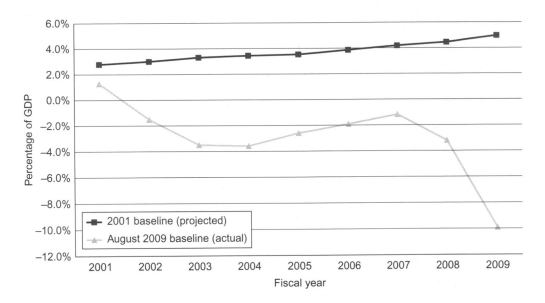

Figure 25.1 Comparison of 2001–09 surpluses/deficits as percentage of GDP projected in 2001 CBO baseline vs actual budget outcomes.
Sources: Congressional Budget Office 2001, 2010; Auerbach and Gale, 2009.

Then came two large Bush Administration tax cuts, new entitlement spending, and the large costs of two extended wars. What many saw as a lack of fiscal restraint by the Bush White House was symbolized by the creation of a prescription drug benefit in the Medicare Modernization Act of 2003 with no attempt to raise revenue to pay for it. As a result, the fiscal outlook became dismal in the short run and dire in the long run. And that was *before* the Great Recession of 2008–09. Figure 25.1 compares those 2001–09 projections with the actual results that ensued. The confluence of the fiscal meltdown of 2008–09 with the long-anticipated demographic shift has thrust the gloomy fiscal forecasts to the top of the policy agenda.

The rapid deterioration of the FY 2009 budget picture is chronicled in CBO's deficit estimates as of September 2008 ($438 billion), January 2009 ($1186 billion), and October 2009 ($1409 billion), which reflects not only the costs of the Troubled Asset Relief Program (TARP) and the ARRA (the President's economic stimulus) but also the cumulative effect of the deepening recession. CBO is required by statute to follow current law in its 10-year budget projections, so it must assume that the Bush Administration tax cuts of 2001 and 2003 will expire at the end of 2010 as scheduled under current law, an assumption that many regard as artificially optimistic. The Obama Administration assumed the expiration of only that portion of the tax cuts

benefiting taxpayers with income of $250 000 or higher, and projected a 10-year deficit of $10.3 trillion (Auerbach & Gale, 2009), while other analysts who assumed the extension of all the Bush Administration tax cuts saw 10-year deficits in the $12 trillion range (Auerbach & Gale, 2009; Peterson-Pew Commission on Budget Reform, 2009; Ruffing et al., 2010).

By comparison with recent tumultuous economic events and rapidly worsening near-term deficits, the looming problems posed by population aging may seem almost quaint. On the contrary, unlike the Great Recession, the pressures of population aging will not quickly subside but rather worsen over time and, without remedial action, contribute to unprecedented deficits and debt that could have severely deleterious, even catastrophic, effects on the American economy (Burman et al., 2010).

The linkages between population aging and the looming fiscal crisis are both direct and indirect. The most direct fiscal impacts of population aging will come in the form of rapidly increasing budget outlays for entitlement programs – those programs that provide automatic benefits to individuals based on statutory eligibility – which constitute the bulk of what CBO calls "mandatory spending." It is not entitlements in general but rather the three largest – Social Security, Medicare, and Medicaid (70% of Medicaid spending goes to elderly and disabled enrollees) (CBO, 2006)) – that pose a severe budgetary and economic threat. The "big three" represent three-quarters of entitlement spending, and their rapid escalation and the age of their beneficiary population have led many to assume that population aging is the chief cause of projected increases in federal outlays. The reality is more complicated. Whereas population aging – specifically the retirement of baby boomers and increased longevity – is the chief cause of projected increases in Social Security spending, Social Security is not a seriously problematic source of future budget pressures. The core of the looming fiscal crisis is the projected escalation in overall national health spending, including Medicare and Medicaid spending. But projected Medicare and Medicaid spending is primarily driven by increasing health care costs per beneficiary *regardless of age*, not by population aging.

The indirect fiscal impacts of aging stem from its effects on the three sources of economic growth: the composition of the workforce, national saving, and productivity. Slower projected growth in those factors means slower future economic growth, which has important impacts on both revenue and spending growth. The next section briefly describes these indirect impacts on the economy and their linkages to fiscal outcomes. The following section discusses the direct impacts of population aging on budget outcomes and the long-term gap between revenues and outlays. Then, we address the causes of this fiscal gap, especially health costs. A final section provides a brief summary.

INDIRECT IMPACTS – DEMOGRAPHIC CHANGE, THE ECONOMY, AND THE BUDGET

Over the next 20 years, a large share of mature workers (the baby boomers) will be gradually exiting the US labor force, and the growth rate in the labor force will slow to 0.5% per year from its average of 1.6% per year from 1950 to 2007 (CBO, 2009b). A declining rate of labor force growth means that the labor supply of American workers may be insufficient to sustain living standards (measured by per capita GDP), assuming the continuation of past patterns of labor force participation by age and gender.

The availability of capital for investment is critical to economic growth, and national saving, which consists of personal, business, and government saving (i.e. the net of the federal, state, and local sectors' surpluses or deficits), must provide much of this capital. Normally, we would expect societies having larger shares of prime-age workers and low dependency ratios – like the US in the late twentieth century – to have higher saving rates. That the US, nevertheless, had a declining personal saving rate for the past two

decades remains a conundrum, despite numerous efforts seeking explanations (Bosworth et al., 1991; Browning & Lusardi, 1996; Gale & Sabelhaus, 1999; Gokhale et al., 1996; Parker, 1999). Large federal budget deficits have also lowered the overall saving rate, except for the late 1990s when the federal government ran surpluses and added to national saving. Business saving was the largest contributor to net national saving for most of the past two decades, becoming a larger share of private saving as the personal saving share shrank. The demographic scenario in the near future is far less rosy for personal saving than in the past, and future federal deficits are likely to depress government saving, so we should expect future saving rates to fall, slowing economic growth and lowering potential output.

Productivity, the third important element of economic growth, is the value of goods and services produced per hour of additional labor. Productivity growth results from two factors: growth in the amount of productive capital per worker and technological advances that increase the amount of goods and services that can be produced by a *given* level of labor and capital. Productivity is the key determinant of the rate of change in hourly wages, and therefore plays a large role in boosting national output. Productivity increases averaged 2.1% annually from 1947–1995, but that average conceals a sharp decline in trend growth, which went from 2.6% during 1947–73 to 1.4% during 1974–95 (CBO, 2007a). After 1995 and again after 2001, however, productivity surged, averaging 2.9% growth over 1996–2006 (CBO, 2007a). Each increase of 0.1 percentage point in the average growth rate of labor productivity would, if sustained for 10 years, raise the level of GDP by roughly 1%, or by about $200 billion (CBO, 2007a). Some analysts have speculated that advances in computer technology may have raised the rate of productivity increase in the US (Jorgenson & Siroh, 2000; Oliner & Sichel, 2000), but rates of productivity growth have slowed, and both the Social Security Trustees and the CBO project rates of productivity growth more in line with historical averages (Board of Trustees, 2009; CBO, 2010).

Under normal conditions, economic expansion promotes budget balance because it has the effect of causing revenues to increase more rapidly and causing expenditures sensitive to business cycles to grow more slowly. On the revenue side, Federal income tax revenues grow faster than the economy because of the progressive income tax rate structure. As taxpayers' incomes increase due to economic growth, they are pushed into higher income tax brackets. Faster growth means faster revenue increases. This works in reverse when the economy slows: incomes decline and tax payments decline as well, leaving more dollars in taxpayers' wallets than they would have had otherwise to help cushion economic downturns. This is good for the economy but bad for budget balance.

On the spending side, economic contractions increase spending for entitlement programs that are explicitly intended to counteract economic cycles – like Unemployment Insurance UI, Temporary Assistance to Needy Families (TANF), and the Supplemental Nutrition Assistance Program (SNAP), formerly known as Food Stamps – as harder economic times cause more people to qualify for benefits. Just the opposite occurs when the economy expands – fewer unemployed and fewer families that are economically pressed mean fewer applicants for UI, SNAP, and TANF. The largest entitlement programs – Social Security, Medicare, and Medicaid – although not primarily intended to offset recessions, nevertheless exhibit these countercyclical patterns as well (Gist, 2009), especially in the period since 1985. These changes are largely automatic (the so-called "automatic stabilizers"), so that much of fiscal policy in the form of deficits or surpluses is actually a reflection of the economy rather than a result of discretionary policy. Of the cumulative 2009–11 projected deficits of nearly $4 trillion, more than one quarter would result from the operation of the automatic stabilizers (CBO, 2009c, 2009d).

Real GDP is projected to grow at only 2.25% per year through to 2083, a full percentage point below the average from 1962–2007. To illustrate the impact of the slower rate of growth on living standards, consider that real per capita GDP was $38 000 in 2007, and would increase to $105 000 per capita by 2050 at a 3.25% growth rate but would reach only $68 000 in 2050 at a growth rate of 2.25%. Despite slower growth, federal revenues would nevertheless increase from about 15% of GDP in 2009 (uncharacteristically low due to the deep recession) to 21.8% by 2035 and 26.1% in 2083 *if* current tax laws were to remain in place during that period (CBO, 2009a). This compares with the long-run (since World War II) average revenue total of 18% of GDP. This automatic growth can occur despite the fact that income tax brackets are indexed for inflation because incomes generally grow faster than inflation, thus increasing revenues as a share of the economy.

Despite the boost to revenues from economic growth, it is not expected to be nearly sufficient over the next 75 years to offset the projected budget increases resulting from the rapid escalation of health care costs. The latter have grown steadily at more than two percentage points faster than the rate of growth of the economy for three decades, and are projected to continue to do so (CBO, 2007b). The consensus among experts is that more rapid economic growth could improve the long-term fiscal outlook, but it would not fundamentally change it. In other words, we cannot grow our way out of our looming fiscal crisis.

BUDGET PROJECTIONS AND THE LONG-TERM OUTLOOK

Budget Sustainability

As discussed above, rapidly increasing health costs, population aging, and slower economic growth will, in the absence of remedial legislative action, drive up Social Security, Medicare, and Medicaid spending in the next few decades, resulting in ever-larger budget deficits and increased government borrowing. Increased borrowing is likely to make capital scarcer and put upward pressure on interest rates, adversely impacting the investment necessary for sustained economic growth. Debt service costs could eventually grow faster than the economy and possibly too fast for the government's capacity to finance them. Foreign lenders to the US might demand a risk premium (higher interest rates) to continue financing our debt, or choose not to purchase it at all. If prolonged, the increased debt burden could create an economic situation as dire as the recent financial crisis, but by then the government might lack the borrowing capacity to bail out the US economy. The use of the term "unsustainable" to describe this scenario has become a cliché, but one that is often not defined. A precise definition of sustainability is offered by the CBO as "for any path of spending and revenues to be sustainable, the resulting debt must eventually grow no faster than the economy" (CBO, 1998). In other words, an unsustainable budget path is one where debt is steadily rising relative to GDP.

The Congressional Budget Office's most recent long-term budget projections are depicted in Figures 25.2 and 25.3, representing two distinct policy scenarios. Although one scenario is more optimistic and one is more pessimistic, *both* ultimately result in unprecedented, unsustainable, and potentially catastrophic levels of public debt. The main difference between the two is on the revenue side. The optimistic projection (depicted in Figure 25.2), which CBO calls the "extended baseline" scenario, starts with the CBO's detailed and neutral 10-year baseline. The baseline assumes the Bush tax cuts expire as scheduled under current law and does not index the Alternative Minimum Tax (AMT) for inflation, so that it will reach many millions more taxpayers in the next few years – 27 million by 2010 and 52 million by 2020 (Lim & Rohaly, 2009) and generate more revenue. The pessimistic "alternative fiscal scenario" (Figure 25.3) assumes that the Bush tax cuts are extended and the AMT parameters are indexed for inflation after 2019. The other revenue difference is that excise, estate, and gift taxes are constant shares of GDP over the long term in the alternative fiscal scenario, but follow current law under the extended baseline. The impact of these assumptions can be seen in the upward slope of the revenue line in Figure 25.2 compared with the flatter revenue line in Figure 25.3.

Spending is slowed somewhat in the optimistic scenario by stricter reimbursement of physicians according to the Medicare "sustainable growth rate" formula (CBO, 2007c; US Department of Health and Human Services, 2006). In the long run, however,

CBO's mandatory spending category (which consists mainly of entitlements) is quite similar in the two scenarios, reaching approximately one-quarter of GDP by 2083. The larger spending difference is in the "other" spending category, three-quarters of which is discretionary spending, in which a short-term reduction occurs through 2011 in the optimistic scenario,

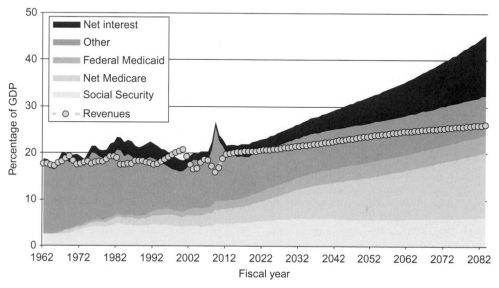

Figure 25.2 Past and projected spending for major entitlement programs, net interest, other programs, and revenues as percentage of GDP, 1962–2083 (CBO optimistic scenario).
Source: Congressional Budget Office, 2009a.

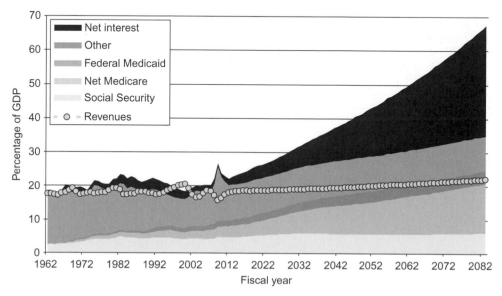

Figure 25.3 Growth in federal spending for major entitlement programs, net interest, and other programs, and revenues as percentage of GDP (CBO pessimistic scenario).
Source: Congressional Budget Office, 2009a.

after which both scenarios assume that discretionary spending is a constant share of GDP.

In the optimistic scenario, federal primary (i.e. non-interest) spending would rise to 32% of GDP by 2083, but revenues would reach only 26% of GDP, a gap of 6% of GDP. Because interest payments would steadily increase as a share of the economy and reach 13% of GDP by 2083 (absorbing half of all revenues), the overall deficit would be 19% of GDP in that year. In the pessimistic scenario, revenues would rise to only 22% and non-interest spending would reach 34% of GDP by 2083, for a deficit *excluding interest* that would be almost twice as large as that projected under the optimistic scenario. But, in the pessimistic scenario, sustained larger deficits cause interest payments on the debt to reach an unimaginable one-third of GDP (almost half of federal spending and 50% more than total revenues) by 2083, so the overall deficit would be 45.4% of GDP, more than twice the level of the optimistic scenario. Public debt would be more than four times GDP by mid-century and would be more than eight times GDP by 2083 (CBO, 2009a). Such levels of debt would over time adversely affect interest rates and economic growth, but macro models such as the one CBO uses to project future budget scenarios require assumptions that interest rates remain relatively stable (Manchester & Schwabish, 2010). Consequently, the models do not allow for unconstrained increases in interest rates, so that even CBO's pessimistic projections may underestimate the negative effects of long-term deficits.

Aside from the limitations of macro models in projecting fiscal effects, a number of analysts regard the policy assumptions of both CBO scenarios as too optimistic (Auerbach & Gale, 2009; Peterson-Pew Commission on Budget Reform, 2009; Ruffing et al., 2010). In particular, the optimistic scenario is seen as unrealistic, albeit one that is consistent with the CBO's 10-year projection required by law. These analysts generally assume that future spending for Social Security, Medicare, and Medicaid will follow current law projections as reported in the Social Security Trustees' reports and assume no changes to those laws that might slow spending growth. On the other hand, they assume that revenues will *not* follow current law; i.e. that taxes will be adjusted by Congress and the president to maintain a lower revenue trajectory, keeping them at about their long-run share of GDP. These assumptions are also unrealistic in that they ignore the fact that spending cuts to Medicare have been consistently proposed and adopted over the past 30 years and that those changes have frequently reduced spending by far more than was expected (Gabel, 2010). They are also unrealistic in assuming that Congress will take affirmative action to reduce taxes when, faced with the prospect of economically harmful (some would say disastrous)

deficits, it would be wiser to do nothing and simply let taxes rise in step with economic growth. The argument for using current law assumptions for both revenue and outlays, aside from being a requirement for CBO, is that it treats revenues and outlays symmetrically. It tells us what things would look like if Congress did nothing.

The Fiscal Gap

One measure of the severity of the imbalance between spending and revenues in the current budget projections is the "fiscal gap," which is a "present value" measure of the long-term deficit. It projects 75-year future imbalances between revenues and outlays and then adjusts those future estimates to their value in today's dollars as a ratio to today's GDP. The CBO's June 2009 *Long-Term Budget Outlook* (CBO, 2009a) estimated the 75-year fiscal gap under the optimistic scenario to be 3.2% of GDP, meaning that spending cuts or revenue increases equal to 3.2% of GDP (approximately $460 billion at 2009 levels of GDP) would have to be enacted immediately *and permanently* to keep the public debt at its current share of GDP. Under the pessimistic scenario, the fiscal gap equals 8.1% of GDP (approximately $1.2 trillion at 2009 levels of GDP). To put this into perspective, under the pessimistic scenario, the *annual* price tag to eliminate the fiscal gap is larger than the *10-year* price tag of the 2009–10 proposals to reform the nation's health care system.

Estimates of the fiscal gap depend on the underlying assumptions, as is apparent from the difference in the CBO's two scenarios. Other analysts project even larger fiscal gaps. Auerbach and Gale (2009) estimate that the long-term fiscal gap is 5–7% of GDP using the CBO baseline assumptions, 7–9% using the Obama Administration assumptions, and 8–10% using the Bush policy baseline (extension of tax cuts and indexing of the AMT). A key difference among these estimates is whether the Bush Administration tax cuts, which have been estimated to cost on the order of 2% of GDP over the long run (Cox & Kogan, 2008), are made permanent, partially extended, or expire.

Estimates of the fiscal gap have fluctuated rather sharply over time as the fiscal picture has brightened (as it did in the late 1990s) or become more dismal, as it is today. In happier fiscal times, the fiscal gap went from 5.4% of GDP in 1996 to less than 1% in both 1999 and 2000, thanks to sharp capital gains revenue increases and much slower growth in health care costs (due by some accounts to the spread of managed care through the health care delivery system). Given the dismal short-term outlook, no such fiscal turnaround seems imminent today, and delay is costly. Under the CBO pessimistic scenario, if remedial actions occurred immediately, changes equal to 8.1% of

GDP would suffice to eliminate the fiscal gap, but, if action were delayed until 2020, necessary reductions would reach 9.7% of GDP, and by 2040 they would cost 15.5% of GDP (CBO, 2009a).

WHAT IS CAUSING THE FISCAL GAP?

Entitlement Spending and Tax Expenditures

Federal policy initiatives requiring a commitment of funds have taken two distinct forms, broadly speaking. The more familiar form consists of direct spending programs that provide benefits to specific constituencies or populations based on eligibility criteria established in law. Many of these programs, including the three largest in the federal budget, are encompassed under the rubric "entitlement authority," which, as defined in the Congressional Budget Reform and Impoundment Control Act of 1974 (P.L. 93–344, 88 Stat. 297, July 12, 1974), provides authority to make payments to individuals without prior appropriations legislation if the government is obligated to make the payments under law to qualified individuals.

A less familiar form of social policy in the US is represented by numerous provisions of the tax code that offer special incentives to individuals and businesses. These "tax expenditures" are also defined in the Congressional Budget Act, as:

> *revenue losses attributable to provisions of the Federal tax laws which allow a special exclusion, exemption, or deduction from gross income or which provide a special credit, a preferential rate of tax, or a deferral of tax liability (P. L. 93–344, sec. 3(3)).*

Tax expenditures increase the deficit in the same way as direct spending, are very large in size, and are, in the words of the Joint Committee on Taxation, "similar to those direct spending programs that are available as entitlements to those who meet the statutory criteria established for the programs" (US Congress, 2010). However, tax expenditures rarely receive an equal level of scrutiny from deficit "hawks," who prefer to focus on spending. Since a dollar of foregone revenue increases the deficit as much as a dollar of added spending, both entitlements and tax expenditures hold equal potential for the deficit reduction needed to bring about long-term federal budget sustainability.

Spending entitlements represented just over half of all federal spending in FY 2008 ($1.6 trillion out of nearly $3 trillion), but concerns about the long-term sustainability of budget policy have generally focused on the largest three – Social Security, Medicare, and Medicaid – which cost $1.3 trillion, or more than three-quarters of all federal entitlement spending. In the early 1960s, before the enactment of Medicare and Medicaid, entitlement spending (half of which was Social Security) was about one quarter of total federal outlays. By the 1990s, the "big three" (net of offsetting receipts, such as Medicare premiums) exceeded 70% of entitlement dollars (see Figure 25.4) and total entitlement spending represented half of all outlays. Projecting 75 years into the future, the "big three" will represent an increasing share of all non-interest spending, although their share of *total* (including net interest) spending will begin to shrink around 2040 because interest on the debt will have become so large and grown so fast by then that it will exceed the growth rate of the largest three entitlements.

The term "entitlement spending" has become synonymous with the "big three" despite the importance of other entitlement programs, such as the aforementioned UI TANF, and SNAP (Food Stamps), as well as federal civilian and military pensions, veterans' benefits, and Supplemental Security Income. Clearly, Social Security, Medicare, and Medicaid as a group are driving up non-interest spending and, unless reined in, may eventually cause interest costs to rise to dangerous levels. These programs have drawn the attention of critics who see the federal budget as too focused on programs for the elderly. They believe these programs are too insulated from congressional scrutiny and need to be subjected to periodic review (Brookings Institution/Heritage Foundation, 2008; Peterson-Pew Commission on Budget Reform, 2009). Such criticism has been challenged by others (Aaron et al., 2008) as misguided or unbalanced, and it fails to recognize the annual review and oversight role played by the Social Security Board of Trustees, composed of the Secretaries of Treasury, Labor, and HHS, together with two independent public trustees. The trustees must provide annual reports to Congress and the public about the fiscal status of the Social Security and Medicare programs.

In contrast, tax expenditures for individuals and businesses draw relatively little attention, despite totaling $1.2 trillion in 2008 (Kleinbard, 2009), an amount equal to all individual income tax revenues today and almost equal to the total spending for Social Security, Medicare, and Medicaid combined (Figure 25.5). The largest tax expenditures are the tax exclusion for employer-provided health insurance ($127 billion); the deferral of tax on employer-provided pensions, 401(k)s, and Keogh plans ($125 billion); and the mortgage interest deduction ($80 billion). The pension and health exclusions are also both payroll tax expenditures; i.e. these contributions are exempt from the payroll tax as well. They have both

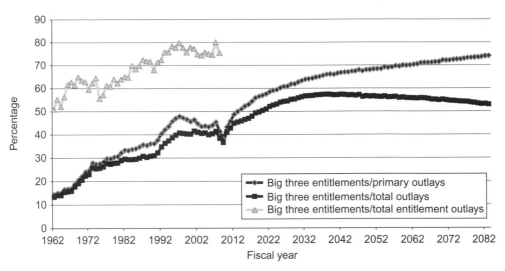

Figure 25.4 Spending for big three entitlements as percentage of total entitlement spending (historical) and projected outlays and non-interest outlays under *CBO* optimistic scenario, FY 1962–2083.
Source: Congressional Budget Office, 2009a.

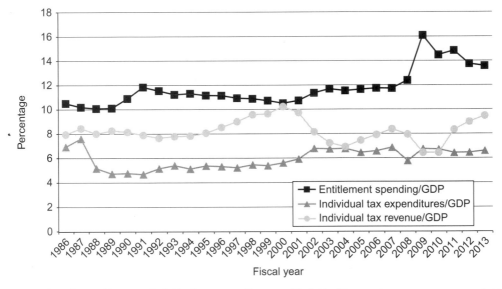

Figure 25.5 Spending entitlements, individual tax expenditures, and individual income tax revenues as percentage of GDP, 1986–2013.
Sources: Congressional Budget Office, 2010; Joint Committee on Taxation, Estimates of Federal Tax Expenditures, various years.

been challenged as inefficient (Gruber, 2010; Munnell, 1991), and the health exclusion in particular has been consistently cited by experts as a cause of rapid growth in health care costs. Unlike entitlements, tax expenditures are highly skewed toward affluent households and toward the working-age population. The highest income quintile taxpayers would experience the largest share of increased taxes from elimination of tax preferences for homeownership (70.9), health expenses and

insurance (41.9%), and retirement saving (79.6%) (Burman et al., 2008; Toder et al., 2009). Moreover, tax benefits are far more concentrated among the population under age 65 than entitlement spending, which is concentrated on the population aged over 65. When combined, a majority of entitlement spending and tax expenditure dollars – 54% overall – flowed to the population aged under 65, while 46% flowed to the population aged over 65 (Gist, 2009).

Social Security

Social Security, the largest entitlement, is often the prime suspect in the alleged deleterious effect of population aging on the federal budget. In fact, Social Security outlays have been a stable share of the economy for more than 30 years (4.2% of GDP in 1975; 4.3% in 2008). Today it represents a smaller share of the economy than in Ronald Reagan's first term. It will grow steadily as a share of GDP for the next two decades, but just how problematic is its growth? In 2031, when the youngest boomer reaches full retirement age (67), Social Security will be 6.0% of GDP, compared with today's 4.3%. It grew faster from 1962 to 1982, a comparable time span (nearly doubling from 2.5% to 4.9% of GDP) without harming the economy. Moreover, it has been shown that Social Security's expansion in benefits between 1967 and 2000 explains the entire 17 percentage point decline in poverty that occurred during that period (Engelhardt & Gruber, 2004).

The growth in Social Security in the next two decades does not constitute a threat to fiscal stability. Its funding needs are well within the parameters of policies recently enacted by the Congress. For example, it represents only slightly more than the increase in defense spending during the George W. Bush administration (which occurred over a much shorter period). The entire cost of Social Security's long-term financing deficit over 75 years is roughly one third as great as George W. Bush's 2001 and 2003 tax cuts projected over the same period (Cox & Kogan, 2008). Beyond 2031, Social Security's cost as a percentage of the economy is remarkably stable, declining from 6.0% of GDP in 2031 to as low as 5.7% of GDP from 2048 to 2053 before rising again to 6.2% of GDP by 2083.

Medicare and Medicaid Growth

If population aging alone were the source of the nation's future fiscal problems, one would expect Social Security and Medicare to exhibit similar patterns of growth over time – but they do not (see Figure 25.6). In its first two decades, Medicare grew at about the same rate as Social Security. From the mid-1980s to the present, Medicare's growth rate was well above that of Social Security, which remained constant as a share of the economy. Medicare's future growth rate also far exceeds that of Social Security, especially after 2030. In 2008, an entitlement milestone of sorts was reached – the two main federal health entitlements (Medicare and Medicaid) together finally reached the same 4.3% share of the economy as Social Security. As the projections in Figure 25.6 show, the combined Medicare/Medicaid and Social Security lines will steadily diverge in the future. By 2030, when the boomers are mostly retired, Medicare *alone* will equal Social Security at

5.9% of GDP. By 2046, combined Medicare (net of offsetting premiums) and federal Medicaid spending will be double that of Social Security, and nearly triple it by 2083. Medicare and Medicaid are projected to account for 80% of the growth in combined "big three entitlement" spending over the next 25 years, and for 90% of that growth by 2080.

Further indication that health spending is the one area of federal spending that poses acute budgetary problems can be seen in Figure 25.7, shows that which, after 2009, all federal non-interest spending other than health care ceases to grow relative to GDP, first declining sharply after the Great Recession and subsequently leveling off as a percentage of GDP through 2083. Meanwhile, Medicare and Medicaid spending exceeds all other non-interest federal spending by 2063. Nevertheless, solving the budget crisis through cuts in these programs alone is not a practicable strategy. Auerbach and Gale (2009) have estimated that the elimination of the long-term fiscal gap through reductions in health care spending growth alone would require that the growth rate of Medicare and Medicaid spending be reduced by 3% of GDP annually over the next 75 years. Federal health expenditures are currently growing at an estimated 2.5% faster than GDP, so a reduction of this magnitude would require that health expenditures would have to immediately and permanently *fall* by 0.5% per capita per year relative to GDP. It is highly unlikely (to say nothing of poor public policy) that we would attempt to eliminate the fiscal gap through either spending cuts alone or higher revenues alone.

On the other hand, a budget strategy that combined cuts in health care costs with increased revenues may be able to address the projected fiscal shortfall. The CBO has estimated that, if health costs were contained to the rate of GDP plus 1% and taxes were allowed to increase in pace with real economic growth, the increased revenues would be enough to finance the increase in health costs (CBO, 2007d).

Sources of Health Spending Growth

The inability to constrain health costs is a systemic problem not unique to government. Overall health spending has far outpaced economic growth for years, and now consumes 17% of GDP. The size and rapid growth of Medicare and Medicaid, and the fact that health spending per capita is higher among older people than younger people, has led many observers to conclude that the aging of baby boomers, larger Medicare and Medicaid beneficiary populations, and longer life expectancies are the factors driving up government health spending. In numerous recent reports, however, the CBO (and other health experts) have demonstrated that population aging is not the most important factor explaining

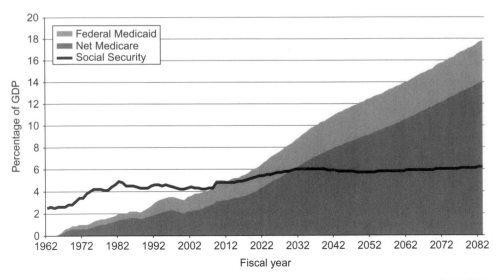

Figure 25.6 Growth in federal spending for social security and health entitlements as a percentage of GDP (CBO optimistic scenario).
Source: Congressional Budget Office, 2009a.

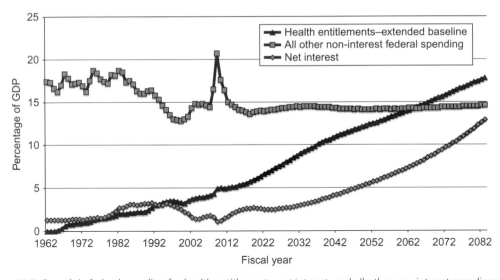

Figure 25.7 Growth in federal spending for health entitlements, net interest, and all other non-interest spending as a percentage of GDP (CBO optimistic scenario).
Source: Congressional Budget Office, 2009a.

the growth in health care costs (Cutler, 2001; Cutler & Sheiner, 1998; Hoover et al., 2002; Lubitz et al., 1995, 2003) and is far less important than proximity to death in explaining increases in Medicare costs (Miller, 2001; Spillman & Lubitz, 2000).

Even if today's population age distribution held constant into the future, health care spending would still grow rapidly because per beneficiary costs are rising faster than per capita gross domestic product, a phenomenon known in the health policy world as "excess cost growth" (ECG). For example, if per capita

GDP grows one percentage point per year above inflation and Medicare costs per beneficiary increase at three percentage points above inflation, ECG is two percentage points. The term "excess cost growth" conveys no value judgment about the utility or desirability of Medicare or other health spending. Several factors are thought to be responsible for the rapid growth in per person health costs: new medical technology, income growth, and health insurance coverage among them. But the consensus is that the advance of technology – the development of new medical

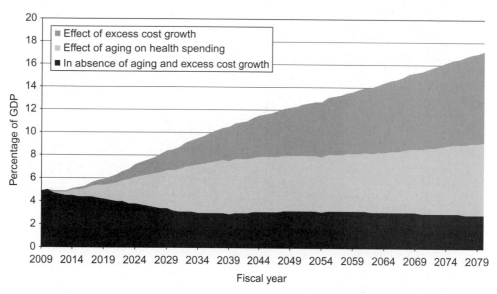

Figure 25.8 Factors explaining the growth in Medicare and Medicaid, allocating the interaction of aging and excess cost to the two factors, as percentage of GDP.
Source: Congressional Budget Office, 2009a.

procedures, drugs, and treatments – is the single most important factor (CBO, 2007b; Newhouse, 1992).

From 1975 to 1990, ECG in national (public and private) health spending was 2.6 percentage points higher than economic growth, while ECG in Medicare and Medicaid during that period were 2.9 and 3.2 percentage points higher, respectively. However, ECG since 1990 has been substantially lower (1.7 percentage points for Medicare, 0.8 percentage points for Medicaid, and 1.4 percentage points for the overall health care system), and it is not a settled question whether the slower growth since 1990 is a result of short-term factors or a true shift in the underlying cost. There is some evidence that a growth rate of 1% in excess of GDP would be a necessary target to achieve fiscal sustainability (CBO, 2009a; Chernew et al., 2003; Follette & Sheiner, 2005).

Although population aging is not included in ECG, the CBO has calculated the share of health spending growth due to each of these two factors in several reports (CBO, 2007b, 2008, 2009a). Aging and ECG interact to drive up health care costs. That is, higher costs per beneficiary will mean higher total costs, even if the number of total beneficiaries remains constant; but, because the total number of beneficiaries also rises, the per beneficiary cost increase is magnified. The CBO isolates the separate effects of aging and ECG by analyzing scenarios where (1) costs per beneficiary are assumed to remain constant (i.e. no ECG exists) but population aging occurs (pure aging effect) and (2) the age composition of the population is constant but ECG continues.

Figure 25.8 shows the projected increases in federal spending on Medicare and Medicaid with the costs allocated to the ECG and age factors. Aging accounts for a larger share in the near term than it does in the long run, but, even during the period from now until 2035, ECG accounts for a larger share of total cost increases (56%) than does aging (44% of cost increases). Over the entire period through 2083, ECG accounts for 70% of health spending increases, whereas aging accounts for only 30%. The importance of aging declines because the impact of new beneficiaries diminishes once the wave of boomers subsides.

Sustainability of Health Costs

Although costs that continually grow faster than the economy are by definition unsustainable because they will inevitably exceed 100% of GDP, some analysts have inquired what level of growth in health costs would be sustainable. For that, a criterion of sustainability is needed. Several studies (CBO, 2009a; Chernew et al., 2003; Follette & Sheiner, 2005) have suggested that health costs are sustainable if they allow for real growth (or at least do not reduce growth) in non-health spending. Chernew et al. (2003) concluded that a rate of GDP plus one percentage point would allow for real growth in non-health spending through a 75-year projection period, but that a rate of GDP plus two percentage points would cause real non-health spending to fall below current levels by 2060 or so. Follette and Sheiner (2005) similarly conclude that a persistent excess growth rate of

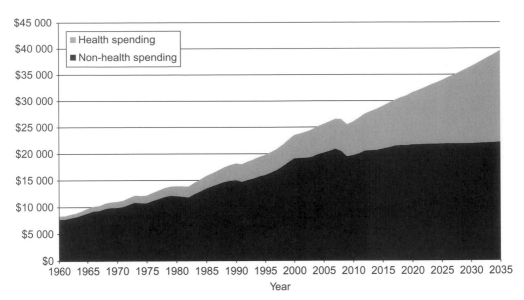

Figure 25.9 Real per capita health and non-health spending (2009 dollars).
Source: Congressional Budget Office, 2009a.

GDP plus 1% would not crowd out non-health spending until about 2090, but that higher rates result in crowd-out within 75 years. The CBO's (2009a) projections assume that ECG only begins to slow from historical rates after 2020. By 2083, Medicare's excess growth rate is assumed to reach 0.9% and Medicaid and private health spending to reach 0.1% (i.e. above GDP growth). The resulting growth in economy-wide per capita private and public health and non-health spending is shown in Figure 25.9, which shows that per capita non-health spending barely grows relative to GDP after 2015.

CONCLUSIONS

Population aging has direct and indirect as well as near-term and long-term fiscal implications. The indirect impacts of aging are longer-term and stem from its effects on the components of macroeconomic growth – the size and composition of the labor force, saving and investment, and productivity. Slower growth in the labor force and lower saving rates will cause the economy to grow more slowly, which will cause revenues to grow more slowly and spending to be higher. Even robust economic growth such as the US enjoyed in the post-World War II era through the 1960s would not be enough by itself to avoid severe fiscal problems in the future. But future economic growth is likely to be slower and make fiscal recovery more difficult.

The most direct fiscal effect is the surge in outlays over the next two decades for the tens of millions of Americans who will become recipients of Social Security, Medicare, and Medicaid benefits. Outlays for those three programs will soar from nearly 10% of GDP today to nearly twice that share of GDP by 2050. Within this period it is health care, especially Medicare, that presents the most serious fiscal challenge. What we have seen from the trends in Social Security and health spending is that aging has manageable direct impacts on spending for Social Security. The direct impacts of aging on health spending are magnified by the interaction between increasing numbers of beneficiaries and the increase in per beneficiary health care costs that exceeds the rate of growth of per capita GDP ("excess cost growth"). Over the next 75 years, well beyond 2030, the impacts of aging become somewhat less pronounced relative to "excess cost growth," and costs per beneficiary (mostly due to medical technology) become paramount, although aging still accounts for 30% of overall rising health costs between now and 2083.

Health care is the single non-interest spending component of the federal budget that grows faster than the overall economy over the next 75 years. The aging of the population without question plays a role in that cost, but the evidence is that the per beneficiary cost of health care, regardless of aging, is the most important factor driving up federal spending. Thus, finding answers to controlling per beneficiary health care costs is the key to a solution to our long-run fiscal problems. Without some success in containing health costs, we face a bleak, perhaps catastrophic, budget future. If health costs can be contained to the rate of GDP plus one percentage point, there is evidence that income tax revenue growth, or perhaps a new revenue source, combined with slower growth in health costs could bring about a sustainable budget future (CBO, 2007d). But, even with some success in controlling costs in the long run, other budgetary measures on both revenue and expenditures sides are likely to be necessary in order to achieve a sustainable fiscal solution.

REFERENCES

Aaron, H., Atlman, N., Apfel, K., Blum, J., DeLong, J. B., Diamond, P., et al. (2008). A balanced approach to restoring fiscal responsibility. July. Retrieved March 6, 2010 from http://www.thefiscaltimes.com/~/media/Fiscal-Times/Research-Center/Budget-Impact/Think-Tanks/2008/07/01/BudgetBrookingsCBPPBalancedApproachtoRestoringFiscalResponsibility07012008pdf.ashx

Auerbach, A., & Gale, W. (2009). The economic crisis and the fiscal crisis: 2009 and beyond. *Tax Notes, October 5*, 101–130.

Board of Trustees (2009). *Annual report of the Board of Trustees of the Federal Old-Age and Survivors Insurance and Federal Disbility Insurance Trust Funds*. Washington, DC: US Social Security Administration.

Bosworth, B., Burtless, G., & Sabelhaus, J. (1991). The decline in saving: Evidence from household surveys. *Brookings papers on economic activity, 22*, 183–256.

Brookings Institution/Heritage Foundation. (2008). *Taking back our fiscal future*. April. Retrieved March 6, 2010 from http://www.brookings.edu/~/media/Files/rc/papers/2008/04_fiscal_future/04_fiscal_future.pdf.

Browning, E., & Lusardi, A. (1996). Household saving: Micro theories and micro facts. *Journal of Economic Literature, 34*, 1797–1855.

Burman, L., Toder, E., & Geissler, C. (2008). *How big are total individual income tax expenditures, and who benefits from them?* Washington, DC: Urban-Brookings Tax Policy

Center, Discussion Paper No. 31, December.

Burman, L., Rohaly, J., Rosenberg, J. & Lim, K. (2010). *Catastrophic budget failure*. Presented at joint Tax Policy Center-University of Southern California conference: "Train Wreck: A Conference on America's Looming Fiscal Crisis." Los Angeles, January 15.

Chernew, M., Hirth, R., & Cutler, D. (2003). Increased spending on health care: How much can the United States afford? *Health Affairs, 22*(4), 15–25.

Congressional Budget Office (1998). *Long-term budgetary pressures and policy options*. Washington, DC: United States Government Printing Office, May.

Congressional Budget Office (2001). *The budget and economic outlook, 2002–2011*. Washington, DC: United States Government Printing Office, January.

Congressional Budget Office. (2007a). *Labor productivity: Developments since 1995*. CBO Paper. Washington, DC: United States Government Printing Office, March.

Congressional Budget Office (2007b). *The long-term outlook for health care spending*. Washington, DC: United States Government Printing Office, November.

Congressional Budget Office. (2007c). *Factors underlying the growth in Medicare's spending for physicians' services*. Background Paper. Washington, DC: United States Government Printing Office, June.

Congressional Budget Office. (2007d) *Financing projected spending in the long run*. Letter to Senator Judd Gregg. Washington, DC: United States Government Printing Office, July 9.

Congressional Budget Office. (2008). *Accounting for sources of projected growth in federal spending on Medicare and Medicaid*. Economic and budget issue brief. Washington, DC: United States Government Printing Office, May 28.

Congressional Budget Office (July 13, 2006). *Medicaid spending growth and options for controlling costs*. Washington, DC: United States Government Printing Office. CBO testimony before the Special Committee on Aging, US Senate

Congressional Budget Office (2009a). *The long-term budget outlook*. Washington, DC: United States Government Printing Office, June.

Congressional Budget Office. (2009b). *How slower growth in the labor force could affect the return on capital*. CBO Background Paper. Washington, DC: United States Government Printing Office, October.

Congressional Budget Office. (2009c). *Measuring the effects of the business cycle on the federal budget (an update)*. CBO Report. Washington, DC: United States Government Printing Office, September 1.

Congressional Budget Office. (2009d). *Measuring the effects of the business cycle on the federal budget*. CBO Report, Washington, DC: United States Government Printing Office, June.

Congressional Budget Office (2010). *The budget and economic outlook: Fiscal years 2010 to 2020*. Washington, DC: US Government Printing Office, January.

Congressional Budget Reform and Impoundment Control Act of 1974 (P.L. 93-344, 88 Stat. 297, July 12, 1974).

Cox, K., & Kogan, R. (2008). *Long-term Social Security shortfall smaller than cost of extending tax cuts for top 1 percent*. Washington, DC: Center on Budget and Policy Priorities, March 31.

Cutler, D. (2001). Declining disability among the elderly. *Health Affairs, 20,* 11–27.

Cutler, D., & Sheiner, L. (1998). *Demographics and medical care spending: Standard and non-standard effects*. Burch Center Working Paper No. B98-3, November. Retrieved March 6, 2010 from http://elsa.berkeley.edu/~burch/web/cutlersheiner.pdf.

Engelhardt, G., & Gruber, J. (2004). *The evolution of elderly poverty*. NBER Working Paper No. 10466. Retrieved March 6, 2010 from http://www.nber.org/papers/w10466.

European Commission. (2006). *The impact of aging on public expenditure*. Report prepared by the Economic Policy Committee and the European Commission. Retrieved March 6, 2010 from http://ec.europa.eu/economy_finance/publications/publication6654_en.pdf.

Follette, G., & Sheiner, L. (2005). The sustainability of health spending growth. *National Tax Journal, 58*(3), 391–408.

Gabel, J. (2010). *Does the Congressional Budget Office underestimate savings from reform? A review of the historical record*. Issue Brief. The Commonwealth Fund, January. Retrieved March 6, 2010 from http://www.commonwealthfund.org/Content/Publications/Issue-Briefs/2010/Jan/Does-the-Congressional-Budget-Office-Underestimate-Savings.aspx.

Gale, W., & Sabelhaus, J. (1999). Perspectives on the household saving rate. *Brookings Papers on Economic Activity, 1,* 181–224.

Gist, J. (2009). Population aging, entitlement growth, and the economy. In R. Hudson (Ed.), *Boomer bust? Economic and political issues of the graying society* (pp. 173–196). Westport, CT: Praeger.

Gokhale, J., Kotlikoff, L., & Sabelhaus, J. (1996). Understanding the postwar decline in U.S. saving: A cohort analysis. *Brookings Papers on Economic Activity, 1,* 315–407.

Gruber, J. (2010) The tax exclusion for employer-sponsored health insurance. NBER Working Paper No. 15766, February. Retrieved March 6, 2010 from http://www.nber.org/papers/w15766

Hoover, D., Crystal, S., Kumar, R., Sambamoorthi, U., & Cantor, J. (2002). Medical expenditures during the last year of life: Findings from the 1992–1996 Medicare current beneficiary survey. *Health Services Research, 37,* 1625–1642.

Jorgenson, D., & Siroh, K. (2000). Raising the speed limit: U.S. economic growth in the information age. *Brookings Papers on Economic Activity, 1,* 125–211.

Kleinbard, E. (2009). How tax expenditures distort our budget and our political processes. *Tax Notes May, 18,* 925–938.

Lim, K., & Rohaly, J. (2009). *The individual alternative minimum tax: Historical data and projections*. Washington, DC: Urban-Brookings Tax Policy Center, October.

Lubitz, J., Beebe, J., & Baker, C. (1995). Longevity and Medicare expenditures. *New England Journal of Medicine, 332,* 999–1003.

Lubitz, J., Cai, L., Kramarow, E., & Lentzner, H. (2003). Health, life expectancy, and health care spending among the elderly. *New England Journal of Medicine, 349,* 1048–1055.

Manchester, J., & Schwabish, J. (2010). *The long-term budget outlook in the United States and the role of health care entitlements*. Los Angeles, CA: Tax Policy Center-University of Southern California conference on long-term fiscal crisis, January 15.

Miller, T. (2001). Increasing longevity and Medicare expenditures. *Demography, 38*(2), 215–226.

Munnell, A. (1991). Are pensions worth the cost? *National Tax Journal, 44,* 393–403.

Newhouse, J. (1992). Medical care costs: How much welfare loss? *Journal of Economic Perspectives, 6*(3), 3–21.

Oliner, S., & Sichel, D. (2000). The resurgence of growth in the late 1990s: Is information technology the story? *Journal of Economic Perspectives, 14*(4), 3–22.

Parker, J. (1999). Spendthrift in America? On two decades of decline in the U.S. saving rate. *NBER macroeconomics annual, 14,* 317–370.

Peterson-Pew Commission on Budget Reform. (2009) *Red ink rising: A call to action to stem the mounting federal debt*. Retrieved March 6, 2010 from http://www.pewtrusts.org/uploadedFiles/wwwpewtrustsorg/Reports/Economic_Mobility/40543%20FR_R1.pdf?n=7003.

Ruffing, K., Cox, K., & Horney, J. (2010). *The right target: Stabilize the federal budget*. Washington, DC: Center on Budget and Policy Priorities, January 12.

Spillman, B., & Lubitz, J. (2000). The effect of longevity on spending for acute and long term care. *New England Journal of Medicine, 342,* 1409–1415.

Toder, E., Harris, B., & Lim, K. (2009). *Distributional effects of tax expenditures*. Washington, DC: The Urban-Brookings Tax Policy Center.

US Congress. (2010). *Estimates of federal tax expenditures for fiscal years 2009–2013*. Joint Committee on Taxation, January 11. Washington, DC: US Government Printing Office.

US Department of Health and Human Services. (2006). *Short-term fixes to the sustainable growth rate process*. Final report to Assistant Secretary for Planning and Evaluation, from National Opinion Research Center, Washington, DC, October 30. Retrieved March 6, 2010 from http://aspe.hhs.gov/health/reports/08/sgr/sgr.pdf

Author Index

Page numbers in *italic* denote references. Page numbers in roman denote citations.

Author Index

Medawar, H., 50, *55*
Medicare Payment Advisory
 Commission (MedPAC), 276,
 278, 297, 301, 302, 304, *307*, 330,
 331, *333*
Melchior, M., 342, *348*
Mellick, D. C., 60, *71*
Menaghan, E. G., 152, *161*
Menard, J. L., 339, *351*
Mendes de Leon, C. F., 123, *134*,
 153, 154, *161*, 211, *219*, 341, 344,
 348
Menken, J., 19, 27, 28, *29*
Menten, J., 238, *247*
Mentnech, R. M., 126, *131*
Merkin, S. S., 68, *71*, 125, *134*
Merli, M. G., 85, *88*
Mermin, G. B. T., 201, *205*
Mero, R. P., 25, *29*, 107, 109, 113,
 116, 122, 125, 126, *132*
Merton, R. K., 109, *116*
Meslé, F., 36, *44*, 84, *88*
Mestelman, S., 166, *172*
Metlife, 299, *307*
Metsemakers, J., 345, *348*
Mettler, S., 267, *278*
Metzner, H. L., 341, *350*
Meulman, J., 343, *349*
Meyers, M., 332, *333*
Mezuk, B., 99, *102*
Michaels, R. T., 178, *190*
Michel, J., 226, *232*
Michel, P. J., 66, *71*
Michel, V., 241, *245*
Michelmore, K., 283, *292*
Michels, K. B., 141, *147*
Miech, R. A., 124, *133*, 153, 154, *161*
Miles, T. P., 93, 98, 100, *101*, *102*,
 123, *132*
Milionis, D., 240, *247*
Milkie, M. A., 325, *332*
Mill, J., 139, 140, *145*
Miller, D., 299, *306*
Miller, G. E., 143, *146*
Miller, L., 346, *351*
Miller, R. A., 48, 52, *55*
Miller, T., 84, *88*, 362, *366*
Miller-Martinez, D., 211, *220*
Milliken, G. A., 24, *29*
Mills, C. W., 4, *16*, 107, *116*
Milner, D., 342, *349*
Miner, C. R., 345, *349*
Miner, J. R., 49, *56*
Minkler, M., 222, 228, *232*
Mirowsky, J., 9, *16*, 107, 115, *116*,
 125, 126, *133*, *134*, 150, 151, *161*
Mitchell, A. M., 243, *247*
Mitchell, J. M., 216, *219*
Mitchell, O. S., 122, *134*, 164, *173*,
 327, 329, *333*
Mitchell, S. L., 242, *247*

Mitford, J., 237, *247*
Mitnitski, A., 61, *71*
Mittleman, M. A., 342, *351*
Miyashita, M., 237, *247*
Modan, B., 226, *233*
Modell, J., 9, *16*
Moen, P., 7, *15*, 324, *333*
Moffit, R., 303, *306*
Moffitt, T. E., 139, 140, *145*
Mohammed, S. A., 94, 95, 98, 99,
 103, 123, *134*
Molfese, D. L., 141, *146*
Mollica, R. L., 215, *219*, 318, *321*
Monteiro, C., 78, *88*
Montgomery, S. M., 124, *132*
Moody, H. R., 213, 214, *219*, 330,
 334
Moon, M., 126, *133*, 296, 297, 298,
 300, 301, 305, *306*, *307*, 328, 330,
 331, *334*
Moore, C. I., 341, *349*
Moore, J. F., 164, *173*
Moore, K. B., 184, 185, *190*
Moore, M., 83, *87*
Moore, W. E., 106, *115*
Moos, B. S., 154, 155, *161*
Moos, R. H., 154, 155, 157, *160*,
 161, 346, *350*
Mor, V., 237, *246*
Morello-Frosch, R. A., 140, *145*
Morenoff, J., 123, *133*
Morenoff, J. D., 211, *217*
Morgan, K. J., 272, *278*
Morgan, L. A., 215, *217*
Morito, T., 237, *247*
Morley, R., 141, *145*
Morris, J. C., 60, *70*
Morrow, J. D., 326, *332*
Morrow-Howell, N., 156, *161*, 226,
 227, 228, *232*
Mortimer, J. A., 345, *351*
Mortimer, J. T., 110, *117*, 123, *133*
Moskowitz, R. W., 60, *70*
Moura, E., 78, *88*
Moustafa, A. A., 138, *145*
Mrc, C., 211, *217*
Mui, A. C., 93, *103*
Mulatu, M. S., 341, *351*
Muldoon, D., 185, 186, 187, *190*,
 283, *293*
Mullan, J. T., 152, *161*
Müller, K., 256, *263*
Muller, R. A., 166, *172*
Mulvey, J., 202, *205*
Munnell, A. H., 163, 164, *173*, 181,
 182, 183, 185, 186, 187, *190*, 196,
 200, 203, *205*, 274, *278*, 283, *293*,
 329, *334*, 360, *366*
Muntaner, C., 123, *131*
Muramatsu, N., 156, *161*, 238, *247*
Murphy, D. J., 241, 242, *246*

Murphy, M., 124, *133*
Murphy, S. T., 241, *245*
Musick, M. A., 225, 226, 230, *232*,
 233
Mutchler, J. E., 123, *133*, 226, *230*,
 231, *232*
Myles, J., 252, 253, 259, *264*
Myrskylä, M., 254, *264*

N

Nabe, C. M., 237, *245*
Naegele, G., 265, *279*
Nagi, S. Z., 59, *70*
Najarian, B., 346, *350*
Nanchahal, K., 110, *116*
Napaporn, C., 86, *88*
Natali, D., 253, 255, 259, *264*
National Academy on an Aging
 Society, 222, 227, *232*
National Alliance for Caregiving,
 325, 326, 330, *334*
National Center for Health Statistics,
 237, *245*, 324, 329, 330, *334*
National Conference on Citizenship,
 223, 224, 225, 230, *232*
National Research Council, 110, *116*
Natividad, J., 40, *44*
Navaie-Waliser, M., 241, *247*, 326, *334*
Naydeck, B. L., 60, *70*
Nazroo, J., 123, *131*
Neels, K., 10, *15*
Negron, A., 345, *351*
Neigh, J. E., 243, *247*
Neighbors, H. W., 93, *102*, 156, *160*
Neimeyer, R. A., 240, *245*
Nelson, C. A. III, 345, *351*
Nelson, E., 216, *217*
Nemeroff, C. B., 139, *145*
Nemetz, P. N., 52, *55*
Nesbit, R., 224, 225, *231*
Nesbitt, C., 339, *351*
Nesse, R., 93, *102*
Nestler, E. J., 141, 142, *147*
Netherlands Ministry of Health,
 Welfare and Sport, 316, *321*
Neugarten, B. L., 42, *44*
Neuman, P., 272, *278*
Neuman, T., 298, 299, *306*, *307*
Neumark, D., 202, *205*
Neve, R. L., 141, 142, *147*
Newhouse, J., 276, *278*, 363, *366*
Ng, D., 127, *133*
Ng-Baumhackl, M., 167, *173*
Nicholls, E. F., 143, *146*
Nicholson, A., 124, *133*
Nieto, J., 123, *131*
Nikolaus, T., 65, *71*
Nissinen, A., 345, *351*
Noke, J. M., 346, *350*

Subject Index